Management of
High-Risk
Pregnancy

THIRD EDITION

Edited by

JOHN T. QUEENAN, M.D.

Professor and Chairman, Department of Obstetrics
and Gynecology,
Georgetown University School of Medicine;
Obstetrician Gynecologist-in-Chief,
Georgetown University Hospital;
Editor-in-Chief, *Contemporary OB/GYN*
Washington, D.C.

Management of
High-Risk
Pregnancy

b

**Blackwell
Science**

Blackwell Science

Editorial Offices:
238 Main Street, Cambridge, Massachusetts 02142, USA
Osney Mead, Oxford OX2 0EL, England
25 John Street, London, WC1N 2BL, England
23 Ainslie Place, Edinburgh EH3 6AJ, Scotland
54 University Street, Carlton, Victoria 3053, Australia
Arnette SA, 1 rue de Lille, 75007 Paris, France
Blackwell Wissenschaft-Verlag GmbH,
    Kurfürstendamm 57, 10707 Berlin, Germany
    Feldgasse 13, A-1238 Vienna, Austria

Distributors:
NORTH AMERICA
Blackwell Science, Inc.
238 Main Street
Cambridge, Massachusetts 02142
(Telephone orders: 800-215-1000 or 617-876-7000)

AUSTRALIA
Blackwell Science Pty Ltd
54 University Street
Carlton, Victoria 3053
(Telephone orders: 03-347-5552)

OUTSIDE NORTH AMERICA AND AUSTRALIA
Blackwell Science, Ltd.
c/o Marston Book Services, Ltd.
P.O. Box 87
Oxford OX2 0DT
England
(Telephone orders: 44-865-791155)

Typeset by The Type Shoppe, Inc., Chestertown, Maryland
Printed and bound by BookCrafters, Ann Arbor, Michigan

© 1994 by Blackwell Science, Inc.

Printed in the United States of America
95 96 97 98 5 4 3 2

Library of Congress Cataloging-in-Publication Data
Management of the high-risk pregnancy / edited by John T. Queenan.—
3rd ed.
    p. cm.
    Includes bibliographical references and index.
    ISBN 0-86542-187-0
    1. Pregnancy—Complications. I. Queenan, John T.
    [DNLM: 1. Pregnancy Complications—therapy. WQ 240 M266]
RG571.M24 1992
618.3—dc20
DNLM/DLC   92-21899
for Library of Congress   CIP

Contents

CONTENTS

CONTENTS

PART SEVEN: Complications of Labor and Delivery

PART EIGHT: Neonatal Considerations

Contributors

J. Antonio Aldrete, M.D., MS
Medical Director
The Destin Center for Pain Management
Destin, Florida

Mohammad R. Alijani, M.D., FACS
Director, Kidney and Pancreas Transplant Service
Associate Professor, Department of Surgery
Georgetown School of Medicine
Washington, D.C.

Marvin S. Amstey, M.D.
Chief of Obstetrics and Gynecology
Highland Hospital
Rochester, New York

David A. Baker, M.D.
Associate Professor
Department of Obstetrics and Gynecology
State University of New York at Stony Brook
School of Medicine
Stony Brook, New York

Tom P. Barden, M.D.
Professor of Obstetrics and Gynecology
University of Cincinnati College of Medicine
Cincinnati, Ohio

Sandra Ann Carson, M.D.
Associate Professor and Chief
In Vitro Fertilization and Embryo Transfer
Division of Reproductive Endocrinology and Infertility
University of Tennessee, Memphis
Memphis, Tennessee

Jane Chueh, M.D.
Assistant Professor
Division of Reproductive Genetics
Department of Obstetrics and Gynecology
University of California, San Francisco
San Francisco, California

Steven L. Clark, M.D.
Department of Obstetrics and Gynecology
University of Utah
Salt Lake City, Utah

CONTRIBUTORS

Daniel Clement, M.D.
Encino-Tarzana Regional Medical Center
Tarzana, California

Hartley Cohen, M.D.
Professor of Medicine
University of Southern California
School of Medicine
Los Angeles, California

Manley Cohen, M.D.
Consultant Gastroenterologist
Long Beach Memorial Women's Hospital
Associate Professor of Medicine
University of California, Irvine
Irvine, California

Joseph V. Collea, M.D.
Professor
Division of Maternal-Fetal Medicine
Department of Obstetrics and Gynecology
Georgetown University School of Medicine
Washington, D.C.

Larry N. Cook, M.D.
Professor and Associate Chairman
Department of Pediatrics
University of Louisville School of Medicine
Louisville, Kentucky

Donald R. Coustan, M.D.
Professor and Chairman
Department of Obstetrics and Gynecology
Brown University School of Medicine
Providence, Rhode Island

Sergio Demarini, M.D.
Children's Hospital Medical Center
University of Cincinnati
Cincinnati, Ohio

Mara J. Dinsmoor, M.D.
Assistant Professor
Department of Obstetrics and Gynecology
Medical College of Virginia
Richmond, VA

Gary S. Eglinton, M.D.
Associate Professor
Division of Maternal-Fetal Medicine
Department of Obstetrics and Gynecology
Georgetown University Hospital
Washington, D.C.

Sherman Elias, M.D.
Professor and Director
Division of Reproductive Genetics
Department of Obstetrics and Gynecology
University of Tennessee
Memphis, Tennessee

Emanuel A. Friedman, M.D., ScD
Professor of Obstetrics and Gynecology
Harvard Medical School
Boston, Massachusetts

Janice I. French, M.D.
Department of Obstetrics and Gynecology
University of Colorado Health Science Center
Denver, Colorado

Steven G. Gabbe, M.D.
Professor and Chairman
Department of Obstetrics and Gynecology
Ohio State University College of Medicine
Columbus, Ohio

Thomas J. Garite, M.D.
Professor and Chairman
Department of Obstetrics and Gynecology
University of California - Irvine Medical Center
Orange, California

Preston Gazaway, M.D.
Director of Obstetrics
Center for Addiction and Pregnancy
Francis Scott Key Medical Center
Obstetrics and Gynecology Office
Baltimore, Maryland

Martin L. Gimovsky, M.D.
Associate Chairman and Director of Education
Department of Obstetrics and Gynecology

Bay State Medical Center
Springfield, Massachusetts

Mitchell S. Golbus, M.D.
Professor of Obstetrics and Gynecology,
   Reproductive Sciences and Pediatrics
University of California at San Francisco Medical Center
San Francisco, California

Roger J. Harris, M.D., DCH
The London Trust
The Royal London Hospital
London, England

Robert H. Hayashi, M.D.
J. Robert Wilson Professor of Obstetrics
Women's Hospital - University of Michigan
Ann Arbor, Michigan

Edgar O. Horger III, M.D.
Professor of Obstetrics and Gynecology
Director of Maternal and Fetal Medicine
University of South Carolina
Columbia, South Carolina

Dorothy M. Horstmann, M.D.
John R. Paul Professor of Epidemiology and
Professor of Pediatrics Emeritus
Department of Epidemiology and Public Health
Yale University School of Medicine
New Haven, Connecticut

Jay Iams, M.D.
Professor of Obstetrics and Gynecology
Ohio State University College of Medicine
Columbus, Ohio

Adrian I. Katz, M.D.
Professor of Medicine
Pritzker School of Medicine
The University of Chicago
Chicago, Illinois

Martin Keszler, M.D.
Associate Professor of Pediatrics
Division of Neonatology

Department of Pediatrics
Department of Obstetrics and Gynecology
Georgetown University School of Medicine
Washington, D.C.

Jeffrey C. King, M.D.
Associate Professor
Division of Maternal-Fetal Medicine
Department of Obstetrics and Gynecology
Georgetown University School of Medicine
Washington, D.C.

David Z. Kitay, M.D.
Director, Division of Women's Health Services
Department of Health and Rehabilitative Services
State of Florida

Neil K. Kochenour, M.D.
Professor and Vice-Chairman
Department of Obstetrics and Gynecology
University of Utah Medical Center
Salt Lake City, Utah

J. Patrick Lavery, M.D.
Perinatologist
Department of Perinatology
Bronson Methodist Hospital
Kalimazoo, Michigan

Marshall D. Lindheimer, M.D.
Professor of Medicine and Obstetrics and Gynecology
Sections of Nephrology and Maternal Fetal Medicine
Pritzker School of Medicine
The University of Chicago
Chicago, Illinois

Armand Lione, PhD
Pharmacologist and Toxicologist
Reproductive Toxicology Center
Columbia Hospital for Women
Washington, D.C.

Charles J. Lockwood, M.D.
Professor of Obstetrics and Gynecology
Mount Sinai College of Medicine
New York, New York

CONTRIBUTORS

James A. McGregor, M.D.
Professor and Vice Chairman
Department of Obstetrics and Gynecology
University of Colorado Health Science Center
Denver, Colorado

Philip B. Mead, M.D.
Clinical Professor
Department of Obstetrics and Gynecology
University of Vermont College of Medicine
Medical Center Hospital of Vermont
Burlington, Vermont

S. Roy Meadow, M.D., DCH
Director of Department of Paediatrics and Childrens Health
St. James University Hospital
Leeds, England

Irwin R. Merkatz, M.D.
Professor and Chairman
Department of Obstetrics and Gynecology
The Albert Einstein College of Medicine of Yeshiva
    University
Bronx, New York

Jorge H. Mestman, M.D.
Professor and Director
USC Center for Diabetes
Los Angeles, California

Carole M. Meyers, M.D.
Division of Reproductive Genetics
Department of Obstetrics and Gynecology
University of Tennessee
Memphis, Tennessee

Howard L. Minkoff, M.D.
Professor of Obstetrics and Gynecology
State University of New York
Health Science Center at Brooklyn
Brooklyn, New York

Houchang D. Modanlou, M.D.
Director, Neonatal-Perinatal Medicine
Miller Children's Hospital
Associate Professor, Pediatrics

University of California
Irvine, California

Deepak Nanda, M.D.
State University of New York
Health Science Center of Brooklyn
Brooklyn, New York

Jennifer R. Niebyl, M.D.
Professor and Head
Department of Obstetrics and Gynecology
University of Iowa Hospitals and Clinics
Iowa City, Iowa

William L. Nyhan, M.D., PhD
Professor
Department of Pediatrics
University of California , San Diego
School of Medicine
La Jolla, California

J. Patrick O'Grady, M.D.
Professor and Chief, Maternal Fetal Medicine
Baystate Medical Center
Tufts University
Springfield, Massachusetts

William Oh, M.D.
Pediatrician-in-Chief
Women and Infants Hospital
Brown University School of Medicine
Providence, Rhode Island

Roy H. Petrie, M.D., Sc.D.
Professor and Chairman
Department of Obstetrics and Gynecology
St. Louis University
St. Louis, Missouri

Richard A. Pircon, M.D.
Division of Maternal-Fetal Medicine
Department of Obstetrics and Gynecology
St. Joseph's Hospital
Whitefish Bay, Wisconsin

John T. Queenan, M.D.
Professor and Chairman

Department of Obstetrics and Gynecology
Georgetown University School of Medicine
Washington, D.C.

Edward J. Quilligan, M.D.
Professor
Department of Obstetrics and Gynecology
University of California - Irvine Medical Center
Orange, California

Robert Resnik, M.D.
Professor and Chairman
Department of Reproductive Medicine
University of California, San Diego
San Diego, California

Pedro Rosso, M.D.
Dean
Catholic University of Chile
Santiago, Chile

Eliahu Sadovsky, M.D.
Professor of Obstetrics and Gynecology
Hadassah University Hospital
Jerusalem, Israel

Evelyn G. Santos, M.D.
Staff Anesthesiologist
Department of Anesthesiology
St. Anthony Medical Center
Crown Point, Indiana

Barry S. Schifrin, M.D.
Director, Maternal-Fetal Medicine
Encino–Tarzana Regional Medical Center
Tarzana, California

Anthony Scialli, M.D.
Associate Professor
Department of Obstetrics and Gynecology
Georgetown University School of Medicine
Washington, D.C.

John W. Seeds, M.D.
Professor and Director, Maternal Medicine
Department of Obstetrics and Gynecology

University of Arizona
Tucson, Arizona

Kyung Seo, M.D.
Department of Obstetrics and Gynecology
University of Colorado Health Science Center
Denver, Colorado

John L. Sever, M.D., PhD
Professor of Pediatrics
Obstetrics and Gynecology and
Microbiology and Immunology
Children's National Medical Center
Washington, D.C.

Frank D. Seydel, PhD
Division of Genetics
Department of Obstetrics and Gynecology
Georgetown University School of Medicine
Washington, D.C.

Baha M. Sibai, M.D.
Division of Maternal-Fetal Medicine
Department of Obstetrics and Gynecology
E.H. Crump Women's Hospital
University of Tennessee, Memphis
Memphis, Tennessee

Joe Leigh Simpson, M.D.
Professor and Chief
Division of Maternal-Fetal Medicine
Department of Obstetrics and Gynecology
E.H. Crump Women's Hospital
University of Tennessee, Memphis
Memphis, Tennessee

Antonio V. Sison, M.D.
Instructor
Division of Gynecology and Obstetrics
Department of Obstetrics and Gynecology
Georgetown University School of Medicine
Washington, D.C.

Robert J. Sokol, M.D.
Dean, School of Medicine
Wayne State University
Detroit, Michigan

CONTRIBUTORS

K.N. Sivasubramanian, M.D.
Professor, Vice Chairman and Director of Neonatology
Department of Pediatrics
Georgetown University School of Medicine
Washington, D.C.

Reginald C. Tsang, M.D.
Executive Director, The Perinatal Research Institute
Childrens Hospital Medical Center
University of Cincinnati
Cincinnati, Ohio

Kent Ueland, M.D.
Professor Emeritus
Department of Gynecology and Obstetrics
Stanford University School of Medicine
Palo Alto, California

Steven L. Warsof, M.D.
Medical Director, Tidewater Perinatal Center

Associate Professor
Eastern Virginia Medical School
Virginia Beach, Virginia

Robert A. Welch, M.D.
Director
Division of Maternal-Fetal Medicine
Providence Hospital
Southfield, Michigan

William C. Wright, M.D.
Anesthesiologist
Cedars-Sinai Medical Center
Los Angeles, California

Frederick P. Zuspan, M.D.
Professor Emeritus
Department of Obstetrics and Gynecology
Ohio State University College of Medicine
Columbus, Ohio

Foreword

TWO decades have passed since the first issue of *Contemporary OB/GYN* was published. Throughout history, the magazine has consistently fulfilled its purpose of presenting state-of-the-art information in the practice of obstetrics and gynecology and keeping practitioners abreast of the latest scientific developments in their specialty. Its success has been reflected by its frequent top ranking in independent reader surveys. The publication has emphasized perinatology and provided a reliable resource for physicians interested in perinatal medicine.

In 1980, editor-in-chief John T. Queenan, M.D., assembled 67 chapters by 73 authors from the pages of *Contemporary OB/GYN* to create the first edition of *Management of High-Risk Pregnancy*. This work has become a classic, not only because of its thorough coverage of the field, but especially because of its timeliness with respect to advances in perinatology.

This third edition has once again brought the latest improvements and discoveries in perinatology from the pages of *Contemporary OB/GYN* to the reader. Under Dr. Queenan's prudent direction, each chapter has been updated by the authors, who are well known authorities in their respective fields. The subjects have been carefully developed to bring clinically relevant facts, techniques, and "how-to" knowledge from the authors to practicing physicians.

The organization of previous editions first focused on factors affecting pregnancy and on genetics, then focused on practical diagnostic techniques, followed by maternal diseases in pregnancy and pregnancy complications, and ended with the delivery process itself, anesthesia, and neonatology. While this format remains essentially unchanged, the third edition presents many new advances in perinatology.

This third edition will be especially valuable to house officers encountering various perinatal problems for the first time. In addition, the book will undoubtedly continue to achieve its primary purpose of providing practicing physicians with a comprehensive, authoritative, practical reference in perinatology.

Roger K. Freeman, M.D.
Professor of Obstetrics and Gynecology
University of California, Irvine
Medical Director, Women's Hospital
Memorial Hospital Medical Center
Long Beach, California

Preface

THE third edition, like its predecessors, is directed to all health professionals involved in the care of women with high-risk pregnancies. It is intended as a resource in perinatal education and as a reference for the diagnosis and management of high-risk pregnancy. The chapters contain important clinical information presented in a clear, concise, and practical manner.

Two series of articles that appeared in *Contemporary OB/GYN* were the inspiration for this work. These primarily clinical articles provided a comprehensive perspective on high-risk pregnancy. By organizing and adding supplemental material to these articles, I was able to create an informative, practical textbook. To ensure accuracy, I asked the authors to update their manuscripts in order to address the rapid advances being made in perinatal medicine.

The first edition of this book had two printings. It was subsequently serialized in 12 modules containing clinical subjects and pertinent questions. These modules were sent to all practicing obstetricians and gynecologists in the United States. A second edition was published in 1985. For this third edition, all of the material is updated to reflect up-to-the-minute practical information from outstanding perinatal experts.

I welcome comments, both laudatory and critical. Your suggestions will help to improve future editions.

John T. Queenan, M.D.

Acknowledgments

I AM fortunate to work in cooperation with a superb editorial staff at Blackwell Scientific Publications, Inc., including Victoria Reeders, Vice President, Editor-in-Chief, and Kathleen Grimes, Books Managing Editor. Their expertise in preparing this book is greatly appreciated. I acknowledge with thanks the skillful efforts of our authors who are outstanding authorities.

Mr. James E. Swan, editor of *Contemporary OB/GYN* almost single-handedly effected the transfer of articles to Blackwell Scientific Publications for chapters of this book. Without his tireless effort and editorial skill, this book would not have been possible. I am indebted to Jim as an editor and friend.

At Georgetown University, I have enjoyed great help and expertise from my colleagues Rene M. Anderson, Regina E. Auth, Christine Colie, Joseph V. Collea, Gary S. Eglinton, Gary D. Helmbrecht, Sharon C. Kiernan, Jeffrey C. King, Shaun G. Lencki, Thomas R. Minner, Thomas L. Pinckert, David W. Rindfusz, Anthony R. Scialli, and Thomas P. Tomai. In addition, I have received excellent editorial help from Laura Gresham.

I wish to thank Carrie Neher Queenan for her valuable editorial assistance, C. Lynne Queenan Beauregard and Drs. John T. Queenan, Jr. and Ruth Anne Queenan for help in the final proofreading of this manuscript. Thanks to Christine McCaffery for her secretarial assistance and the many others who helped complete this book.

Introduction

A HIGH-RISK pregnancy is any pregnancy in which there is a maternal or fetal factor that may adversely affect the outcome of pregnancy. Fortunately, the vast majority of pregnancies are low-risk and have favorable outcomes. Although the mother may experience unpleasant symptoms, physical problems, or minor difficulties with labor and delivery, she usually has a full recovery and a healthy baby.

Predictably, a high-risk pregnancy considerably lessens the likelihood of a positive outcome. In order to improve the outcome of a high-risk pregnancy, a system that identifies risk factors and mitigates problems in pregnancy and labor must be employed. Many conditions lend themselves to this system of management. Rh immunization, diabetes, and epilepsy, for instance, can usually be identified before pregnancy or early in the perinatal period. Accordingly, appropriate diagnostic workups can be performed and the pregnancy managed in an effort to minimize the risks of mortality and morbidity to the mother and baby. Other conditions, such as multiple pregnancies, preeclampsia, and premature rupture of the membranes, usually cannot be predicted. Since these problems are identifiable only with the progression of pregnancy, the clinician must continually be alert to detect and manage these challenging situations.

Prior to the 1950s, newborn care was the responsibility of the delivering physician and nursing staff. Perinatal mortality and morbidity statistics were very poor. Then, in the 1950s, the decade of neonatal awareness, pediatricians began appearing in the newborn nursery, assuming responsibility for their patients at the moment of birth. That decade hosted advances that greatly improved neonatal outcome.

In the 1960s, the decade of fetal medicine, many scientific breakthroughs were directed toward the evaluation of fetal health and disease. Early in that decade, the identification of patients with the risk factor of Rh immunization led to the prototype of the high-risk pregnancy clinic. Rh-negative patients were screened for antibodies. If none were detected, they were managed as normal or "low-risk" patients. If they developed antibodies, they were enrolled in a high-risk pregnancy clinic, where they could be carefully followed by specialists with expertise in Rh immunization. In subsequent years, scientific advances like amniotic fluid analysis, intrauterine transfusion, and finally, Rh immune prophylaxis helped make this kind of systematic manage-

sion, and finally, Rh immune prophylaxis helped make this kind of systematic management of a specific high-risk pregnancy a success story.

The pediatrician and obstetrician combined forces to continue improving perinatal survival in the 1970s, the decade of perinatal medicine. The accompanying table lists some of the most significant perinatal advances, with the approximate dates when they became available. Where appropriate, the table also lists the investigators' names commonly associated with these advances.

The 1980s, the decade of progress, marked many significant changes, including: the comprehensive evaluation of fetal condition with the biophysical profile, cordocentesis for diagnosis and therapy, the development of neonatal surfactant therapy, and major advances in genetics and assisted reproduction. The decade's technological progress suggests that the nineties will bring many new "high tech" advances at a time when the specialty realizes that "high touch" advances are also extremely important for the emotional and developmental well-being of the baby and the parents.

The future will bring better methods of determining fetal jeopardy and health. Continuous readout of fetal conditions will be possible during labor in high-risk pregnancies. New technology will increase the demand for trained workers in the health care industry. The perinatal professional team will expand to emphasize the importance of social workers, nutritionists, child development specialists, and psychologists. New developments will create special ethical issues. Finally, enlightened attitudes toward reproductive awareness and family planning will help to prevent unwanted pregnancies.

Milestones in Perinatology.

Before 1950s	**Neonatal care by obstetricians and nurses**
1950s—Decade of Neonatal Awareness	**Pediatricians entered nursery**
1950 Allen and Diamond	Exchange transfusions
1953 du Vigneaud	Oxytocin synthesis
1954 Patz	Limitation of O_2 to prevent toxicity
1955 Mann	Neonatal hypothermia
1956 Tjio and Levan	Demonstration of 46 human chromosomes
1956 Bevis	Amniocentesis for bilirubin in Rh immunization
1958 Donald	Obstetric use of ultrasound
1958 Hon	Electronic fetal heart rate evaluation
1959 Burns, Hodgman, and Cass	Gray baby syndrome
1960s—Decade of Fetal Medicine	**Prototype of the high-risk pregnancy clinic**
1960 Eisen and Hellman	Lumbar epidural anesthesia
1962 Saling	Fetal scalp blood sampling
1963 Liley	Intrauterine transfusion for Rh immunization
1963 Greene and Touchstone	Urinary estriols and placental function
1964 Wallgren	Neonatal blood pressure
1965 Steele and Breg	Culture of amniotic fluid cells
1965 Mizrahi, Blanc, and Silverman	Necrotizing enterocolitis
1966 Parkman and Myer	Rubella immunization
1967	Neonatal blood gases
1967	Neonatal transport
1967 Jacobsen	Diagnosis of cytogenetic disorders in utero
1968 Dudrick	Hyperalimentation
1968 Nadler	Diagnosis of inborn errors of metabolism in utero
1968 Stern	Neonatal intensive care unit's (NICU) effectiveness
1968 Freda, Gorman, Pollack, and Clarke	Rh prophylaxis

INTRODUCTION

1970s—Decade of Perinatal Medicine		**Refinement of NICU**
		Regionalization of high-risk perinatal care
1971	Gluck	Lecithin/Sphingomyelin (L/S) ratio and respiratory distress syndrome
1972	Brock and Sutcliffe	α-fetoprotein and neural tube defects
1972	Liggins and Howie	Betamethasone for induction of fetal lung maturity
1972		Neonatal temperature control with radiant heat
1972	Quilligan	Fetal heart rate monitoring
1972	Dawes	Fetal breathing movements
1972	Ray and Freeman	Oxytocin challenge test
1972	American Board of Obstetrics and Gynecology (ABOG)	Maternal-Fetal Medicine Boards
1973	Sadovsky	Fetal movement
1973		Real-time ultrasound
1973	Hobbins and Rodeck	Clinical fetoscopy
1975	American Board of Pediatrics (ABP)	Neonatology Boards
1976	Schifrin	Nonstress test
1977	March of Dimes	*Towards Improving the Outcome of Pregnancy I*
1977	Kaback	Heterozygote identification (Tay-Sachs disease)
1978	Bowman	Antepartum Rh prophylaxis
1978	Steptoe and Edwards	In vitro fertilization
1979	Boehm	Maternal transport
1980s—Decade of Progress		**Technological progress**
1980	Bartlett	ECMO
1980	Manning and Platt	Biophysical profile
1981	Fujiwara, Morley, and Jobe	Neonatal surfactant therapy
1982	Harrison and Golbus	Vesicoamniotic shunt for fetal hydronephrosis
1983	Kazy, Ward, and Brambati	Chorionic villus sampling
1984	Buster and Bustillo	Embryo transfer
1985	Daffos	Cordocentesis
1986		DNA analysis
1990s—Current Decade		
	March of Dimes	*Towards Improving the Outcome of Pregnancy II*
	Preimplantation genetics	
	Fetal therapy	

PART ONE Factors of High-Risk Pregnancy

1

Maternal Nutrition and Fetal Development

Carol West Suitor, D.Sc., R.D.
Pedro Rosso, M.D.

SUBSTANTIAL evidence supports the widely held belief that maternal nutrition influences fetal growth. The woman's energy and nutrient stores upon entering pregnancy and her intake of food and supplements during pregnancy may affect fetal growth and development. Because both stores and current intake are involved, however, there are many uncertainties regarding the consequences, if any, of prenatal exposure to nutrient deficiency.

Historically, two discrepant concepts emerged concerning the regulation of maternal-fetal exchange of nutrients. One concept suggests that nutrients preferentially go to the fetus even when the mother has a mild to moderate nutritional deficiency. The other concept suggests that the fetus can be adversely affected by maternal deficiency of any degree. In fact, maternal-fetal nutrient exchange is a complex process that differs for various nutrients. Moreover, the mixture of fuels, amino acids, vitamins, and minerals in the blood can be influenced by such factors as the mother's intake of food and vitamin-mineral supplements; her nutrient stores; use of cigarettes, alcoholic beverages, and other legal and illicit drugs; physical activity; and state of health.

This chapter briefly summarizes evidence concerning relationships between maternal nutrition and fetal growth and development, and then addresses nutritional management during pregnancy.

Energy, Protein and Body Weight

The first data clearly linking maternal undernutrition and reduced mean birthweight, published following the end of World War II, reported observations made during siege conditions in Holland and Leningrad (1). In both populations, at the beginning of the siege there was a sharp increase in the incidence of low-birthweight babies and a significant decrease in mean body weight in term infants. The effect was more marked in Leningrad, where the mean birthweight was reduced by 529 g in boys and 542 g in girls, compared with a drop averaging approximately 250 g in Holland.

The differences in mean birthweights between these two studies can be attributed to a better nutritional status of the Dutch women prior to the famine and to the fact that, in Holland, the famine lasted for a shorter period of time.

When nutritional conditions in the Dutch cities improved, mean birthweight returned to the previous range, even in infants of mothers whose diets had been restricted during the first 28 weeks of pregnancy.

From the fact that famine conditions in previously well-nourished women were followed by a relatively small reduction in mean birthweight, some infer that less extreme conditions would cause unapparent and probably negligible reductions in birthweight. This idea ignores the lack of reliable data on spontaneous abortions as well as the wide variation around the lower mean birthweight. Furthermore, studies indicate that the quantity of maternal body stores (as reflected by weight-to-height ratios) is directly associated with the birthweight of the offspring (see Figure 1). Thus, a massively obese woman with a low caloric intake may deliver a baby of average weight. In contrast, a thin, underweight woman with a low caloric intake is likely to deliver a baby whose weight is considerably below average.

The joint influence of prepregnancy weight and weight gain during pregnancy on birthweight reflects the importance of maternal body mass on fetal growth. Apparently, more important than weight gain per se is the body mass, in relation to height, of the mother near term. After controlling for other factors that influence birthweight, the risk of delivering infants who are small for gestational age appears to be minimized for women whose body mass at delivery is approximately 120% of their desirable prepregnant weight. Average birthweight of infants born to these women is approximately 3,450 g (2, 3).

Among adolescents, low weight gain (less than 4.3 kg by 24 weeks' gestation) has been associated with increased risk of delivering an infant who is small for gestational age—even if total weight gain was within the recommended range (4). Similarly, fat gain before week 30 of pregnancy was directly associated with fetal growth in a Guatemalan study (5).

The influence of obesity on the outcome of pregnancy has been a rather neglected area. Although mean birthweight is higher for obese women than for women of normal weight, data from the 1980 U.S. National Natality Survey demonstrate that over 10% of the obese women who delivered term infants weighing between 3,000 and 4,000 g either lost weight or gained no weight during pregnancy

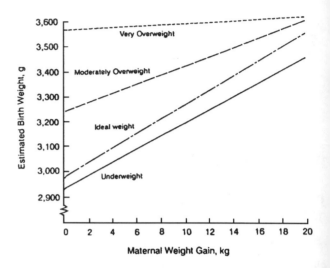

Figure 1.1   Birthweight as a function of maternal weight and prepregnancy weight for height.

(Reprinted with permission from Nutrition during pregnancy. Copyright 1990 by the National Academy of Sciences. Published by the National Academy Press, Washington, D.C.)

(6). It is not known to what extent unfavorable pregnancy outcomes were associated with lack of weight gain by these obese women. Three published reports suggest that the obese gravida tends to have a high percentage of complicated pregnancies and deliveries (7–9). A more recent case-control study concluded that massively obese women (those weighing more than 300 lbs [136.3 kg]) are at increased risk of delivering an infant with intrauterine growth retardation or macrosomia. These increased risks, however, appeared to be related to medical complications of obesity (hypertension and diabetes mellitus, respectively) rather than to obesity per se.

Deficits of Vitamins and Minerals

Considerable effort has been devoted to studying the roles of maternal deficits of vitamins and minerals—especially of folic acid, iron, and zinc. Because of findings from both physiologic and epidemiologic studies, folic acid deficiency has been a prime suspect as a cause of neural tube defects. For example, administration of valproic acid (an anticonvulsant found to interfere with folic acid metabolism) in early pregnancy led to a 20-fold excess risk of neural tube defects (11), which was reduced by administration of folinic acid, the metabolically active form of folic acid. Initially, epidemiologic studies focused on the role of multivitamin supplements rather than just folic acid in the prevention of spina bifida and other neural tube defects (12–15); one study (16) focused on dietary folate. All but one of these studies (12) provided evidence in support of the importance of adequate folic acid intake for the prevention of neural tube defects. The one study that was a double-blind, randomized, controlled clinical trial (17) clearly demonstrated a protective effect for high-dose folic acid. In particular, when 4 mg of folic acid was given daily beginning three months prior to conception and continuing throughout the first trimester of pregnancy, the risk that the fetus would develop a neural tube defect was greatly reduced (but not completely eliminated).

A large percentage of women have low iron stores at the beginning of pregnancy, and many of them develop some degree of iron deficiency anemia during pregnancy. The Institute of Medicine (IOM) recommends that measures be taken to prevent and treat maternal iron deficiency primarily to benefit the mother (18). The effects of maternal iron deficiency on the fetus are still a subject of controversy. There is little or no laboratory evidence that maternal iron deficiency leads to reduced iron stores in the newborn (18). A growing number of studies, however, have been identifying possible links between maternal anemia and adverse outcomes such as low birthweight, prematurity, and perinatal mortality (18, 19). The most convincing of these studies indicates that iron deficiency anemia at entry to prenatal care triples the risk of low birthweight and more than doubles the risk of preterm birth (19).

The zinc deficiency that is associated with inadequate treatment of acrodermatitis enteropathica (a heredity condition in which zinc absorption is impaired) has been linked with a high risk of major obstetric complications and congenital malformations in the offspring (20). No conclusive evidence has been obtained from studies conducted to determine the effects of zinc supplementation for women believed to have low zinc intake (21–23).

Studies in animals and in developing nations where malnutrition is a problem provide evidence that the mother's intake and stores of other vitamins and minerals affect the growth and development of the fetus. Among the most notable examples are iodine, thiamine, and vitamins A and D. Maternal iodine deficiency during pregnancy causes endemic cretinism, congenital anomalies, spontaneous abortions, and other adverse outcomes (24–26). In the United States, usual iodine intake is considerably higher than that needed to avoid deficiency. In some areas of Africa, Asia, South America, and Europe, iodine deficiency remains a public health problem. In regions where endemic goiter persists, preventive measures such as iodination of salt are needed to reduce the risk of goiter and of adverse pregnancy outcomes.

Maternal thiamine deficiency in asymptomatic women causes acute, in most cases fatal, congestive heart failure of the newborn (27). This congenital beriberi can be cured or prevented by prompt administration of thiamine to the neonate.

Adverse effects linked with maternal vitamin A deficiency include preterm birth and intrauterine growth retardation (28). Animal studies provide further support for the role of vitamin A in promoting fetal growth (29–31).

Maternal deficiency of vitamin D could result either from inadequate dietary intake (primarily from vitamin D-fortified foods such as milk) or from inadequate exposure to sunlight. Such deficiency may affect both the fetus and the mother: it has been linked with neonatal hypocalcemia and tetany (32), tooth enamel hypoplasia (33), and maternal osteomalacia (34).

Excessive Intake of Vitamins and Minerals

In the United States, the widespread practice of taking vitamin or mineral supplements, or both, raises concerns about possible harmful effects. Sustained intake of very high doses of preformed vitamin A (retinol) is known to be toxic, and considerable evidence suggests that excessive intake of this vitamin early in pregnancy is teratogenic (35). Such adverse outcomes as obstructive lesions of the ureters and fetal hydronephrosis have been reported. Carotene, the form of vitamin A found in such plant foods as carrots, appears to be neither toxic nor teratogenic.

Vitamin D is potentially toxic to the fetus if large doses of the vitamin are given during pregnancy (18).

Among the adverse effects reported are mental and physical growth retardation and hypercalcemia. The minimum toxic dose to the mother varies considerably.

The safety of large doses of vitamins during pregnancy has not been evaluated systematically, and information about adverse effects of vitamins E and K and the water soluble vitamins is extremely limited. For example, it is anecdotal data (36) that have been used to support the widely disseminated claims that excessive maternal intake of vitamin C leads to increased susceptibility to scurvy in the offspring (18). Large doses of folic acid appear to inhibit the absorption of certain other nutrients, such as zinc (37). For most water-soluble vitamins, such as folic acid, active placental transport leads to fetal plasma and erythrocyte levels of the vitamin that are several times higher than those in the mother. This characteristic of nutrient transport raises questions about the possibility that taking high doses of vitamins might harm the fetus (18).

Nutritional Problems Related to Health Problems

A number of health problems can lead to nutritional problems and thus call for special attention in preparation for and during pregnancy (38). Health problems that may be accompanied by very low or unbalanced dietary intake include eating disorders, surgical treatment to correct obesity (e.g., gastric banding), and serious chronic gastrointestinal disorders such as Crohn's disease, celiac disease, or liver disorders. The amino acid imbalance characteristic of untreated maternal phenylketonuria poses a high risk of microcephaly and mental subnormality for the infant (39). If maternal blood glucose is poorly controlled very early in pregnancy, preexisting diabetes mellitus increases the risk of congenital anomalies (40).

Nutritional Management During Pregnancy

In 1990, the IOM released a report that includes recommendations for weight gain and other aspects of nutritional management during pregnancy. The range of weight gain to be recommended depends principally on the woman's prepregnancy weight for height, as expressed in terms of

Table 1.1 Recommended Total Weight Gain Ranges for Pregnant Women

Prepregnancy weight-for-height category	Recommended total gain	
	lb	kg
Low (BMI <19.8)	28–40	12.5–18
Normal (BMI 19.8 to 26)	25–35	11.5–16
High (BMI >26.0 to 29.0)	15–25	7.0–11.5
Obese (BMI >29.0)	≥15	≥7.0

For singleton pregnancies. The range for women carrying twins is 35 to 45 lbs (16 to 20 kg). Young adolescents (<2 years after menarche) and African-American women should strive for gains at the upper end of the range. Short women (<2 in or <157 cm) should strive for gains at the lower end of the range.

(Reprinted with permission from Nutrition during pregnancy and lactation. Copyright 1992 by the National Academy of Sciences. Published by the National Academy Press, Washington, D.C.)

the body mass index (BMI, or weight in kilograms divided by the square of the height in meters). Figure 2 provides a simple method for estimating the BMI weight category to which the woman belongs. Table 1 gives the recommended weight gain ranges for pregnancy, based on prepregnancy BMI. During the second and third trimesters of pregnancy, these weight gain recommendations translate to approximately 1 lb (0.4 kg) per week for thin and normal-weight women and approximately 0.5 to 0.75 lbs (0.3 kg) per week for overweight and obese women. For obese women, the emphasis should be on diet quality rather than quantity. It is recommended that young adolescents and African-American women gain at the upper end of the weight gain range for their BMI group and that short women (those less than 157 cm or 62 inches tall) gain at the lower end of the range.

According to a study that examined the IOM recommendations, maternal weight gain that falls within these recommended ranges is associated with fewer infants who were either small or large for gestational age and with fewer cesarean deliveries than were found for weight gain outside the recommended range (41).

The IOM recommends a total gain of 35 to 45 lbs for women carrying twins. Data on which to base separate recommendations by prepregnancy BMI were insufficient.

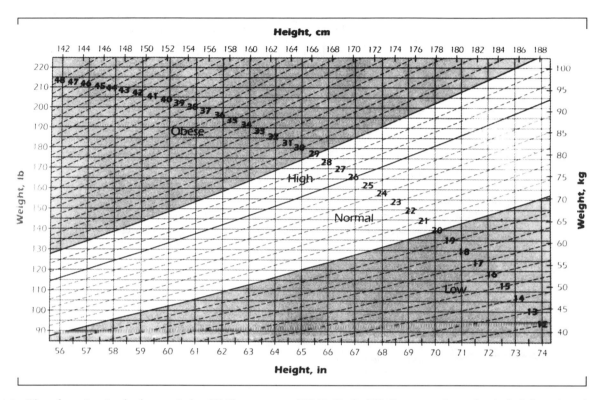

Figure 1.2   Chart for estimating body mass index (BMI) category and BMI. To find BMI category (e.g., obese), find the point where the woman's height and weight intersect. To estimate BMI, read the bold number on the dashed line that is closest to this point.

(Reprinted with permission from Nutrition during pregnancy and lactation. Copyright 1992 by the National Academy of Sciences. Published by the National Academy Press, Washington, D.C.)

In a follow-up publication, the IOM proposed a chart to monitor weight gain during pregnancy (42) (Figure 3). To avoid overinterpretation of normal variations in gain, gentle slopes depict recommended weight gain in these charts. This is a change from the steep slopes that have been typical of previous weight gain charts.

The IOM also recommended routine assessment of dietary practices for all pregnant women. This assessment is to be followed by nutrition education, dietary counseling, vitamin-mineral supplementation, and/or referral to food programs or other sources of assistance, as necessary (42).

To prevent the development of iron-deficiency anemia, routine supplementation of all pregnant women with low-dose (30 mg) iron in the ferrous form is recommended beginning in the second trimester (18). Routine supplementation of all women with other vitamins and minerals

is not recommended. Low-dose vitamin-mineral supplements are indicated, however, along with efforts to improve diet, for women who are found to be at risk of inadequate intakes because of poor dietary practices. Low-dose vitamin-mineral supplements are also indicated for women whose nutrient needs are increased because of multiple gestation, heavy cigarette smoking, or alcohol abuse. Complete vegetarians need a source of vitamin B-12 and often of vitamin D, and those who consume no calcium-rich milk products may benefit from a calcium supplement and vitamin D.

In 1991, the Centers for Disease Control (CDC) recommended that if a woman has had a pregnancy involving a fetus or an infant affected with a neural tube defect, she should consult her physician as soon as she plans a pregnancy. "Unless contraindicated, [women] should be advised to

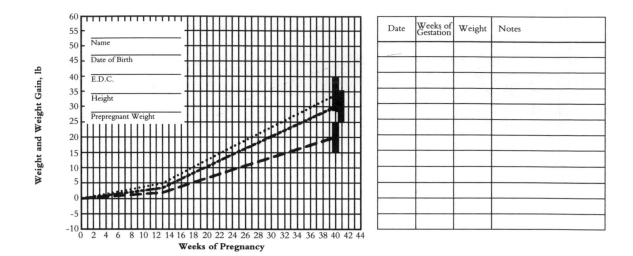

Figure 1.3 Prenatal weight gain chart. Prepregnancy BMI < 19.8 (· · · · · ·); Prepregnancy BMI 19.8–26.0 (Normal Body Weight) (– – – – –); Prepregnancy BMI > 26.0 (— — — —).

(Reprinted with permission from Nutrition during pregnancy and lactation. Copyright 1992 by the National Academy of Sciences. Published by the National Academy Press, Washington, D.C.)

take 4 mg per day of folic acid starting at the time they plan to become pregnant. Women should take the supplement from at least 4 weeks before conception through the first three months of pregnancy. The dose should be taken only under a physician's supervision" (43). Since the specified 4-mg daily dose of folic acid may pose some risks, the recommendation was accompanied by guidelines for physicians. There is some controversy surrounding the recommended dosage, which is 10 times the recommended dietary allowance for pregnant women and 4 times the maximum available dosage unit in the United States.

In 1992, CDC further recommended that "all women of childbearing age in the United States who are capable of becoming pregnant should consume 0.4 mg of folic acid per day for the purpose of reducing their risk of having a pregnancy affected with spina bifida or other [neural tube defects] (44)." A preferred method of meeting this recommendation (i.e. dietary, food fortification or supplements), was not specified.

Conclusion

Even though it is not currently possible to predict the degree of deficiency that is needed to manifest overt problems in the newborn infant, a well-balanced diet is beneficial to the health of both the pregnant woman and her fetus. Women who enter pregnancy with low nutrient stores, at low weight for height, or with certain health problems need to be identified early and given assistance to ensure an adequate supply of nutrients for fetal growth and development as well as for maintenance of the mother's health. Although nutrient stores may be protective to both the fetus and the mother, even previous well-nourished women may need encouragement or direct assistance in achieving a nutrient intake sufficient to support optimal fetal development and growth. This is especially true if factors such as gastrointestinal problems, concern about gaining weight, or lack of financial resources lead to a prolonged period of low food intake.

References

1. Bergner L, Susser MW. Low birth weight and perinatal nutrition: an interpretive review. Pediatrics 1970;46;946.

2. Rosso P. A new chart to monitor weight gain during pregnancy. Am J Clin Nutr 1985;41:644–52.

3. Rosso P. Prenatal nutrition and fetal growth development. Ped Ann 1981;10:430.

4. Scholl TO, Hediger ML, Khoo CS, et al. Maternal weight gain, diet and infant birth weight: correlations during adolescent pregnancy. J Clin Epidemiol 1991;44:123–8.

5. Villar J, Cogswell M, Kestler E, et al. Effect of fat and fat-free mass deposition during pregnancy on birth weight. Am J Obstet Gynecol 1992;167:1344–52.

6. Kleinman JC. Maternal weight gain during pregnancy: determinants and consequences. NCHS Working Paper Series No. 33. Hyattsville, MD: National Center for Health Statistics, Public Health Service, U.S. Department of Health and Human Services, 1990.

7. Emerson G. Obesity and its association with the complication of pregnancy. Br Med J 1962;2:516.

8. Travers CK. Obesity and pregnancy: a review. Obesity/Bariatric Med 1976;5:172.

9. Abrams B, Parker J. Overweight and pregnancy complications. Int J Obes 1988;12:293–303.

10. Perlow JH, Morgan MA, Montgomery D, et al. Perinatal outcome in pregnancy complicated by massive obesity. Am J Obstet Gynecol 1992;167:958–62.

11. Lammer EJ, Sever LE, Oakley GP Jr. Teratogen update: valproic acid. Teratology 1987;35:465–73.

12. Mills JL, Rhoads GG, Simpson JL, et al. The absence of a relation between the periconceptional use of vitamins and neural-tube defects. N Engl J Med 1989;321:430–5.

13. Milunsky A, Jick H, Jick SS, et al. Multivitamin/folic acid supplementation in early pregnancy reduces the prevalence of neural tube defects. JAMA 1989;262:2847–52.

14. Mulinare J, Cordero JF, Erickson JD, et al. Periconceptional use of multivitamins and the occurrence of neural tube defects. JAMA 1988;260:3141–5.

15. Smithells RW, Nevin NC, Seller MJ, et al. Further experience of vitamin supplementation for prevention of neural tube defect recurrences. Lancet 1983;1:1027–31.

16. Bower C, Stanley FJ. Dietary folate as a risk factor for neural tube defects: evidence for a case-control study in Western Australia. Med J Aust 1989;150:613–9.

17. MRC Vitamin Study Research Group. Prevention of neural tube defects: results of the Medical Research Council Vitamin Study. Lancet 1991;338:131–7.

18. Institute of Medicine. Nutrition during pregnancy: weight gain, nutrient supplements. Committee on Nutritional Status During Pregnancy and Lactation, Food and Nutrition Board. Washington, D.C.: National Academy Press, 1990.

19. Scholl TO, Hediger M, Fischer RL, et al. Anemia vs. iron deficiency: increased risk of preterm delivery in a prospective study. Am J Clin Nutr 1992;55:985–8.

20. Hambidge KM, Neldner KH, Walravens PA. Zinc, acrodermatitis enteropathica, and congenital malformations. Lancet 1975;1:577–8.

21. Cherry F, Sandstead H, Bazzano G, et al. Zinc nutriture in adolescent pregnancy: response to zinc supplementation. Fed Proc, Fed Am Soc Exp Biol 1987;46:748.

22. Hunt IF, Murphy NJ, Cleaver AE, et al. Zinc supplementation during pregnancy in low-income teenagers of Mexican descent: effects on selected blood constituents and on progress and outcome of pregnancy. Am J Clin Nutr 1985; 42:815–28.

23. Mahomed K, James DK, Golding J, et al. Zinc supplementation during pregnancy: a double blind randomized controlled trial. Br Med J 1989;299:826–30.

24. Anonymous. From endemic goiter to iodine deficiency disorders. Lancet 1983;2:1121–2.

25. Hetzel BS. Iodine deficiency disorders (IDD) and their eradication. Lancet 1983;2:1126–9.

26. Matovinovic J. Endemic goiter and cretinism at the dawn of the third millennium. Annu Rev Nutr 1983;3:341–412.

27. King EQ. Acute cardiac failure in the newborn due to thiamin deficiency. Exp Med Surg 1967;25:173.

28. Shah RS, Rajalakshmi R. Vitamin A status of the newborn in relation to gestational age, body weight, and maternal nutritional status. Am J Clin Nutr 1984;40:794–800.

29. Khanna A, Reddy TS. Effect of undernutrition and vitamin A deficiency on the phospholipid composition of rat tissues at 21 days of age. Liver, spleen, and kidney. Int J Vitam Nutr Res 1983;53:3–8.

30. Sharma HS, Misra UK. Postnatal distribution of vitamin A in liver, lung, heart, and brain of the rat in relation to maternal vitamin A status. Biol Neonate 1986;50:345–50.

31. Takahashi YI, Smith JE, Winick JE, et al. Vitamin A deficiency and fetal growth and development in the rat. J Nutr

1975;105:1299–310.

32. Paunier L, Lacourt G, Pilloud P, et al. 25-hydroxyvitamin D and calcium levels in maternal, cord and infant serum in relation to maternal vitamin D intake. Helv Paediatr Acta 1978;33:95–103.

33. Cockburn F, Belton NR, Purvis RJ, et al. Maternal vitamin D intake and mineral metabolism in mothers and their newborn infants. Br Med J 1980;281:11–14.

34. Brooke OG, Brown IR, Bone CD, et al. Vitamin D supplements in pregnant Asian women: effects on calcium status and fetal growth. Br Med J 1980;280:751–4.

35. Teratology Society. Teratology Society position paper: recommendations for vitamin A use during pregnancy. Teratology 1987;35:267–75.

36. Hanck A. Tolerance and effects of high doses of ascorbic acid. Doses facit venenum. Int J Vit Nutr Res 1982;suppl 23: 221–38.

37. Ghishan FK, Greene HL. Fetal alcohol syndrome: failure of zinc supplementation to reverse the effect of ethanol on placental transport of zinc. Pediatr Res 1983;17:529–31.

38. Institute of Medicine. Nutrition services in perinatal care, second edition. Committee on Nutritional Status During Pregnancy and Lactation, Food and Nutrition Board. Washington, D.C.; National Academy Press, 1992.

39. Committee on Genetics, American Academy of Pediatrics. Maternal phenylketonuria. Pediatrics 1991;88:1284–5.

40. Langer O. Critical issues in diabetes and pregnancy: early identification, metabolic control, and prevention of adverse outcome. In: IR Merkatz and JE Thompson, eds. New Perspectives on Prenatal Care. New York: Elsevier, 1990, pages 445–60.

41. Parker JD, Abrams B. Prenatal weight gain advice: an examination of the recent prenatal weight gain recommendations of the Institute of Medicine. Obstet Gynecol 1992;79: 664–9.

42. Institute of Medicine. Nutrition during pregnancy and lactation: an implementation guide. Subcommittee for a Clinical Application Guide, Committee on Nutritional Status During Pregnancy and Lactation, Food and Nutrition Board. Washington, D.C.: National Academy Press, 1992.

43. Centers for Disease Control. Use of folic acid for the prevention of spina bifida and other neural tube defects, 1983–1991. Morbid Mortal Weekly Rep 1991;40:513–6.

44. Centers for Disease Control. Recommendations for the use of folic acid to reduce the number of cases of spina bifida and other neural tube defects. Morbid Mortal Weekly Rep 1992:41:(RR–14);1–7.

2

Risks of Alcohol Consumption

Robert A. Welch, M.D.
Robert J. Sokol, M.D.

DESPITE recognized hazards, consumption of alcoholic beverages has long been an established social custom. Excess fetal and infant mortality related to heavy alcohol drinking was described during the London "gin epidemic" of 1720 to 1750 (1). Even with adequate wages, abundant food, and freedom from infectious epidemics, there was a decline in the birth rate and an increase in the fetal and newborn death rate. A series of inconclusive reports followed these assertions linking alcohol and reproduction.

In the United States, it wasn't until the latter part of this century that prenatal growth deficiencies were recognized in children of alcoholic mothers. This finding ultimately guided investigators to the association with other newborn malformations now referred to as the fetal alcohol syndrome (FAS) (2). Only recently have these revelations heightened public awareness about the risks of alcohol consumption during pregnancy and prompted legislation requiring the following label on alcoholic beverages as of October 1989:

Government Warning:
1. According to the Surgeon General, women should not drink alcoholic beverages during pregnancy because of the risk of birth defects.
2. Consumption of alcoholic beverages impairs your ability to drive a car or operate machinery, and may cause health problems (3).

Reproductive Causality

A continuum is suggested by the effects of alcohol on the fetus. The most severe complications of alcohol are abortion and stillbirth, followed in decreasing severity by fetal alcohol syndrome and alcohol-related birth defects, including abnormal neurobehavioral development and growth alterations. The complex of newborn findings characterizing the diagnosis of fetal alcohol syndrome was established in 1980 by the Research Society on Alcoholism (Table 2.1) (4).

Diagnosis requires the presence of characteristic manifestations in three areas: prenatal and/or postnatal growth retardation, central nervous system involvement, and characteristic facial dysmorphology (Figures 2.1 and 2.2).

Table 2.1 Components of Fetal Alcohol Syndrome

Prenatal or postnatal growth retardation (below the 10th per
 centile)
Central nervous system perturbations
  Tremulousness, poor sucking reflexes, abnormal muscle tone,
    hyperactivity, attentional deficits, or mental impairment
At least two characteristic facial anomalies (dysmorphology)
  Narrow eye width, ptosis, a thin upper lip, a short upturned
    nose with underdevelopment of the groove between the
    base of the nose to the top of the upper lip (philtrum), and
    general underdevelopment (hypoplasia) of the midfacial area

Alcohol-related birth defects are congenital anomalies
attributable to alcohol but not meeting the criteria for fetal
alcohol syndrome. Confounding conditions that may

account for these birth defects must be ruled out.

Prevalence of Disorders

Fetal alcohol syndrome surpasses Down syndrome and spina
bifida as the leading cause of known mental retardation,
with an estimated worldwide incidence of 1.9 cases per
1,000 live births (5). Older siblings have an incidence of
fetal alcohol syndrome and alcohol-related birth defects of
170 and 417 cases per 1,000 live births, respectively;
younger siblings have an incidence of 771 and 886 cases
per 1,000 live births, respectively. Other associated factors
are black race, frequent beer drinking, lower maternal
weight and weight gain, low socioeconomic status, and
being part of a Southwest Plains Indian culture.

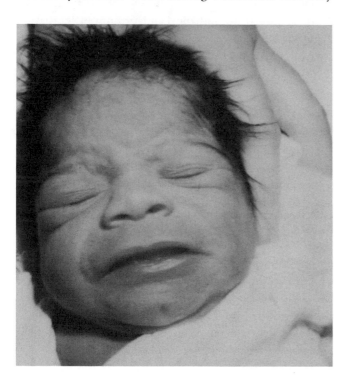

Figure 2.1 In this frontal view of a newborn with fetal alcohol
syndrome, characteristic features are evident: a long simple (flat)
philtrum (area between base of nose and upper lip), thin vermillion (upper lip), short upturned nose, and short palebral fissures as
well as hirsutism. Facial features not evident here are strabismus
and eyelid ptosis.

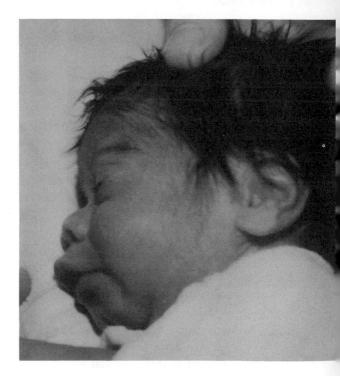

Figure 2.2 In the profile of the same baby, the hirsute appearance
is marked. Long hair partially hides the low-set ears and prominent crus across the concha. A scooped-out nasal bridge and short
upturned nose are also apparent. The relatively small mandible
accentuates the long philtrum, thin vermillion, and protruding
upper lip.

The societal cost of both disorders is difficult to estimate. Exclusive of the more poorly defined costs of lowered productivity and disruption of personal and family lives, one team calculated that treating fetal alcohol syndrome costs the nation nearly a third of a billion dollars yearly ($321 million); and fetal alcohol syndrome-related mental retardation accounts for more than a tenth (10.6%) of the total cost for residential treatment of mental retardation in the United States. Given current levels of federal support for fetal alcohol syndrome-related research ($2.9 million in 1985), a single year of treatment for one patient could support research on this subject for an entire century (6).

Recognized Thresholds

Alcohol is now recognized as a potent teratogen. The anatomic abnormalities detectable in the neonate are related in a clear dose-response fashion to prenatal alcohol exposure, and, as would be expected embryologically, the critical period for precipitating these abnormalities is in the early first trimester. Consumption of more than 1.5 oz. of absolute alcohol per day (that is, three cans of beer, glasses of wine, or mixed drinks) greatly increases the risk of alcohol teratogenicity (7). A precise intake threshold has not been established, however, and lower doses are still related to an increased incidence of craniofacial and neurobehavioral abnormalities.

Women contemplating reducing or stopping alcohol consumption during pregnancy may become aware of conception too late to avoid fetal alcohol syndrome or the risks for alcohol-related birth defects. Typical periconceptional drinking, the period of maximum vulnerability for anatomic defects, has been revealed to be nearly as heavy as that in the nonpregnant state. Thus, women attempting to conceive are advised to refrain from alcohol consumption. Those who conceive involuntarily are advised to stop alcohol consumption as soon as they become aware of pregnancy.

Identifying Drinkers at Risk

Seeking information about the use of tobacco, drugs, and alcohol is considered part of the "social history" portion of the intake history and physical. Typically, physicians ask their patients questions about smoking cigarettes and even about marijuana use. Alcohol consumption questions are often neglected or asked in a manner that conveys lack of concern, which may be due to the fact that alcohol problems are not considered "medical" by many physicians. Often, aware of the stigma associated with heavy drinking, physicians are afraid to evoke patients' anger by delving too deeply into their drinking behavior.

Nonetheless, there are ways to address the patient's drinking history that can be comfortable for both the patient and the physician. The place to start may be asking about a family history of alcohol problems. Besides providing useful information concerning alcoholism, a disease now recognized as having an important genetic component, this helps to identify drinking alcohol as an important concern for the patient and one of interest to her health care professionals. After obtaining other "social history" information, the physician may return to the alcohol history by asking the patient if she has ever had a drink of alcohol. If she responds "no," that is all that is necessary since it is unlikely that she has an alcohol problem. If she responds "yes," the next question should explore how old she was when she first had a drink of alcohol. Usually, this will be sometime during the teenage years. She should then be asked what she preferred as a teenager (beer, wine, or liquor) and when she first got drunk. Posing the query in this way conveys the notion that physicians recognize inebriation as a common experience and that admitting that one has been drunk is "okay."

After establishing a level of comfort with the patient, the physician should move on to a few key questions:

- How many drinks did it take to make you feel high when you were a teenager?
- What's your current alcohol preference, in terms of beer, wine, or liquor?
- How many cans (glasses) of beer (wine, liquor) does it take to make you feel high now?

It appears that eight or nine out of ten people will indicate that they feel high after a maximum of two drinks; that is, two cans of beer, two glasses of wine, or two mixed drinks, all of which contain approximately the same amount of absolute alcohol. If a patient indicates that it takes more than two drinks to make her feel high, this suggests that her drinking behavior needs further exploration. Seeking evidence of alcohol tolerance is a more effective way of obtaining an alcohol consumption history than merely asking a patient how much she drinks. Denial is a large component of alcohol dependence and abuse.

Some Useful Tests

Since a reliable laboratory test has not been developed to identify drinkers at risk, formal questionnaires have been devised to aid in identifying this group. The gold standard questionnaire has been the Michigan Alcoholism Screening Test (MAST), a 25-question data collection instrument widely used in alcohol research. Recognizing that the clinician does not have the time or office staff to administer such a detailed test, simpler, briefer questionnaires have been developed. The efficacy of these miniquestionnaires has not been widely evaluated in pregnant women but they appear to hold some promise.

One such test is the CAGE questionnaire (Table 2.2). When recently comparing this test with the MAST in 1,497 consecutive new prenatal clinic registrants, five or six out of ten risk-drinkers were identified (8). Although the CAGE misses nearly half of risk-drinkers, the test constitutes a very simple screening technique. It takes from 30 seconds to 1 minute to administer, is reasonably efficient, and fits well into many clinical settings.

To improve the sensitivity of the CAGE questionnaire, T-ACE was developed through stepwise linear discriminant analysis of the responses of 971 pregnant risk-drinkers and 929 pregnant women not at risk (9). When none of the answers to these questions is positive, the prob-

Table 2.2   CAGE Questions

C Have you ever felt you should **C**ut down on your drinking?
A Have people **A**nnoyed you by criticizing your drinking?
G Have you ever felt bad or **G**uilty about drinking?
E Have you ever taken a drink first thing in the morning (**E**ye opener) to steady your nerves or get rid of a hangover?

Table 2.3   T-ACE Questions

T How many drinks does it **T**ake to make you feel high (tolerance)?
A Have people **A**nnoyed you by criticizing your drinking?
C Have you felt you ought to **C**ut down your drinking?
E Have you ever had a drink first thing in the morning to steady your nerves or get rid of a hangover (**E**ye opener)?

ability that an individual is a risk-drinker is 1.5% (Table 2.3). If the patient answers the *Tolerance* question alone, the probability of risk-drinking is increased 8.5-fold to 11.7%. Should all four questions be answered positively, there is a 62.7% likelihood of risk drinking. A score of 2 was assigned to the *Tolerance* question and a score of 1 to all others. A T-ACE score of 2 or greater is considered positive for risk drinking.

When compared with other questionnaires, including the Michigan Alcoholism Screening Test, the T-ACE appears to be superior, identifying seven out of ten risk-drinkers during pregnancy. The key appears to be the *Tolerance* question that resists the denial component inherent in problem drinking. These preliminary findings need further verification and possible adjustment for socioeconomic statuses and racial compositions. T-ACE may be used in most clinical practices. It holds great promise for better risk identification, prevention efforts, and improved pregnancy outcomes for offspring at risk from heavy prenatal alcohol exposure.

Suggesting Interventions

Clinicians frequently wonder about their role in intervening to reduce maternal alcohol consumption. It is clear that warnings by clinicians can make an impact on reducing alcohol intake in many. Counseling heavy drinkers may require more time than many busy obstetricians are able to provide. But ignoring these women's drinking may result in marked morbidity in the newborn. The addition of a team approach of psychiatrist, psychologist, and other psychosocial workers may improve the outcome in these cases.

Clinicians may also be approached by women fearing that they have "damaged" their fetus by consuming alcohol early in their pregnancy. In some cases, since decreased fetal growth is a major component of fetal alcohol syndrome, serial ultrasound may be beneficial in suggesting growth abnormalities. We have seldom recommended abortion based on a history of alcohol consumption. The majority of fetal alcohol syndrome infants are born to chronic, heavy alcohol users, a group of women who rarely seek counseling.

The Value of Screening Efforts

Alcohol is a human teratogen capable of producing a variety of defects ranging from abortion and stillbirth to birth defects that are less easily identified. Most obstetricians lack the formal medical training necessary to be able to recognize the risk-drinkers in their practice. However, there are some basic screening techniques that obstetricians can use to identify risk-drinkers in the clinical setting. The results of these screening techniques may lead to secondary prevention efforts and improved pregnancy outcomes for the offspring at risk for fetal alcohol syndrome and alcohol-related birth defects.

References

1. Coffeey TG. Beer Street: Gin Lane: some views of 18th century drinking. QJ Stud Alcohol 1966;27:669.
2. Jones KL, Smith DW, Ulleland CN, et al. Pattern of malformations in offspring of chronic alcoholic mothers. Lancet 1973;7815:1267.
3. Alcoholic Beverage Labeling. 100th Congress, Report 100-596, 1988.
4. Rosett HL. A clinical perspective on the fetal alcohol syndrome (Editorial). Alcohol Clin Exp Res 1980;4:119.
5. Abel EL, Sokol RJ. Fetal alcohol syndrome is now leading cause of mental retardation. Lancet 1986;8517:1222.
6. Abel EL, Sokol RJ. Incidence of fetal alcohol syndrome and economic impact of FAS-related anomalies. Drug Alcohol Depend 1987;19:51.
7. Sokol RJ, Bottoms SF. How successful is the CAGE in identifying excessive female drinkers. Medical Aspects of Human Sexuality 1988:105.
8. Jacobson J, Jacobson S, Sokol RJ, et al. Teratogenic effects of alcohol on infant development. Alcohol Clin Exp Res 1993;17:174.
9. Sokol RJ, Martier SS, Ager J. The T-ACE questions: practical prenatal detection of risk-drinking. Am J Obstet Gynecol 1989;160:863.

3

Substance Abuse and Pregnancy

Preston Gazaway, M.D.

SUBSTANCE abuse is defined as a pathological pattern of use that results in some form of occupational or social impairment lasting longer than one month. Typically, dependence has been reserved for drugs in which a physiologic need can be demonstrated, manifested as either tolerance or withdrawal. Tolerance is the requirement of ever-greater quantities of a drug to produce the desired effect, while withdrawal is the development of a substance-specific syndrome upon the cessation or reduced use of a substance. Alcohol, barbiturates and other similar sedative hypnotics, opioids, amphetamines, and cannabis all have dependence syndromes. Hallucinogens, phencyclidine, and cocaine were initially believed to be associated only with abuse syndromes. However, many researchers felt that such a syndrome would emerge for cocaine if it become readily available. In the mid-1980s, as cocaine became available in greater quantity and better quality, its potential for dependence was realized.

The onset of drug use typically predates pregnancy, and many women are able to discontinue drug use once a gestation is established. However, if a woman continues to use drugs once she has discovered that she is pregnant, such use is considered pathologic if she has been informed of the potential harm to her fetus. If she is aware of the potential damage to the fetus, yet is unable to cease using drugs, she needs outside help to achieve abstinence, regain control of her life, and achieve a good pregnancy outcome.

Cocaine

Cocaine (benzylmethyl ecognine) is an acceptable psychoactive drug for many people because injection is not required, its widespread availability does not require the user to frequent less desirable parts of town, and "crack" (smokable cocaine base) costs as much as modest amounts of alcohol but yields a much greater euphoria. These factors contribute to cocaine being the drug of choice for many people (1). Obstetricians and gynecologists must realize that a large percentage of women who present for health care may be abusing cocaine. A survey of women at the University of Miami found 12% of pregnant women in the prenatal clinic used cocaine. All cocaine-abusing women were probably not detected in this survey, and the actual percentage may be much higher.

Cocaine produces a magnification of pleasurable activities, an increased sense of well-being, increased mental acuity, and an increased capacity for physical work. It lowers anxiety and social inhibitions, heightens self-esteem, sexuality, and other feelings aroused by interpersonal experiences. Although cocaine magnifies all these feelings, it does not distort them as do hallucinogens (3). The physiologic effects of cocaine include increased blood pressure, tachycardia, and a mild temperature elevation. These effects are ephemeral, persisting for only 30 to 45 minutes. The use of cocaine is often followed by a "crash" associated with irritability, depression, dysphoria, and physical discomfort. If no limits are placed, tolerance may occur, with larger and larger amounts of cocaine being ingested with increased frequency; dependence ensues. Cocaine use is self-reinforcing. When rats were given unlimited access, they erratically ingested cocaine in amounts up to 250 mg/kg per day, causing a 90% death rate within 30 days. In contrast, rats who were provided heroin under similar conditions had stable rates of ingestion which averaged 10 mg/kg per day, and about 40% died (4). Similar reactions occur in humans. However, not everyone who tries cocaine becomes dependent. Factors that predict susceptibility to cocaine dependence are presently unknown.

Despite assertions to the contrary, cocaine is not a drug that can be taken with impunity. The most commonly quoted lethal dose is 1.2 g; however, death has occurred with the ingestion of as little as 20 mg. Though the risk of sudden cardiac death is cocaine's most sobering effect, this drug may affect any organ system and is responsible for many other ailments that range from minor to life-threatening (Figure 3.1).

Identifying the Cocaine Abuser

Health care professionals have to be suspicious and willing to investigate potential substance abuse. The simplest, although not the most reliable, method is to ask the patient about the way she uses drugs. It helps to start with a socially acceptable drug such as alcohol and then progress to the illicit drugs such as marijuana, cocaine, and opiates (Table 3.1).

Drug use may be suspected in women who have difficulty keeping their prenatal appointments, who have a disheveled appearance, whose appearance or hygiene deteriorates, who are chronically fatigued, or whose financial status declines. Similarly, women who are irritable or emotionally labile may also be abusing cocaine, as well as other drugs.

These nonspecific symptoms may indicate underlying conditions other than drug abuse, but, regardless of the cause, these symptoms need to be addressed. Careful, nonjudgmental questioning should be used to differentiate between a history of drug abuse and an underlying non-drug-related psychosocial difficulty. The drug-abusing patient often has plausible explanations for her shortcomings, but clinicians should remain skeptical.

Obstetric complications may also be a clue to women who are abusing cocaine. Women who present for prenatal care after 20 weeks, have a hemoglobin reading below 10 mg/dL, have no weight gain or weight loss, or have evidence of intrauterine growth retardation should be evaluated.

Past obstetric history may also reveal drug use and predict current drug abuse. A history of a small-for-gestational-age infant, unexplained vaginal bleeding, abruption, or emergency cesarean delivery for fetal distress may have been associated with drug use during that pregnancy. Similarly, an unusually prolonged neonatal stay without obvious medical complications of a baby who died because of sudden infant death syndrome may be evidence of drug withdrawal or drug effect and should raise suspicions of drug abuse (1–4).

Table 3.1 Substance Dependence Criteria

Continued use despite disorder or problem
Efforts to cut down or control use
Given up activities for substance
Impaired when expected to fulfill obligations
Preoccupation with substance seeking or taking
Taking in larger doses/longer than intended
Tolerance
Used to avoid withdrawal
Withdrawal

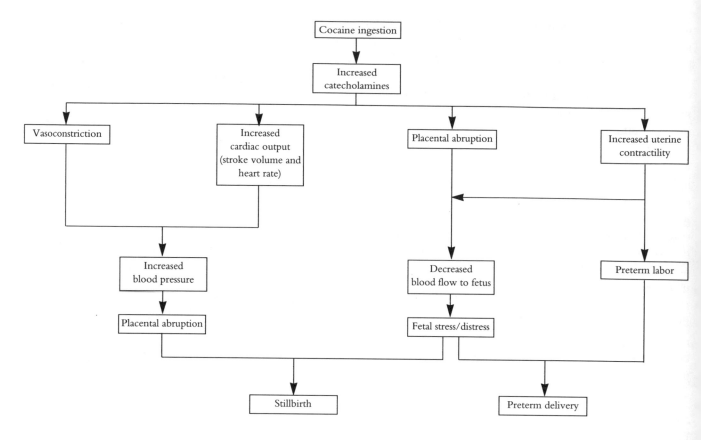

Figure 3.1 Cascade of cocaine effects.

Physical stigmata of cocaine use are rare. A chronic user of intranasal cocaine often has persistent rhinorrhea, edematous and inflamed turbinates, or an ulcerated nasal septum. In severe cases, a perforated septum may be present. A simple screening test is to squeeze the nasal alae together and compress the septum. This maneuver elicits pain because of the inflammation caused by the repeated ischemia of the septum associated with cocaine sniffing (snowbird sign). There are no consistent physical signs in cocaine smokers (Table 3.2).

Close scrutiny is required to discover intravenous (IV) injection sites, since most women attempt to hide IV use. The most commonly seen surreptitious injection sites are the inner thigh, upper arm, and breasts. Look for a puncture site within any area of bruising, especially in locations commonly used for injection. Any area of ecchymosis war-

rants further investigation, since the woman may be the victim of abuse.

Once drug abuse has been established, the specific drug or drugs should be identified, as well as the frequency, amount, and route of administration. A complete urine toxicology screen should also be obtained to confirm all types of drugs abused. Polysubstance abuse is frequent. Cocaine-dependent women frequently use other drugs to temper the effects of cocaine.

In women who presented at Francis Scott Key Medical Center in Baltimore for treatment because of cocaine abuse or dependence and who were not opiate dependent, urine screening showed that 76% had evidence of one illicit drug and 15% of two illicit drugs in addition to cocaine. Opiates were found in 62%, sedative hypnotics in 15%, and alcohol in 8%. Similarly, 62% of pregnant opioid-dependent, methadone-maintained women met lifetime criteria for cocaine dependence, and 40% of their urine tests were positive for cocaine and 15% were positive for sedative hypnotics.

Since cocaine is rapidly metabolized, it is detected in the urine for only three to six hours after ingestion. For this reason, the cocaine metabolites, benzoylecognine and ecognine methylester, which remain in the urine for 40 to 60 hours after ingestion, are usually what is detected, depending on the sensitivity of the test and the quantity of cocaine consumed. Theoretically, cocaine and its metabolites may persist in the urine longer during pregnancy because the concentration of plasma and liver esterases, which are the primary means of cocaine metabolism, are decreased during pregnancy. The resulting prolonged half-life may be counteracted by the increased glomerular filtration rate in pregnancy.

However, no studies have been conducted to determine the process of elimination of cocaine during pregnancy. One study described two heavy cocaine users who had detectable cocaine metabolites for five weeks after their last ingestion (5). If cocaine is persistently detected in the urine, the patient is probably continuing to abuse cocaine. If abstinence must be confirmed, mass spectrography and gas chromatography will document a steady decline in the quantity of cocaine metabolites excreted in the urine.

Central Nervous System Effects

Central nervous system (CNS) complications are potentially life threatening. Seizures are frequent in the heavy cocaine user. In our group of pregnant, cocaine-dependent women, 20% admitted having had a seizure associated with cocaine use. All these women admitted to using more than $100 worth of cocaine daily. None had sought medical treatment for their seizures.

In a survey of teenagers, light users reported a 7% incidence of seizures, and heavy users a 27% incidence. The time between cocaine use and seizure occurrence ranged from a few minutes to up to 12 hours after ingestion (6). Many cocaine users also complain of migraine like headaches after use. These headaches appear to be the result of

Table 3.2 Abnormalities in Substance Abusers

Dermatologic	Cardiovascular
Abscesses	Cardiomegaly
Cellulitis	Murmurs indicative of endocarditis, pulmonary hypertension, or valvular disease
Ecchymosis	
Icterus	**Gastrointestinal**
Madarosis	
Thrombosed veins	Abdominal pain
	Diarrhea
Otolaryngologic	Guaiac-positive stools
	Hepatomegaly
Excoriated or ulcerated nasal septum	
Rhinitis	**Musculoskeletal**
Sinusitis	
	Brawny edema
Respiratory	Myalgias
	Pitting edema
Adventitious breath sounds	
Interstitial lung disease	**Genitourinary**
Obstructive lung disease	
	Pelvic infection
	Presence of sexually transmitted disease
	Trauma

cerebral vasospasm and generally disappear once cocaine is discontinued.

Hyperthermia or pyrexia may also be associated with seizures in acute cocaine intoxication. The increased temperature is centrally mediated and further increased by vasoconstriction and increased muscular activity. Those who inject cocaine may have a febrile episode soon after injection. Pyrogens in the material used to filter the drugs cause an acute elevation in temperature that may persist for several hours. This is known as "cotton fever" among IV drug users.

Neurovascular complications are likely to be devastating. Of 3,712 drug abusers admitted to one hospital over a three-year period, 13 (0.35%) had neurologic deficits attributable to cocaine use; five users (31%) were an average age of 30.6 years (7). In a similar study, 0.94% of hospital admissions precipitated by cocaine use were secondary to neurologic sequelae, and 42% of this sample were women (8). Both ischemic and hemorrhagic events were discovered. There was no predilection for any particular region of the brain. Rupture of cerebral aneurysms and arteriovenous malformations, intracranial hemorrhages, as well as cortical, thalamic, and basal ganglia bleeds were diagnosed.

Cardiovascular Effects

Cocaine has been temporally associated with myocardial infarction. Although an exact pathophysiologic correlation has not been established, the underlying cause appears to be a sudden increase in myocardial oxygen demand accompanied by coronary artery vasospasm that prevents adequate oxygenation. Ischemia and infarction subsequently occur. Only 10% to 20% of patients with myocardial infarction associated with cocaine use reported in the literature are women. The preponderance of males may reflect their predominance in the cocaine-abusing population. In the literature concerning myocardial infarction associated with cocaine use, preexisting cardiac disease was not universally documented. The inciting dose ranged from 140 mg to 20 g. Remarkably, 55.5% of the myocardial infarctions were associated with intranasal use (9).

Acute and subacute bacterial endocarditis is a problem among IV cocaine abusers. Unlike heroin, cocaine is freely water soluble and not heated prior to injection. IV drug users, therefore, expose themselves to a solution with a greater load of pathogenic organisms. This, coupled with more frequent injection, confers a greater risk of infection.

Respiratory System Problems

Abnormalities arise within the respiratory system regardless of the route of ingestion. Those who sniff cocaine are prone to aspiration pneumonia because of paralysis of the glottis. Sniffers are prone to sinusitis with such bacteria as Clostridium botulinum (10). Crack and freebase smokers are susceptible to a "crack lung" syndrome that includes fever, leukocytosis, hypoxemia, and respiratory distress. The chest x-ray generally reveals pulmonary infiltrates. Once the diagnosis is confirmed and corticosteroids are instituted, rapid improvement usually ensues (11, 12). This syndrome appears to be dramatically altered by pregnancy. An epidemic of a similar syndrome occurred in pregnant women at Harlem Hospital Center, New York City: 42 women were admitted with this syndrome over a six-month period; 53% required admission to the intensive care unit (ICU), and 35% died (13).

Psychiatric Complications

Often, patients will meet criteria for many psychiatric diagnoses, from acute anxiety to frank psychosis with hallucinations. Cocaine may also precipitate or exacerbate such preexisting psychiatric disorders as mania, manic depression, and psychosis. There is also the danger of suicide.

Of 80 people who came to one emergency room with psychiatric problems secondary to cocaine abuse, 57% of crack smokers, 43% of IV abusers, 37% of intranasal abusers, and 26% of freebase smokers displayed suicidal tendencies at the time of evaluation. Almost one-quarter of these people had actually made a suicide attempt (14).

In another review, 63% of patients were found to have mood disorders (15). The most common was major depression (present in 20% of the total group), followed by cyclothymic disorder (17%) and bipolar disorder (6%). This incidence was significantly higher than that of patients dependent upon opiates or depressants. These researchers also found a 28% incidence of borderline personality disorder, a 23% incidence of narcissistic personality disorder, and a 17% incidence of histrionic personality disorders.

Effect upon Pregnancy

The pharmacologic effects of cocaine counter the physiologic changes necessary for successful pregnancy. Cocaine potentiates the response of sympathetically innervated organs to epinephrine and norepinephrine. This effect is caused by blocking the reuptake of the catecholamines at the adrenergic nerve terminal (16–18). The ingestion of cocaine begins a cascade of effects that end in preterm labor or delivery or, in severe cases, an intrauterine fetal demise.

Theoretically, small placental infarctions or recurrent abruptions impair nutrient transfer to the fetus and decrease fetal reserves and growth. Hence, the abuse of cocaine during pregnancy has a deleterious effect upon the developing fetus, pregnancy outcome, and neonatal outcome. This negative effect is over and above any compromise that can be attributed to race, cigarette smoking, or socioeconomic status.

Uteroplacental insufficiency, intrauterine growth retardation, microcephaly, placental abruption, premature labor, and premature delivery have all been associated with cocaine use. Since cocaine is also a powerful anorectic, many dependent pregnant women are malnourished because they have neither the desire nor the money to eat well.

Several reports have described placental abruption soon after cocaine ingestion. These abruptions generally occur after either IV injection or smoking. Both routes provide for a rapid rise in plasma concentrations and a particularly intense physiologic response. The abrupt onset and pronounced rise in blood pressure associated with these modes of ingestion probably cause placental abruption. One group has also noted an increased rate of spontaneous abortion in cocaine users (19). This increase is most likely an earlier manifestation of the same physiologic effects that cause abruptions. Unfortunately, even though a woman stops using cocaine early in pregnancy, her risk of abruption does not return to normal and she is still at risk for preterm labor.

Women who are cocaine dependent rarely obtain prenatal care. In a retrospective survey of unregistered patients, investigators found that these patients accounted for 8% of all deliveries, but 36% of these women had cocaine or its metabolites in their urine at the time of delivery. These women also had a significantly increased incidence of low birthweight and prematurity (20). Similar results have been found elsewhere, with up to 60% of cocaine-abusing women having had no prenatal care.

Novel ways of using cocaine have proven lethal. One case report described intravaginal application of approximately 1.5 g of cocaine during pregnancy that led to the eventual death of both the mother and the fetus (21). An acute cardiac event precipitated by the "sex-cocaine syndrome" again led to the death of mother and fetus at 32 weeks. In this syndrome, sex-induced cardiodynamic surges, vasoactive stresses of high levels of catecholamines, and the hyperdynamic circulation of pregnancy lead to malignant arrhythmia, cardiac failure, and death (2).

Neonatal Effects

The neonatal consequences of maternal cocaine abuse are a major concern. Most of the emphasis has been on the acute presentation of these cocaine-affected infants. However, cocaine abuse during pregnancy has both short-term and long-term effects.

Every organ system in the neonate may be affected by prenatal exposure. Cocaine-affected infants have tremors, tachypnea, hypertonia, poor feeding, abnormal sleep patterns, and, occasionally, seizures. A recurring defect is microcephaly, a defect whose long-term implications are uncertain.

Defects of the neonatal skull ranging from exencephaly to delayed ossification of the calvarium have also been described (22). In one case, an antepartum cerebral vascular accident occurred in a child born of a cocaine-abusing mother (23). Of neonates exposed to cocaine in utero, 87% displayed CNS irritability, and 45% had abnormal electroencephalograms. No correlation existed among abnormal neurologic examinations, Apgar scores, head circumference, route of cocaine ingestion, birthweight or EEG abnormalities.

The abnormalities were transient and resolved within three to 12 months (24). The EEG abnormalities eventually resolved, but the effect upon the maturation of the neonatal EEG and the subsequent intellectual and social development has not been established.

Substance abuse has been implicated as an etiologic factor in sudden infant death syndrome (SIDS). Infants of opiate-dependent mothers have a higher risk for this syndrome. In Chicago, the rate of SIDS in the general population was 0.27% and 0.83% in preterm births. However, during the same period, the infants of methadone-using mothers had a rate of 4%, and the offspring of cocaine-dependent mothers had an incidence of 15% (25). Others, however, have not found such a dramatic increase in the incidence of SIDS among the offspring of cocaine-abusing mothers.

Treating Cocaine Dependence

Frequently, the cocaine-dependent woman's first medical contact is when she appears in labor. She is usually tachycardic, agitated, garrulous, irritable, and hypervigilant. However, if the cocaine ingestion was not recent, she may be lethargic.

The most frequent reason for the visit is the onset of regular uterine contractions after ingesting cocaine. Up to 17% of women with preterm labor have been found to have illicit drugs in their urine (26). Cocaine-induced contractions are usually transient and gradually resolve as the effects of cocaine abate. If the contractions persist, or if preterm labor is well established, magnesium sulfate is the agent of choice for tocolysis. The interactions between the mimetic effects of cocaine and the mimetic effects of ritodrine or terbutaline are unknown. In sheep, pretreatment with magnesium attenuated the cardiovascular response to cocaine, decreased the incidence of seizures, and prevented fetal distress (27).

The patient may also complain of an acute onset of abdominal pain, with or without vaginal bleeding. In this event, both mother and fetus must be closely monitored. An abruption may be present or the mother may be experiencing visceral angina because of bowel ischemia. These two syndromes may be differentiated by fetal monitoring and lab testing.

The rare patient may seek medical attention because of hypertension, and she may have had a seizure. It's important to establish whether the patient is preeclamptic, eclamptic, or is suffering from a cocaine overdose. All initial efforts should be directed towards stabilizing the mother.

In the event that a cocaine overdose is diagnosed, high-flow oxygen should be instituted after establishing a patent airway to prevent cerebral anoxia. The increased anaerobic metabolism should be treated secondary to muscle hyperactivity, hyperthermia, and seizures. An arterial blood gas reading must be obtained to determine the patient's acid-base status and facilitate interpretation of the fetal monitoring.

IV access with 5% dextrose and normal saline should be established. Laboratory studies should include a complete blood count, electrolytes, coagulation studies, and cardiac and liver enzymes. The creatinine phosphokinase may be elevated because of cardiac injury or myonecrosis. Similarly, a mild elevation of alanine amino transferase and aspartate amino transferase may be a result of drug abuse.

Close monitoring of urine output and vital signs, including an accurate core temperature, is necessary since rapid deterioration may occur. Hyperthermia can be life threatening in cocaine overdose. Continuous cardiac monitoring can diagnose any life-threatening arrhythmias.

If the patient is obtunded, a 4-mg ampule of naloxone may be administered since cocaine and opiates (speedball) are frequently injected together. Rapid administration may precipitate a sudden withdrawal and yield a wide-awake, but combative and uncontrollable patient.

Severe hypertension can be treated with sodium nitroprusside, although some advocate propranolol or phentolamine. Valium or magnesium sulfate may overcome seizures. If intubation and paralysis are required for intractable seizures, a nondepolarizing agent should be given to avoid fasciculations that could cause or aggravate hyperthermia.

Once the obstetric and medical problems have been resolved, the patient should be referred to a drug abuse program. Most obstetricians have neither the time nor the expertise to address the multitude of problems that this group of patients presents.

Treatment of cocaine dependence during pregnancy

requires an integrated and coordinated program to help the cocaine-dependent pregnant woman abstain. The life of the cocaine-abusing patient is often in such disarray that she will need social service intervention to provide social support. Her needs may vary from emergency housing or financial assistance to legal aid.

Clinicians have to develop an expertise in the treatment of substance abuse and social services. Because the drug-dependent woman is frequently impatient and impulsive, every effort must be made to provide easy access to care if any of the interventions are to succeed. It's important that such agencies inform the clinician of the patient's progress in treatment as well as substantive treatment concerns.

Hospitalization for two to four weeks is often required. This period allows the drug effect to resolve and permits physicians to evaluate the patient for any stigmata of drug use and any concurrent psychiatric disorders. Further, the patient should also be observed for substance withdrawal syndromes. Treatment for withdrawal from other drugs should be instituted before discharge.

Underlying psychiatric disorders should also be treated, since this type of regimen may decrease the craving for cocaine and facilitate a patient's ability to maintain abstinence. Counseling is unlikely to be effective if the patient continues to use cocaine and remains drug affected.

A physician should see the patient frequently throughout her pregnancy. Liberal use of ultrasound confirms appropriate fetal growth and allows the mother to bond prenatally with her developing child. Urine toxicology screens at each visit confirm abstinence. If continued drug use is detected, more intensive intervention measures and rehospitalization for acute detoxification may be considered.

Antepartum fetal heart rate monitoring should commence at 32 weeks to ascertain whether any compromise to the pregnancy has occurred. Nonstress testing results may be abnormal. These generally consist of a hypervariable or saltatory tracing.

In one study, abnormal biophysical profiles were seen in 65% of patients examined. The affected fetuses most often had hyperflexion, persistent sucking behavior, and excessive movement in response to stimulation. Recurrent yawning and sustained hyperpneic breathing movements were long-term effects. These changes correlated with the amount and duration of cocaine abuse (28).

Complete abstinence is unlikely after a single hospitalization. Like alcoholism, drug abuse is a chronic relapsing disease. Because the patient has taken several months to several years to arrive at her present situation, abstinence is unlikely to be achieved immediately. Nevertheless, abstinence from cocaine abuse should be the primary goal of treatment, and all efforts should be directed toward this end.

References

1. Keith LG, MacGregor S, Friedell S, et al. Substance abuse in pregnant women: recent experience at the perinatal center for chemical dependence of Northwestern Memorial Hospital. Obstet Gynecol 1989;73:715.

2. Burkett G, Bandstra ES, Cohen J, et al. Cocaine-related maternal death. Am J Obstet Gynecol 1990,163.40.

3. Gawin FH, Ellinwood EH. Cocaine and other stimulants: actions, abuse, and treatment. N Engl J Med 1973;318:18.

4. Bozarth MA, Wise RA. Toxicity associated with long term intravenous heroin and cocaine self administration in the rat. JAMA 1985;254:81.

5. Weiss RD, Gawin FH. Protracted elimination of cocaine metabolites in long-term, high dose cocaine abusers. Am J Med 1988;85:879.

6. Schwartz RH. Seizures and syncope in adolescent cocaine abusers. Am J Med 1988;85:462.

7. Jacobs IJ, Roszler MH, Kelly JK, et al. Cocaine abuse: neurovascular complications. Radiol 1989;170:223.

8. Lowenstein DH, Massa SM, Rowbotham MC, et al. Acute neurologic and psychiatric complications associated with cocaine abuse. Am J Med 1987;83:841.

9. Isner JM, Estes NAM, Thompson PD, et al. Acute cardiac events temporally related to cocaine abuse. N Engl J Med 1986;315:1438.

10. Kudrow DB, Henry DA, Haake DA, et al. Botulism associated with *Clostridium botulinum* sinusitus after intranasal cocaine abuse. Ann Int Med 1988;109:984.

11. Kissner DG, Lawrence D, Selis JE, et al. Crack lung: pulmonary disease caused by cocaine abuse. Am Rev Resp Dis 1987;136:1250.

12. Patel RC, Dutta D, Schofeld SA. Free-base cocaine use associated with bronchiolitis obliterations organizing pneumo-

nia. Ann Int Med 1987;107:186.

13. Brown GM. Pneumonia associated with crack use in pregnancy (abstract). Pregnant and hooked on cocaine and other drugs. New York: Columbia University College of Physicians and Surgeons, 1989.

14. Honer WG, Gewirtz G, Turey M. Psychosis and violence in cocaine smokers. Lancet 1987; 2:451.

15. Weiss RD, Mirin SM, Michael JL, et al. Psychopathology in chronic cocaine abusers. Am J Drug Alcohol Abuse 1986; 12(1):17.

16. Woods JR, Plessinger MA, Clark KE. Effect of cocaine on uterine blood flow and fetal oxygenation. JAMA 1987; 257:957.

17. Dolkart LA, Plessinger MA, Woods JR. Effect of alpha 1 receptor blockade upon maternal and fetal cardiovascular responses to cocaine. Obstet Gynecol 1990;75:745.

18. Woods JR, Plessinger MA. Pregnancy increases cardiovascular toxicity to cocaine. Am J Obstet Gynecol 1990;162:529.

19. Neerhoff MG, MacGregor SN, Retzky SS, et al. Cocaine abuse during pregnancy: peripartum prevalence and perinatal outcome. Am J Obstet Gynecol 1989;161:633.

20. Chouteau M, Namerow PB, Leppert P. The effect of cocaine abuse upon birth weight and gestational age. Obstet Gynecol 1988;72:351.

21. Greenland VC, Delke I, Minkoff HL. Vaginally administered cocaine overdose in a pregnant woman. Obstet Gynecol 1989;74:476.

22. Bingol N, Fuchs M, Diaz V, et al. Teratogenicity of cocaine in humans. J Pediatr 1987;110:93.

23. Chasnoff IJ, Burns WJ, Savich R, et al. Perinatal cerebral infarction and maternal cocaine use. J Pediatr 1986;108: 456.

24. Doberczak TM, Shanzer S, Senie RT, et al. Neonatal neurologic and electroencephalographic effects of intrauterine cocaine exposure. J Pediatr 1988;113:354.

25. Chasnoff IJ, Hunt CE, Kletter R, et al. Prenatal cocaine exposure is associated with respiratory pattern abnormalities. Am J Dis Child 1989;143:583.

26. Ney JA, Dooley SL, Keith LG, et al. The prevalence of substance abuse in patients with suspected preterm labor. Am J Obstet Gynecol 1990;162:1562.

27. Weaver K, Merrell CL, Griffin G. Effect of magnesium on cocaine-induced, catecholamine mediated platelet and vascular response in term pregnant ewes. Am J Obstet Gynecol 1989;161:1331.

28. Hume RF, O'Donnell KJ, Stanger CL, et al. In utero cocaine exposure: observations of fetal behavioral state may predict outcome. Am J Obstet Gynecol 1989;161:685.

4

Environmental Toxicants and Adverse Pregnancy Outcome

Anthony R. Scialli, M.D.
Armand Lione, Ph.D.

DESPITE the difficulties inherent in reproductive epidemiology, some environmental pollutants have been identified as important reproductive hazards in humans (1–4). Others, because of their prevalence in the environment and their general potential for toxicity in biologic systems, are viewed with concern, although they are not proven hazards in humans.

Lead

While lead toxicity has been recognized for centuries, the usefulness of various forms of lead has kept it widely available. In the recent past, the burning of lead alkyl additives in gasoline constituted the largest and most widespread exposure. Federal guidelines now prohibit this use of lead, lowering atmospheric exposures substantially but leaving residual soil contamination and a large variety of alternative sources. These include lead solders, pipes, storage batteries, construction materials (for example, lead-based paints), dyes, and wood preservatives.

Although most lead exposure was formerly associated with atmospheric exposure, lead intake may now occur from variable and, at times, insidious sources. For example, growth retardation and neurologic deficits were found in a newborn whose lead exposure was traced to the chronic use of "moonshine" whiskey by the mother. The equipment used to distill the whiskey was found to contain lead solder, which contaminated the liquor (5). Animal and human studies indicate that lead can be readily transferred across the placenta to the fetus (6). In humans, this transfer takes place as early as the twelfth week of gestation (7). Generally, the alkyl lead salts (such as tetraethyl lead) have not been associated with teratogenic effects (8, 9).

Inorganic lead salts have been associated with malformations of the central nervous system (CNS) and cleft palate in mice, tail defects in hamsters, and hydronephrosis and skeletal defects in rats (10–12). Although postnatal behavioral studies in rats have given contradictory results (13, 14), sheep experiments indicated that maternal blood levels of 34 µg/dL induced learning defects in newborn lambs (15). Over 100 years ago, the toxic effects of lead on human pregnancy were suspected in women who worked with lead salts contained in pottery glazes and other substances. Stillbirths and miscarriages were also recognized as common in this population (16). Lead salts were considered to be abortifacients (17, 18). Modern industrial hygiene has markedly limited occupational exposures to lead. Whenever possible, however, women at risk of lead exposures in the workplace should be monitored for blood lead levels before becoming pregnant.

If the blood lead level is elevated (>30 µg/dL), pregnancy should be postponed until chelation therapy and reduced exposures prove effective. Currently, there is intense interest in identifying the possible behavioral and developmental toxicity of low levels of blood lead (< 35 µg/dL). In one report, umbilical cord blood lead levels between 8.7 and 35.1 µg/dL were associated with a variety of minor fetal anomalies, including hemangiomas, lymphangiomas, hydrocele, skin tags, papillae, and undescended testicles (19). Because no pattern was evident in the anomalies detected, these findings can be alternatively interpreted as indicative of more serious malformations (19, 20) or discounted as inadvertently associated with fetal lead.

Another report suggests that measurable deficits in early cognitive development can be correlated with prenatal exposure as measured by more than 10 µg/dL in umbilical cord blood (21). The variations reported are small and demonstrable only when sophisticated behavioral and statistical analyses are applied to the available clinical data. This study was supported by the finding that decrements in the Bayley Mental Developmental Index correlated with increasing measures of intrauterine exposure to lead, even at maternal blood lead levels less than 30 µg/dL (22).

These findings suggest that the current standards for blood lead levels in young children may be inadequate for fetuses and newborns. The data do not establish, however, that low-level lead exposures, such as might occur in a typical urban environment, pose a formidable health risk to newborns. While avoidance of fetal lead exposure seems desirable, there are no data showing that elaborate alterations in the diet or health care of otherwise healthy pregnant women to minimize lead intake would markedly benefit fetal development.

Mercury

Mercury has had a long history as a potential reproductive toxicant. It was noted many years ago that pregnant women treated with mercurials had a high incidence of spontaneous abortion (23). More recent mercury effects became publicized after an outbreak of cerebral palsy and microcephaly in the fishing village of Minimata, Japan (24, 25). This was traced to methyl mercury contamination of fish eaten by the population.

A similar incident involved the poisoning of an Iraqi population by grain contaminated with methyl mercury (26, 27). Infants exposed in utero demonstrated psychomotor retardation and cerebral palsy. Similar congenital neurologic disease has been reported in other instances of methyl mercury food contamination (28). The risk, if any, for women exposed to commonly found levels of mercury contamination in the environment is unknown. Because organic mercurials have polluted a large proportion of the earth's waterways, some authorities have suggested limiting the intake of fish during pregnancy to 350 g/week or less (29).

Polychlorinated Biphenyls

There are a group of more than 200 lipid-soluble chemicals used extensively in industry. Most of the polychlorinated biphenyls (PCBs) available commercially are not single chemical compounds but mixtures of several compounds, a fact that greatly complicates investigations into their reproductive effects. Environmental contamination with these agents has been extensive; most fish, birds, mammals, and humans now have measurable levels of PCBs in their tissues.

PCBs are not teratogenic in most animal species, although intrauterine growth retardation is sometimes seen (30). An impairment of reproductive function in rodents may occur after intrauterine exposure to large doses of these chemicals (31, 32). It is clear from animal work that different PCBs have varying degrees of toxicity. Some PCBs are mutagenic and probably carcinogenic (30). In humans, the most extensive information on the effects of PCB exposure during pregnancy was derived from two episodes of PCB poisonings of rice oil in Japan in 1968 and in Taiwan in 1979. In both cases, cooking oil was accidentally contaminated with large amounts of PCBs and with smaller amounts of other toxicants. In the 1968 incident, 13 exposed pregnant women were delivered of two stillborn and 11 live babies (33).

Abnormalities associated with these poisoning episodes included gray-brown discoloration of the skin, gingiva, and nails; parchmentlike skin with desquamation; conjunctivitis; and low birthweight (34–40). Nearly all the exposed mothers exhibited evidence of poisoning as well. Postnatally, the babies demonstrated "catch-up" growth, and skin discoloration slowly disappeared.

One recent study attempted to define the reproductive effects of PCB exposure from eating fish caught in contaminated waterways, such as Lake Michigan and the St. Lawrence Seaway (41). Mothers were classified as having significant PCB intake if they recalled eating 11.8 kg or more of Lake Michigan fish during the six years before delivery. Infants classified by this system as having been exposed to PCBs were 160 to 190 g lighter and had smaller head sizes than nonexposed infants. In the affected infants, head circumference was disproportionately small in relation to birthweight and gestational age. These findings on reduced birth size in association with PCB exposure are consistent with experimental studies in rhesus monkeys and data collected from the Japanese intoxications (36, 42, 43). The data also suggested that, at low levels of exposure, the threat to the fetus is based more on gradual long-term bioaccumulation than on acute exposures during pregnancy (41).

PCBs are excreted very efficiently in the fat portion of milk. Analytical determinations of PCB levels in fetal and neonatal rats indicate a greater transfer of PCBs during lactation than during gestation (44). Toxemia of pregnancy and breastfeeding seem to mobilize residual PCBs stored in fat tissues (45, 46). Women who are occupationally exposed to PCBs or who eat large quantities of game fish caught in contaminated waterways are likely to have elevated levels of PCBs in their tissues and breast milk. Such women should be informed that, if they choose to breastfeed, they will probably pass PCBs to their newborns. In general, women have higher levels at first lactation. Levels decline with time spent breastfeeding and with number of children nursed (46).

Pesticides

Pesticides include a large number of diverse agents used to control unwanted plants and animals. Because these agents are widely used, human exposure to them is commonplace. Although all pesticides are toxic in biologic systems in sufficient doses, it is unclear whether any of these agents poses a hazard to human reproduction in the doses usually encountered in the environment.

There is considerable concern about a particular group of pesticides: the organochlorine insecticides, which include DDT, chlordane, heptachlor, lindane, and others. Organochlorine insecticides are very lipid soluble and persist in the environment for many years. Because of toxicity issues, DDT was banned from use some years ago, and other agents of this class became more widely used. Of these, heptachlor and chlordane were among the most common. There are few studies on possible teratogenic effects of heptachlor or its metabolite, heptachlor epoxide. One multigeneration rat study found an increase in cataracts associated with heptachlor exposure (47). During the early 1980s, the entire milk supply of the island of Oahu, Hawaii, was contaminated with heptachlor.

One examination of birth defect rates on Oahu used as controls the rate of defects on other Hawaiian islands, in the entire United States, and during the immediate preexposure years on Oahu. No increase in total defects or in the incidence of any of 23 individual defects was identified (48). The exposure of pregnant women to heptachlor could not be quantitated in the study or control groups. Although this report cannot prove that heptachlor is not teratogenic, the negative findings in this very large survey are reassuring.

Chlordane is not teratogenic in rats (49). Studies in mice have shown impaired cellular or humoral immune response in offspring exposed antenatally to this insecticide (50-53). Human reproductive consequences of chlordane exposure are unknown.

Reproductive Epidemiology

As it began to be recognized that environmental pollution adversely affected the health of plants and animals, concern increased that some pollutants might also harm human reproduction. Some comments in the lay press might suggest that virtually all adverse reproductive outcomes are caused by poisoning from medications or insidious environmental factors. Yet, even under the best of circumstances, the risk is about 20% for spontaneous abortion, 10% for preterm delivery, and 5% for congenital anomalies. Few of these adverse effects are known to be caused by environmental agents.

It has been estimated, for example, that only 3% to 5% of birth defects are caused by teratogens such as drugs or chemicals in the environment. Two-thirds of birth defects have no known cause. Therefore, it is frequently difficult to counsel concerned patients about the potential risk of exposure to our complex environment.

Although animal and in vitro studies are useful in characterizing the effects of toxicants on reproduction and embryonic development, doses used in such studies tend to be very high, and routes of administration may not be relevant to human exposure. Currently, we rely on epidemiologic studies of exposed populations to identify possible reproductive hazards in the environment. The difficulty of controlling confounding variables has been a major problem in designing such studies and interpreting their results.

An important example is the effort to identify a cause of neural tube defects in the United Kingdom, where some areas have an incidence of these abnormalities ten times that found among whites elsewhere in the world. At first, it might appear that there is a teratogenic agent localized to the United Kingdom. In the early 1970s, it was proposed that the eating or handling of blighted potatoes was responsible for producing these abnormalities. The potato blight theory, subsequently discredited by other investigations,

illustrates the tendency to explain geographic variability in defects by invoking environmental exposures as causes. It is now believed to be more likely that the incidence of neural tube defects in the United Kingdom is related to a genetic predisposition that is perpetuated in the population.

Differences among people in characteristics important to reproductive outcome may confound the investigation of seemingly straightforward toxicants. Lead exposure, for example, has long been suspected to be capable of interfering with fetal neurologic development. The evaluation of the offspring of women exposed to lead in drinking water, however, is hampered by the association of leaded pipes with old plumbing and, therefore, old housing and low socioeconomic status.

Low socioeconomic status may also be associated with cigarette smoking and with deficiencies in diet and prenatal care, which have adverse effects on pregnancy outcome. Identifying lead exposure as an independent factor in pregnancy outcome requires special expertise. Modern statistical analyses, often aided by computer programs, have improved investigators' ability to identify reproductive outcomes associated with such isolated variables as exposure to an environmental agent. No statistical test, however, can compensate for deficiencies in study design that cause the study results to be biased.

In a study on the reproductive effects of air pollution from a smelter in Sweden, for example, an association was found between low birthweight at high parity and residence close to the smelter. The study design did not include a determination of socioeconomic status, which certainly influences the place of residence. Failure to collect data on such an important variable makes it unlikely that these data will give meaningful information about the effect of smelter pollution on reproductive outcome.

Determinants of Pollutant Toxicity

The lack of definitive information on the safety or lack of safety of most of the many thousands of chemicals in our environment is discouraging to many practitioners and their patients. The need to make decisions about environmental exposures in the absence of conclusive data requires that health professionals who counsel women of reproductive age be guided by general principles of reproductive toxicology. The relevant principles are those that determine access of the potential toxicant to the developing conceptus (54).

The safest course of action for women, then, is to avoid exposure to chemicals in the environment, whether by oral ingestion, inhalation, or dermal contact. Avoidance of exposure may not be possible for ubiquitous pollutants such as PCBs. In some instances, however, minimizing exposure to environmental chemicals is as simple as washing one's hands before eating, washing produce before eating it, and not smoking cigarettes, which contain a number of pollutants in themselves.

An additional reassuring principle of reproductive toxicology is that most chemicals tested for embryotoxicity in animals are harmful mainly at doses that also cause maternal illness. Serious damage to the conceptus without maternal toxicity is the exception rather than the rule. Therefore, an environment that promotes health in the mother is likely to be compatible with a good pregnancy outcome.

References

1. Shepard TH. Teratogenesis: general principles. In: Fabro S, Scialli AR, eds. Drug and chemical action in pregnancy. New York: Marcel Dekker, 1986:237–50.

2. Renwick JH. Anencephaly and spina bifida are usually preventable by avoidance of a specific but unidentified substance present in certain potato tubers. Br J Prev Soc Med 1972;26:67.

3. End of the potato avoidance hypothesis (unsigned). Br Med J 1975;4:308.

4. Nordstrom S, Beckman L, Nordenson I. Occupational and environmental risks in and around a smelter in northern Sweden. I. Variations in birth weight. Hereditas 1978; 88:43.

5. Palmisano PA, Sneed RC, Cassady G. Untaxed whiskey and fetal lead exposure. J Pediatr 1969;75:869.

6. McClain RM, Becker BA. Teratogenicity, fetal toxicity, and placental transfer of lead nitrate in rats. Toxicol Appl Pharmacol 1975;31:72.

7. Barltrop D. Transfer of lead to the human foetus. In: Barltrop D, Burland WL, eds. Mineral metabolism in pediatrics. Oxford, England: Blackwell Scientific Publications, 1969: 135–51.

8. McClain RM, Becker BA. Effects of organolead compounds on rat embryonic and fetal development. Toxicol Appl Pharmacol 1972;21:265.

9. Kennedy G, Arnold D, Keplinger ML, et al. Mutagenic and teratogenic studies with lead acetate and tetraethyl lead. Toxicol Appl Pharmacol 1971;19:370.

10. Murakami U, Kameyama Y, Kato T. Basic processes seen in disturbances of early development of the central nervous system. Nagoya J Med Sci 1954;17:74.

11. Ferm VH, Carpenter SJ. Developmental malformations resulting from the administration of lead salts. Exp Mol Pathol 1967;7:208.

12. McClain RM, Becker BA. Placental transport and teratogenicity of lead in rats and mice. Fed Proc 1970;29:347.

13. Tesh J, Pritchard A. Lead and the neonate. Teratology 1977; 15:23A.

14. Minsker DH, Moskalski N, Peter CP, et al. Exposure of rats to lead nitrate in utero or postpartum: effects on morphology and behavior. Biol Neonate 1982;41:193.

15. Carson TL, Van Gelder GA, Karas GG, et al. Development of behavioral tests for the assessment of neurologic effects of lead in sheep. Environ Health Perspect 1974;7:233.

16. Scanlon JW. Dangers to the human fetus from certain heavy metals in the environment. Rev Environ Health 1975; 2:39.

17. Pindborg S. Om salvergladfargiftning i Danmark. Ugeskr Laeg 1945;107:1.

18. Rom WN. Effects of lead on the female and reproduction: a review. Mt Sinai J Med 1976;43:542.

19. Needleman HL, Rabinowitz M, Leviton A, et al. The relationship between prenatal exposure to lead and congenital anomalies. JAMA 1984;251:2956.

20. Marden PM, Smith DW, McDonald MJ. Congenital anomalies in the newborn infant, including minor variations. J Pediatr 1964;62:357.

21. Bellinger D, Leviton A, Waternaux C, et al. Longitudinal analyses of prenatal and postnatal lead exposure and early cognitive development. N Engl J Med 1987;316:1037.

22. Dietrich KN, Krafft KM, Bornschein RL, et al. Low-level fetal lead exposure effect on neurobehavioral development in early infancy. Pediatrics 1987;80:721.

23. Alfonso J, DeAlvarez R. Effects of mercury on human gestation. Am J Obstet Gynecol 1960;80:145.

24. Matsumoto H, Koya G, Takeuchi T. Fetal Minimata disease. J Neuropathol Exp Neurol 1965;24:563.

25. Muramaki U. The effect of organic mercury on intrauterine

life. Adv Exp Med Biol 1972;27:301.

26. Marsh DO, et al. Fetal methylmercury poisoning: clinical and toxicological data on 29 cases. Ann Neurol 1980;7:348.

27. Amin-Zaki L, Elhassani S, Majeed MA, et al. Perinatal methylmercury poisoning in Iraq. Am J Dis Child 1976; 130:1070.

28. Snyder RD. Congenital mercury poisoning. N Engl J Med 1971;284:1014.

29. Koos BJ, Longo LD. Mercury toxicity in the pregnant woman, fetus, and newborn infant. Am J Obstet Gynecol 1976;126:390.

30. Barlow SM, Sullivan FM. Reproductive hazards of industrial chemicals. London: Academic Press, 1982:455–82.

31. Kihlstrom JE, Lundberg C, Orberg J, et al. Sexual functions of mice neonatally exposed to DDT or PCB. Environ Physiol Biochem 1975;5:54.

32. Gellert RJ, Wilson C. Reproductive function in rats exposed prenatally to pesticides and polychlorinated biphenyls (PCB). Environ Res 1979;18:437.

33. Kuratsune M, Yoshimura Y, Matsuzaka J, et al. Epidemiologic study on yusho, a poisoning caused by ingestion of rice oil contaminated with a commercial brand of polychlorinated biphenyls. Environ Health Perspect 1972;1:119.

34. Miller RW. Congenital PCB poisoning: a reevaluation. Environ Health Perspect 1985;60:211.

35. Kodama H, Ota H. Studies on the transfer of PCB to infants from their mothers. Jap J Hygiene 1977;32:567.

36. Funatsu I, Yamashita F, Ito Y, et al. Polychlorbiphenyls (PCB)-induced fetopathy. Kurume Med J 1972;19:43.

37. Overmann SR, Kostas J, Wilson LR, et al. Neurobehavioral and somatic effects of perinatal PCB exposure in rats. Environ Res 1987;44:56.

38. Kato T, Yakushiji M, Tsuda H, et al. Polychlorobiphenyls (PCB) induced fetopathy. Kurume Med J 1972;19:53.

39. Taki I, Hisanaga S, Amagase Y. Report on Yusho (chloro-biphenyls poisoning) in pregnant women and their fetuses. Fukuoko Igaku Zasshi 1969;60:471.

40. Yamashita F. Clinical features of polychlorbiphenyls (PCB)-induced fetopathy. Paediatrician 1977;6:20.

41. Fein GG, Jacobson JL, Jacobson SW, et al. Prenatal exposure to polychlorinated biphenyls: effects on birth size and gesta-tional age. J Pediatr 1984;105:315.

42. Barsotti DA, Marlar RJ, Allen JR. Reproductive dysfunction in rhesus monkeys exposed to low levels of polychlorinated biphenyls (Arochlor 1248). Food Cosmet Toxicol 1976; 14:99.

43. Allen JR, Barsotti DA. The effects of transplacental and mam-mary movement of PCBs on infant rhesus monkeys. Toxicology 1976;6:331.

44. Overmann SR, Kostas J, Wilson LR, et al. Neurobehavioral and somatic effects of perinatal PCB exposure in rats. Environ Res 1987;44:56.

45. Wassermann M, Bercovici B, Cucos S, et al. Storage of some organochlorine compounds in toxemia of pregnancy. Environ Res 1980;22:404.

46. Rogan WJ, Gladen BC, McKinney JD, et al. Polychlorinated biphenyls (PCBs) and dichlorodiphenyl dichloroethene (DDE) in human milk: effects of maternal factors and pre-vious lactation. Am J Public Health 1986;76:172.

47. Ruttkay-Nedecka K, Cerey K, Rosival L. Evaluation of the chronic toxic effects of heptachlor. Kongr Chem Polno-hospd, 1972. Cited by Schardein JL. Chemically induced birth defects. New York: Marcel Dekker, 1985:599.

48. Marchand LL, Kolonel LN, Siegel BZ, et al. Trends in birth defects for a Hawaiian population exposed to heptachlor and for the United States. Arch Environ Health 1986; 41:145.

49. Ingle L. Chronic oral toxicity of chlordane to rats. Arch Ind Hygiene Occup Med 1952;6:357.

50. Cranmer JS, Avery DL, Barnett JB. Altered immune compe-tence of offspring exposed during development to the chlo-rinated hydrocarbon pesticide chlordane. Teratology 1979; 19:23A.

51. Spyker-Cranmer JM, Barnett JB, Avery DL, Cranmer MF. Immunoteratology of chlordane: cell-mediated and hu-moral immune responses in adult mice exposed in utero. Toxicol Appl Pharmacol 1982;62:402.

52. Barnett JB, Holcomb D, Menna JH, et al. The effect of pre-natal chlordane exposure on specific anti-influenza cell-mediated immunity. Toxicol Lett 1985;25:229.

53. Barnett JB, Solderberg LS, Menna JH. The effect of prenatal chlordane exposure on the delayed hypersensitivity re-sponse of BALB/c mice. Toxicol Lett 1985;25:173.

54. Scialli AR. A clinical guide to reproductive and developmental toxicology. Boca Raton: CRC Press, 1992.

5

Medications in Early Pregnancy

Neil K. Kochenour, M.D.

A RECENT study performed in Utah determined that, on the average, each woman included took nearly four drugs while pregnant, 25% took five or more, almost 10% took eight or more, and only 4% took none. Extent of responsibility of such drug use for congenital anomalies is uncertain (Table 5.1). Approximately 4% of newborns have an anomaly requiring medical attention, one third of which are life threatening. With increasing age, an additional number of defects—functional or behavioral as well as structural—are found. Ultimately, incidence of congenital defects may approach twice the number initially detected.

Nature of Teratogens

Teratogens are substances that prevent a developing organism from reaching its full genetic potential. They include viruses (rubella), chemical compounds (methyl mercury), and medications (thalidomide). Environmental factors (hyperthermia) can also act teratogenically, as can irradiation.

Indications of teratogenicity may include prenatal-onset growth deficiency, alterations in morphogenesis or central nervous system (CNS) function, infertility, or fetal wastage. In some instances, a teratogen's effect may not be apparent until the exposed person attempts reproduction.

An example is in utero exposure to diethylstilbestrol (DES), which, by altering the anatomy and function of the uterus, leads to increased pregnancy wastage. Although nearly all drugs are safe during pregnancy, one should always weigh benefits against possible adverse effects.

Table 5.1 Causes of Human Birth Defects

Mendelian, single gene (cystic fibrosis, Tay-Sachs, congenital deafness) (20%)

Chromosomal (10%)

Environmental (5%)
    Infections (rubella, cytomegalovirus) (<1%)
    Maternal (diabetes, phenylketonuria, hyperthermia) (2%)
    Radiation (<1%)
    Drugs, chemical (thalidomide, alcohol, methyl mercury) (2%)

Unknown, multifactorial (65%)

Table 5.2 Human Embryonic/Fetal Development in Days Post Conception

Blastula (5–6)	Upper limb bud (27–28)
Implantation (6–7)	Posterior neuropore closed (26–27)
Primitive streak (16–18)	Lung bud appears (28)
Neural plate (18–20)	Lower limb bud appears (29–30)
First branchial arch (20)	Herniation of gut (34)
Heart first beats (22)	Ossification begins (40–43)
Pronephros (22)	Müllerian duct appears (40)
Oral plate perforation (24)	Testes, histologic differentiation (43)
Anterior neuropore closed (24–25)	Heart septation complete (46–47)
	Palate closed completely (56–58)
Mesonephic duct to cloaca (26)	Herniation of gut reduced (60)
	Urethral groove closed (male) (90)
Thyroid appears (27)	

Determining Teratogenicity

Animal experiments have shown that very large quantities of most agents can cause some embryo teratogenicity. A clear example is radiation. However, some agents, such as thalidomide, are highly teratogenic even in normal doses if exposure occurs at a critical time in pregnancy.

Time of Exposure

Most organ systems in the human fetus develop during the first trimester of pregnancy (Table 5.2). However, some, such as the CNS, continue to evolve throughout pregnancy and after birth. For an agent to have a teratogenic effect on a particular organ or system, it must be taken at a time when that organ or system is still immature. Therefore, although the greatest risk of exposure occurs during the first trimester, the CNS is susceptible to adverse effects throughout gestation.

Similarly, thalidomide, one of the most potent human teratogens, is teratogenic only during a very specific period in pregnancy when the face, limbs, and ears are developing (Table 5.3). When taken at other times, this drug appears to involve no increased risk for birth defects.

Duration of Exposure

Some agents, such as androgens, if taken only once or twice at a critical time (when the genitals are forming), are teratogenic, even though duration of use is short. Others appear to embody a higher risk for birth defects if taken for longer periods. Alcohol can have an adverse effect on the developing fetus both when large amounts are drunk during a short interval (binge drinking) and when smaller amounts are ingested chronically.

Route of Administration

Because most agents are transmitted to the fetus through the maternal bloodstream, the amount of exposure will depend on maternal blood level, which, in turn, depends on route of administration and on maternal metabolism. Many drugs are absorbed differently during pregnancy. For example, hydantoin is absorbed less during pregnancy. A dose given orally to a pregnant woman will result in a lower blood level than the same dose given orally to a nonpregnant woman. The same dose given intravenously (IV) will result in a much higher—hence fetal—blood level.

Species Susceptibility

An agent may be very teratogenic to one species and harmless to another. For instance, thalidomide, a potent human teratogen, had no teratogenic effect on many of the animals in which it was tested. Other agents, teratogenic in animals, have not proved so in humans. For this reason, usefulness of animal experimentation in investigating teratogenicity in humans is limited.

Table 5.3 Thalidomide Teratogenicity Sensitivity Times

Anotia (34–38)★
Aplasia of thumb (38–40)
Amelia of arms (38–43)
Dislocation of hips (38–48)
Phocomelia of arms (38–47)
Deformity of ears (39–43)
Ectromelia of arms (39–45)
Amelia of legs (41–45)
Phocomelia of legs (45–47)
Ectromelia of legs (45–47)
Triphalangism of thumbs (46–50)

★Days after last menstrual period.

Concurrent Exposure to Other Agents

Exposures to teratogens in pregnancy frequently do not occur in isolation. A pregnant woman who takes an aspirin tablet may also drink alcohol, be exposed to chemical solvents at work, smoke cigarettes, or use other chemicals around her garden and house. Therefore, it is difficult, often impossible, to determine which exposure might have caused a birth defect. Simultaneous exposure can both increase and decrease the teratogenic potential of a given drug.

Individual Maternal Metabolism

Because different people metabolize the same substance at different rates and occasionally have different end products, it is very difficult to determine thresholds of safety in pregnancy for any agent. For example, a level of alcohol use that may consistently lead to the birth of alcohol-syndrome-affected children in one pregnant woman may result in normal children in another.

Placental Transport

To have a teratogenic effect, an agent must reach the fetus. Although most agents found in maternal blood will cross the placenta, the rate at which they cross and the amounts that reach the fetus vary widely. In general, molecules of low weight and ionization and high fat solubility pass rapidly. Thus, if anticoagulation is required, it is important to realize that large heparin molecules will not cross the placenta freely, whereas smaller warfarin (Coumadin) molecules will.

Individual Fetal Metabolism

A fetus's distinct genotype determines its metabolism and susceptibility to a given agent. Because of differences in pH, protein binding, and other factors, some substances are concentrated in fetal circulation and actually have higher levels than in maternal circulation.

Clinical Consistency of Effect

True teratogens produce characteristic patterns of abnormalities. For example, the pattern of malformations seen in fetuses adversely affected by isotretinoin is specific. An agent may not always produce every effect on every infant. Nevertheless, the spectrum of abnormalities that an agent can cause is consistent.

A single abnormality is not always specific for one teratogen. For example, intrauterine growth retardation can be caused by ionizing radiation, rubella, or alcohol.

Known Human Teratogenic Medications

At least ten agents used as medications have been shown to cause specific defects.

Thalidomide

Although a potent teratogen in humans, the sedative thalidomide doesn't affect all species equally. Mouse and rat embryos are relatively insensitive to it, whereas monkeys and rabbits respond more like humans. In the monkey, a single dose of 10 to 20 mg/kg on the 25th or 30th day produces thalidomide syndrome.

In humans, defects correlate well with time of treatment. The critical period for development of limb defects is 16 days (between days 34 to 50 after LMP). Administration between days 34 and 45 is associated most often with arm defects only, whereas that between days 41 to 47 causes leg deformities, with less involvement of arms. Defects of the external ears (between about days 34 to 38) are the earliest anomalies.

Thalidomide sales correlate very closely with incidence rates of phocomelia. Over 5,000 cases were found in Germany, whereas only 17 were found in the United States, where the drug was not permitted on the market.

DES

The female exposed in utero to the synthetic estrogen DES has a higher-than-normal incidence of precancerous vaginal adenosis and of clear-cell adenocarcinoma, particularly if exposed early in gestation. Among women exposed before week 9, 70% show evidence of vaginal adenosis, compared with only 7% of those exposed after week 17. The reproductive potential of these women is also markedly impaired, as shown by an increased incidence of spontaneous abortions and preterm deliveries.

Coumarin Derivatives

The adverse effects of coumarin and its derivatives (warfarin and phenindione) include nasal hypoplasia and calcific stippling of the secondary epiphyses when exposure occurs in the first trimester. Numerous infants with CNS defects have been born to women exposed to these substances during the second and third trimesters.

Hydantoin

Approximately 10% of infants exposed to diphenylhydantoin in utero show evidence of fetal hydantoin syndrome, and as many as three times that number reveal some stigmata of the syndrome. Manifestations include nondeforming changes in the face, growth retardation, underdeveloped fingernails and toenails, microcephaly, and impaired neurologic (especially intellectual) performance. Also found is depletion of fetal vitamin K, needed for clotting.

Research into the teratogenicity of anticonvulsant medications has been complicated because many epileptic women take more than one agent. Background risk may also be elevated since epileptics have a greater incidence of malformations even when they are not taking anticonvulsants. Frequent folic acid deficiency in epileptics may further contribute to teratogenicity.

Valproic Acid

Investigations have shown an association between prenatal valproate exposure and spina bifida. Risk of exposure during early pregnancy is uncertain but appears to be in the 1% to 2% range.

Trimethadione

Defects arising from trimethadione exposure early in gestation include developmental delay, cleft palate, V-shaped eyebrows, and low-set ears. The folic acid antagonist aminopterin is associated with spontaneous abortions. In survivors, there are growth and mental retardation, low-set ears, palate defects, irregular teeth, V-shaped eyebrows, and speech disturbances.

Tetracycline

Evidence shows staining of a baby's teeth when tetracycline is used by the mother after the fourth month. Generally, only deciduous teeth are involved. However, administration close to term may cause staining of permanent crowns.

Isotretinoin

When taken early in pregnancy, isotretinoin is associated with a high risk of spontaneous abortion and congenital malformations. Anomalies include small, malformed, or absent ears, atretic ear canals, cleft palate, cortical blindness, severe congenital heart disease primarily involving the great vessels, interrupted aortic arch, and CNS malformations, including hydrocephalus, decreased cerebral tissue, and posterior fossa cysts.

Lithium

Ebstein's anomaly, a cardiac malformation consisting of a defective tricuspid valve, often accompanied by an atrial septal defect, appears to occur frequently among fetuses exposed to lithium, commonly used to treat manic-depressive disorders. Estimated risk is about 7% to 8%.

Also, since lithium can accumulate in the fetus, toxicity may result. Therefore, infants whose mothers used lithium throughout pregnancy or near term should be closely monitored for such possible toxic effects as tremors, reduced muscle tone, and enlarged thyroid.

Hormonal Agents

When pregnant women ingest androgenic hormones, masculinization of the female fetus can involve clitoral enlargement, with or without labial scrotal fusion. The critical time appears to be the first 10 weeks after conception, especially week 8. In male offspring, no convincing evidence exists that progestins cause hypospadia by interfering with urethral fold fusion. Although some have associated late administration of exogenous hormones with cardiovascular, limb reduction, and CNS defects, data are not convincing. Oral contraceptives do not appear to be teratogens. Nevertheless, it is advisable, when possible, to avoid unnecessary exposure to hormones during early pregnancy.

Summary

Probably the vast majority of medications are safe for use during pregnancy. However, individual differences in metabolism and susceptibility, as well as possible adverse interactions with other medications and with environmental exposures, make it impossible to state that a given medication poses no risk.

Therefore, medications should be used during pregnancy only when potential benefit outweighs potential risk. When several available agents appear equally effective, select that with the least potential risk to the fetus and record of greatest experience during pregnancy.

SUGGESTED READING

Benke PJ. The isotretinoin teratogen syndrome. JAMA 1984; 251:3267.

Briggs GG, Freeman RK, Yaffe SJ. Drugs in pregnancy and lactation, ed 2. Baltimore: Williams & Wilkins, 1986.

Hall JG, Pauli RM, Wilson KM. Maternal and fetal sequelae of anticoagulation during pregnancy. Am J Med 1980;68:122.

Hanson JW. Teratogen update: fetal hydantoin effects. Teratology 1986;33:349.

Herbst AL, Anderson S, Hubby MM, et al. Risk factors for the development of diethylstilbestrol-associated clear cell adenocarcinoma: a case-control study. Am J Obstet Gynecol 1986;154:814.

Kallen B, Tandbert A: Lithium and pregnancy. Acta Psychiatr Scand 1983;68:134.

Kelly TE: Teratogenicity of anticonvulsant drugs. I. Review of the literature. Am J Med Genet 1984;19:413.

Lenz W. A short history of thalidomide embryopathy. Teratology 1988;38:203.

Linden S, Rich CL. The use of lithium during pregnancy and lactation. J Clin Psychiatry 1983;44:358.

Ludmir J, Landon MB, Gabbe SG, et al. Management of the diethylstilbestrol-exposed pregnancy patient: a prospective study. Am J Obstet Gynecol 1987;157:665.

Senekjian EK, Potkul RK, Frey K, et al. Infertility among daughters either exposed or not exposed to diethylstilbestrol. Am J Obstet Gynecol 1988;158:493.

Shepard TH. Catalog of teratogenic agents, ed 5. London: Johns Hopkins Press Ltd, 1986.

Tein I, MacGregor DL. Possible valproate teratogenicity. Arch Neurol 1985;42:291.

Warkany J. Teratogen update: lithium. Teratology 1988;38:593.

Weinbaum PJ, Cassidy SB, Vintzileos AM, et al. Prenatal detection of a neural tube defect after fetal exposure to valproic acid. Obstet Gynecol 1986;67:31S.

Zackai EH, Mellman WJ, Neiderer B, et al. The fetal trimethadione syndrome. J Pediatr 1975;87:280.

6

Medications in Late Pregnancy and Lactation

Jennifer R. Niebyl, M.D.

THE term "placental barrier" is truly a contradiction. Actually, the placenta allows passage of many drugs (Table 6.1). For this reason, medications should be used only when absolutely necessary.

The first trimester is the critical period of organogenesis. Teratogens ingested at this time cause malformations that are usually recognized at birth. However, drugs also may affect the fetus in the second and third trimesters, although the effects may not be recognized until later. For example, some of the anomalies of the uterus and vagina that resulted from exposure to diethylstilbestrol (DES) occurred in the second trimester and were not recognized until after puberty. The fetal brain continues to develop throughout pregnancy and the neonatal period, and disorders such as fetal alcohol syndrome may occur with chronic exposure to alcohol in later stages of pregnancy. This type of abnormality may not be recognized at birth. As long-term effects on the fetus may not become apparent for many years, cautious drug use is warranted throughout pregnancy.

The amount of drug in breast milk is proportional to the maternal oral dose. The dose to the infant is usually subtherapeutic—approximately 1% to 2% of the maternal dose—so no adverse effects are noted. Drugs may appear in

---

Table 6.1 Effects on Fetus of Maternal Drugs

Potential Fetal Toxicity
Antineoplastics
Antithyroid drugs
Benzodiazepines
Coumadin anticoagulants
Lithium
Immunosuppressants

Little or No Documented Fetal Toxicity
Analgesics
Antiasthmatics
Antibiotics
Antihistamines
Antihypertensives
Decongestants

Note: The amount of drug in breast milk is proportional to the maternal oral dose. The dose to the infant is usually subtherapeutic, so no adverse effects are noted.

higher concentrations in the milk only if the mother has unusually high blood concentrations, such as occur with increased dosage or decreased renal function.

In the case of toxic drugs, however, any exposure may be inappropriate. It is also possible that the infant may develop an allergy to a drug. Long-term effects of even small doses of new drugs may be discovered in the future. Also, infants eliminate drugs more slowly because of their immature enzyme systems. However, the benefits of breast-feeding are well known, so the risk of drug exposure must be weighed against them.

During the few days postpartum, before lactation is fully established, the infant receives only a small volume of colostrum. It is helpful to allay fears of patients undergoing cesarean section that analgesics or other drugs administered at this time will have no adverse effect on their infants.

For drugs requiring daily dosing during lactation, knowledge of pharmacokinetics in breast milk may minimize the dose to the infant. For example, nighttime dosing after nursing will decrease exposure in infants who nurse less frequently overnight. In general, medications should be taken after breast-feeding, and long-acting preparations should be avoided.

Antineoplastic Drugs and Immunosuppressants

Methotrexate (Folex, Methotrexate, Mexate), a folic acid antagonist, is a human teratogen in the first trimester. In the later trimesters, eight normal infants have been delivered to seven women treated with methotrexate in combination with other agents (1).

Azathioprine (Imuran) was used in 42 patients with renal transplants or systemic lupus erythematosus. Two infants had leukopenia, one was small for gestational age, and the other 39 were normal (1).

Four cases have been reported in which cyclosporine (Sandimmune) was used for immunosuppression in renal transplant recipients (2). Cord blood values of 14% and 57% of maternal values of the drug were found at delivery. No adverse effects on the infants were noted.

During lactation, these drugs and other cytotoxic agents might cause immune suppression in the infant, but data are limited. In general, the drugs' potential risks outweigh the benefits of nursing.

Anticonvulsants

Epileptic women taking anticonvulsants during pregnancy have approximately double the risk of malformations of the general population, which is 2% to 3% (3). The risk for epileptic women is about 5%, especially for cleft lip, with or without cleft palate, and congenital heart disease. Recently, it has been recognized that valproic acid (Depakene) carries approximately a 1% risk of neural tube defects and possibly others as well, so α-fetoprotein screening is appropriate for these patients (4).

Women with a convulsive disorder have an increased risk of birth defects, even when they take no anticonvulsant drugs. Possible causes of malformations include the disease itself, a genetic predisposition to epilepsy and malformations, genetic differences in drug metabolism, the specific drugs themselves, and deficiency states induced by drugs such as decreased serum folate (5). Phenytoin decreases absorption of folate and lowering of the serum folate has been implicated in birth defects in animals. A combination of more than three drugs or a high daily dose increases the chance of malformations (6).

Fewer than 10% of offspring show the fetal hydantoin syndrome (7). It consists of microcephaly, growth deficiency, developmental delays, mental retardation, and dysmorphic craniofacial features. Carbamazepine (Epitol, Tegretol) has also been reported to cause a similar syndrome (8).

Some women taking anticonvulsants have had no recent reevaluation of the need for continuation. If a patient with idiopathic epilepsy has been seizure-free for two years and has a normal electroencephalogram, it may be safe to try withdrawing her medication before she attempts pregnancy (9). Most authorities agree that the benefits of anticonvulsant therapy outweigh the risks of discontinuing the drug if the patient is already pregnant when seen for the first time. The blood level of the drug should be monitored, preferably monthly, to assure a therapeutic level but minimal dosage.

Most sedatives and anticonvulsants appear to have no adverse effect on nursing infants. Patients may be reassured that, in normal doses, carbamazepine, phenytoin (Dilantin), and magnesium sulfate cause no obvious adverse effects on neonates (10). The dose detectable in the breast milk is about 1% to 2% of the mother's dose, which is sufficiently low to have no pharmacologic activity. However, the infant eliminates phenobarbital and diazepam slowly, so accumulation may occur. Women consuming barbiturates or benzodiazepines while breast-feeding should observe their infants for sedation. Accumulation does not seem to occur with carbamazepine (11).

Anticoagulants

Warfarin sodium (Coumadin, Panwarfin, Warfarin) has been associated with chondrodysplasia punctata, similar to the genetic Conradi-Hünermann syndrome. This syndrome includes nasal hypoplasia and bone stippling (found on x-ray); it also may involve ophthalmologic abnormalities such as bilateral optic atrophy and mental retardation. These abnormalities presumably are caused by microhemorrhages during development. Ophthalmologic abnormalities and mental retardation may occur even when warfarin is used only after the first trimester.

The alternative drug, heparin, a large molecule with a strong negative charge, does not cross the placenta. As it has no adverse effect on the fetus, it should be the drug of choice for patients requiring anticoagulation. However, some evidence suggests that therapy with 20,000 U/day for more than 20 weeks may result in bone demineralization. It should be used for prolonged periods only when clearly necessary (12).

The risks of full anticoagulation during pregnancy may not be justified in patients with nothing more than a history of thrombosis. Certainly, conservative measures such as wearing elastic stockings and avoiding prolonged sitting or standing should be recommended. Patients who have cardiac valve prostheses need full anticoagulation. In one study of 35 mothers, low-dose heparin resulted in three valve thromboses (two fatal) (13).

Most mothers requiring anticoagulation may continue to nurse. Heparin does not cross into milk and is not active orally, in any case (14). In one study of seven patients, no warfarin was detected in breast milk or plasma at a maternal dose of 5 to 12 mg/day, probably because this drug is 98% protein bound. Thus, 1 L of milk would contain a maximum of 20 g, an amount too insignificant to have an anticoagulant effect (14). Dicumarol (formerly known as bishydroxycoumarin), an oral anticoagulant, was given to 125 nursing mothers, with no effect on the infants' prothrombin times and no hemorrhages. Thus, with careful monitoring of maternal prothrombin time (so the dosage is minimized) and neonatal prothrombin times (to assure lack of drug accumulation), it is safe to administer warfarin to nursing mothers.

This safety does not apply to all oral anticoagulant drugs, however. In one case, an infant whose nursing mother was taking phenindione (Heduli, Indon) underwent surgical repair of an inguinal hernia at five weeks of age. He developed a large hematoma, and his prothrombin time was found to be elevated.

Effects of Lithium

Because lithium (Eskalith, Lithane, Lithobid) is excreted more rapidly in pregnancy, serum levels should be monitored. Fetal exposure to lithium during the first trimester may cause cardiovascular anomalies (15) although the risk is low. However, 60 infants unaffected by heart disease who were followed up to age five had no more mental or physical abnormalities than their unexposed siblings. Adverse perinatal effects include hypotonia, lethargy, and poor feeding. Also, complications in newborns similar to those seen in adults taking lithium include goiter and hypothyroidism and nephrogenic diabetes insipidus.

To avoid fetal drug exposure, a change in therapy is usually recommended for pregnant women. However, there is a 70% chance of a relapse of the affective disorder within a year after therapy is discontinued, while women who continue to take lithium have only a 20% chance of a relapse. Thus, the risk/benefit ratio of lithium therapy in later pregnancy should be weighed.

Breast-milk levels of lithium are about half maternal serum levels, and the serum levels of nursing infants are much lower than if they were exposed in utero. However, nursing infants of mothers taking lithium have been reported to be hypotonic and flaccid. Thus, women who must take lithium probably should not nurse their infants.

Thyroid and Antithyroid Drugs

Both propylthiouracil (PTU) and methimazole (Tapazole) cross the placenta and may cause fetal goiter. However, because the thyroid hormones triiodothyronine (T_3) and thyroxin (T_4) cross the placenta poorly, giving the mother thyroid hormone cannot correct fetal hypothyroidism produced by antithyroid drugs. Thus, to minimize fetal drug exposure, the goal of antithyroid therapy during pregnancy is to keep the mother slightly hyperthyroid. As methimazole has been associated with scalp defects in infants, PTU is the drug of choice (16). Free T_4 should be checked monthly as pregnancy advances, and the dose of PTU should be adjusted accordingly.

Propylthiouracil is found in breast milk only in small amounts. If the mother takes 200 mg three times a day, the child would receive 149 μg daily; that is the equivalent of a 70-kg adult receiving 3 mg a day. One infant studied for five months showed no changes in thyroid values, including thyroid-stimulating hormone. Lactating mothers taking PTU can continue nursing, provided that their infants are supervised closely (17).

Benzodiazepines

Reports of the possible teratogenicity of the various tranquilizers are conflicting. Recently, a fetal benzodiazepine syndrome was reported in seven infants of 36 mothers who regularly took one of these drugs (Librium, Serax, Valium) during pregnancy (18). These infants had growth retardation, dysmorphism, and central nervous system dysfunction. In most clinical situations, the risk/benefit ratio does not justify the use of benzodiazepines in pregnancy or lactation. Perinatal use of diazepam has been associated with hypotonia, hypothermia, and respiratory depression.

Antihistamines and Decongestants

If clinicians can convince patients that these drugs only treat symptoms of the common cold but have no influence on the course of the disease, patients may be receptive to the

recommendation of such remedies as use of a humidifier, rest, and fluid intake. If medications are necessary, combinations of two or more drugs should not be used if only one is needed. If the problem is an allergy, an antihistamine will suffice. When a decongestant is needed, topical nasal sprays subject the fetus to lower doses than systemic medication does. Although these drugs are not known to be teratogenic, pregnant women should be discouraged from using over-the-counter drugs for trivial indications. The long-term effects, especially of chronic use, are unknown.

Although studies are limited, these drugs appear to have no harmful effects during lactation. Women who are having trouble with their milk supply, however, should avoid decongestants.

Effects of Analgesics

Pregnant patients should be encouraged to use nonpharmacologic remedies such as local heat and rest for aches and pains. Aspirin (Bayer, Bufferin, Ecotrin), which inhibits prostaglandin synthesis, has marked perinatal effects. It also decreases uterine contractility. Patients taking aspirin for analgesia have delayed onset and longer duration of labor and an increased risk of prolonged pregnancy.

Because therapeutic doses of aspirin also decrease platelet aggregation, there is increased risk of antepartum, as well as intrapartum, bleeding. Platelet dysfunction has been described in newborns five days after their mothers ingested aspirin. Since prostaglandin synthetase in platelets is inhibited, the baby's bone marrow must produce more platelets.

Prostaglandins also mediate neonatal closure of the ductus arteriosus. In one case, aspirin ingestion close to the time of delivery presumably was related to closure of the ductus in utero (19).

On the plus side, low-dose aspirin (approximately 80 mg), which improves the thromboxane/prostacyclin ratio, may ultimately prove of benefit in preventing preeclampsia or fetal wastage associated with autoimmune disease. When patients who had positive angiotensin II infusion tests were given low-dose aspirin therapy, their incidence of preeclampsia was lower than that of a placebo group (20). Prednisone (DeltaDome, Deltasone, Meticorten), 40 to 60 mg/day, and low-dose aspirin improved fetal outcome in patients with lupus anticoagulant and fetal wastage (21).

Aspirin is transferred in small amounts into breast milk. There is risk only when maternal dosages exceed sixteen 300-mg tablets/day. Then, the infant's serum levels may become high enough to affect platelet aggregation.

Acetaminophen (Datril, Phenaphen, Tylenol) inhibition of prostaglandin synthesis is reversible, so platelet aggregation returns to normal once the drug has cleared. The drug does not prolong the bleeding time in pregnant patients, and it is not toxic to newborns. Thus, if a mild analgesic or antipyretic is indicated during pregnancy, acetaminophen is preferred over aspirin. The absorption and disposition of acetaminophen is not altered by pregnancy. It is found in small amounts in breast milk, and no harmful effects have been noted.

When mild analgesia is needed, propoxyphene (Darvon, Dolene, Wygesic) is an acceptable alternative. However, it should not be used for trivial indications, as it has potential for narcotic addiction. Evidence of risk in late pregnancy comes from case reports of infants of mothers who were addicted to propoxyphene and had typical narcotic withdrawal in the neonatal period.

Codeine can cause addiction and newborn withdrawal symptoms if used in the perinatal period. There is no documented adverse effect of its use or that of propoxyphene during lactation.

Antibiotics and Antiinfective Agents

Pregnant patients are particularly susceptible to vaginal yeast infections, and antibiotics should be used only when clearly indicated. Therapy with antifungal agents may be necessary during or after the course of antibiotic therapy.

Penicillin and its derivatives, such as ampicillin, are safe in pregnancy and lactation, as are erythromycin and the cephalosporins. Sulfonamides have not been associated with any particular risk except when given to premature infants. Then, the drugs compete with bilirubin for albumin-binding sites and increase the risk of hyperbilirubinemia. Thus, they are not a first choice in the third trimester, especially if the mother is at risk for preterm labor. Most sulfonamides appear in small amounts in breast milk and are not contraindicated, as the infant receives less than 1% of the maternal dose. However, the drug is best avoided during the first five days of life or in premature infants, when hyperbilirubinemia may be a problem. Sulfasalazine (Azulfidine) is poorly absorbed orally and, in one study, was undetectable in all milk samples (22).

Tetracyclines (Tetracyn, Pannmycin, Steclin) bind to developing enamel, discoloring the teeth. The drug affects deciduous teeth between 26 weeks of development and six months of age, and the permanent teeth if given to children between the ages of six months and five years. Since the tetracyclines also deposit in developing osseous sites and inhibit bone growth, alternate drugs are preferable during pregnancy. Tooth staining and delayed bone growth from tetracycline have not been reported when the drug is taken by nursing mothers. This is probably because the high binding of the drug to calcium and protein limits absorption from the milk.

Nitrofurantoin (Macrodantin) causes no adverse affects to the fetus during lactation. It can induce hemolytic anemia in G6PD (glucose-6-phosphate dehydrogenase)-deficient patients. Since the newborn's red cells are deficient in reduced glutathione, the label carries a warning against use of the drug at term. However, hemolytic anemia in the newborn after exposure before birth has not been reported to date.

Aminoglycosides do cross the placenta, and a rate of ototoxicity of 3% to 11% has been reported in children of mothers who received prolonged streptomycin (Streptomycin, Strycin) treatment for tuberculosis during pregnancy (23). Although the hearing loss appears to be dose-related, these agents should be used only if absolutely necessary. When they are required for serious infections, their use should be restricted to a short course, and maternal serum levels should be monitored to minimize fetal exposure.

Antituberculosis drugs—isoniazid (Dinacrin, INH, Isolyn), rifampin (Rifadin, Rifamate, Rimactane), and ethambutol (Myambutol)—should be used when indicated. No adverse effects on infants have been reported. Their use is considered compatible with breast-feeding. Because they may be associated with hemorrhagic disease of the newborn, prophylactic vitamin K is recommended.

Metronidazole (Flagyl, Metric, Protostat) was shown

to be positive in the Ames test, which correlates with carcinogenicity in animals. However, the doses were far greater than those used clinically. Of 880 infants exposed during pregnancy, no difference in frequency of any adverse outcome was noted compared with controls (24). Because of the controversy surrounding metronidazole, deferring therapy until after the first trimester is probably wise, and it should be given then only for clear-cut indications. The minimal (2 g) dose reduces the risk for carcinogenesis. After single-dose therapy, interruption of lactation for 12 to 24 hours results in negligible exposure to the infant.

Lindane (Kwell, Scabene) is a potent neurotoxin. Toxicity in humans after use of topical 1% lindane has been observed almost exclusively after misuse and overexposure. After application to the skin, about 10% of the dose used can be recovered in the urine. Use of lindane during pregnancy or lactation should be limited to two doses, even though there is no evidence of specific reproductive damage. Pregnant women should be cautioned to wear gloves while shampooing their children's hair. Absorption could easily occur across the skin of the mother's hands. Pyrethroids with piperonyl butoxide (Pronto, R&C, Rid), which is poorly absorbed topically, is considered preferable for treatment of lice during pregnancy.

Antiasthmatics

Theophylline and aminophylline are safe to use during pregnancy for treatment of asthma. Terbutaline (Brethaire, Brethine, Bricanyl), which has been widely used during preterm labor, is more rapid in onset and has a longer duration of action than epinephrine (Bronkaid). It is often preferred for treatment of asthma in pregnant patients. Long-term use has been associated with an increased risk of glucose intolerance (25).

Cromolyn sodium (Intal, Nasalcrom, Opticrom) may be administered in pregnancy, and the systemic absorption is minimal. When isoproterenol (Isuprel, Norisodrine, Vapo-Iso) and metaproterenol (Alupent, Metaprel, Metaproterenol) are given as topical aerosols, the total dose absorbed usually is not significant. However, with oral or IV doses, the cardiovascular effects may decrease uterine blood flow,

so they should be used with caution.

Maximum milk concentrations of aminophylline are achieved between one and three hours after an oral dose. It has been calculated that the nursing infant receives less than 1% of the maternal dose, and no adverse effects have been cited (26).

Prednisone (Deltasone, Prednisone, Sterapred) and prednisolone (Prednisolone, Prelone) are inactivated by the placenta, so the concentration of active compound in the fetus is less than 10% of that in the mother. Thus, these are the drugs of choice for treating medical diseases such as asthma. When a corticosteroid effect is desired in the infant for lung maturity, betamethasone (B-S-P, Celestone) and dexamethasone (Decadron, Decaspray, Hexadrol) are preferred, as these drugs readily cross the placenta.

The levels of prednisone achieved in breast milk are less than 1% of the maternal dose and less than 10% of the infant's endogenous cortisol, even at 80 mg/day. Thus, corticosteroids are not contraindicated during lactation.

Iodide, such as that found in a saturated solution of potassium iodide expectorant (Elixophyllin-KI, Mudrane, SSKI), crosses the placenta and may cause a very large fetal goiter, enough to produce respiratory obstruction in the newborn. Thus, before advising a patient to take cough medicine, the clinician should make sure that it does not contain iodide. As iodide is concentrated in breast milk, such medications should be avoided during lactation.

Antihypertensive Drugs

Alpha-methyldopa (Aldomet, Methyldopa) has been widely used for treatment of chronic hypertension in pregnancy. Although postural hypotension may occur, no unusual fetal effects have been noted. Hydralazine (Apresoline) is usually reserved for treatment of severe preeclampsia.

Propranolol (Inderal), a sympathetic blocking agent, has been widely used for a variety of indications during pregnancy with no recognized adverse effects. Bradycardia has been reported in a newborn as a direct result of the mother's injestion of the drug within two hours of delivery (27). Studies suggest improved outcome with the use of atenolol (Tenormin) to treat chronic hypertension during pregnancy and do not suggest any of the adverse effects reported in the United States in isolated cases.

Propranolol and atenolol are excreted in breast milk in low doses. The infant receives a dose of about 1% of the therapeutic dose. This amount of drug is unlikely to cause any adverse effect (27).

Conclusions

Although most of the drugs discussed are reasonably safe during pregnancy, it is always advisable to use nonpharmacologic remedies whenever possible. Most drug therapy does not require the mother to stop breast-feeding. The amount excreted into breast milk is so small that it is pharmacologically insignificant.

References

1. Buscema J, Stern JL, Johnson TRB. Antineoplastic drugs and pregnancy. In: Niebyl JR, ed. Drug use in pregnancy. Philadelphia: Lea & Febiger, 1988;89.

2. Burrows DA, O'Neil TJ, Sorrells TL. Successful twin pregnancy after renal transplant maintained on cyclosporine A immunosuppression. Obstet Gynecol 1988;72:459.

3. Speidel BD, Meadow SR. Maternal epilepsy and abnormalities of the fetus and newborn. Lancet 1972;2:839.

4. Robert E, Guibaud P. Maternal valproic acid and congenital neural tube defects (Letter). Lancet 1982;2:937.

5. Shapiro S, Hartz SC, Siskind V, et al. Anticonvulsants and parental epilepsy in the development of birth defects. Lancet 1976;1:272.

6. Nakane Y, Okuma T, Takahashi R, et al. Multi-institutional study on the teratogenicity and fetal toxicity of antiepileptic drugs: a report of a collaborative study group in Japan. Epilepsia 1980;21:663.

7. Hanson JW, Smith DW. The fetal hydantoin syndrome. J Pediatr 1975;87:285.

8. Jones KL, Lacro RV, Johnson KA, et al. Pattern of malformation in the children of women treated with carbamazepine during pregnancy. N Engl J Med 1989;320:1661.

9. Callaghan N, Garrett A, Goggin T. Withdrawal of anticonvulsant drugs in patients free of seizures for two years. N Engl J Med 1988;318:942.

10. Briggs GG, Freeman RK, Yaffe SJ. Drugs in pregnancy and lactation, 2nd ed. Baltimore: Williams and Wilkins, 1986: 256–7.

11. Pynnonen S, Sillanpaa M. Carbamazapine and mother's milk. Lancet 1975;2:563.

12. deSwiet M, Ward PD, Fidler J, et al. Prolonged heparin therapy in pregnancy causes bone demineralization. Br J Obstet Gynaecol 1983;90:1129.

13. Iturbe-Alessio I, Fonseca MC, Mutchinik O, et al. Risks of anticoagulant therapy in pregnant women with artificial heart valves. N Engl J Med 1986;315:1390.

14. deSwiet M, Lewis PJ. Excretion of anticoagulants in human milk (Letter). N Engl J Med 1977;297:1471.

15. Prospective multicentre study of pregnancy outcome after lithium exposure during the first trimester. Lancet 1992; 339:530.

16. Mujtaba Q, Burrow GN. Treatment of hyperthyroidism in pregnancy with propylthiouracil and methimazole. Obstet Gynecol 1975;46:282.

17. Cooper DS. Antithyroid drugs: to breast-feed or not to breast-feed. Am J Obstet Gynecol 1987;157:234.

18. Laegreid L, Olegard R, Wahlstrom J, et al. Abnormalities in children exposed to benzodiazepines in utero (Letter). Lancet 1987;1:108.

19. Arcilla RA, Thilenius OG, Ranniger K. Congestive heart failure from suspected ductal closure in utero. J Pediatr 1969; 75:74.

20. Wallenburg HC, Dekker GA, Makovitz JW, et al. Low-dose aspirin prevents pregnancy-induced hypertension and preeclampsia in angiotensin-sensitive primigravidae. Lancet 1986;1:1.

21. Lubbe WF, Butler WS, Palmer SJ, et al. Lupus anticoagulant in pregnancy. Br J Obstet Gynaecol 1984;91:357.

22. Foster FP. Excretion of sulfanilamide in breast milk: report of a case. Proc Staff Meet Mayo Clin 1939;14:153.

23. Robinson GC, Cambon KG. Hearing loss in infants of tuberculous mothers treated with streptomycin during pregnancy. N Engl J Med 1964;271:949.

24. Morgan IFK. Metronidazole treatment in pregnancy International Congress and Symposium series. Roy Soc Med 1979;18:245.

25. Main EK, Main DM, Gabbe SG. Chronic oral terbutaline tocolytic therapy is associated with maternal glucose intolerance. Am J Obstet Gynecol 1987;157:644.

26. Yurchak AM, Jusko WJ. Theophylline secretion into breast milk. Pediatrics 1976;57:518.

27. Pruyn SC, Phelan JP, Buchanan GC. Long-term propranolol therapy in pregnancy: maternal and fetal outcome. Am J Obstet Gynecol 1979;135:485.

PART TWO Procedures

7

Chorionic Villus Sampling

Sherman Elias, M.D.
Joe Leigh Simpson, M.D.

AVAILABLE for two decades, amniocentesis remains the most common technique for prenatal diagnosis of genetic disorders (1, 2). Because amniocentesis is generally performed after 14 to 15 weeks' gestation, results are not usually available before 18 weeks' gestation. Therefore, couples awaiting results experience considerable psychologic stress. Moreover, if a fetal abnormality is diagnosed and the couple elects to terminate the pregnancy, abortion at midtrimester carries greater morbidity and mortality risks than first-trimester termination (3). Accordingly, there is a strong impetus to develop a method for first-trimester prenatal diagnosis, not only to allow pregnancy termination early in gestation, but also to enhance patient privacy. Early diagnosis may also be required for prenatal treatment. For example, in our own center, virilization has been prevented in a female fetus affected with 21-hydroxylase deficiency by administering dexamethasone to the mother (4).

Chorionic villus sampling (CVS) permits first-trimester diagnosis of genetic disease, usually beginning at 10–12 weeks' gestation. Under direct guidance, chorionic villi are aspirated via a catheter placed transcervically or a needle inserted transabdominally into the developing placenta. Use of chorionic villi for various genetic studies is possible because, shortly after fertilization, the zygote differentiates first into the blastocyst, which contains an inner cell mass that develops into the fetus, and an outer trophoblastic layer that develops into nonfetal structures such as amnion, chorion, and placenta. The genetic complement of the outer cell mass nearly always reflects the genetic constitution of the inner cell mass (that is, the fetus) because both are derived from the same zygote. It follows that cytogenetic, DNA, or biochemical analysis on trophoblast cells should provide information comparable with that obtained from cultured amniotic fluid cells.

Indications for CVS

Cytogenetic indications include 1) advanced maternal age, (usually ±35 years), 2) previous offspring with a chromosome abnormality, 3) balanced structural chromosome rearrangement in a parent, and 4) fetal sex determination in X-linked recessive disorders for which a specific prenatal diagnostic test is not yet available (5).

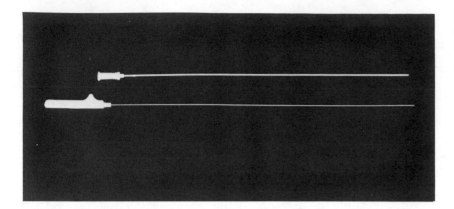

Figure 7.1   For sampling villi, the 26-cm CVS catheter (above) and the metal obturator (below) are used.

(Portex Inc., Wilmington, Mass.)

Indications for prenatal diagnosis of mendelian disorders are increasing. Usually a couple is recognized to be at increased risk because a previous child or relative had a detectable disorder. Cystic fibrosis, α or β thalassemia, sickle cell anemia, hemophilia, Tay-Sachs disease, and Duchenne /Becker's muscular dystrophy are among the most common conditions. Couples at risk for the hemoglobinopathies or Tay-Sachs disease may be identified through screening programs to identify heterozygotes. Either enzymatic analysis or DNA analysis may be required, depending on the specific disorder.

Patients at increased risk for disorders in which amniotic fluid liquor is needed to obtain a prenatal diagnosis— specifically α-fetoprotein analysis for fetal neural tube defects—are not candidates for CVS, but rather should be offered amniocentesis

Transcervical Sampling

Prior to chorionic villus sampling, fetal viability and normal fetal growth must be confirmed by ultrasound. The optimal time for transcervical sampling is 10 to 12 completed gestational weeks. The procedure is commonly performed with either the Portex catheter (Portex Inc., Wilmington, Massachusetts) or a device of comparable diameter (1.5 mm). These devices are characterized by a plastic cannula that encloses a metal obturator extending just distal to the catheter tip. Absolute contraindications include maternal blood group sensitization and active cervical pathology (for example, herpes); relative contraindications include leiomy-

omata obstructing the cervical canal, multiple gestation, bleeding from the vagina within one week of CVS, and a markedly retroverted, retroflexed uterus (6).

For transcervical CVS, the patient is placed in the lithotomy position. After insertion of a vaginal speculum, the vagina is cleansed with povidone-iodine solution. Usually, a tenaculum is placed on the anterior lip of the cervix, after which a catheter with encased obturator (Figure 7.1) is introduced transcervically under concurrent ultrasonographic visualization. The device is directed into the placenta, parallel to the long axis and away from either gestational sac or maternal decidua (Figure 7.2). Once within the placenta, the obturator is withdrawn and the catheter connected to a 20- or 30-mL syringe containing approximately 5 mL of tissue culture medium and heparin. Chorionic villi are then obtained by multiple, rapid aspirations of the syringe plunger up to 20- or 30-mL negative pressure (depending on syringe size). The catheter is withdrawn under continuous maximum negative pressure (6). An adequate sample is at least 5 mg, but a sample of 10 to 25 mg is preferred.

Adequacy of sample should be confirmed immediately by visualization under a dissecting microscope. Our unit is housed in a room contiguous to the ultrasound suite where sampling is performed. If a second attempt to obtain villi is required, a new sampling instrument is used. Villi are transferred immediately to the laboratory, where they are dissected free of decidua and blood clots using fine forceps. Cytogenetic studies are performed either by direct harvest (cytotrophoblast cells) after an overnight incubation or after

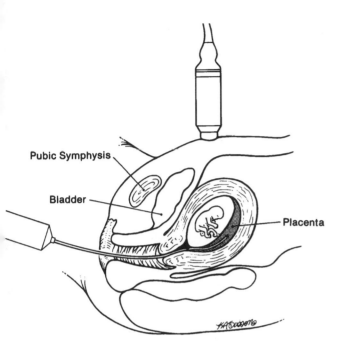

Figure 7.2   The CVS procedure here is performed transcervically.

establishment of in situ cultures (mesenchymal core cells) that are harvested at five to eight days. Chorionic villi can also be processed for DNA or enzymatic analyses.

Following CVS, fetal heart activity is verified by ultrasonography. Patients are observed for any untoward effects for approximately 30 minutes. Unsensitized Rh-negative patients are given Rh-immune globulin. Maternal serum α-fetoprotein screening for fetal neural tube defects is necessary at 15 to 18 weeks' gestation.

Transabdominal Sampling

Described more recently than transcervical CVS, transabdominal CVS is proving a useful complementary technique (7). Placentas especially amenable to this approach include those located in the fundus or anteriorly in a slightly anteflexed uterus. Transabdominal CVS may also permit sampling in circumstances in which transcervical CVS is contraindicated (for example, herpes or chronic cervicitis). Other women likely to benefit from transabdominal CVS include those with cervical leiomyomata or with a long,

narrow, or angulated endocervical canal. A transabdominal approach may also be preferable to transcervical CVS in nulliparous women.

The patient is placed in the supine position. A needle insertion site is selected by ultrasonographic examination, the abdominal skin cleansed with povidone-iodine solution, and the abdominal area draped in a fashion similar to amniocentesis. Skin is infiltrated with 2 mL of 1% xylocaine, and an 19- or 20-gauge spinal needle with stylet is inserted percutaneously through the maternal abdominal wall and myometrium. The tip is advanced into the long axis of the chorion frondosum under concurrent ultrasound monitoring (Figure 7.3).

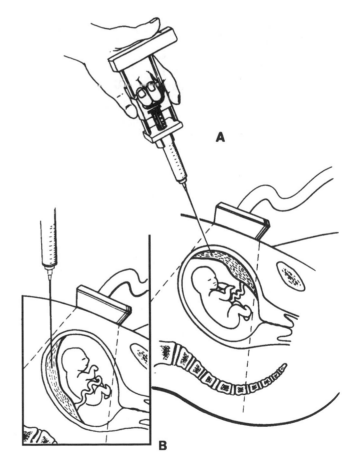

Figure 7.3   In these transabdominal CVS procedures, (A) is an anterior and (B) a posterior placenta.

The stylet is withdrawn and a 20- or 30-mL syringe containing media and heparin is attached to the needle. Many centers perform transabdominal CVS with a syringe attached to an aspiration device, most commonly a biopsy aspiration device (Cameco syringe pistol, Precision Dynamics Inc., San Fernando California), which facilitates one-handed aspiration (Figure 7.4). Chorionic villi are obtained, as in transcervical CVS, by repeated (15 to 20), rapid aspirations of the syringe plunger to 20- or 30-mL negative pressure (depending on syringe size). Simultaneously, the needle is redirected within placental sub-stance to sample different sites. The needle is then withdrawn under continuous maximum negative pressure. In our experience, the amount of villi obtained by transabdominal CVS (mean ± SD, 12.1 mg ± 8.4) is about half of that usually obtained by transcervical CVS (mean ± SD, 23.4 mg ± 15.2) (7). Such smaller amounts are, however, still adequate for diagnostic testing. If a repeat sampling is required, a new needle is used.

Other investigators have proposed variations in technique for transabdominal CVS. In addition to our "free-hand technique" using a 19-gauge needle, others have used needles with cutting abilities and double-needle systems with an 18-gauge thin-walled outer needle guide and a 20-gauge sampling needle. Smidt-Jensen and colleagues use a stereotaxic device (guide needle) to define an exact site and angle for needle insertion (8). However, we and apparently others find these devices cumbersome and unnecessary.

Transabdominal CVS may also prove useful in the late second and third trimesters for obtaining rapid fetal karyotypes, offering an alternative to cordocentesis and late amniocentesis. Transcervical CVS cannot be used for this purpose.

Transvaginal Sampling

Occasionally, a patient has such a markedly retroflexed and retroverted uterus with a predominantly posterior placenta that there is no facile approach for either transcervical or transabdominal CVS. In such cases, we have performed transvaginal CVS.

The patient is prepared in the same fashion as for transcervical CVS. However, a tenaculum is placed on the posterior lip of the cervix. Vaginal mucosa overlying the expected site of entry into the cul-de-sac is infiltrated with 5 mL of 1% xylocaine. The speculum is then removed, and a vaginal ultrasound transducer with needle guide affixed to its side is inserted into the vagina. Under continuous ultrasound guidance, a 35-cm, 18-gauge needle with stylet is introduced through the transvaginal transducer needle guide and passed sequentially through the cul-de-sac and uterine myometrium into the placenta. The stylet is withdrawn, and a 20-mL syringe containing 5 mL of medium

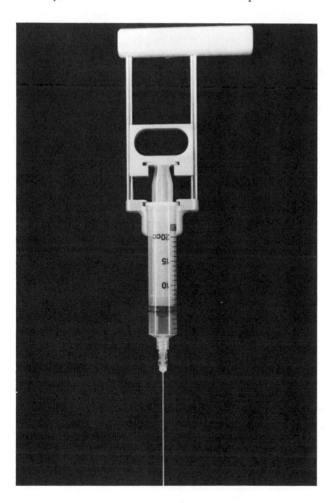

Figure 7.4   The photo shows the Cameco syringe pistol aspiration device.

(Precision Dynamics Inc., San Fernando, California.)

and medium housed in the same biopsy aspiration device used for transabdominal CVS is attached to the needle. Villi are obtained by repeated, rapid aspirations up to 20-mL negative pressure.

Safety Comparisons

Data concerning the risks for transcervical CVS have recently been reported from two large prospective trials. Transcervical CVS and transabdominal have proved comparable in safety to amniocentesis. (Despite ultrasound advances, amniocentesis should be considered to carry a fetal loss rate of about 0.5% above background (2).)

The National Institute of Child Health and Development (NICHD) studies involved seven US centers, including our own (9). A total of 2,278 women selected transcervical CVS; 671 women recruited in the first trimester selected amniocentesis. (Randomization did not prove possible.) After statistical adjustment for differences in maternal age and gestational age between the two groups, the excess loss rate in the CVS group was 0.8% (80% confidence limits 0.6% to 2.2%; not statistically significant). If transcervical CVS carries higher risk of fetal loss than amniocentesis, the difference is thus only slight. Further, there were no differences in gestational age at delivery and birthweights between the two groups. One or more pregnancy complications (hypertension, placental abruption, and necessity for labor induction) were slightly more common in the amniocentesis group; however, in all other obstetric respects, patients in the two groups were not statistically different. Logically, procedures requiring more than one pass of the catheter to obtain chorionic villi were associated with a higher loss rate than single-pass procedures. Eight U.S. centers, including our own, then participate in a NICHD-sponsored collaborative study to address relative safety of transcervical CVS and transabdominal CVS. Subjects in whom either procedure is technically feasible were randomized into transabdominal and transcervical arms. Loss rates were nearly identical in the two groups (10). Further, with availability of both transcervical and transabdominal CVS, loss rates decreased over the rate when only transcervical CVS was available.

The Canadian Collaborative CVS-Amniocentesis Trial Group evaluated 2,787 women (11). They were randomized either to transcervical CVS (1,391 subjects) or amniocentesis (1,396); women were excluded after randomization if they showed a nonviable fetus, multiple gestation, infection, or pregnancy advanced beyond 12 completed gestational weeks. Comparison of total losses (spontaneous abortions and induced abortions and losses ≥ 20 weeks' gestation) revealed the CVS group to be 0.6% higher (7.6% versus 7.0%; however, the difference was not statistically significant). There was a tendency to later losses in the CVS group, but no specific event appeared to be responsible for this observation. Mean birthweights for each week of gestation, proportion of preterm births, percentage of growth-retarded infants, and maternal morbidity were similar for both groups. The investigators concluded that these data " . . . may reassure women on the safety of first trimester CVS " (11).

In contrast to amniocentesis, a relatively easy procedure, considerable variation seems to exist among centers with respect to CVS safety. Despite two reported clusters of limb reduction defects (LRD), the World Health Organization tabulated that in experienced centers LRD following CVS was virtually identical (6.0/10,000 based upon 80,051 cases) to population expectations (5.4/10,000) (12). Loss rates in CVS are generally higher in centers that perform fewer procedures, suggesting that inexperience could be related to LRD (12). For example, in the one U.S. center reporting a LRD cluster, the loss rate using a 1.9 mm transcervical catheter was 10.9% (20/183); the rate reached 21% (7/33) when two attempts were required (13). Following CVS at 10–12 weeks, LRD are thus probably not increased in experienced hands; however, patients should nonetheless be appraised of the controversy, and CVS should not generally be performed earlier than 9 weeks (12).

Although we and others have performed transvaginal CVS, numbers of cases are far too few to make any statements concerning success either in obtaining adequate specimens or safety of this procedure.

Cytogenetics

Analysis of either chorionic villi or amniotic fluid cells has pitfalls that should be recognized by the obstetrician

(14–16). First, cells may not grow, or growth may be insufficient to perform analyses. Although failure of amniotic cell cultures are now uncommon, failures still occur. Chorionic villus cultures are likewise usually successful and, in fact, may require fewer days for growth than amniotic fluid cell cultures. In addition, chorionic villus trophoblasts divide so rapidly that metaphases can be accumulated within hours or overnight. Such "direct" analysis provides rapid answers, but metaphases are usually of poorer quality than those obtained by culture methods. Thus, for cytogenetic analysis, most centers perform standard tissue culture analysis using mesenchymal core cells.

Inadvertent inclusion of maternal cells (so-called "maternal cell contamination") is a potential concern of CVS. The frequency of this error in CVS is still being determined, although, in our experience, it is rare. In CVS, decidua can be readily identified under the dissecting microscope. Moreover, when maternal cell contamination occurs, it can be recognized readily; amniocentesis is not usually required. In neither the U.S. nor the Canadian trials did maternal cell contamination lead to a diagnostic error (9, 11).

In the study, the rate of aneuploid fetuses in the CVS group (1.8%) was only slightly higher than in the amniocentesis group (1.4%) (10). No aneuploid fetuses were missed and there were no errors in the determination of fetal sex in the CVS group. The only difference arose in the frequency of mosaicism. Of relevance is that detection of chromosome abnormalities in villi does not always signify abnormal fetal status. Aberrations like tetraploidy, certain lethal trisomies (for example, trisomy 16) and monosomy X may occur in chorionic villi preparations but not in embryonic tissue (14). This holds especially for direct cytogenetic analysis. Recall, moreover, that in vitro chromosome aberrations may arise in amniotic fluid or villus cultures (16). In fact, cells containing at least one additional structurally normal chromosome are detected in 1% to 3% of all amniotic cell cultures (16). If such cells are confined to a single culture flask or clone, the phenomenon is termed "pseudomosaicism" and is not considered clinically important. If a chromosome abnormality is detected in more than one flask or clone, "true mosaicism" is said to exist, and is considered clinically significant. True mosaicism occurs in 0.25% of amniotic cell cultures and is confirmed in 70% to 80% of abortuses or live births (16).

In CVS, discrepancies are documented between either direct (cytotrophoblast) and culture (mesenchymal core) techniques and between either abortus or live birth (9, 11, 15). Because of these potential discrepancies, interpretation of cytogenetic results for CVS may be more difficult than for amniocentesis (15). However, in both the Canadian and U.S. collaborative studies, a definitive diagnosis could be reached in all cases by using amniocentesis to follow up cases of ambiguous cytogenetic results from CVS. Thus, patients who undergo CVS must be aware that amniocentesis may occasionally (<1%) be required to clarify cytogenetic results obtained from CVS.

In contrast with the U.S. study, the Canadian study revealed a significantly higher rate of aneuploidy in the CVS group (4.5% versus 2.4%; $P < 0.01$) (11). The more frequent false-positive results are likely explained by two factors: 1) a higher rate of "false-positive" diagnoses (2.5% versus 0.3%; $P < 0.001$), and 2) a higher rate of true aneuploidy (2.1% versus 1.0%; $P < 0.05$). False-positive results were defined as cytogenetic abnormalities detected at prenatal diagnosis but not found at time of follow-up (amniocentesis, abortus, or infant). With four exceptions, all "false-positive" CVS results requiring amniocentesis showed that CVS diagnosis was correct. The increased rate of true aneuploidy in the CVS group could have been due to early diagnosis of aneuploidy in fetuses, some of which would probably have aborted spontaneously had terminations not been performed.

The accuracy of transabdominal CVS is comparable to that in transcervical CVS as shown in the most recent analysis of the NICHD (17).

Enzymatic and DNA Analyses

Enzymatic or DNA analyses of chorionic villi may be used to detect the same genetic disorders as are detectable using amniotic fluid cells. Although most enzymatic or DNA analyses using chorionic villi have been accurate, no large studies are yet available. Potential pitfalls include maternal cell contamination, failure to optimize conditions for chorionic villi analyses (for example, appropriate controls matched for gestational age), or investigator inexperience with a particular assay.

Conclusions

Results of the U.S. and Canadian collaborative trials indicate that transcervical chorionic villus sampling is a safe and effective method for the first-trimester, prenatal diagnosis of genetic disorders, comparable with amniocentesis. Although the safety and accuracy of transabdominal CVS remains to be elucidated, initial reports indicate that the outcome of transabdominal CVS is comparable with transcervical CVS. On the other hand, technical aspects of obtaining villi and performing villus cytogenetic analyses place a greater burden on physicians, cytogeneticists, and genetic counselors than amniocentesis does. This added responsibility is best handled with a team approach to CVS, in which all aspects of CVS, including training of personnel, counseling, technical aspects of procedure, performance, interpretation of diagnostic studies, and postprocedure counseling are handled by a team of specialists who are in constant communication with each other.

References

1. Nadler HL, Gerbie AB. Role of amniocentesis in the intrauterine detection of genetic disorders. N Engl J Med 1970; 282:596.

2. Elias S, Simpson JL. Amniocentesis. In: Milunsky A, ed. Genetic disorders of the fetus: diagnosis, prevention and treatment. New York: Plenum Press, 1986:31–52.

3. Castodot RG. Pregnancy termination: techniques, risks and complications and their management. Fertil Steril 1986; 45:5.

4. Speiser PW, Laforgia N, Kato K, et al. First trimester prenatal diagnosis and molecular genetic diagnosis of congenital adrenal hyperplasia (21-hydroxylase deficiency). J Clin Endo Metab 1990;60:838.

5. Elias S, Annas GJ: Reproductive genetics and the law. Chicago: Year Book Medical Publishers, 1987:121–42.

6. Elias S, Simpson JL, Martin AO, et al. Chorionic villus sampling for first trimester prenatal diagnosis: Northwestern University Program. Am J Obstet Gynecol 1985;152:204.

7. Elias S, Simpson JL, Shulman LP, et al. Transabdominal chorionic villus sampling for first-trimester prenatal diagnosis. Am J Obstet Gynecol 1989;160:879.

8. Smidt-Jensen S, Hahnemann N, Hariri J, et al. Transabdominal chorionic villus sampling for first trimester fetal diagnosis. First 26 pregnancies followed to term. Prenat Diag 1986; 6:125.

9. Rhoads GG, Jackson LG, Schlesselman SE, et al. The safety and efficacy of chorionic villus sampling for early prenatal diagnosis of cytogenetic abnormalities. N Engl J Med 1989; 320:609.

10. Jackson LG, Zachary JM, Fowler SE, et al. A randomized comparison of transcervical and transabdominal chronic villus sampling. N Engl J Med 1992;327:594.

11. Canadian Collaborative CVS–Amniocentesis Clinical Trial Group. Multicentre randomised clinical trial of chorion villus sampling and amniocentesis. First report. Lancet 1989; 1:1.

12. World Health Organization/European Regional Office (WHO/EURO): Risk evaluation of CVS. WHO/EURO: Copenhagen, Denmark, 1992.

13. Burton BK, Schulz CJ, Burd LI: Limb anomalies associated with chorionic villus sampling. Obstet Gynecol 1992;79: 726.

14. Tharapel AT, Elias S, Shulman LP, et al. Resorbed co-twin as an explanation for discrepant chorionic villi results: nonmosaic 47, XX, +16 in villi (direct and culture) with normal (46, XX) amniotic fluid and neonatal blood. Prenat Diagn 1989;9:1.

15. Ledbetter DH, Gilbert F, Jackson L, et al. Cytogenetic results of chorion villus sampling: high success rate and diagnostic accuracy in the U.S. collaborative study. Am J Obstet Gynecol 1990;162:495.

16. Hsu LYF, Perlis TE. United States survey on chromosome mosaicism and pseudomosaicism in prenatal diagnosis. Prenat Diagn 1980;4:97.

17. Ledbetter DH, Zachary JM, Simpson JL, et al. Cytogenetic results from the U.S. Collaborative study on CVS. Hematol Diag 1992;12:317.

8

Amniocentesis

John T. Queenan, M.D.

AMNIOCENTESIS began to be used routinely after 1956, when Bevis demonstrated that third-trimester amniocentesis was helpful in managing the Rh-immunized pregnancy (1). Shortly thereafter, Liley and others developed systems for analyzing amniotic fluid to determine fetal condition in erythroblastosis fetalis (2–6). Second-trimester amniocentesis became common after it was demonstrated that Down syndrome could be diagnosed by genetic amniocentesis.

What Are the Indications for Early Amniocentesis?

Most amniocenteses performed between 15 and 17 weeks' gestation are for genetic indications. Chromosome or biochemical studies are done on cultured cells from the amniotic fluid. The indications for genetic amniocentesis are as follows:

- Maternal age 35 years or greater
- Parent with a chromosome abnormality
- Previous child with chromosome abnormality
- Carrier state for a metabolic disorder
- Previous child with a neural tube defect (NTD)
- Elevated maternal serum α-fetoprotein (MSAFP)
- Low MSAFP
- Abnormal MSAFP, estriol and BHCG screen
- Abnormal fetal anatomy

The ideal time for genetic amniocentesis is from 15 to 17 weeks. Technically, the procedure can be done as early as 14 weeks, provided the uterus is well above the pubic symphysis. However, after 14 weeks, amniotic fluid volume

Table 8.1 Typical Increases in Amniotic Fluid

Gestation (weeks)	Fluid volume (mL)
12	50
14	100
16	150
18	200
20	250

increases rapidly, making the procedure easier to perform (Table 8.1). There are reports of performing amniocentesis from 10 to 14 weeks, but this is still experimental and the risks are not fully known (7–9).

Doing the procedure between 15 and 17 weeks allows enough time for cell cultures and laboratory tests before it is too late to consider pregnancy termination if the fetus is abnormal. In most cases, abortion can be done by 20 weeks' gestation. The risk of fetal loss is 0.5% to 1.0% (10–11).

Placental size is also a consideration in timing amniocentesis. During early pregnancy, the placenta is relatively large compared with the uterus, fetus, and amniotic fluid volume. Because there can be placenta covering two-thirds of the uterine cavity surface, it may be difficult to obtain fluid without piercing the placenta. Later in pregnancy, after the uterus has grown considerably, the placenta, while also larger, appears to cover a smaller proportion of the uterine cavity. A placenta-free window is usually easy to find.

What Are the Indications for Later Amniocentesis?

Diagnostic amniocentesis is performed in the second half of pregnancy to determine fetal condition in Rh disease or other blood group immunizations (but not ABO incompatibility). It is also used to determine fetal maturity and to check for infection and maturity in the setting of premature rupture of the membranes. On rare occasions, diagnostic amniocentesis may be done in the second half of pregnancy for genetic reasons, or if structural abnormalities are noted.

A Guide to Technique

The following protocol may be helpful in performing amniocentesis (12).

As a preliminary step, use ultrasound scanning to:
- Document fetal life.
- Document gestational age.
- Evaluate the fetus for gross malformations.
- Detect multiple gestation.

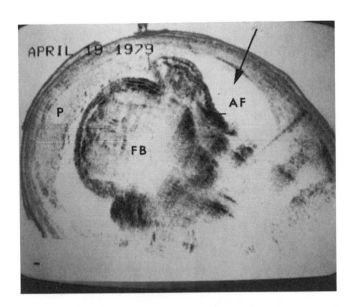

Figure 8.1　Transverse ultrasound scan demonstrating a pocket of amniotic fluid (AF). Arrow indicates site for insertion of needle. Placenta (P) is located on patient's right. Fetal body (FB) is outlined.

- Locate pockets of amniotic fluid (Figure 8.1).
- Guide the needle insertion to avoid the placenta and fetus and facilitate aspiration of amniotic fluid (AF).
- Prep the abdomen three times with povidone-iodine (Betadine) solution.
- Drape the abdomen.
- Local anesthetic is an option but it increases the number of needle insertions.
- Insert the ultrasound transducer in a sterile sheath.
- Alert the patient that there will be a needle stick.
- Insert the needle briskly under ultrasound guidance.
- Remove the stylet.
- Observe for a drop of AF. If none appears, rotate the needle 90 degrees and again observe for a drop of fluid. If still none appears, advance the needle briskly a short distance under ultrasound guidance. (Generally, AF is obtained upon insertion, not withdrawal, of the needle.)
- When fluid appears, discard the first few drops to decrease risk of maternal r.b.c. contamination, then attach syringe.
- Aspirate AF.

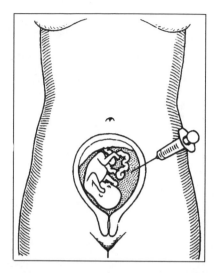

Figure 8.2   Diagram demonstrating genetic amniocentesis.
(Reproduced with permission, from Queenan JT. Intrauterine diagnosis of Down's syndrome. Annals of the New York Academy of Science 1970; 171:617.)

- Disengage the syringe.
- Withdraw the needle. It is not necessary to reinsert the stylet.

    If the patient is Rh-negative, unimmunized:
- Following genetic amniocentesis, give 300 micrograms of Rh-immune globulin intramuscularly.
- Proceed as with "two-dose regimen" (as outlined in Chapter 48, Rh and Other Blood Group Immunizations).
- If the Rh-negative, unimmunized patient is undergoing an amniocentesis closer to term, for example, for amniotic fluid maturity studies, prophylactic Rh-immune globulin would also be indicated.

    See Figures 8.2–8.4 for illustration of the procedure.

How to Approach Problem Taps

Abdominal Scars

The presence of abdominal scars should suggest the possibility of adhesions. The history of an abdominal operation, in itself, is not a contraindication to amniocentesis. How-

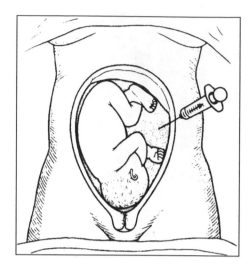

Figure 8.3   Diagram demonstrating amniocentesis in the area of the fetal small parts.
(Reproduced with permission, from Queenan JT. Amniocentesis and transamniotic fetal transfusion for Rh disease. Clin Obstet Gynecol 1966: 9:491.)

ever, certain procedures often produce multiple abdominal adhesions, for example, appendectomy for a ruptured appendix. Watch out particularly for evidence of a drain site and proceed with caution. Surgery for endometriosis or pelvic inflammatory disease can be associated with multiple adhesions. Cholecystectomy can also cause postoperative adhesions, although these are usually higher in the abdomen.

Anterior Placenta

When the placenta is in this position, it is more likely to be pierced, causing hemorrhage and other related complications. The clinician can avoid placental trauma by scanning with ultrasound to find a placenta-free window. If the placenta is implanted over the entire anterior uterine wall, careful ultrasound scanning should be used to select the thinnest part of the placenta to traverse. The clinician should take special care to avoid the area of umbilical cord insertion because this area contains the highest concentration of blood vessels on the chorionic plate (Figure 8.5).

Uterine Rotation

When marked, it means that the uterine artery and vein are

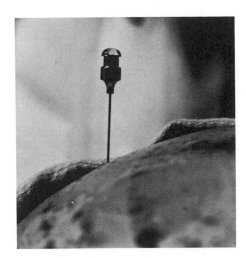

Figure 8.4   Following insertion, observe the end of the needle for a drop of amniotic fluid.

rotated from a lateral to an anterior position. These vessels are then more vulnerable to trauma by amniocentesis, particularly if the patient has severe pelvic varicosities and if the suprapubic approach is used.

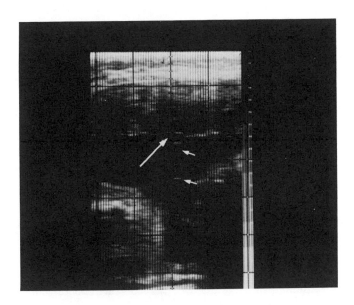

Figure 8.5   Real-time ultrasound demonstrating an anteriorly implanted placenta. Large arrow points to cord insertion into the placenta. Small arrows indicate cord echoes.

Obesity

This condition presents a problem in that the needle must traverse the thick abdominal wall as well as the uterine wall. It may be necessary to change from the standard $3^{1}/2$ inch needle to one that is 5 or 7 inches.

Hydropic Placenta

If the placenta is massively enlarged, there may be mechanical difficulty in obtaining AF. If the needle tip often becomes lodged in the substance of the edematous placenta, neither blood nor AF can be aspirated. But by using ultrasound to locate pockets of fluid, it is usually possible to avoid this problem.

Oligohydramnios

A pathologically decreased volume of AF may make successful amniocentesis very difficult. Pockets of fluid can be located by ultrasound (Figure 8.6). These pockets may be small and virtually inaccessible to the amniocentesis needle, but it is very rare that no fluid is recoverable.

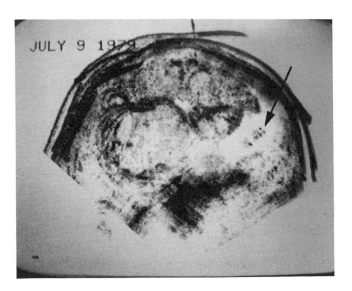

Figure 8.6   Ultrasound scan demonstrating the localization of a pocket of amniotic fluid (AF) in cases of reduced volume of AF.

Special Clinical Situations

Various factors can affect the performance of the amniocentesis. The operator performing the procedure should be particularly alert to the following possibilities.

Multiple Gestation

When there is more than one fetus, be sure to enter each sac when technically feasible so that tests are specific for each fetus. Sonography is helpful in determining the confines of the sac by identifying the membranes separating the sacs. If indigo carmine is instilled into the first sac, the operator can be certain when the second is entered by aspirating AF with no dye. If a fetus must be identified after delivery, injection of 10–15 mL of Hypaque-M 15 (diazotriazoate, meglumine) into the AF will facilitate such identification. The ingested contrast media may be visualized in the newborn gastrointestinal tract two to three weeks later by abdominal roentgenogram.

Rh Immunization

When the mother is immunized to the Rh or other blood group factors, it is critically important to avoid piercing the placenta. A transplacental hemorrhage during amniocentesis may further increase the level of immunization or produce fetal anemia. Rh-immunized patients usually require serial amniocentesis. Sonographic guidance is essential to avoid the placenta.

Postmaturity

Amniocentesis is important in managing suspected postmaturity. Besides obtaining AF for fetal maturity studies, the clinician may wish to look for meconium in the AF. Because fluid volume is often decreased in the postmature pregnancy, the amniocentesis can be difficult but sonographic guidance assures recovery of AF.

Congenital Malformations

Commonly, malformations are associated with either increased or decreased AF. A pathologic increase, or polyhydramnios, facilitates amniocentesis. Certain central nervous system or gastrointestinal tract malformations are often associated with polyhydramnios. CNS malformations usually are severe and may be incompatible with life. Gastrointestinal malformations are often amenable to surgical correction. Chromosome abnormalities may be present with polyhydramnios and/or omphalocoele.

A pathologic decrease in AF, or oligohydramnios, is frequently seen with such disorders as Potter syndrome, which includes renal agenesis, low-set ears, and other major malformations. It is also encountered in fetuses with bilateral obstructive uropathy.

Premature Rupture of the Membranes (PROM)

When faced with PROM, the clinician may want to perform amniocentesis for fetal maturity studies or to look for white blood cells or bacteria. PROM does not make amniocentesis impossible, but decreased fluid will, of course, make it more difficult. The operator should use ultrasound to locate pockets of fluid after placing the patient in slight Trendelenberg position.

Problems in Handling the Specimen

Normal Precautions

These basic steps are necessary if the test is to be valid:

- Protect the specimen from sunlight. Analysis for Rh immunization entails a spectrophotometric scan. Exposure to sunlight decreases the spectrophotometric levels of bilirubin in the fluid and leads to a false-low reading due to a change in absorbance at 450 mμ.
- Protect the specimen from bacterial contamination. Fluid submitted for genetic studies usually will be cultured. Bacterial contamination prevents proper growth of the cells. The clinician must use meticulous aseptic technique.
- Protect the fluid from contamination with blood. If the specimen is contaminated with maternal blood, the maternal white blood cells may grow in the cell culture, yielding the maternal karyotype rather than the desired fetal karyotype. Fetal studies such as those for α-fetoprotein (AFP) are markedly altered if the specimen is contaminated with fetal blood. Fetal concentration of AFP is many times that in AF or mater-

nal serum. Even if the fetal red blood cells are removed from the sample immediately by centrifugation, the fetal AFP remains in the specimen because only particulate matter can be centrifuged out.

Turbidity

This condition is normal in later pregnancy. But it will affect the spectrophotometric scan of the fluid by increasing the absorption of light. Rarely, turbid fluid may have to be filtered before spectrophotometry.

Contamination with Blood

Probably no aspect of amniocentesis is more poorly defined in the medical literature than is the bloody tap. Blood may be obtained on every amniocentesis simply by inserting the needle as far as the myometrium and stopping. Because of the large number of venous sinuses in the myometrium, blood can always be aspirated. If the needle traverses the abdominal wall and uterus and enters the amniotic sac, then no blood is obtained. To be valid, any study of the incidence of bloody taps must answer the following questions:

- Was blood obtained on insertion?
- Was blood present in the fluid?
- Was blood encountered upon withdrawal of the needle?
- Was there sonographic evidence of bleeding after withdrawal of the needle?
- Was the blood fetal or maternal, or both?

If blood is present, this fact should be recorded, along with data on when blood was encountered. The source of the blood is extremely important. Maternal blood is obtained when the needle pierces a vessel in the abdominal wall or, more commonly, comes to rest in a venous sinus in the myometrium. It may also be obtained by piercing the placenta. Fetal blood is encountered if the needle stops in the substance of the placenta. The needle causes an interruption in the fetal circulation that promptly becomes a microhematoma. The fetal blood can then be aspirated slowly from the hematoma. More often, fetal blood appears at the hub of the needle but cannot be aspirated. There is a danger that the needle may pierce the fetal heart or a major vessel, but not if the procedure is done with proper skills

utilizing ultrasound guidance.

Meconium Contamination

Occasionally, meconium stains the specimen, giving it an opaque greenish tinge. Meconium increases absorbance at the lower spectrophotometric wavelengths (Figure 8.7).

Urine Aspiration

If a patient has a full bladder and the needle is inserted into its lumen, urine may be aspirated which has an appearance similar to AF. But it is easy to identify because it does not demonstrate characteristic ferning and it will have a typical spectrophotometric scan, shown in Figure 8.8. Absorbance at the lower wavelengths will be increased. A rapid test of aspirated fluid with nitrazine paper will determine the source because AF is alkaline and urine is usually acidic.

Dealing with Complications

Bloody Amniotic Fluid

One of the most common complications of amniocentesis, blood contamination of the AF, usually occurs in the first portion of the specimen, when the operator readjusts the needle. If small amounts of blood continue to contaminate the fluid, the specimen should be centrifuged to remove the particulate matter. The serum will not be removed.

If there is continued difficulty in obtaining a clear specimen, syringes should be changed frequently so that the whole 10-mL specimen is not contaminated with a drop of blood.

Maternal Hemorrhage

Although maternal bleeding must occur fairly often in amniocentesis, it is rarely clinically evident. In over 7,000 diagnostic amniocenteses, admission to the hospital was necessary only once. On that occasion, a maternal hemorrhage was suspected but, after careful evaluation, was found not to be occurring. Still, it is easy to imagine amniocentesis producing hematomas in the uterine or abdominal walls. But these appear not to be clinically significant unless the mother has a bleeding disorder.

Fetal Hemorrhage

Rarely, the operator may pierce fetal vessels or the umbili-

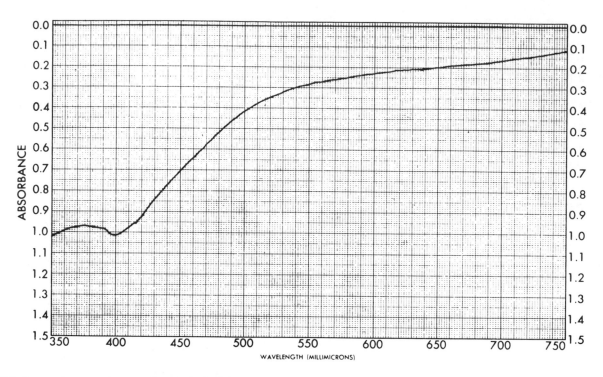

Figure 8.7 Spectrophotometric scan of amniotic fluid (AF) contaminated with meconium. Note increased absorbance in shorter wavelengths.

(Reproduced, with permission, from Queenan JT. Modern management of the Rh problem. 2nd ed. Hagerstown, MD: Harper & Row, 1977.)

cal cord. This produces hemorrhage into the AF and could cause fetal distress. There is no question that such an accident is a potential hazard of amniocentesis. If the procedure is done skillfully, however, the risk is minimal.

Maternal Immunization

Numerous studies have shown that transplacental hemorrhages occur in the wake of an amniocentesis that traverses the placenta. Since as little as 0.3 mL of fetal blood is all it takes to immunize the mother, amniocentesis obviously can cause isoimmunization. If the mother already has a low level of Rh immunization, a transplacental hemorrhage caused by amniocentesis may produce an anamnestic response such that the level of immunization will subsequently be very severe. Queenan and Adams showed this in 1964, and the finding has also been confirmed by other investigators (13, 14).

Premature Rupture of the Membranes

When an operator uses a 20-gauge needle, the likelihood of

causing PROM is extremely small. An unskilled operator who makes several needle insertions to obtain fluid increases the risk of PROM; doing the procedure in the lower portion of the uterus possibly increases the risk of PROM.

Premature Labor

There is no evidence that amniocentesis done skillfully will cause premature labor. Over 7,000 patients who had amniocentesis had an incidence of spontaneous premature labor no higher than that in the general population.

Infection

It can be said categorically that amniocentesis done properly is not a source of infection. If the patient's membranes have ruptured prematurely, amniocentesis may be valuable to detect amnionitis.

Fetal Trauma

Amniocentesis certainly can injure the fetus, but sonographic guidance minimizes the risks of fetal trauma. It is

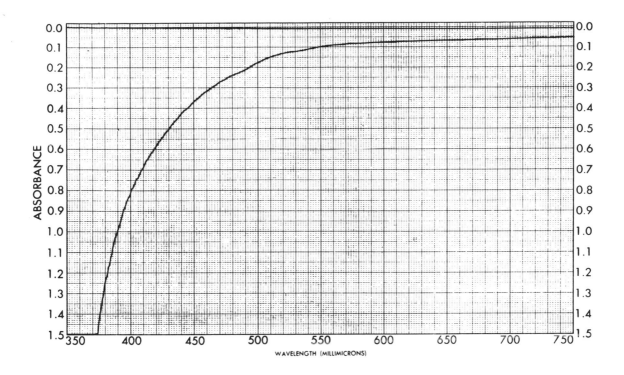

Figure 8.8 Spectrophotometric scan of urine. Note increased absorbance at shorter wavelengths.

(Reproduced, with permission, from Queenan JT. Modern management of the Rh problem. 2nd ed. Hagerstown, MD: Harper & Row, 1977.)

always possible to stick a moving fetal limb inadvertently, but this is of little or no clinical significance; it would amount to no more trauma than giving a newborn an injection of vitamin K.

Recording the Procedure

Adequate records must be kept of the amniocentesis procedure. Sample diagrams that graphically demonstrate the important points for each amniocentesis are shown in Figure 8.9. Placental location, where the needle entered relative to the fetus, whether blood was encountered, fetal heart observation after the procedure, whether there is bleeding at the tapsite, and if Rh-immune globulin was indicated and administered should be recorded.

Therapeutic Amniocentesis

The only recognized indication for therapeutic amniocentesis is polyhydramnios so severe that the mother has car-

diorespiratory distress. Such underlying causes of polyhydramnios as Rh disease, multiple gestation, diabetes, and congenital malformations should be ruled out.

If the acute polyhydramnios is idiopathic and not associated with the complications cited, it may be managed by repeated amniocenteses to alleviate extreme maternal symptoms and prevent premature labor. Aspiration of amniotic fluid will relieve symptoms almost immediately.

There are several case reports in the literature of pregnancies that would have terminated in the second trimester had not therapeutic amniocentesis allowed the fetus to become viable in utero (15, 16). In a series of 243 patients with polyhydramnios, Queenan and Gadow found only one who required therapeutic amniocentesis (17). Other reports in the literature also suggest that the procedure is rarely indicated.

Where We Stand Today

A procedure that was at one time considered daring and

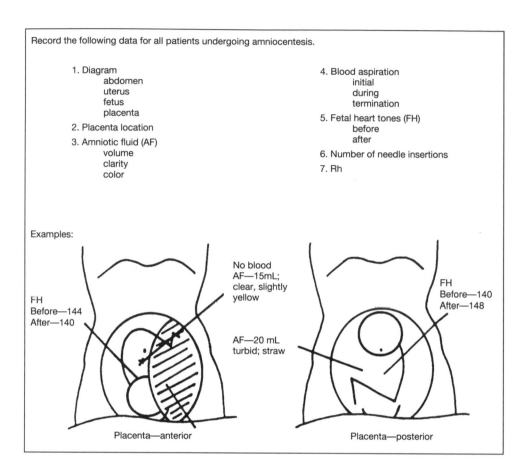

Record the following data for all patients undergoing amniocentesis.

1. Diagram
   abdomen
   uterus
   fetus
   placenta
2. Placenta location
3. Amniotic fluid (AF)
   volume
   clarity
   color

4. Blood aspiration
   initial
   during
   termination
5. Fetal heart tones (FH)
   before
   after
6. Number of needle insertions
7. Rh

Examples:

FH
Before—144
After—140

No blood
AF—15mL;
clear, slightly
yellow

AF—20 mL
turbid; straw

Placenta—anterior

FH
Before—140
After—148

Placenta—posterior

Figure 8.9 Diagram demonstrating data recorded following amniocentesis procedure.

risky, is now routine in approximately 15% of pregnancies. With careful consideration of the indications, the benefits of amniocentesis far outweigh the risks. Amniocentesis is safe when careful judgment and skill are used. Scanning the pregnancy prior to amniocentesis provides necessary knowledge about the pregnancy before the procedure. Sonographic guidance for needle insertion is now the standard of care in the United States.

This procedure belongs solely to our specialty. With the advent of ultrasound, the safety of amniocentesis should have increased markedly. Unfortunately, such is not the case. It is hoped that the technique of amniocentesis will be better understood and physicians will be trained extensively in this important obstetrical tool.

There has been a deficiency in residency training pro-

grams with respect to this common obstetrical procedure, which is probably the most poorly taught. As the teaching of ultrasonography becomes more established in residency training programs, the education of young physicians with respect to the indications and proper technique of amniocentesis should follow. It should also be stressed that, if obstetricians are going to perform the technique of amniocentesis, they should perform the procedure often enough so that their skills remain sharp.

We have good information concerning the risks and benefits of CVS and 15–17 week amniocentesis and more is being learned about the safety of 11–14 week amniocentesis. To date, it appears to have comparable efficacy as far as quality of the specimen but slightly higher pregnancy loss than 15–17 week amniocentesis. If future studies confirm a good safety record, then earlier amniocentesis could be a major competitor to CVS.

References

1. Bevis DC. Blood pigments in haemolytic disease of the newborn. J Obstet Gynaecol Br Emp 1956;63:68.

2. Liley AW. Liquor amnii analysis in management of the pregnancy complicated by rhesus sensitization. Am J Obstet Gynecol 1961;82:1359.

3. Freda VJ. The Rh problem in obstetrics and a new concept of its management using amniocentesis and spectrophotometric scanning of amniotic fluid. Am J Obstet Gynecol 1965; 92:341.

4. Whitfield CR. A three-year assessment of an action line method of timing intervention in rhesus isoimmunization. Am J Obstet Gynecol 1970;108:1239.

5. Queenan JT, Goetschel E. Amniotic fluid analysis for erythroblastosis fetalis. Obstet Gynecol 1968;32:120.

6. Queenan JT. Modern management of the Rh problem. 2nd ed. Hagerstown, MD: Harper & Row, 1977.

7. Assel BG, Lewis SM, Dickerman LH, et al. Single operator comparison of early and mid-second-trimester amniocentesis. Obstet Gynecol 1992;79:940.

8. Penso CA, Sandstrom MM, Garber MF, et al. Early amniocentesis: report of 407 cases with neonatal follow-up. Obstet Gynecol 1990;76:1032.

9. Hanson FW, Happ RL, Tennant FR, et al. Ultrasonography-guided early amniocentesis in singleton pregnancies. Am J Obstet Gynecol 1990;162:1376.

10. NICHD National Registry for amniocentesis study group. Mid-trimester amniocentesis for prenatal diagnosis, safety and accuracy. JAMA 1973;236:1471.

11. Tabor A, Madsen M, Obel E, et al. Randomized controlled trial of genetic amniocentesis in 4606 low risk women. Lancet 1986;6:1287.

12. Queenan JT. Genetic amniocentesis. In: Queenan JT, Hobbins JC, eds. Protocols for high-risk pregnancies. Oradell, NJ: Medical Economics Books, 1982.

13. Queenan JT, Adams DW. Amniocentesis: A possible immunizing hazard. Obstet Gynecol 1964;24:530.

14. Zipursky A, Pollock J, Chown B, et al. Transplacental fetal hemorrhage after placental injury during delivery or amniocentesis. Lancet 1963;2:493.

15. Pitkin R. Acute polyhydramnios recurrent in successive pregnancies: Management with multiple amniocentesis. Obstet Gynecol 1976;48:42.

16. Queenan JT. Recurrent acute polyhydramnios. Am J Obstet Gynecol 1970;106:625.

17. Queenan JT, Gadow EC. Polyhydramnios: Chronic versus acute. Am J Obstet Gynecol 1970;108:349.

9

Direct Umbilical Fetal Blood Sampling: Cordocentesis

John W. Seeds, M.D.

DIRECT fetal blood sampling using an ultrasonically guided transabdominal needle has rapidly become an important tool in the assessment of the fetus (1–4). A pure sample of fetal blood enables the performance of a rapid fetal karyotype, as well as fetal blood typing, antibody testing, acid-base assessment, and precise evaluation of isoimmune hemolytic anemia (3). In addition, clotting factor deficiencies, thrombocytopenia, and hemoglobinopathies may be diagnosed with fetal blood (2). This technique is commonly referred to as percutaneous umbilical blood sampling (PUBS), cordocentesis, and, more recently, as funipuncture (5). Funipuncture is derived from the Latin roots *funis*, meaning cordlike structure, and *punctura*, meaning to pierce or to penetrate, and has been recently promoted as a more precise and appropriate name for this new technique.

Compared to previous methods for sampling fetal blood, including placentocentesis and fetoscopy, cordocentesis is more direct, simpler, and apparently safer in the hands of experienced operators (4). Placentocentesis is imprecise and impractical because of a high rate of contamination with maternal blood and/or amniotic fluid, while fetoscopy imposes a 4%–5% risk of pregnancy loss, has limited availability, and is technically restricted to gestations under 26 weeks' gestation (3, 6, 7).

Direct umbilical vein blood sampling was first described by Beng in 1982 (8). He reported the successful intravenous intrauterine transfusion of a fetus with severe hemolytic anemia using a narrow-gauge needle sonographically guided to the umbilical vein within the fetal liver. Daffos, in 1983, described 66 patients from whom he successfully obtained fetal blood from the umbilical vein, also using a percutaneous needle (1). Later, he reported 606 patients sampled for a variety of indications across a wide spectrum of gestational age (4). This remains the largest reported series, and it includes 394 patients under 24 weeks' gestational age at the time of sampling. The rate of pregnancy loss in this subgroup was 0.8%. The rate of procedure-related pregnancy loss in more recent reports appears to confirm this low level of risk. In addition to fetal blood sampling, many investigators have documented the use of this new technique for the direct intravascular transfusion of blood into the anemic fetus (3, 9–13). Furthermore, resolution in utero of severe hydrops due to Rh iso-immunization after intravascular transfusion has been described (10).

Although many previous indications for fetal blood sampling are detectable through DNA fragmentation analysis of either chorionic villus material or amniotic fluid fibroblasts, many uses for fetal blood sampling remain. In the case of a late prenatal registrant or late identification of high-risk status for an aneuploid fetus, fetal blood sampling enables preparation of a rapid karyotype from fetal lymphocytes. Furthermore, fetal blood component analysis is only possible with a sample of fetal blood (14, 15).

The technique of percutaneous umbilical blood sampling is remarkably simple. Using high-resolution, dynamic image ultrasound, the umbilical vein is identified and an aspiration site selected. Within a sterile field, a narrow gauge needle is guided percutaneously to the umbilical vein by ultrasound, and fetal blood is aspirated. If indicated, donor blood is infused.

We will review the range of indications for fetal blood sampling, then examine in greater detail the sampling procedure itself, and finally look at intrauterine intravascular fetal blood transfusions. Appropriate training pathways will also be discussed.

Indications

Indications for cordocentesis include all indications for fetal karyotype, analysis of fetal blood components, and evaluation and possible treatment of fetal hemolytic anemia (see Table 9.1).

The assessment of fetal platelet count in a case of immunological thrombocytopenic purpura, or the evaluation of possible fetal infection by measuring the level of disease-specific fetal IgM may also be accomplished using a sample of fetal blood. In the case of severe intrauterine growth retardation not in labor, or questionable fetal heart rate evidence of distress in early labor, fetal blood sampling and respiratory gas analysis or assessment of acid base balance may only be done with a pure sample of fetal blood.

In the case of maternal-fetal blood incompatibility, percutaneous blood sampling offers several specific advantages (16, 17). If the father of the pregnancy is established to be heterozygous for the antigen in question, a single funipuncture done early in gestation will establish fetal antigen status and, with an antigen-negative infant, serial amniocenteses for optical density studies can be avoided. This possibility can lead to substantial savings of both risk and cost. Second, a fetal blood sample can establish the precise degree of hemolysis, and the technique enables direct intravascular transfusion earlier in gestation than intraperitoneal transfusion was previously possible. Third, reversal in utero of hydrops fetalis after direct intravascular transfusion has been reported (10, 16, 17). Direct intravascular fetal blood transfusion is considered by some to be the treatment of choice in the case of hydrops fetalis resulting from isoimmunization.

Fetal Blood Sampling: Technique

The technique of fetal blood sampling includes site selection, preparation of a sterile field, selection of appropriate equipment, actual needle placement, sample aspiration, therapeutic infusion, if appropriate, and, finally, blood origin confirmation (Table 9.2).

Table 9.1 Possible Indications for Cordocentesis

Fetal Karyotype—Late Gestation
Increased maternal age
Low maternal serum alphafetoprotein
Previous aneuploid fetus
Parental translocation
Sonographic dysmorphology

Blood Component
Coagulation factors
Hemoglobin composition
Platelets
Respiratory gases
IgM-specific antibody testing
Drug level

Isoimmunization
Fetal blood type and Rh status
Coombs antibody testing
Complete blood count
Transfusion of compatible donor blood

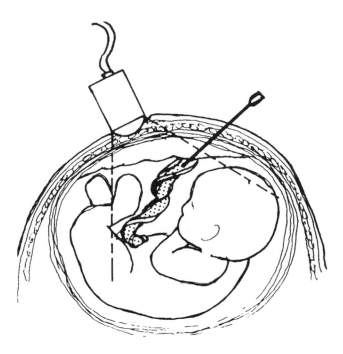

Figure 9.1   The potential needle track approaching the umbilical vein at its insertion on an anterior placenta.

Table 9.2   Fetal Blood Sampling Technique

Location
Clean, traffic-controlled room (funipuncture)
Operating room (intravascular transfusion)

Equipment
Linear or sector scanner
Amniocentesis tray
20- or 22-gauge needle (10–17 cm)

Procedure
Prescan
Sterile field
Rescan
Aspiration site selection
Local anesthesia to maternal skin
Insertion and guidance of needle to UV
Aspiration of blood
Testing of blood
   Modified Apt test
   Corpuscular volume analysis
   Kleihauer-Betke

Site Selection

Aspiration site selection begins with the preprocedure ultrasound examination to locate the placenta and umbilical cord insertion site. Possible aspiration sites include the cord insertion on an anterior or a posterior placenta (Figures 9.1 and 9.2), the cord at the fetal umbilicus (Figure 9.3), a free loop of cord, or the umbilical vein within the fetal liver (Figure 9.4). A cord insertion on an anterior placenta allows the needle to approach the umbilical vein without passing through the amniotic cavity. Such an approach decreases needle vulnerability to fetal movement but limits lateral mobility of the needle, requiring either a perfect initial entry angle or multiple attempts with multiple transplacental needle passes.

Crossing the amniotic cavity, although offering considerably more lateral needle mobility and reducing the need for perfect initial surface angle placement, makes the needle vulnerable to fetal movement and either displacement from the aspiration site or laceration of the umbilical vein, with severe consequences. Therefore, if such vulnerability to movement is present, the administration to the fetus of either an intramuscular or intravenous paralytic agent (curare or pancuronium) to temporarily prevent such movement is considered a necessary safety measure (18).

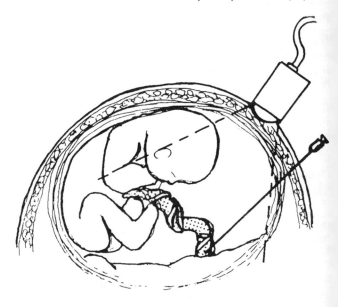

Figure 9.2   The needle track to the insertion on a posterior placenta.

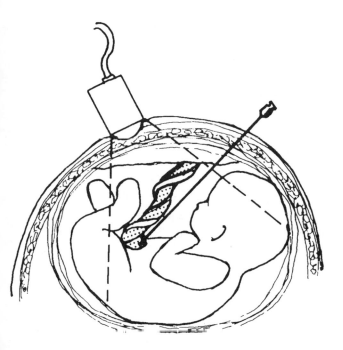

Figure 9.3 The aspiration needle might approach the umbilical vein at the umbilicus in this way.

Equipment Considerations

The Ultrasound Machine: A high-resolution ultrasound machine is necessary for the accurate guidance of a narrow-gauge needle to an umbilical vein that measures only 6–10 mm diameter and may be located 10–12 cm deep. The thickness of the sonographic slice (azimuthal plane) of tissue included in the on-screen image (Figure 9.5) is critical. If an ultrasound machine derives its image from a very thick slice of anatomy, both the needle and the vein could be seen simultaneously on screen but not be truly coplanar. A missed approach would therefore be more likely. This possibility underscores the need for good-quality imaging equipment.

The Needle: Narrow needles, including 20-, 22-, and 25-gauge have been used successfully by investigators performing fetal blood sampling (1, 3, 4, 10). Either a 10-cm or a 17-cm length needle may be used. The longer needle offers the advantage of a greater length extending beyond the skin surface for attachment and change of syringe (10).

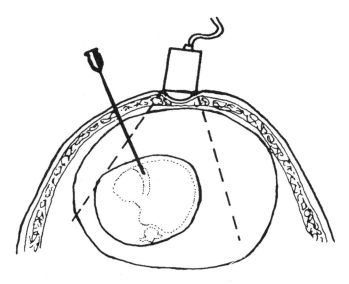

Figure 9.4 A possible aspiration needle approaching the umbilical vein within the fetal liver.

Aspiration Syringes: To facilitate fetal blood aspiration through a narrow-gauge needle, 1- or 2-cc syringes are recommended. The use of larger syringes makes aspiration difficult and increases the possibility of failure. The syringes may be easily rinsed with the anticoagulant of choice.

Needle Guide: The use of a needle guide is a matter of personal preference. A needle guide attachment to the ultrasound transducer may be helpful during a clinician's early experience. Many observers find, however, that such a device limits flexibility in needle manipulation and may increase the risk of a break in sterile technique, and therefore prefer a freehand technique (19, 20).

Amniocentesis Tray: A standard amniocentesis tray contains everything necessary for fetal blood sampling, although it is not sufficient to support a fetal blood transfusion. The only additional components that might be required for blood sampling would be a longer needle, if desired, the required number of anticoagulated 1-cc syringes, and a paralytic drug, if considered necessary.

Sampling Procedure

Sterile Field: A wide field of the maternal abdomen is

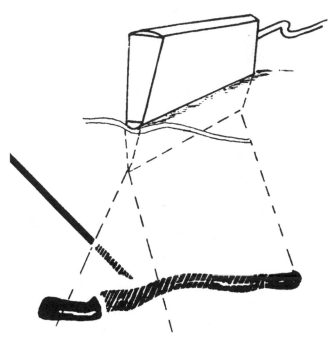

Figure 9.5 Three-dimensional view of the azimuthal plane of an ultrasound scan plane. Divergence of scan beam in this plane results in greater slice thickness at greater depths. The vein and the needle could both be on screen without being coplanar.

cleansed with antiseptic solution, and a sterile drape is placed. The ultrasound transducer is covered with a sterile glove or appropriate sterile cover.

Needle Placement: After final site selection, local anesthetic is infiltrated. The aspiration needle may be placed either in a transplanar or a coplanar (Figure 9.6) relationship to the scan plane. If the coplanar technique is chosen, the needle track will be seen as the needle advances from the skin surface in the plane of the ultrasound (Figure 9.7). The use of a needle guide, as noted above, is a personal choice.

Fetal Paralysis: If the needle path appears to require fetal paralysis, this may be accomplished either with intramuscular injection before final needle placement, or intravenous injection just after vein entry. Intravenous injection avoids the obligate need for two needle passes, but there is the slight risk of damage from fetal movement before paralysis is accomplished.

Aspiration: Fetal blood aspiration is easily accomplished using 1-cc syringes until the total volume required is obtained (Figure 9.8).

Analysis of Blood Origin: After a sample of blood is obtained, it may be necessary to confirm fetal origin. The risk of contamination with maternal blood exists anytime the aspiration site is near the chorionic plate. If the aspiration site is a free loop of cord, the cord at the umbilicus, or the umbilical vein within the fetal liver, laboratory confirmation of fetal origin should not be necessary.

Fetal origin may be established by biochemical means or by cell size analysis. A Kleihauer–Betke acid elution test will identify fetal red cells and, if mixed with maternal cells, can precisely measure the differential proportions. The test, however, takes several hours. An automatic cell size analyzer will display and print a histogram of cell volume as a function of cell count, as well as calculate the mean corpuscular volume for the sample (Figure 9.9). Since the mean corpuscular volume (MCV) of adult blood ranges from 78 to 98 µL, and the MCV of fetal blood varies from 118 to 135 µL, fetal origin may therefore be confirmed. Cell size analysis, however, is not sensitive to minor degrees of maternal red cell mixture.

The easiest and fastest method for confirming fetal origin is to perform a modified Apt test with a few drops of the blood (21). A test tube is filled with tap water. Six drops of 10% KOH are added, and then four drops of the blood sample in question. Fetal blood will produce and maintain a pink color over two minutes, while adult blood will instead change to a brown-green color. It is helpful to test a known adult control side by side. If there is any chance of partial contamination, a Kleihauer–Betke test is recommended.

Intravascular Transfusion

The administration of donor blood through the same needle used to aspirate a diagnostic sample is accomplished using a similar technique to that described above, but with important differences. It is recommended that intrauterine transfusions be done in an operating room. All technical preparations for the transfusion should be complete, including the complete filling of the tubing with donor blood

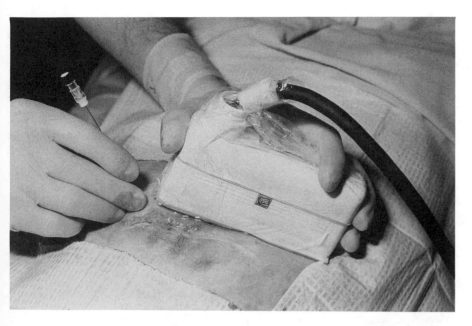

Figure 9.6(*A*) This operator is holding the aspiration needle in a coplanar relationship with the transducer. Note the sterile plastic cover on the transducer.

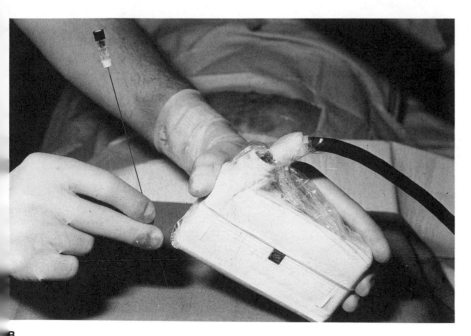

Figure 9.6(*B*) Here, during an aspiration, the operator is advancing the needle in a coplanar fashion. Note the sterile cover and the sterile field. Local anesthetic has already been infiltrated.

before needle placement. Skilled assistance is necessary, as the operator must maintain undivided attention to needle stability and ultrasound surveillance throughout the procedure.

Tightly packed, washed, irradiated, antigen-negative red cells are first passed through a microfilter to remove debris, then through a blood warmer to raise the blood to body temperature, and on to a three-way stopcock. A 3-cc

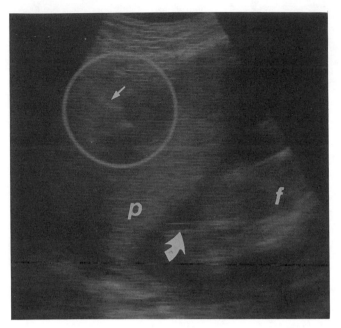

A

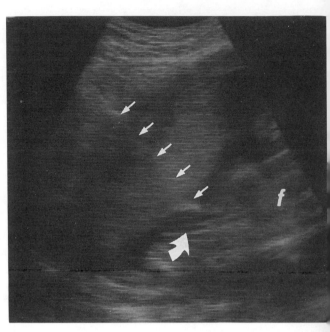

B

Figure 9.7(*A*) This sonogram shows the advancing aspiration needle. The small arrow indicates the needle within the circle. The large arrow indicates the umbilical cord near its insertion (p = placenta, f = fetus).

Figure 9.7(*B*) Here, the entire needle length is seen (small arrows) approaching the cord (large arrow).

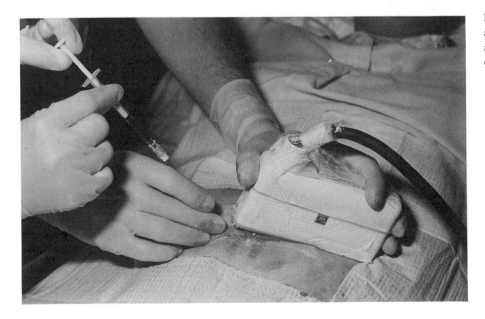

Figure 9.8   As the operator stabilizes the aspiration needle, an assistant attaches and aspirates fetal blood. The syringes may be easily attached and changed.

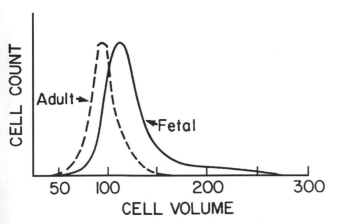

Figure 9.9   This histogram of red cell volume as a function of cell count illustrates the volume distribution of fetal blood compared to adult blood. Such an analysis may be used to differentiate fetal from maternal blood.

syringe is filled with donor blood at one of the outlets, and the third outlet feeds the blood to tubing to the operative needle. Such a system allows the smooth sequential injection of donor blood, with minimal disturbance of the operator or the needle.

The blood may be injected at a comfortable rate. On the ultrasound screen, with the initiation of injection, echogenic turbulance seen within the umbilical vein confirms proper needle placement. This turbulance may arise from tiny gas bubbles suspended in nonvacuum-deaerated blood, and their presence is useful confirmation of correct placement throughout the transfusion (22). If, during injection, these swirl patterns are lost, further injection should be temporarily delayed and needle placement evaluated. Improper placement or needle tip migration could result in blood being injected improperly and either maternal or fetal complications (23).

The volume of blood that may safely be injected at a single transfusion is not clearly established. Early reports limited the volume to a 20% fetal volume expansion, but greater volumes have been given safely (6, 10). Using funipuncture techniques, the fetal blood volume, including placenta, has been estimated to be 94 cc per kg (24). The estimated fetal blood volume and the initial hematocrit must be used to estimate the volume of donor blood required to raise the fetal hematocrit to between 35% and 40%.

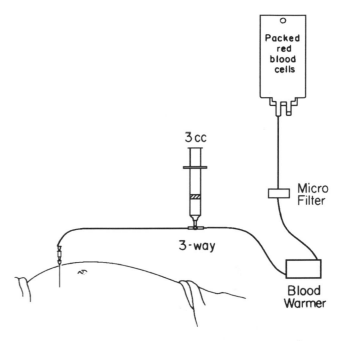

Figure 9.10   Schematic drawing of the blood tubing system well-suited to intrauterine intravascular transfusions. This system should be completely prepared prior to needle placement.

Training: PUBS

As simple as percutaneous umbilical blood sampling appears to be, the safe and successful application of this technique is possible only after considerable experience with sonographically guided invasive procedures. The need to maintain the advancing needle in the scan plane is a critical element of success. It is possible to practice this technique by routinely using ultrasound to guide the needle at the time of amniocentesis, but the ideal method for acquisition of this skill is to observe and perform such aspirations under the direction of someone skilled in the procedure. Alternative training methods have been described using water bath models, with simulated experience performing funipuncture on suspended umbilical cords obtained postpartum (25).

Safety and Utilization

Although since the report by Beng, many investigators have reported consistent success both with transfusion and blood sampling, the growing but limited number of reported procedure events allows only an estimate of safety and the rate of complications from percutaneous fetal blood sampling and intravenous transfusion (19, 26). The rate of procedure-related pregnancy loss associated with funipuncture appears to be at or near 1%. However, it is important to remember that reports to date originate from investigators with considerable experience with sonographically guided invasive procedures. It is therefore probable that the risk reported is lower than that to be expected from operators with less experience. Complications reported include amnionitis, transient and sustained fetal bradycardia, and fetal death (27–30).

The ability to directly evaluate fetal hemolysis and administer blood intravascularly using this technique is an important development. Early experience with intravascular transfusion, especially in cases of severe isoimmunization with hydrops, supports the method as a superior treatment when compared to intraperitoneal transfusion (31, 32). There appears to be a lower rate of procedure-related loss when compared to intraperitoneal transfusion and a higher rate of therapeutic success. As popular as this new technique has become, however, it is still a relatively new development, and the accumulation of experience with risks and benefits is ongoing.

References

1. Daffos F, Capella-Pavlovsky M, Forestier F. Fetal blood sampling via the umbilical cord using a needle guided by ultrasound. Prenatal Diagnosis 1983;3:271–7.
2. Hsieh F, Chang F, Ko T, Chen H. Percutaneous ultrasound guided fetal blood sampling in the management of non-immune hydrops fetalis. Am J Obstet Gynecol 1987; 157(1):44–9.
3. Hobbins JC, Grannum PA, Romero R, Reece EA, Mahoney MJ. Percutaneous umbilical blood sampling. Am J Obstet Gynecol 1985;152(1):1-6.
4. Daffos F, Capella-Pavlovsky M, Forestier F. Fetal blood sampling during pregnancy with use of a needle guided by ultrasound: a study of 606 consecutive cases. Am J Obstet Gynecol 1985;153(6):655–60.
5. Pastorek JG. Funipuncture: a rose by any other name. . . Obstet Gynecol 1988;71:646–7.
6. Rodeck CH, Nicolaides KH, Warsof SL, et al. The management of severe rhesus isoimmunization by fetoscopic intravascular transfusions. Am J Obstet Gynecol 1984;150(6): 769–74.
7. Valenti C. Antenatal detection of hemoglobinopathies: a preliminary report. Am J Obstet Gynecol 1973;115(5):851–3.
8. Beng J, Bock JE, Trolle D. Ultrasound guided fetal intravenous transfusion for severe rhesus haemolytic disease. Br Med J 1982;284:373.
9. Ch de Crespigny L, Robinson HP, Quinn M, et al. Ultrasound-guided fetal blood transfusion for severe rhesus isoimmunization. Obstet Gynecol 1985;66:529–32.
10. Seeds JW, Bowes WA. Ultrasound-guided fetal intravascular transfusion in severe rhesus immunization. Am J Obstet Gynecol 1986;154(5):1105–7.
11. Copel JA, Scioscia A, Grannum PA, et al. Percutaneous umbilical blood sampling in the management of Kell isoimmunization. Obstet Gynecol 1986;67:288–90.
12. Benacerraf BR, Barss VA, Saltzman DH, et al. Acute fetal distress associated with percutaneous umbilical blood sampling. Am J Obstet Gynecol 1987;156(5):1218–20.
13. Berkowitz RL, Chitkara U, Goldberg JD, et al. Intrauterine intravascular transfusions for severe red blood cell isoimmunization ultrasound-guided percutaneous approach. Am J Obstet Gynecol 1986;155(3):574–81.
14. Daffos F, Forestier F, Kaplan C, Cox W. Prenatal diagnosis and management of bleeding disorders with fetal blood sampling. Am J Obstet Gynecol 1988;158:939–46.
15. Moise KJ, Carpenter RJ, Cotton DB, et al. Percutaneous umbilical cord blood sampling in the evaluation of fetal platelet counts in pregnant patients with autoimmune thrombocytopenia purpura. Obstet Gynecol 1988;72:346–50.
16. Barss VA, Benacerraf BR, Frigoletto FD, et al. Management of isoimmunized pregnancy by use of intravascular techniques. Am J Obstet Gynecol 1988;159:932–7.
17. Reece EA, Copel JA, Scioscia AL, et al. Diagnostic fetal umbilical blood sampling in the management of isoimmunization. Am J Obstet Gynecol 1988;159:1057–62.
18. Seeds JW, Corke BC, Spielman FJ. Prevention of fetal movement during invasive procedures with pancuronium bromide. Am J Obstet Gynecol 1986;155(4):818–19.
19. Weiner CP. Cordocentesis for diagnostic indications: two year's experience. Obstet Gynecol 1987;70:664–7.
20. Ney JA, Fee SC, Dooley SL, et al. Factors influencing hemostasis after umbilical vein puncture in vitro. Am J Obstet Gynecol 1989;160:424–6.
21. Apt L, Downey WS. "Melena" neonatorum: the swallowed

blood syndrome. A simple test for the differentiation of adult and fetal hemoglobin in bloody stools. J Ped 1955; 47:6–12.

22. Seeds JW, Bowes WA, Chescheir NC. Echogenic venous turbulence is a critical feature of successful intravascular intrauterine transfusion. Obstet Gynecol 1989;73:488–9.

23. Seeds JW, Chescheir NC, Bowes WA, Owl-Smith FA. Fetal death as a complication of intrauterine intravascular transfusion. Obstet Gynecol 1989;74:461–3.

24. MacGregor SN, Socol ML, Pielet BW, et al. Prediction of fetoplacental blood volume in isoimmunized pregnancy. Am J Obstet Gynecol 1988;159:1493–7.

25. Angel JL, O'Brien WF, Michelson JA, et al. Instructional model for percutaneous fetal umbilical blood sampling. Obstet Gynecol 1989;73:669–71.

26. Bovicelli L, Orsini LF, Grannum PAT, et al. A new funipuncture technique: two-needle ultrasound and needle biopsy-guided procedure. Obstet Gynecol 1989;73:428–31.

27. Wilkins I, Mezrow G, Lynch L, et al. Amnionitis and life-threatening respiratory distress after percutaneous umbilical blood sampling. Am J Obstet Gynecol 1989;160:427–8.

28. Pielet BW, Socol ML, MacGregor SN, et al. Cordocentesis: an appraisal of risks. Am J Obstet Gynecol 1988; 159:1497–500.

29. Hogge WA, Thiagarajah S, Brenbridge AN, Harbert GM. Fetal evaluation by percutaneous blood sampling. Am J Obstet Gynecol 1988;158:132–6.

30. Foley MR, Sonek J, Paraskos J, et al. Development and initial experience with a manually controlled spring wire device ("cordostat") to aid in difficult funipuncture. Obstet Gynecol 1991;77:471–5.

31. Weiner CP, Weinstrom KD, Sipes SL, Williamson RA. Risk factors for cordocentesis and fetal intravascular transfusion. Am J Obstet Gynecol 1991;165:1020–5.

32. Weiner CR, Williamson RA, Wenstrom KD, et al. Management of fetal hemolytic disease by cordocentesis. II. Outcome of treatment. Am J Obstet Gynecol 1991;165:1302–7.

10

Ultrasonography

John T. Queenan, M.D.
Steven L. Warsof, M.D.

THE impact of diagnostic ultrasound in perinatal management has been monumental. Within the past two decades, we have seen two-dimensional real-time imaging move from the research laboratory into the clinician's office. Ultrasound has become an integral part of perinatal medicine. Included among its many uses are determining gestational age and presentation, detecting multiple gestations, establishing early fetal life by the detection of fetal heartbeat and movement, diagnosing fetal congenital abnormalities, locating the placenta, monitoring fetal growth and determining well-being by the biophysical profile, confirming fetal maturity, and enhancing parental bonding. New technical developments have been introduced rapidly. Transvaginal scanning has greatly improved our ability to zoom in on the first-trimester fetus and has greatly increased our ability to examine other pelvic structures. Doppler sonography has given the clinician a new way to study not only fetal growth but physiology as well.

Two-dimensional scanning was originally performed with static B-scanners. Gray-scale scan converters, developed in the early 1970s, enhanced the clarity of the output. Serial static scans in transverse and longitudinal axes were then done to obtain a composite image. This technique has been replaced by real-time technology.

Real-time ultrasound has been a major advance in perinatal medicine. Using gray-scale, linear-array, or sector imaging, continuous cross-sectional motion pictures of internal structures are produced. The scan takes a fraction of the time required with the static modality. Because of its versatility, real-time ultrasound has become the workhorse of perinatal medicine. Its portability allows the instrument to be brought to the patient, whether in the office or on the labor and delivery floor. Its ease of operation makes this diagnostic technique potentially available to all pregnant patients. With a large selection of transducers from linear, sector, curvilinear, or vaginal, and with a range of frequencies from 3.5 to 7.5 MHz, the operator can enhance the ability for visualization dramatically.

Real-time scanning is rapid and provides immediate feedback to both the obstetrician and the patient. Amniotic fluid provides an excellent interface to produce a good image. With digitalization of output and electronic focusing, the resolution is remarkably clear. Table 10.1 reviews

Table 10.1 Evolution of Diagnostic Ultrasound Technology

	1970	1980	1990
Technology	Primitive A & B mode scans	Early real-time	Modern real-time, gray scale
Picture Quality	Abstact art form, poor	Markedly improved	Excellent
Trained Person	Limited to perinatal centers	Most major medical centers	Widespread; most doctor's offices
Training	Self-taught	Some training programs	Part of most obstetrical and radiology residencies
Equipment Cost	Prototypes	Expensive	High-quality equipment at wide range of prices

the evolution of obstetrical sonography over the past 20 years.

Dating the Pregnancy

The single most important task of the obstetrician is the accurate establishment of gestational age and estimated date of confinement (EDC). Virtually all obstetrical problems and clinical judgments are based on this knowledge, yet prior to the use of ultrasound, pregnancy dating was frequently erroneous.

It is anticipated that 85% of patients will deliver within ±2 weeks of their expected date of confinement as derived by Nagele's rule from the last menstrual period (LMP). This system, however, may be greatly in error when patients provide an inadequate menstrual history, have amenorrhea or oligomenorrhea prior to conceiving, or conceive within a short interval after pregnancy, while lactating, or within two months of discontinuation of birth control pills. Our recent experience in a middle class population indicates that 45% of patients have questionable menstrual histories (Figure 10.1) (1). In indigent patients, unreliable menstrual his-

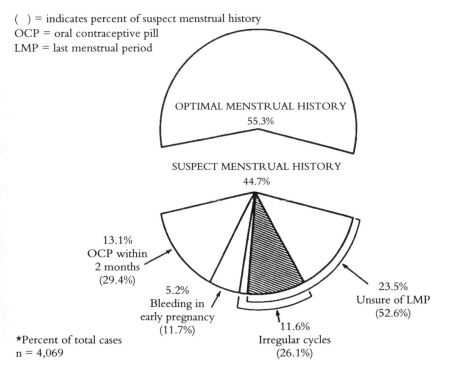

( ) = indicates percent of suspect menstrual history
OCP = oral contraceptive pill
LMP = last menstrual period

OPTIMAL MENSTRUAL HISTORY
55.3%

SUSPECT MENSTRUAL HISTORY
44.7%

13.1%
OCP within
2 months
(29.4%)

5.2%
Bleeding in
early pregnancy
(11.7%)

11.6%
Irregular cycles
(26.1%)

23.5%
Unsure of LMP
(52.6%)

*Percent of total cases
n = 4,069

Figure 10.1   Distribution of menstrual histories.*

Adapted with permission from Campbell S, Warsof S, Little D, Cooper DJ. Routine ultrasound screening for the prediction of gestational age. Obstet Gynecol 1985; 65:613.

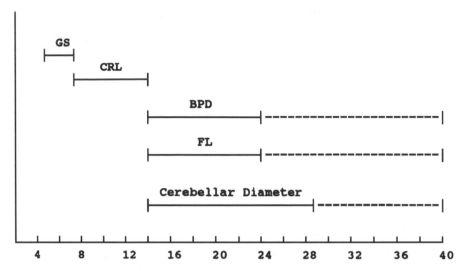

Figure 10.2 Appropriate methods of determining gestational age for various stages of pregnancy. GS = gestational sac diameter; CRL = crown-rump length; BPD = biparietal diameter; FL= femur length.

tories occur in 90%-100% of gravidas. In patients with questionable histories, as well as those with high-risk factors, or for those requiring elective deliveries either by induction or cesarean section, ultrasound scanning should be performed at the most optimal time for dating, which is prior to the twentieth week of gestation.

A number of ultrasound measurements can be used to determine gestational age: gestational sac diameter, crown-rump length (CRL), biparietal diameter (BPD), femur length (FL), and cerebellar diameters (Figure 10.2). Other fetal parameters have been used for dating gestations, but have been found to be less accurate.

The gestational sac diameter correlates well with the gestational age in patients between five and eight weeks' gestation (see Figures 10.3, 10.4) (2). After that date, the gestational sac may no longer be round so that the measurements are no longer valid. Furthermore, this technique is limited as it gives no information on the viability and number or morphology of the fetus.

The crown-rump length correlates excellently with

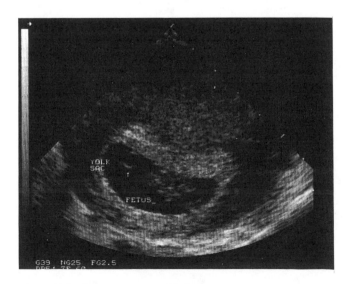

Figure 10.3 Pregnant uterus with fetus.

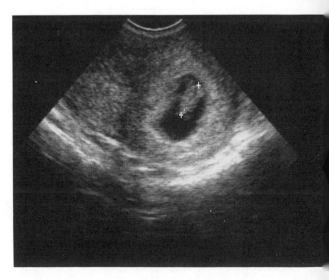

Figure 10.4 Early pregnancy with fetus and yolk sac.

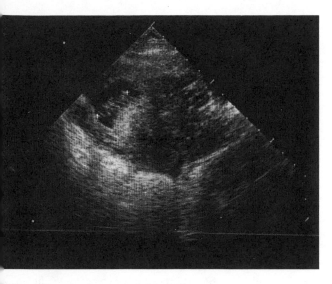

Figure 10.5   Crown-rump determination.

he gestational age from eight to 14 weeks (Figure 10.5)
3) After that date, it is difficult to get a good crown-rump
measurement, as the fetus becomes increasingly mobile in a
arge fluid-filled amniotic cavity. Fetal flexion and exten-
ion can also cause erroneous measurements. This tech-

Table 10.2   BPD versus Weeks' Gestation

Week	BPD Composite Mean (cm)	Week	BPD Composite Mean (cm)
14	2.8	28	7.2
15	3.2	29	7.5
16	3.6	30	7.8
17	3.9	31	8.0
18	4.2	32	8.2
19	4.5	33	8.5
20	4.8	34	8.7
21	5.1	35	8.8
22	5.4	36	9.0
23	5.8	37	9.2
24	6.1	38	9.3
25	6.4	39	9.4
26	6.7	40	9.5
27	7.0		

Based on table presented in Sabbagha RE, Hughey M. ACOG Technical
Bulletin No. 63, October 1981. Diagnostic ultrasound in obstetrics and
gynecology.

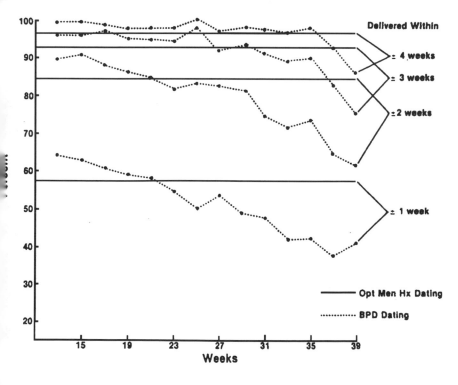

Figure 10.6   Comparison of ultrasonic
and clinical estimated dates of confinement
and percent of patients delivering within
one, two, three, and four weeks from prediction. Note that BPD dating is more
accurate in predicting EDC than optimal
menstrual histories prior to 20 weeks, with
its accuracy falling throughout gestation.

Reproduced with permission from
Goldkrand JW, Benjamin DS, Canton
DM. Role of ultrasound in obstetric man-
agement. J Clin Ultrasound 1986;14:589.

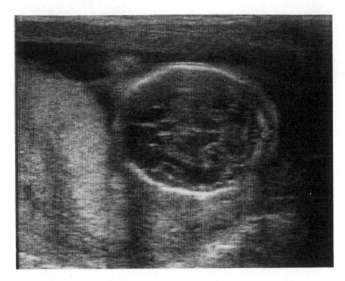

Figure 10.7   Orientation of fetal head for biparietal and head circumference measurements.

nique is suboptimal in this time period, as the fetus is too small to review fetal anatomy.

The BPD can be measured accurately from 14 weeks onward in gestation. But, since maximum growth occurs early in gestation, the BPD corresponds best to gestational age from 15 to 24 weeks, during which time it is accurate (±10 days). A single BPD measurement obtained late in pregnancy, e.g., 30 weeks, is not a very accurate indicator (±3 weeks) of gestational age (Table 10.2). It has been our experience that ultrasound dating prior to 24 weeks' gestation has virtually eliminated the problem of iatrogenic prematurity at the time of planned delivery and has reduced the confusion from false-positive studies for possible growth retardation. The falling accuracy of BPD measurements for the determination of gestational age throughout pregnancy can be seen in Figure 10.6.

The BPD is the most commonly used method for dating gestations. The image of the fetal skull should be elliptical with the midline structures, including the thalami and septum pellucidum cavum, visualized (Figure 10.7). The edges of the skull should be a crisp image. The most commonly used measuring technique determines the distance from the outer edge of the anterior skull table to the inner edge of the posterior skull echo. This is the so-called "leading edge" or "outer-to-inner" technique. There are other

acceptable techniques, so one must be careful to use the identical technique employed in the determination of the BPD growth curves.

Later in pregnancy, the BPD determination becomes more difficult due to molding and descent of the fetal head deep into the pelvis. In addition, positions such as occiput anterior and posterior make it difficult to obtain accurate BPDs. These unfavorable positions increase later in pregnancy. These factors, as well as the increasing biological variation, make gestational age determinations less accurate (±3 weeks) in the third trimester. The clinician must remember that a single determination of the BPD indicating a 38-week gestation could actually be obtained on a 35-week-old fetus. Obviously, delivery of such a fetus could cause problems due to prematurity. When a BPD is unobtainable due to a persistent occiput posterior position, it may be helpful to perform alternative measurements, such as the femur length, cerebellar diameters (4), or orbital diameters (5), to date the pregnancy. Additionally, fetal head circumference may be a more accurate indicator as pregnancy progresses to avoid error due to dolichocephaly or brachycephaly. Dating pregnancies in the third trimester is hazardous because of the diminished accuracy of the third-trimester scan and increasing biological variability.

The femur length has also been shown to be a very accurate parameter for gestational dating (Figures 10.8, 10.9) (6). Like the BPD, the predictive accuracy of the FL is greatest in the first half of gestation. Uniform growth is, however, better maintained in the FL as it is not affected by molding. FL has become an arbiter when BPD and menstrual dating are at odds, and it is our impression that it is a more accurate predictor of gestational age than the BPD in the last trimester. Growth curves have also been determined for other fetal long bones (Figure 10.10). These may be of some assistance when the femur is unobtainable or when skeletal dysplasia is suspected.

The cerebellar diameter measurement has been recently introduced as a fetal dating parameter (4). Similar to the BPD and FL, it is most accurate in the second trimester with unproven accuracy in the third trimester. This measurement has a practical advantage as its measurements in millimeters directly correspond with weeks of gestation, thus diminishing the need for growth tables. The cerebe-

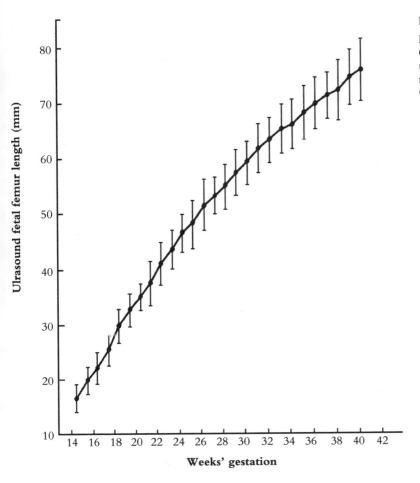

Figure 10.8   Femur length growth curve.

Reproduced with permission from O'Brien GD, Queenan JT. Growth of the ultrasound fetal femur length during normal pregnancy. Part I. Am J Obstet Gynecol 1981;141:833.

lum is easily found by rotating the transducer slightly into the posterior fossa from the typical BPD view (Figure 10.11).

Studies have shown that, in patients with questionable menstrual histories, as many as two-thirds had their dates adjusted by two weeks or more by early second-trimester scans. Even in patients with optimal histories, 5% have their dates adjusted by two weeks or more (7).

Determining Fetal Presentation

Although presentation is determined absolutely at delivery, during the prenatal course, it is not always known for certain. Textbooks contain information concerning the frequency of abnormal presentation at various weeks of gestation. Because these data were obtained by abdominal palpation or from pre-

mature deliveries, they are not necessarily accurate. Ultrasound studies on our normal patients indicate that the incidence of changes in fetal presentation is significant. Figure 10.12 shows that the incidence of abnormal lies is between 17 and 42 weeks. The peak incidence of abnormal lies is 34% at 24 weeks. It decreases to approximately 22% at 28 weeks and 4% at term. Similar information for presentation in twin deliveries are seen in Figure 10.13. Vertex-vertex becomes the most common presentation after 20 weeks. This, along with vertex-breech and vertex-transverse, make up over 80% of presentations in twins after 20 weeks (8). Prior to the performance of a cesarean section for a suspected abnormal presentation, the abnormal lie should be confirmed by ultrasound, and the possibility of a major fetal, placental, or uterine anomaly should be evaluated as the cause of the abnormal presentation.

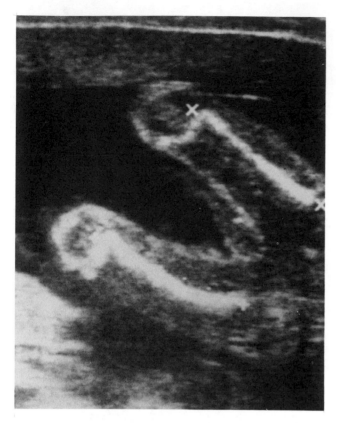

Figure 10.9 Fetal femur bone length measure.

Multiple Gestations

Obstetricians have long sought techniques to diagnose multiple gestations. Prior to ultrasound scanning, as many as 58% of cases of multiple gestations were undetected until the onset of labor, and, in 31%, the diagnosis was not made until after delivery of the first baby (9). The detection of multiple gestations is important, for, although its incidence is approximately 1%, twins comprise 10%–15% of all perinatal mortalities. This morbidity and mortality can be caused by premature births, intrauterine growth retardation, an increased incidence of congenital anomalies, placental problems, preeclampsia, and malpresentation. Early detection of multiple gestation should decrease these complications by closer antenatal surveillance, intensive intrapartum management, and the liberal use of cesarean deliveries. Ultrasonography has had a dramatic effect on this problem.

Twin gestations can be determined quickly and easily at any time after 10 weeks' gestation by meticulously performed scanning. When twins are seen, care should be taken to assure that three or more fetuses are not present. Prior to 10 weeks, it is more common to miss multiple gestations. Scanning prior to seven weeks' gestation may reveal two gestational sacs. Occasionally, at follow-up scans, only a single fetus is noted, and it is concluded that one of the sacs was blighted. The frequency of this occurrence is much higher than previously expected.

In a recently published randomized prospective study utilizing routine scanning (10), all sets of twins were diagnosed at the first scan, prior to 20 weeks. In the selectively scanned group, only 35% were diagnosed before 20 weeks, and 20% were not diagnosed until after 32 weeks. In a second study, using selective scanning (11), 8% of twins were not diagnosed until delivery. There was a significantly lower incidence of low-birthweight infants (22% versus 49%) and prematurity (25% versus 43%) in the routinely scanned group. The incidence of unfavorable perinatal outcome, as defined by stillbirth, depressed Apgar score, low birthweight, small for gestational age, or prematurity under 37 weeks, was 71% in the selectively scanned population and only 25% in the routinely scanned one. These improved results were due to the early diagnosis allowing for a better management of the pregnancy. Similar results have been shown in other studies.

With ultrasound, it is also possible to detect monoamniotic twins and discordant fetal growth. These are extremely high-risk situations which require the closest of obstetrical surveillance to avoid untoward outcomes.

Abnormalities of Early Pregnancy

Abnormalities of early gestation, such as missed abortions, blighted ova, ectopic gestations, or hydatidiform moles, affect as many as one-third of all conceptions.

Most early pregnancy abnormalities are suspected by first-trimester bleeding or a lack of fundal growth. If the pregnancy is progressing normally, a well-formed sac should be seen after 5 1/2 weeks of gestation, embryonic echoes by 7 weeks, and fetal heartbeat and fetal movements can be detected by ultrasound by the eighth week of gestation.

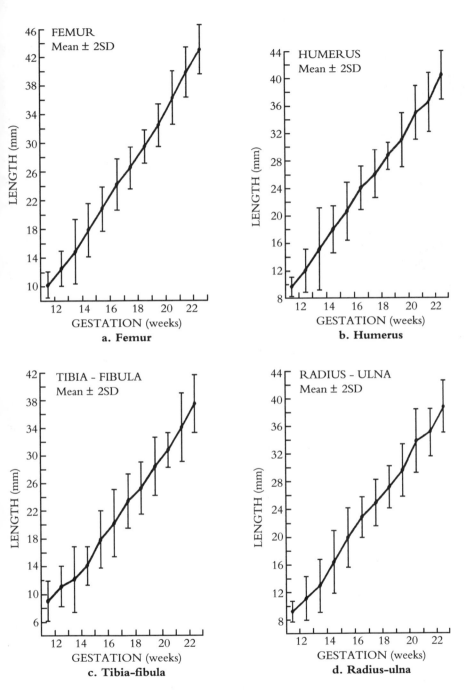

Figure 10.10   Long bone growth curves.

Reproduced with permission from Queenan JT, O'Brien GD, Campbell S. Ultrasound measurement of fetal limb bones. Am J Obstet Gynecol 1980; 138:297.

These findings can be seen 1-2 weeks earlier with vaginal scanning. Lack of these findings, however, is frequently not diagnostic and may require a follow-up scan in one to two weeks to establish exactly how the pregnancy is progressing.

Serial scans in the first trimester are important to evaluate fetal development and to exclude a missed abortion.

A molar gestation is easily diagnosed, as the uterus will be completely filled with high-density echoes rather than

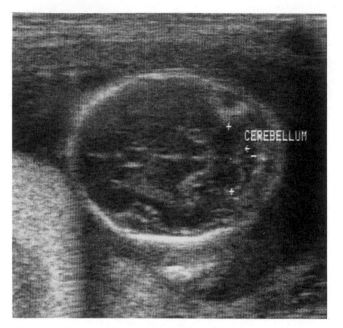

Figure 10.11   Technique for measuring cerebellum.

the expected fetus and amniotic fluid. Ectopic gestations frequently cannot be definitely diagnosed by ultrasound, but the presence of a normal intrauterine pregnancy essentially excludes an ectopic gestation. The incidence of pregnancies occurring spontaneously in both the uterus and the tube is 1:20,000. This may be greater with ovulation induction. With vaginal scanning, intact ectopic pregnancies can occasionally be seen in the tubes. Early detection and removal of the pregnancy has been shown to be the best technique to preserve fertility.

Although ultrasonic evaluation cannot detect an incompetent cervix, cervical dilatation and length can be measured by scans. When cervical cerclage is anticipated, ultrasound plays an important role by precise dating of the pregnancy and assuring the fetal viability prior to suture placement. Following cerclage placement, serial ultrasonic evaluation of the cerclage, cervix and fetus, would replace the necessity for repeated internal pelvic examinations.

Detecting Congenital Malformations

Congenital fetal anomalies are one of the leading causes of perinatal morbidity and mortality. Major anomalies occur in approximately 5% of liveborn infants. Early detection of these anomalies would permit formulation of short- and

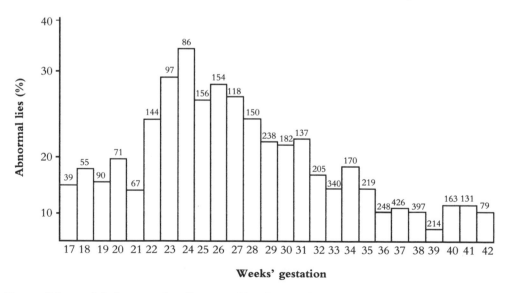

Figure 10.12   Incidence of abnormal fetal presentation (determined by ultrasound).

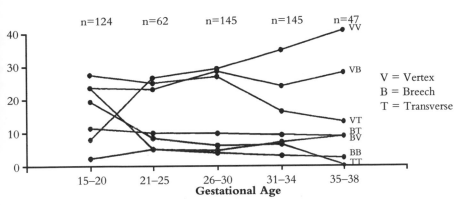

Figure 10.13 Incidence of various presentations throughout pregnancy in twin pregnancies.

V = Vertex
B = Breech
T = Transverse

long-term prognoses and recurrence risks, with better parental counseling. The optimal mode, time, and location of the delivery can be determined, and decisions regarding expectant management, in utero intervention, or pregnancy termination can be made. Although certain patients are known to be at risk for congenital anomalies (Table 10.3), recurrence is usually low. Furthermore, 90% of congenital abnormalities occur in pregnancies with no identifiable risk factors.

In order to detect fetal anomalies by ultrasound, every scan should be done in a thorough systematic fashion, with a morphologic evaluation of all the major fetal organ systems. In many areas, this type of scan is reserved for only a few high-risk patients. This type of thorough detailed scan must be done for all patients. Failure to scan in this way will lead to many missed diagnoses.

Congenital anomalies should be suspected in cases with oligo- or polyhydramnios. Oligohydramnios should alert the clinician to the possibility of renal anomalies such as polycystic kidney disease (PCKD), renal agenesis (Potter syndrome), or obstructive uropathies such as found with the posterior urethral valve syndrome. The kidneys will appear as large solid masses in PCKD, while, in Potter syndrome, the kidneys are absent. In both instances, the bladder will not be visualized, and there will be oligohydramnios in the second trimester. With posterior urethral valve syndrome, the bladder and ureters will be markedly dilated.

Polyhydramnios is commonly associated with neurologic or gastrointestinal malformations. Some of these, such as anencephaly and hydrocephaly, are easily detectable. Gastroschisis and omphalocele are diagnosed by a protrusion of the fetal viscera from the anterior abdominal wall. Gastrointestinal (GI) obstructions are noted by single or multiple loops of fluid-filled dilated bowel. Refinements in ultrasound have virtually eliminated the need for amniography and fetoscopy.

Table 10.4 lists the various fetal anomalies that have been detected by ultrasound over a four-year period at the Eastern Virginia Medical School. It should be noted that fetal anomalies tend to cluster. Identification of a single anomaly should intensify an evaluation for others. In addition, fetuses with a structural anomaly are also at risk for a chromosomal anomaly. Therefore, prenatal karyotyping should be offered to all mothers of fetuses with a major anomaly.

Ultrasound for Evaluation of MSAFP

In the last five years, maternal serum alpha-fetoprotein (MSAFP) screening has been introduced into obstetrical care in the United States. It has proved to be a useful tool to help detect open neural tube and ventral wall defects and

---

Table 10.3 High-Risk Factors for Congenital Fetal Anomalies

Oligohydramnios or polyhydramnios
Family history of congenital anomalies
Abnormal MSAFP
Multiple gestation
Maternal diabetes mellitus
Medication or drug exposure
Inadvertent exposure to diagnostic or therapeutic radiation
Documented maternal viral infection early in gestation

Table 10.4 Congenital Anomalies Detected at Eastern Virginia Medical School, July 1, 1985–June 30, 1989

Central Nervous System	**101**
Neural tube	
Spina bifida	28
Encephalocele	8
Anencephaly	23
Hydrocephaly	
Hydranencephaly	23
Holoprosencephaly	4
Others	15
Cardiac	**47**
Hypoplastic ventricle	6
ASD or VSD	15
Arrhythmia	19
Ectopia Cordis	2
Others	5
Gastrointestinal	**49**
Ventral wall defect	30
Omphalocele	21
Gastroschisis	9
Obstruction (T–E fistula,	
duodenal atresia etc.)	13
Diaphragmatic hernia	5
Others	1
Renal	**98**
Renal agenesis	
Unilateral	5
Bilateral	2
Multicystic kidney	
Unilateral	14
Bilateral	2
Polycystic dysplasia	2
Obstruction-hydronephrosis	43
Megacystis	4
Miscellaneous	**88**
Skeleton	18
Nonimmune hydrops	19
Abdominal mass	7
Cystic hygroma	23
Cleft lip	7
Conjoint twins (sets)	2
Cloacal extrophy	9
Amniotic band (and defects)	3

ASD = atrial septal defect; VSD = ventricular septal defect.

chromosomal aneuploidies. Unexplained high levels may also predict high perinatal morbidity in the third trimester.

The American College of Obstetrics and Gynecology (ACOG) recommends that MSAFP screening be offered to all obstetrical patients (Figure 10.14) (12). Since normal values for MSAFP vary with gestational age, the most accurate knowledge of the gestational age is necessary to best interpret the MSAFP value. This can best be done with simultaneous ultrasound examinations for determining the gestational age. The high incidence of false positives and false negatives that are seen with this screening technique can be virtually eliminated when scans are performed in conjunction with the MSAFP. Thorough scanning in conjunction with MSAFP testing will also detect most major neural tube and ventral wall defects. Furthermore, the scan can detect multiple gestations, other fetal anomalies, and fetal death, all of which can cause an abnormal MSAFP. A tentative MSAFP screening protocol is seen in Figure 10.15.

Adjunct to Amniocentesis and Other Procedures

Amniocentesis has become a widely available clinical tool for prenatal diagnosis of chromosomal and biochemical disorders. To assure the safety of this procedure, ultrasound is a necessary adjunct (see Chapter 8).

Early Amniocentesis

Amniocentesis for genetic diagnosis is usually performed between 15 and 18 weeks' gestation, but at times can be performed as early as 12 weeks' or as late as 24 weeks' gestation. Ultrasound scanning is essential to rule out multiple gestations, confirm fetal life and gestational age, and determine the location of the placenta, which occupies a larger portion of the uterine cavity at this stage than it does later.

Real-time imaging gives clinicians a visual guide to pockets of amniotic fluid. By inserting a finger between the transducer and the maternal skin surface, the clinician can determine the exact site and depth to insert the needle. Although many clinicians remove the scanner at the time of the actual procedure, it is preferable to maintain the scanner

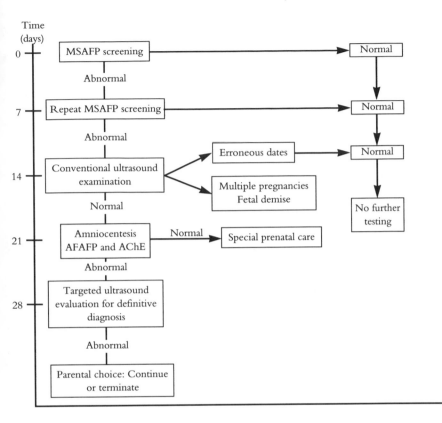

Figure 10.14 The American College of Obstetrics and Gynecology protocol for maternal serum α–fetoprotein (MSAFP) screening. AFAFP = amniotic fluid α–fetoprotein; AChE = acetylcholinestrase. Note: 1) On average, there are more than 28 days from initial MSAFP to definitive diagnosis; 2) no back-up testing for false negatives.

on the field throughout the procedure so that the needle can be followed during the entire procedure. Fetal positioning can change rapidly in utero, so, in this way, the operator can continually guide the needle to the best fluid pocket and avoid inadvertent puncture of important fetal or maternal structures.

If the placenta is anterior and the operator is unable to find a placenta-free area, the needle may have to be inserted through the placenta. In such instances, ultrasound scanning is important to locate the cord insertion on the chorionic plate. This area must be avoided during amniocentesis because of the large number of fetal blood vessels radiating from the cord insertion. Using ultrasound guidance for amniocentesis decreases the number of fetomaternal hemorrhages and bloody taps resulting from pierced placentas. Even when it is impossible to avoid the placenta, the real-time display makes the procedure safer and more efficient

by showing the exact location of the placenta and the location of the amniotic fluid pockets.

Late Amniocentesis

For Rh disease and fetal maturity determinations, amniocentesis is performed between 18 weeks' gestation and term. Sonography is essential to avoid the placenta and the fetus and to locate areas that contain amniotic fluid. Two recently introduced clinical techniques require close ultrasound guidance.

Chorionic Villus Sampling (CVS)

CVS can be performed either transabdominally or transcervically, usually from 8–12 weeks. In both cases, ultrasound is mandatory to guide the CVS catheter or needle to its precise location in the placental substance. In this fashion, a fetal karyotype can be obtained in the first trimester.

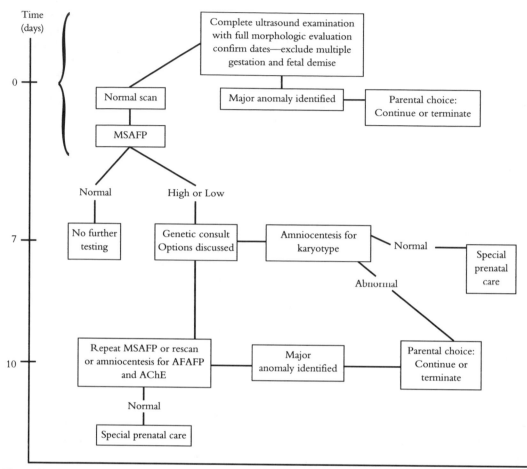

Figure 10.15   Eastern Virginia Medical School's protocol for MSAFP testing. Note how 1) false negatives are very low as all patients have ultrasonic confirmation of dates, 2) most major anomalies are identified at first ultrasound visit, 3) evaluation time is compressed from 20 to 10 days, and 4) there is rare need for repeat MSAFP testing.

Percutaneous Umbilical Blood Sampling (PUBS)

PUBS also requires continuous real-time ultrasound guidance. With ultrasound, the needle can be directed at the placental insertion of the umbilical cord, and a pure fetal blood sample can be obtained for chromosomal, genetic, biochemical, hematologic, or acid-base evaluation. Direct intravascular fetal blood transfusions can also be performed in cases of severe fetal anemia.

Placentography

The implantation of any part of the placenta in the lower uterine segment is not only dangerous to the patient, but also medically expensive. Ultrasound can detect or rule out this complication. Often, in early pregnancy, the placenta is close to or covers the cervix, but, as pregnancy advances, the placenta moves a significant distance from the cervical os. The reason for this apparent "migrating placenta" is that the uterus is some 40 times larger at term than in its nonpregnant state. With this uterine growth, the placenta is carried upward on the uterine wall away from the os. As the lower uterine segment develops, the distance of the placenta from the os increases still further.

If a low-lying placenta is noted in an early scan, the patient is made aware of the potential problem, but no further diagnostic or therapeutic precautions are undertaken unless bleeding is noted. If a complete previa, which has little chance of "migrating," is noted, then the patient is placed on pelvic rest with full explanation of the problem. Confirmation of the diagnosis of placenta previa must be made prior to an operative delivery.

It has been recently recognized that, throughout gestation, the placenta undergoes ultrasonically detectable maturational changes. These changes have been well described by Grannum et al (13). Cases of premature placental maturity require close antenatal surveillance. Unfortunately, this technique cannot be used reliably for determination of fetal pulmonary maturity (14).

Determination of Fetal Sex

Starting at approximately 16 to 18 weeks, the fetal sex may be determined by scanning the perineal region (15). The diagnosis of a male is made by visualizing the scrotum and penis (Figure 10.16). Formerly, the diagnosis of a female infant was made by nonvisualization of these organs. This can sometimes be misleading. The diagnosis of the female sex should be made by visualization of the labia and introitus (Figure 10.17). Sex determination can be clinically important in many X-linked genetic conditions. Sex determination should never be used for selective pregnancy termination.

Assessing Fetal Growth and Development

The clinical evaluation of fetal growth and well-being by either symphysis-fundal height measurement, clinical estimation of fetal weight, or maternal weight gain is fraught with inaccuracy. Fifty percent of cases of intrauterine growth retardation (IUGR) are not suspected on the basis of clinical evaluation until delivery (16). The major reason for this is miscalculation of gestational age by clinical techniques. The key to the diagnosis of IUGR or macrosomia is the accurate knowledge of gestational age. This can best

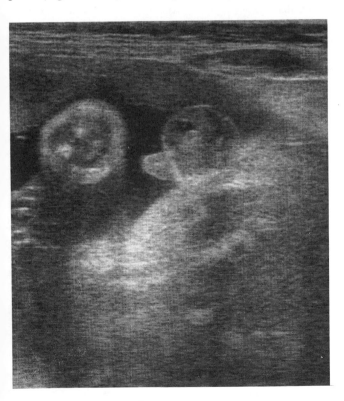

Figure 10.16   Male genitalia.

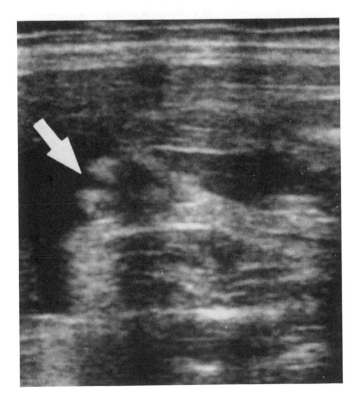

Figure 10.17   Female genitalia. The arrow points to the labia.

be determined by ultrasound evaluation in the early second trimester.

Ultrasound with direct measurement of the fetus plays an essential role in monitoring normal and abnormal fetal growth. Abnormal fetal growth can best be documented by a combination of measurements of fetal parameters. Although no single measurement is fully reliable, fetal weight seems to correlate best with fetal abdominal circumference (AC) (Figure 10.18). Although this is true, to estimate fetal weight accurately, a combination of BPD and AC measurements are most predictive (17). Many obstetricians prefer working with a single, familiar fetal parameter, weight, rather than with unfamiliar parameters such as AC or BPD. With accurate knowledge of both fetal weight and gestational age, fetal growth can be plotted on standard growth curves. If gestational age is questionable, then serial scans may be needed in 2 to 3 weeks to document interval fetal growth. If this interval growth is adequate, the problem may

be only in dating. If, however, interval growth is poor and the picture is complicated by oligohydramnios, then one can be confident with the diagnosis of IUGR. For a more thorough discussion, the reader is referred to Chapter 47.

Evaluation of Fetal Condition

Presently, there are many tests of fetal well-being. The most reliable are biophysical in nature. The oldest parameter is maternal perception of fetal activity. The mother is simply asked to monitor fetal movements. This is commonly referred to as kick counts. Other biophysical tests available are the nonstress test (NST), oxytocin challenge test (OCT), and the now more commonly used biophysical profile (BPP). Many advocate the BPP as the most reliable technique to monitor fetal well being (18). This is a combination of a NST with a thorough ultrasonic evaluation, including observation of fetal breathing and body movements, amniotic fluid volume, and fetal tone (Table 10.5). There have been several adaptions to this biophysical profile. One of the most predictive includes the amniotic fluid index (AFI) by which, instead of measuring a single pocket of fluid, the amniotic fluid is assessed in all four quadrants of the uterus (19). This score is then included in the BPP.

Doppler Ultrasound

Recently, Doppler evaluation of the flow velocity wave profile has been used to evaluate fetal well-being (Figure 10.19). Using simple ratios of peak systolic to diastolic (S/D) flow, fetal well-being can be assessed. Flow is determined both by pressure and "downsteam resistance." In the case of the umbilical artery, the downstream resistance is the placenta. This should be a low-resistance system, thus promoting large volumes of forward flow in both systole and diastole, leading to gas and metabolic exchange. In abnormal situations, the placenta has increased resistance, as evidenced by decreasing diastolic flow leading to an increased S/D ratio. In the worst scenario, there is either absent or reverse diastolic flow (20). It is generally recommended that a fetus in this situation needs to be delivered or assessed very closely. The precise clinical role of Doppler sonography remains to be determined.

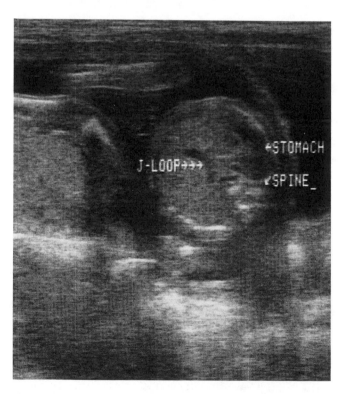

Figure 10.18   Proper orientation of fetal abdomen for measuring abdominal circumference.

Table 10.5 Fetal Biophysical Profile Score

Variable	Score 2	Score 0
Fetal breating movements (FBM)	The presence of at least 30 seconds of sustained FBM in 30 minutes of observation	Less than 30 seconds of FBM in 30 minutes
Fetal movements	Three or more gross body movements in 30 minutes of observation (simultaneous limb and trunk movements are counted as a single movement)	Two or fewer gross body movements in 30 minutes of observation
Fetal tone	At least one episode of motion of a limb from a position of flexion to extension and a rapid return to flexion	Fetus in a position of simi- or full-limb extension with no return to flexion with movement (absence of fetal movement is counted as absent tone)
Fetal reactivity	The presence of two or more fetal heart rate accelerations of at least 15 bpm and lasting at least 15 seconds, and associated with fetal movement in 40 minutes	No acceleration or fewer than two accelerations of the fetal heart rate in 40 minutes of observation
Qualitative amniotic fluid volume	A pocket of amniotic fluid that measures at least 1 cm in two perpendicular planes	Largest pocket of amniotic fluid measures 1 cm in two perpendicular planes
Maximal score	10	—
Minimal score	—	0
Score		

       8–10: Reassuring
       4–6: Repeat
       0–2: Deliver

Reproduced with permission from Manning FA, Basket TF, Morrison I, et al. Fetal biophysical profile scoring: a prospective study on 1184 high-risk patients. Am J Obstet Gynecol 1982;142:47.

Evaluation of Amniotic Fluid

The amniotic fluid (AF) in the gestational sac is the first visualized aspect of a pregnancy. Normally, AF volume increases until 32 to 35 weeks' gestation and then slowly falls toward term and after the EDC is passed. Although difficult to quantitate, the appearance of oligohydramnios should alert the sonographer to the possibility of growth retardation or a fetal malformation of the urinary tract. The amniotic fluid index is a useful technique to evaluate AF volume. Excessive AF, polyhydramnios, although frequently idiopathic, has at least a 20% fetal abnormality rate. In this case, the malformations are usually GI or central nervous system (CNS) in origin.

Parental Bonding

Another positive aspect of ultrasound scanning that is often overlooked is the tremendous emotional impact and psychological lift that the parents obtain upon visualizing their fetus (Figures 10.20, 10.21). For most women, the first half of pregnancy is fraught with malaise, fatigue, and nausea. Ambivalence about the pregnancy may be high, and compliance with obstetrical care poor. For the parents, ultrasonic visualization of the fetus, fetal movement, and fetal heart activity may start the process of maternal bonding prior to delivery and encourage compliance to rest and restriction of alcohol, tobacco, or drug consumption (21).

Safety

A frequently asked question is whether ultrasound has been proven to be safe in pregnancy. Ultrasound must be differentiated from x-ray or radioisotope studies which are known to have potentially harmful effects in pregnancy. The latter requires the transfer of ionizing energy to create

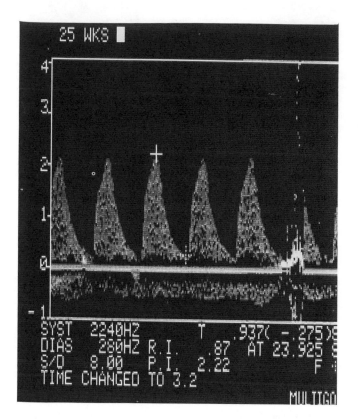 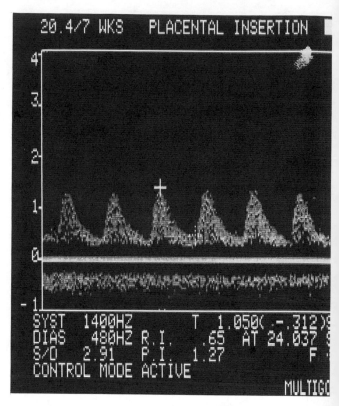

Figure 10.19 Examples of Doppler measurement of fetal blood flow.

images, while ultrasound imaging relies solely on mechanical energy. Because of its widespread use in pregnancy, no other diagnostic technique has been as thoroughly tested or scrutinized prior to its use on humans. Ultrasound has been tested in vivo and in vitro. The effects on animals, organs, tissues, cells, and subcellular particles have been investigated. Even the ultrasonic effect on chromosomes, genes, and DNA has been tested for structural changes and breaks in the genetic material.

Although there have been scattered reports of an ultrasonic effect at greater intensities and frequencies than used in diagnostic ultrasound, none of these reports are reproducible or have been independently verified. Although the effect of ultrasound on multiple generations of animals has been tested, the effect on subsequent generations in humans remains to be determined. The effect on future generations or in ways still untested remains open, and, for this reason, the prudent physician should not "guarantee" the safety of ultrasound.

Despite over 25 years of clinical use and numerous epidemiologic studies, no reproducible biological hazard in a mammalian system has ever been attributed to ultrasonic imaging at the intensities and frequencies employed in obstetrical diagnostic equipment. The American Institute of Ultrasound in Medicine Bio-Effects Committee stated in 1984 that "in the low megahertz frequency range there have been (as of this date) no independently confirmed significant biological effects in mammalian tissues exposed to intensities (SPTA) below 100 mW/cm^2. Furthermore, such effects have not been demonstrated even at higher intensities when the product of intensity and exposure time is less than 50 joules/cm" (21, 22). These conclusions were endorsed by the European Federation for Ultrasound in Medicine and Biology and the British Medical Ultrasound Society Report on the Safety of Diagnostic Ultrasound (23). To some, however, the lack of finding a hazard is dis-

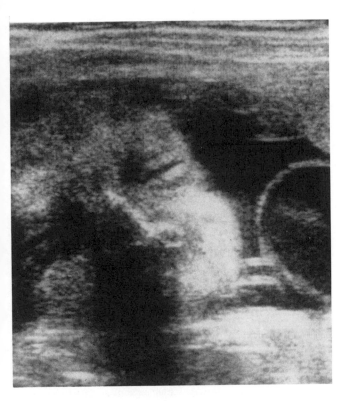

Figure 10.20   Fetal face.

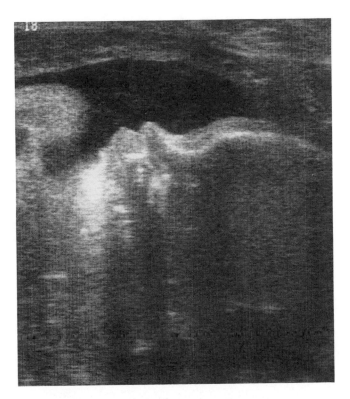

Figure 10.21   Fetal face in profile.

tinctly short of proving the safety of ultrasound. For this reason, ongoing continued surveillance and studies are recommended (24).

Routine Scanning

One of the most important issues that faces the obstetrical community is how to best utilize ultrasound in obstetrical care. Should an ultrasonic evaluation be routine in all pregnancies or performed in a selective fashion, only when there is a clinical indication?

In February 1984, the National Institutes of Health (NIH) convened their Consensus Development Conference on the use of diagnostic ultrasound imaging in pregnancy (25). They concluded that ultrasound improved pregnancy management and outcome only when an acceptable indication existed and that the value of routine scanning of the entire obstetrical population had not been proven. Many argued that the NIH could not advocate routine

scanning as it was felt that it would set a national standard of care, making practitioners who either chose not to scan their patients or those working in areas with inadequate facilities open to litigation. Furthermore, the cost of a mandatory scanning program was judged prohibitive in a time of escalating health costs.

In Great Britain, the Royal College of Obstetricians and Gynaecologist's policy on routine scanning was reviewed in December 1984 (23). Using the exact same data that were available to the NIH, they concluded that the potential diagnostic benefits of routine ultrasound far outweighed the theoretical and yet unproven potential risks of the procedure. Therefore, in direct contrast to the NIH, a routine ultrasound scan between 16 and 20 weeks' gestation was strongly endorsed.

Since that time, there have now been five randomized prospective studies performed in Europe whose results have been published (10). The largest involved over 7,000 patients. Each study has shown definite benefits by routine scanning.

Conclusion

Prior to ultrasound, obstetrics was a field of surprises, such as undiagnosed twins, unanticipated pre- and postmaturity and fetal anomalies. Today, these surprises are not necessary. The weight of evidence has shown that a complete routine scan done between 16 and 20 weeks' gestation is most effective for assigning dates, MSAFP screening, diagnosing multiple gestations and major fetal anomalies in a timely fashion, and evaluating the amniotic fluid and the placenta. It also has been shown to provide a tremendous psychologic benefit to pregnant families. Selective scanning is frequently performed too late. When a problem becomes clinically evident, mothers and their physicians are frequently denied appropriate choices. Diagnostic ultrasound, although not proven safe, has yet to be associated with any biological hazards. Therefore, every physician will have to answer the question of how to best utilize obstetrical ultrasound, either routinely or selectively. It is our feeling that, in communities with appropriate expertise and with the realities of clinical practice in the United States, routine ultrasound should be utilized. In view of the medical-legal climate that exists today and the anticipation of every parent to have a "perfect" child, the question should not be "Can we afford the ultrasound?," but "Can we afford not to perform the scan?."

References

1. Campbell S, Warsof S, Little D, Cooper DJ. Routine ultrasound screening for the prediction of gestational age. Obstet Gynecol 1985;65:613.
2. Robinson HP. Gestational sac volume as determined by sonar in the first trimester of pregnancy. Br J Obstet-Gynaecol 1975;82:100.
3. Robinson HP, Fleming JEE. A critical evaluation of sonar crown-rump length measurements. Br J Obstet-Gynaecol 1975;82:702.
4. Goldstein I, Reece E, Pilu G, et al. Cerebellar measurements with ultrasonography in the evaluation of fetal growth and development. Am J Obstet Gynecol 1987;156:1065.
5. Jeanty P, Dramaix-Wilmet M, Van Gansbeke D, et al. Fetal ocular biometry by ultrasound. Radiology 1982;143:513.
6. O'Brien GD, Queenan JT, Campbell S. Assessment of gestational age in the second trimester by real time ultrasound measurements of the femur length. Am J Obstet Gynecol 1981;139:540.
7. Goldkrand JW, Benjamin DS, Canton DM. Role of ultrasound in obstetric management. J Clin Ultrasound 1986;14:589.
8. Santolaya, J, Sampson M, Abramowicz JS, Warsof SL. Twin pregnancy: ultrasonographically observed changes in fetal presentation. J Rep Med 1992;37:328–30.
9. Farooqui MD, Grossman JH, Shannon RA. A review of twin pregnancies. Obstet Gynecol Surveys 1973;28:144.
10. Waldenstrom U, Axelsson O, Nilsson S, et al. Effects of routine one-stage ultrasound screening in pregnancy: a randomized controlled trial. Lancet 1988;2:585.
11. Hughey MJ, Olive DL. Routine ultrasound scanning for the detection of a management of twin pregnancies. J Reprod Med 1985;30:427.
12. Prenatal Detection of Neural Tube Defect. ACOG Technical Bulletin Number 99, Washington DC. December 1986.
13. Grannum PAT, Berkourtz RL, Hobbins JC. The ultrasonic changes in the maturing placenta and their relation to fetal pulmonic maturity. Am J Obstet Gynecol 1979;113:915.
14. Quintan RW, Cruz AC, Buhi WC, et al. Changes in placental ultrasonic appearance. Incidence of grade III changes in the placenta in correlation to fetal pulmonary maturity. Am J Obstet Gynecol 1982;144:468.
15. Birnholz J. Determination of fetal sex. N Engl J Med 1983;309:942.
16. Rosenberg K, Grant JM, Hepburn M. Antenatal detection of growth retardation. Actual practice in a large maternity hospital. Br J Obstet Gynaecol 1982;89:212.
17. Shepard MJ, Richards VA, Berkowitz RL. An evaluation of two equations for predicting fetal weight by ultrasound. Am J Obstet Gynecol 1982;142:47.
18. Manning FA, Basket TF, Morrison I, et al. Fetal biophysical profile scoring: a prospective study on 1184 high-risk patients. Am J Obstet Gynecol 1982;142:47.
19. Rutherford SE, Phelan JP, Smith CV, Jacobs N. The four quadrant assessment of amniotic fluid volume: an adjunct to antepartum fetal heart rate testing. Obstet Gynecol 1987;70:353.
20. Shulman H. The clinical implications of doppler ultrasound analysis of the uterine and umbilical arteries. Am J Obstet Gynecol 1987;156:889.
21. Campbell S, Reading AE, Cox DN, et al. Short term psychological effect of early ultrasonic scanning in pregnancy. J

Psychosomatic Obstet Gynecol 1982;1:57.

22. Safety Considerations for Diagnostic Ultrasound. The Bio-effects Committee of the American Institute of Ultrasound in Medicine. Bethesda, MD: AIUM Publication #316, 1984.

23. Report of the RCOG Working Party on Routine Ultrasound Examination in Pregnancy. Royal College of Obstetricians and Gynaecologists. London: Chameleon Press Ltd., 1984.

24. Meire HR. The safety of diagnostic ultrasound. Br J Obstet Gynecol 1987;94:1121.

25. Diagnostic Ultrasound Imaging in Pregnancy. Report of a Consensus Development Conference. Sponsored by the National Institute of Child Health and Human Development. Bethesda, MD: NIH Publication #84-557, February 6–8, 1984.

PART THREE Genetics

11

Genetic Screening for Mendelian Disorders

Carole M. Meyers, M.D.
Sherman Elias, M.D.

GENETIC screening is a ". . . search in a population for persons possessing certain genotypes that are already associated with disease or predisposed to disease, may lead to disease in their descendents, or may produce other variations not known to be associated with disease"(1).

Genetic screening can be performed on several different groups with whom obstetrician-gynecologists have direct or indirect contact. Therefore, it is important that clinicians be familiar with the indications, techniques, requirements, and responsibilities for all types of genetic screening.

Technologic advances in detecting and treating diseases have created pressure for use of genetic screening. But increased demand and limited resources are forcing decisions about who should be screened and how the choice of diseases to be screened should be made. Important factors include: frequency and severity of the condition; availability of a therapy of proven efficacy; extent to which detection by screening improves the outcome; validity and safety of the screening tests; adequacy of resources to assure effective screening and follow-up; costs; and acceptance of the screening program by the community, including both patients and practicing physicians (2).

The optimal genetic program would be initiated only after adequate public education, with community support and involvement in the program. Those screened would be informed of the purpose, give consent, and would be assured about confidentiality. Results would be conveyed through nondirective counseling. Screening tests would be inexpensive, simple, and accurate. There would be sufficient qualified personnel and laboratory facilities for required follow-up, and the program would provide a means of self-assessment.

Pedigree Analysis

Taking an accurate family history is the single most important step in genetic screening and should be a routine part of a patient's complete evaluation. This information can be summarized simply in the form of a pedigree. Figure 11.1 lists the commonly used symbols for pedigree construction. Minimum information for an uncomplicated family history should include three generations; complicated ones require extended pedigrees. All first-degree relatives of the proband

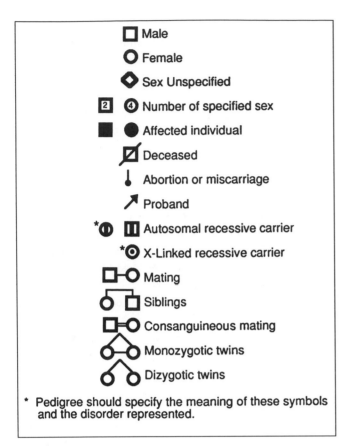

Figure 11.1 Pedigree symbols.

should be listed, and their state of health noted. The number, sex, and state of health of second-degree relatives should also be recorded. A history of the more common specific genetic diseases should be routinely sought, and a history of rare genetic disorders obtained when relevant. Questionnaires are available for identifying patients in whom more detailed information or further counseling is indicated (3). Genetic diagnoses suggested by the pedigree must be confirmed by review of the medical records whenever possible.

Mendelian Inheritance

Most mendelian, or single-gene, disorders are uncommon, usually occurring in one in 10,000 to 50,000 births, or fewer. Although individually rare, mendelian disorders in aggregate occur in approximately 1% of all live births McKusick's catalogue lists 2,208 disorders with confirmed mendelian inheritance and 2,136 additional disorders suggestive of mendelian inheritance (4). While it is not expected that clinicians be familiar with every mendelian disorder a general approach to screening for these disorders, as well as familiarity with some of the more common mendelian disorders, is appropriate.

Mendelian disorders result from the transmission of a mutant gene at a single locus, as opposed to polygenic disorders, which involve genes at many loci. Mendelian disorders show four patterns of inheritance: 1) autosomal dominant; 2) autosomal recessive; 3) sex-linked dominant; or 4 sex-linked recessive. Genes are situated on chromosomes a a given locus. Each gene has an allele that occupies the same locus on the other member of the chromosome pair If the alleles are different, the individual is heterozygous fo that gene. If the alleles are identical, the person is homozygous for that gene.

If the effects of an abnormal gene are evident when the gene is present in a single dose, then the gene is said to be dominant. If the disorder occurs only when the abnormal gene is present in a double dose, the gene is said to be recessive. Because the mutant gene may be located on the autosomal chromosomes or on the sex chromosomes, the inheritance is further described as autosomal or sex-linked respectively. Pedigree analysis is important in determining the type of inheritance of a given mendelian disorder.

Each type of mendelian inheritance—autosomal dominant, autosomal recessive, sex-linked dominant, and sex linked recessive—shows characteristic pedigree patterns The mode of inheritance is important when counseling fo mendelian disorders. Figure 11.2 shows characteristic pedi grees for each mode of inheritance.

Autosomal Dominant Disorders

These can occur in one of two ways: the gene can be inherited from an affected parent, or the abnormal gene may arise as a new mutation in an affected individual. Pedigree analysis is essential in differentiating these patterns. Differentiation is important because the recurrence risk for other family members can vary from zero, if the index case is new mutation, to 50%, if the gene has been inherited.

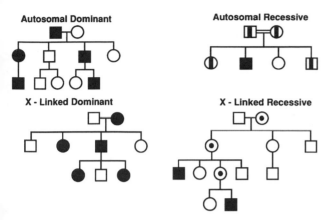

Figure 11.2   Patterns of mendelian inheritance.

Pedigree analysis can be complicated in dominant disorders by incomplete penetrance and variable expressivity. Complete penetrance exists when every individual carrying a given gene manifests the phenotype of that gene. Some dominant genes display incomplete penetrance; some individuals who carry the gene (as determined by pedigree analysis) do not express the phenotype. For example, a grandparent and grandchild have polydactyly, yet the child's mother does not. Expressivity refers to the extent to which a person carrying a dominant gene is affected. For example, an individual with neurofibromatosis may have only a few café au lait spots, or he or she may have large, disfiguring neurofibromas.

For dominant disorders, the offspring of an affected individual will have a 50% chance of inheriting the mutant gene from the affected parent and thus have the disorder, assuming complete penetrance. Unaffected individuals will have unaffected offspring, under the same assumptions.

Autosomal Recessive Disorders

These are rare in the population, and generally occur by the mating of two phenotypically normal individuals, each of whom carries the same autosomal recessive gene. Pedigree analysis typically shows only siblings to be affected. Each offspring of parents heterozygous for the same autosomal recessive gene has a 25% chance of having the disorder, a 50% chance of being a phenotypically normal heterozygote (like the parents), and a 25% chance of being a phenotypically normal homozygote. There are frequently consan-

guineous matings (between relatives) in the history of individuals with autosomal recessive disorders. The rarer the mutant gene in the population, the more often the parents of affected individuals are likely to be related. Inbreeding does not increase the frequency of the gene in the population, but it does increase the frequency of homozygotes, and thus the number of clinically affected individuals.

Sex-linked Inheritance

This is unique, since females have two X chromosomes and males only one. Males are hemizygous for genes on the X chromosome. Therefore, any gene carried on the X chromosome will be expressed in males. If a female heterozygous for a gene on the X chromosome does not express the gene, the gene is sex-linked (or X-linked) recessive. Typically, only males are affected, having received the mutant gene from their heterozygous, but unaffected mothers. A son of a heterozygous (carrier) female has a 50% chance of inheriting the mutant gene and having the disorder, or he has a 50% chance of inheriting the normal gene and being unaffected. Of her daughters, 50% have a chance of being carriers like the mother, and 50% have a chance of being homozygous normal for the gene

Affected males transmit the gene to all of their daughters, all of whom are carriers, but transmit it to none of their sons. Unaffected males do not carry the gene, and therefore have only unaffected offspring. It is important to realize, however, that the mother of a child with an X-linked recessive mutation cannot necessarily be assumed to be heterozygous; the child may represent a new mutation in a maternally derived X chromosome. If the trait is lethal with respect to fertility and if no other relatives are affected, the likelihood of a new mutation can be shown to be one-third.

Likewise, if a female heterozygous for a gene on the X chromosome does express the disorder, then the gene is X-linked dominant. The frequency of affected females is twice that of affected males. Females, however, are usually less severely affected. Indeed, some X-linked dominant disorders are lethal in males: for example, incontinentia pigmenti. With X-linked dominance, all the daughters, but none of the sons, of an affected male manifest the disorder. X-linked dominant disorders are rare.

Carrier Screening

From a clinical standpoint, "carrier screening" generally refers to identification of heterozygotes (that is, carriers) for an autosomal or X-linked recessive disorder. The most common indication for carrier screening in obstetric practice is to provide prospective parents with reproductive alternatives, such as prenatal diagnosis with possible termination of affected fetuses, artificial insemination, or deferral of childbearing.

Screening all individuals for carrier status, regardless of their family history or ethnic background, would be impossible. The decision of who should be screened is generally based on such criteria as availability of a simple, accurate, inexpensive test for the identification of carriers; an ethnic, racial, or geographic heritage associated with an increased risk for that specific genetic disorder; and treatment or reproductive options for identified individuals.

In the United States, three disorders currently meet the criteria for routine genetic screening in obstetric practice: Tay-Sachs disease, sickle cell anemia, and the thalassemias. For other diseases not routinely screened, carrier detection can sometimes be performed if the family history indicates an increased risk. An example would be a pregnant woman with a brother affected with Duchenne muscular dystrophy. Molecular techniques can usually substantially alter her empiric risk (50% risk of carrying the Duchenne gene), sometimes obviating the need for invasive prenatal diagnostic procedures. Carrier testing for a growing number of diseases, including cystic fibrosis and Huntington disease, is available when indicated by a positive family history. Participation of multiple family members, including affected individuals, is usually required for the most accurate risk assessment.

Sickle Cell Anemia

Sickle cell disease is the most common mendelian disorder in African-Americans, occurring in about one in 400 U. S. African-Americans. The disease is inherited as an autosomal recessive disorder (that is, individuals with sickle cell disease are homozygous for the mutant gene), while the trait is inherited as an autosomal dominant (individuals with the trait are heterozygous). The underlying abnormality is a single nucleotide substitution (GAG to GTG) in the sixth codon of the β-globin gene. This mutation leads to the transcription of the amino acid valine, instead of the amino acid glutamic acid, which results in the formation of an abnormal hemoglobin molecule. Sickle cell disease is characterized by a chronic, severe, hemolytic anemia. Red blood cells tend to become distorted, or "sickle shaped," under conditions of lowered oxygen tension. This abnormal shape results in increased blood viscosity, capillary stasis, vascular occlusion, and infarction of tissues such as bone, lungs, and spleen (a sickle "crisis"). About 10% of sickle cell anemia patients born in the United States die by the age of 10. Newborn screening for sickle cell disease has recently been recommended because prophylactic antibiotics can decrease the incidence of infection, often an inciting event in the sickle crisis (5). Carrier screening is available by hemoglobin electrophoresis, which shows approximately 50% sickle hemoglobin in carriers. Prenatal diagnosis is available through the direct analysis of the DNA encoding for the abnormal sickle hemoglobin.

Tay-Sachs Disease

Tay-Sachs disease occurs in approximately one in 3,600 infants of Ashkenazi Jewish parents. It is inherited as an autosomal recessive disorder. The biochemical abnormality is the absence of the enzyme hexosaminidase A, which is involved in the metabolism of a class of nervous system lipids called gangliosides. Accumulation of gangliosides in the brains of affected individuals causes motor weakness, psychomotor retardation, generalized spasticity, deafness, blindness, and convulsions. Death from bronchopneumonia usually occurs by age three. Accurate carrier detection is possible by demonstrating intermediate reduction of hexosaminidase A activity in serum. Of importance to the obstetrician, however, are observations that serum hexosaminidase A decreases during pregnancy relative to total hexosaminidase. Pregnant women may, therefore, be diagnosed erroneously as heterozygotes. Leukocyte assays, which are not altered during pregnancy, are routinely recommended whenever pregnant women are tested. Since many noncarriers have been found with reduced hex osaminidase A on serum testing (values in the inconclusive or heterozygous range), leukocyte assays are again specifically recommended. Prenatal diagnosis is available by assay of hexosaminidase A activity in cultured cells from amniotic fluid or chorionic villi.

Thalassemias

The thalassemias are a heterogeneous group of hereditary anemias in which the common feature is diminished synthesis of hemoglobin. The α-thalassemias involve mutations that result in the deletion of from one to four genes, at the same loci on homologous chromosomes, which code for the two chains in the hemoglobin molecule. The disorder is most common in Southeast Asia. Individuals may be missing from zero to four genes coding for the four chains. If no genes are deleted, the individual is unaffected. If one or two of the genes are deleted, the individual will have α-thalassemia minor, which is usually asymptomatic. Deletion of three genes results in hemoglobin H disease, which is a more severe anemia than α-thalassemia minor. A fetus with deletions of all four α-chain genes can only make an unstable hemoglobin (hemoglobin Barts), develops hydrops fetalis, and dies in utero.

The β-thalassemias are associated with a defective β-chain synthesis, and fall into two general groups. In the β^+ group, reduced amounts of mRNA are produced because of incomplete suppression of the β gene. In the β^0 group, mRNA for the β chain is absent or nonfunctional. β-thalassemia is present in all populations, but is more common in Mediterranean countries, the Middle East, Southeast Asia, and parts of India and Pakistan.

The heterozygous (carrier) state for β-thalassemia (thalassemia minor) is not usually associated with clinical disability, except in periods of stress. Homozygous β-thalassemia (thalassemia major or Cooley's anemia) is characterized by failure to thrive, hepatosplenomegaly, growth retardation, and bony changes secondary to marrow hypertrophy. Unless maintained on an adequate transfusion program, the affected person usually dies in childhood. Medical complications are common, even with transfusions.

Screening for carriers of both α-thalassemia and β-thalassemia is possible by evaluation of the red cell indices. A mean corpuscular hemoglobin value of 20–22 pg and mean corpuscular volume values of 50 to 70 fL suggest the diagnosis of thalassemia minor. Confirmation is by demonstration of elevated levels of hemoglobin A_2 by electrophoresis. Prenatal diagnosis for both α-thalassemia and β-thalassemia is possible by molecular techniques. However, accurate characterization of the hemoglobin defect involved is essential.

Disorders Associated with Pregnancy Complications

In patients identified by pedigree analysis or carrier screening to be at increased risk for having an offspring with a mendelian disorder, prenatal diagnosis is often available by chorionic villus sampling, amniocentesis, fetal skin or blood sampling, or ultrasound examination. Not every mendelian disorder is detectable prenatally, but many of the more common disorders are, and the number of disorders detectable prenatally is increasing rapidly. The incidence, inheritance, and availability of prenatal diagnosis of several mendelian disorders that occur frequently in the general population are summarized in Table 11.1.

It should not be forgotten that pregnant patients may themselves have a mendelian disorder. The risk of the fetus inheriting the disorder must be determined accordingly. In addition, these disorders may be of clinical importance for pregnancy management of the affected patient. For example, patients with Marfan and Ehlers-Danlos syndromes are at risk of aortic dissection during pregnancy.

A woman with phenylketonuria may have been treated successfully with dietary restriction of phenylalanine in childhood, but unless phenylalanine levels are strictly controlled during pregnancy (and optimally prior to pregnancy), severe mental retardation and somatic abnormalities in her offspring are the rule. There are many other genetic disorders compatible with fertility yet associated with pregnancy complications. In any case, women with genetic disorders should receive genetic counseling about the risks of transmission of the disorder to their offspring and the availability of prenatal diagnosis, as well as input from geneticists or other appropriate specialists for pregnancy management, when indicated.

Table 11.1 Selected Mendelian Disorders

Disorder	Incidence	Inheritance	Prenatal Diagnosis
Tay-Sachs (GM$_2$ gangliosidosis)	1/3,600 Ashkenazic Jews and French Canadians; 1/400,000 other populations	Autosomal recessive	Hexosaminidase A levels in cultured amniotic fluid cells (AFC) or chorionic villi (CV)
Cystic fibrosis	1/1,500 white population	Autosomal recessive	Molecular techniques* on AFC or CV, microvillar intestinal enzyme (amniotic fluid)
Duchenne muscular dystrophy	1/3,300 male births	X-linked recessive	Molecular techniques on AFC or CV
Hemophilia A	1/8,500 male births	X-linked recessive	Molecular techniques on AFC or CV, rarely fetal blood sampling
Congenital adrenal hyperplasia	1/10,000	Autosomal recessive	Molecular techniques on AFC or CV; prenatal therapy available
Homozygous α- and β-thalassemia	Varies widely, but present in most populations	Autosomal recessive	Molecular techniques on AFC or CV
Sickle cell anemia	1/400 U. S. Blacks	Autosomal recessive	Direct DNA analysis on AFC or CV

*See Reference 6 for a discussion of molecular techniques for prenatal diagnosis.

Reprinted with permission from Simpson JL, Elias S. Prenatal diagnosis of genetic disorders in: Creasy R, Resnick R, eds. Maternal fetal medicine: principles and practice, ed 2. Orlando, Florida: W.B. Saunders, 1989.

Newborn Screening

Genetic screening of the newborn is possible for a variety of diseases. The selection of diseases for screening has been controversial. Currently, for newborn screening to be justified, the disorder in question should cause severe impairment if it is left untreated. In addition, the method for diagnosis must be definitive. Finally, treatment for the disorder must be available and must be of benefit to the patient.

Table 11.2 summarizes the incidence, biochemical abnormality, and screening and diagnostic tests for some mendelian disorders for which newborn screening can be performed. This is not to imply that all newborns are routinely tested for all these disorders or that screening for each of the disorders is warranted, but only to indicate the large number of disorders for which screening is technically possible. Prenatal diagnosis is potentially available for all the disorders that have been included in Table 11.2.

Newborn screening for most mendelian disorders is performed by collecting capillary blood from a heel puncture onto a filter paper. Specimens are then sent to a reference laboratory where they are assayed for the specified diseases. Abnormal screening tests must be confirmed with more sensitive diagnostic tests. Assays for multiple disorders can be performed on an individual specimen. This makes screening for some rare disorders (such as maple syrup urine disease) worthwhile, when it would not be cost effective to screen for these disorders individually.

Donor Screening

Recently developed techniques for noncoital reproduction such as artificial insemination by donor, embryo transfer, and use of donor oocytes, raise questions concerning the appropriate genetic screening for genetic donors. The American Fertility Society has published guidelines for the

Table 11.2 Selected Mendelian Disorders for which Newborn Screening is Available

Disorder*	Incidence (Average)	Inheritance	Screening Test (Dried Blood Spot)	Diagnostic Test
Biotinidase deficiency	1/70,000	Autosomal recessive	Biotinidase activity	Biotinidase activity in serum
Branched chain ketoaciduria (maple syrup urine disease)	1/275,000	Autosomal recessive	Leucine level	Quantitative leucine, isoleucine, valine
Congenital adrenal hyperplasia	1/12,000	Autosomal recessive	17-hydroxy-progesterone level	Quantitative 17-hydroxy-progesterone in plasma
Congenital hypothyroidism	1/4,300 by screening	Varies with etiology, rare autosomal recessive	T_4 and/or TSH level	Quantitative T_4 and TSH
Cystic fibrosis	1/2,000 white	Autosomal recessive	Immunoreactive trypsin	Sweat test
Duchenne muscular dystrophy	1/4,000 male births	X-linked recessive	Creatine kinase level	Creatine kinase, SGOT, SGPT, LDH, aldolase, muscle biopsy, electromyography
Galactosemia	1/70,000	Autosomal recessive	Galactose level or enzyme activity	Quantitative galactose, galactose-1-phosphate and transferase activity
Homocystinuria	1/100,00	Autosomal recessive	Methionine level	Quantitative methionine and homocysteine
Phenylketonuria	1/17,500	Autosomal recessive	Phenylalanine level	Quantitative phenylalanine, tyrosine, urinary pteridines, dihydropteridine reductase
Sickle cell disease	1/400 U. S. African-Americans	Autosomal recessive	Hemoglobin electrophoresis	Hemoglobin electrophoresis and parental testing

*Listing of a disorder does not imply that all newborns are routinely tested for all these disorders, or that screening for each of the disorders is warranted, but only indicates the large number of disorders for which screening is technically possible.

Reprinted with permission from The American Academy of Pediatrics, Committee of Genetics. Newborn screening fact sheets. Pediatrics 1989; 83:449.

minimal genetic screening of donors, which include mendelian disorders (7).

Legal Issues

Genetic screening has given rise to some legislation of varying quality. The specific requirements for screening vary widely with regard to the responsibility for administration of the mandated program.

A major legal issue in all types of genetic screening is whether the program should be voluntary or mandatory. The National Academy of Sciences, in 1975, recommended that "participation in a genetic screening program should not be mandatory by law, but should be left to the discretion of the person tested or, if a minor, of the parents or legal guardian"(1). In 1983, the President's Bioethics Commission endorsed voluntary screening, but noted that mandatory programs "requiring the performance of low-risk, minimally intrusive procedures may be justified if voluntary testing would fail to prevent an avoidable, serious injury to people—such as children—who are unable to protect themselves" (8). However, the vast majority of newborn genetic screening programs remain mandatory.

The confidentiality of genetic screening results is a second major legal issue. In 1983, the President's Bioethics Commission underlined the importance of confidentiality in genetic testing by recommending, along with other things, that:

- Genetic information should not be given to unrelated third parties, such as employers, without the explicit and informed consent of the person screened or a surrogate for that person;

- Private and governmental agencies that use data banks for genetic-related information should require that sorted information be coded whenever that is compatible with the purpose of the data bank (8).

In view of the history of genetic screening and the possible stigma that can result from the possession even of a recessive gene, the recommendations for such screening seem minimal and should be followed. In addition, the Commission recommended that screening programs should not be undertaken at all unless the results that are produced could be routinely relied upon, and a full range of pre-screening and follow-up services for the population to be screened should be available before a screening program is introduced. We believe that these recommendations are reasonable and should be followed.

References

1. National Academy of Sciences. Genetic screening: programs principles and research. Washington, DC: National Academy of Sciences, 1975.
2. Holtzman NA. Newborn screening for genetic-metabolic diseases: progress, principles and recommendations. US Dept of Health, Education, and Welfare, Publication No (HSA) 78–5207, 1977.
3. ACOG Technical Bulletin. Antenatal diagnosis of genetic disorders. 1987;108.
4. McKusick VA. Mendelian inheritance in man, 8th ed. Baltimore: The Johns Hopkins University Press, 1988.
5. Sickle cell disease—consensus conference: newborn screening for sickle cell disease and other hemoglobinopathies. JAMA 1987;258:9.
6. Elias S, Annas GJ. Reproductive genetics and the law. Chicago Year Book Medical Publishers, 1987.
7. American Fertility Society. New guidelines for the use of semen donor insemination. Fertil Steril 1986;46(suppl 2):4.
8. President's Commission for the Study of Ethical Problems in Medicine and Biomedical and Behavioral Research. Screening and counseling for genetic conditions. Washington D.C.: US Government Printing Office, 1983.

12

Maternal Serum Screening

Gary S. Eglinton, M.D.
Frank D. Seydel, Ph.D.

NEURAL tube defects (NTDs) are among the most common major birth defects, with a frequency of 1–2/1,000 births in the United States. Although NTDs may occur in association with other specific defects with different inheritance patterns, the vast majority of NTDs are of unknown cause and follow a multifactorial inheritance pattern. The risk varies by ethnic origin and geographic region in the United States. Rates decline from east to west, and are higher among Caucasians than among African-Americans. The highest frequency in the developed world is in the United Kingdom, with an average of 4.5/1,000, over twice the rate in the United States (Table 12.1 and Figures 12.1 and 12.2) (1, 2). Although the risk in the United Kingdom for recurrence is 5% after one affected child and 9% after two, the recurrence risk in the United States is lower (Table 12.2). Couples who have a known recurrence risk can have prenatal diagnosis in subsequent pregnancies, but 90% of the mothers delivering infants with NTDs have no history placing them at high risk.

Approximately 18 days after fertilization, the neural groove forms in the primitive neural plate, surrounded by the lateral neural folds. The folds fuse in the midline over the groove in the cervical region initiating formation of the neural tube, and fusion progresses cephalad and caudad simultaneously, closing the anterior neuropore at 24 days

Table 12.1 Incidence of Neural Tube Defects in Various Geographical Areas

	Spina Bifida Incidence per 1,000 Births	Anencephaly Incidence per 1,000 Births
South Wales	4.1	3.5
Southampton	3.2	1.9
Birmingham, UK	2.8	2.0
Charleston		
White	1.5	1.2
Black	0.6	0.2
Alexandria	2.0	3.6
Japan	0.3	0.6

Modified from Brocklehurst. In: Vinken PJ, Bruyn GW, eds. Handbook of clinical neurology, vol 32. Amsterdam: Elsevier/North Holland Biomedical Press, 1978:519–578.

Table 12.2 Estimated Incidence of Neural Tube Defects Based on Specific Risk Factors in the United States

Population	Incidence/1,000 Live Births
Mother as Reference	
General incidence	1.4–1.6
Women undergoing amniocentesis for advanced maternal age	1.5–3.0
Women with diabetes mellitus	20
Women on valproic acid in first trimester	10–20
Fetus as Reference	
1 sibling with NTD	15–30
2 siblings with NTD*	57
Parent with NTD	11
Half sibling with NTD	8
First cousin (mother's sister's child)	10
Other first cousins	3
Sibling with severe scoliosis secondary to multiple vertebral defects	15–30
Sibling with occult spinal dysraphism	15–30
Sibling with sacrococcygeal teratoma or hamartoma	≤ 15–30

*Risk is higher in British studies. Risk increases further for three or more siblings or combinations of other close relatives.

Reprinted with permission from Main DM, Mennuti MT. Neural tube defects: issues in prenatal diagnosis and counselling. Obstet Gynecol 1986; 67:1.

and the posterior neuropore at 26 days, respectively, after fertilization. Thus, the neural tube ordinarily closes prior to six weeks after the first day of the last menstrual period (3). This ends the period of neurulation. Failure of fusion of the anterior neuropore leads to anencephaly. Failure of fusion of the posterior neuropore leads to spina bifida, which may be open (meninges exposed) or closed (skin–covered). Anencephaly is universally fatal, but, with early aggressive neurosurgical care, survival with spinal defects can be excellent (Table 12.3). Postneurulation defects may develop, but they are skin–covered and may escape detection using biochemical methods.

In 1972, Brock and Sutcliffe first suggested the possibility for prenatal diagnosis of open NTDs when they demonstrated elevated amniotic fluid α–fetoprotein (AFP) in the stored frozen amniotic fluid from affected pregnan-

cies (4). AFP is a glycoprotein similar in molecular weight (70,000) to albumin. The fetus synthesizes it in the yolk sac, gastrointestinal tract, and liver. Its level in fetal plasma peaks at about 12 weeks' gestation and then declines exponentially. It normally passes into the fetal urine and then into the amniotic fluid, where its levels roughly parallel fetal serum, but are two orders of magnitude lower. AFP normally leaks across the placenta in small amounts (from both amniotic fluid and fetal serum), leading to levels in the maternal serum that rise through the first 30 weeks of gestation but, again, at orders of magnitude lower than in the amniotic fluid (Figure 12.3) (5). When a fetal anomaly occurs that presents greater exposure of fetal capillaries to the amniotic fluid (such as anencephaly, open spina bifida, omphalocele, gastroschisis, etc.), higher AFP levels result in the fluid and in the maternal serum.

Maternal serum AFP (MSAFP) screening developed in the United Kingdom during the 1970s and spread to this country during the 1980s. The U.K. Collaborative Study of MSAFP retrospectively reported results for 18,684 singleton and 163 twin pregnancies without fetal NTDs and 301 singleton pregnancies with fetal NTDs (6). The authors felt that they had identified all NTD births during the period of the study. They assayed maternal serum specimens from these pregnancies and from a sampling of the non-NTD

Table 12.3 Results of Aggressive Treatment of 171 Consecutive Infants With Meningomyeloceles in the 1960s

Level of Lesion	Percent with this Level of Lesion	Mortality (%)	IQ>80 (%)	Able to Walk† (%)	Able to Walk Without Appliance (%)
Thoracolumbar	37	35	44	71	0
Lumbosacral	59	11	65	81	16
Sacral	4	0	100	100	83

*Three- to eight-year follow-up.
†Many of the children, particularly those with higher lesions, can walk with braces and other supports in the first decade of life but lose this ability in adolescence.

Reprinted with permission from Main DM, Mennuti MT. Neural tube defects: issues in prenatal diagnosis and counselling. Obstet Gynecol 1986;67:

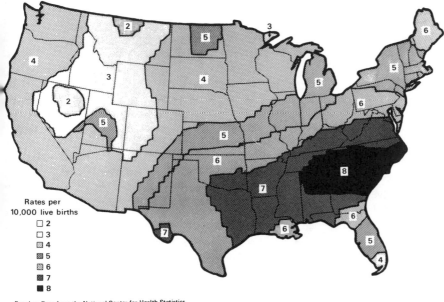

Figure 12.1 Estimates of birth prevalence rates of spina bifida for white births in the United States from computer-generated maps.

Reproduced with permission from Greenberg F, James LM, Oakley GP Jr. Estimates of birth prevalence rates of spina bifida in the United States from computer-generated maps. Am J Obstet Gynecol 1983;145:570.

Rates per 10,000 live births
☐ 2
☐ 3
▨ 4
▧ 5
▨ 6
▨ 7
■ 8

Based on Data from the National Center for Health Statistics

births. They determined that, at the time of their study, 16–18 weeks' gestation was the optimal time for serum screening, and they introduced the concept of using multiples of the median (MoM), rather than percentiles or standard deviations, to report results. The value of the multiple of the median for a sample is the ratio of the specimen value to the population median value at the same gestational age. Calculation of a MoM value permits comparisons among laboratories with disparate assay accuracies and precisions. In the initial experiences with MSAFP assays in

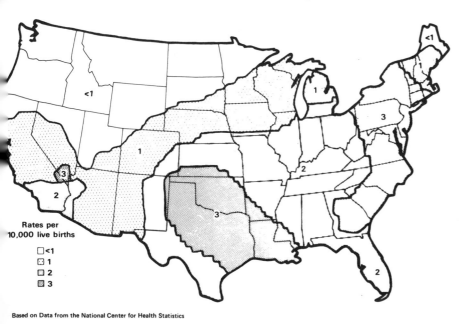

Figure 12.2 Estimates of birth prevalence rates of spina bifida for black births in the United States from computer-generated maps.

Reproduced with permission from Greenberg F, James LM, Oakley GP Jr. Estimates of birth prevalence rates of spina bifida in the United States from computer-generated maps. Am J Obstet Gynecol 1983;145:570.

Rates per 10,000 live births
☐ <1
☐ 1
☐ 2
▨ 3

Based on Data from the National Center for Health Statistics

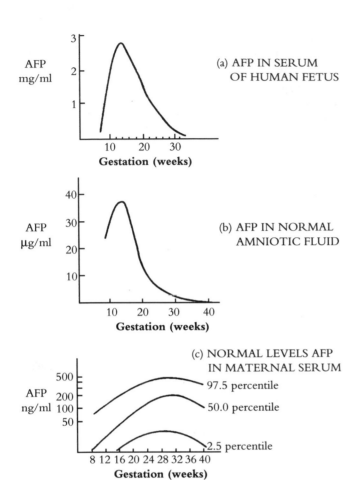

Figure 12.3 Approximate relationship between α-fetoprotein values in a) fetal serum, b) amniotic fluid, and c) maternal serum. Note different units for each graph.

Reproduced with permission from Habib A. Maternal serum alpha-fetoprotein: its value in antenatal diagnosis of genetic disease and in obstetrical-gynecological care. Acta Obstet Gynecol Scand Suppl 1977;61:14.

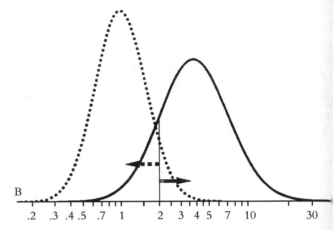

Figure 12.4 Distribution of MSAFP (as MoM) in open spina bifida (solid line) and unaffected pregnancies (dotted line). Arrows indicate the most probable direction of a repeat sample with an initial MoM of 2.1 (light vertical line).

Reproduced with permission from Knight GJ, Palomaki GE, Haddow JE. Use of maternal serum alpha-fetoprotein measurements to screen for Down's syndrome. Clin Obstet Gynecol 1988;31:306.

multiple laboratories, the absolute value of AFP concentrations varied by a factor of 2, and interassay coefficients of variation ranged to 20%.

Defining the desired sensitivity and specificity of the serum screening sets the critical MoM value (Table 12.4). In turn, the MoM of a single sample result determines the odds of an individual pregnancy's being affected by an NTD (Table 12.5). At 16–18 weeks of gestation, if 2.5 MoM is the cutoff level indicating further action, assay pre-

Table 12.4 Percentage of Pregnancies with Maternal Serum AFP Levels at 16–18 Weeks of Gestation Equal to o Greater than Specified Multiples of the Normal Median

	Cut-off Level (Multiple of the Normal Median)				
Pregnancy	2.0	2.5	3.0	3.5	4.0
Singleton NTD pregnancies					
Anencephaly	90.0	88.0	84.0	82.0	76.0
Open spina bifida	91.0	79.0	70.0	64.0	45.0
All spina bifida	83.0	69.0	60.0	55.0	38.0
Singleton non-NTD pregnancies	7.2	3.3	1.4	0.6	0.3
Twin non-NTD pregnancies	47.0	26.0	19.0	13.0	11.0
All non-NTD pregnancies (assuming 1 in 80 is a twin pregnancy)	7.7	3.6	1.6	0.8	0.4

Reprinted with permission from UK Collaborative Study on Alpha-fetoprotein in Relation to Neural Tube Defects. Maternal serum alpha-fetoprotein measurement in antenatal screening for anencephaly and spina bifida in early pregnancy. Lancet 1977;1:1323.

Table 12.5 Odds of Women with Serum AFP Levels Equal to or Greater than Specified Cut-off Levels at 16–18 Weeks of Gestation Having a Fetus with an NTD or Open Spina Bifida (Multiple Pregnancy Having Been Excluded by Ultrasonography)

Cut-Off Level (Multiple of Normal Median)	All NTDs, with Incidence (per 1,000 Births) of:					Open Spina Bifida, with Incidence (per 1,000 Births) of:				
	2	4	6	8	10	1	2	3	4	5
	1:41	1:21	1:14	1:10	1:8	1:79	1:40	1:26	1:20	1:16
.5	1:21	1:10	1:7	1:5	1:4	1:42	1:21	1:14	1:10	1:8
	1:10	1:5	1:3	1:2	1:2	1:20	1:10	1:7	1:5	1:4
.5	1:4	1:2	2:3	1:1	1:1	1:9	1:5	1:3	1:2	1:2
	1:3	1:1	1:1	3:2	2:1	1:7	1:3	1:2	2:3	1:1

Note: In the calculations, an average assay precision is assumed.

Reprinted with permission from UK Collaborative Study on Alpha-feto-protein in Relation to Neural Tube Defects. Maternal serum alpha-feto-protein measurement in antenatal screening for anencephaly and spina bifi-da in early pregnancy. Lancet 1977; 1:1323.

...sion contributes only 10% of the variation in result, while ...dividual patient variation contributes about one third of the ...ariation in result. Therefore, improved assay precision or ...peating the assay of the same specimen will not potential-... reduce the proportion of misidentified unaffected preg-...ancies as greatly as will a repeat sample from the patient. ...he authors speculated that repeating the serum sample for ...ose patients with a result within 20% of the 2.5 MoM ...2.5–3.0 MoM) cutoff and then using the mean of the two ...ight decrease the number of unaffected pregnancies iden-...fied for further study by one third without significantly ...creasing the detection rate. Figure 12.4 illustrates the sta-...stical reason for this: Because of the tendency for regres-...on toward the mean, repeated sampling from separate but ...erlapping populations will tend to produce results closer ... the mean of the population from which the sample orig-...ates (7).

MSAFP screening is not a diagnostic test. Figure 12.5 ...ustrates the reason for this: There is a significant overlap ... expected AFP levels among unaffected pregnancies and ...nong those affected by open spina bifida or anencephaly

(8). Follow-up is necessary, with counseling, ultrasonography, and amniocentesis for amniotic fluid AFP (AFAFP) testing. The second report from the U.K. Collaborative Study detailed findings related to AFAFP levels for 13,105 singleton pregnancies without fetal NTDs and for 385 with fetal NTDs (222 with anencephaly, 152 with spina bifida, of which 123 were open, and 11 with encephalocele)(9). Again, the AFAFP level is not diagnostic, and varying the cutoff MoM that indicates further action affects the sensitivity and specificity of the assay. The authors chose specified cutoffs from 2.5–4.0 for advancing gestational ages (Table 12.6). Even these cutoffs resulted in a small false-positive rate. Analogous to the case for MSAFP, the authors felt that borderline positive samples could be repeated, which would further reduce the false-positive rate without seriously affecting the detection rate. Also, analogous to the case for MSAFP, the study's results permitted calculation of odds of having a fetus with open spina bifida based on AFAFP and other criteria (Table 12.7).

Screening in the United States may not be cost effective, since the frequency of NTDs is so much lower than in the United Kingdom, but medicolegal pressures are among the considerations that have spurred the spread of MSAFP

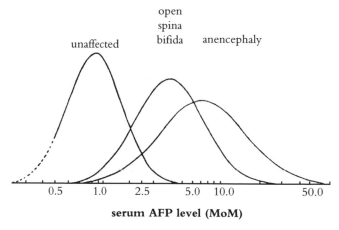

Figure 12.5 AFP levels in maternal serum at 16–18 weeks of gestation in singleton pregnancies. MoM = multiples of normal median.

Reproduced with permission from Wald NJ, Cuckle HS, Catz C, et al. Alpha-fetoprotein screening and diagnosis of fetal open neural tube defects: the need for quality control. Am J Obstet Gynecol 1981;141:1.

Table 12.6 Singleton Pregnancies: Practical False–Positive and Detection Rates at Different Weeks of Gestation and Different Cut-off Levels, Among Clear Amniotic Fluid Samples and Among All Samples

Gestation (Completed Wks)			Total No. Pregnancies*	No.(%) Equal to or Greater than Cut-off Levels† (Multiples of Normal Median)			
				Specified	Specified +0.5	Specified +1.0	Specified +1.5
				2.5	3.0	3.5	4.0
13–15							
	Clear samples:	Non-NTD	2,938	9 (0.31)	2 (0.07)	1 (0.03)	1 (0.03)
		Anencephaly	16	16 (100)	16 (100)	16 (100)	16 (100)
		OSB	20	19 (95)	19 (95)	17 (85)	17 (85)
	All samples:	Non-NTD	3,171	14 (0.44)	4 (0.13)	1 (0.03)	1 (0.03)
		Anencephaly	21	21 (100)	21 (100)	21 (100)	21 (100)
		OSB	23	22 (96)	21 (91)	20 (87)	19 (83)
				3.0	3.5	4.0	4.5
16–18							
	Clear samples:	Non-NTD	7,009	17 (0.24)	7 (0.10)	6 (0.09)	3 (0.04)
		Anencephaly	59	58 (98)	58 (98)	58 (98)	58 (98)
		OSB	60	60 (100)	55 (92)	51 (85)	47 (78)
	All samples:	Non-NTD	7,701	32 (0.42)	17 (0.22)	15 (0.19)	9 (0.12)
		Anencephaly	97	96 (99)	96 (99)	96 (99)	96 (99)
		OSB	74	73 (99)	68 (92)	64 (86)	60 (81)
				3.5	4.0	4.5	5.0
19–21							
	Clear samples:	Non-NTD	1,343	4 (0.30)	2 (0.15)	0	0
		Anencephaly	39	38 (97)	38 (97)	38 (97)	37 (95)
		OSB	19	18 (95)	18 (95)	16 (84)	13 (68)
	All samples:	Non-NTD	1,530	10 (0.65)	5 (0.33)	1 (0.07)	1 (0.07)
		Anencephaly	70	69 (99)	69 (99)	69 (99)	68 (97)
		OSB	21	20 (95)	20 (95)	18 (86)	15 (71)
				4.0	4.5	5.0	5.5
22–24							
	Clear samples:	Non-NTD	335	1 (0.30)	1 (0.30)	1 (0.30)	1 (0.30)
		Anencephaly	23	22 (96)	22 (96)	21 (91)	21 (91)
		OSB	2	2 (100)	2 (100)	2 (100)	2 (100)
	All samples:	Non-NTD	402	5 (1.24)	5 (1.24)	4 (1.00)	3 (0.75)
		Anencephaly	34	32 (94)	32 (94)	31 (91)	31 (91)
		OSB	5	5 (100)	5 (100)	5 (100)	4 (80)
13–24							
	Clear samples:	Non-NTD	11,625	31 (0.27)	12 (0.10)	8 (0,07)	5 (0.04)
		Anencephaly	137	134 (98)	134 (98)	133 (97)	132 (96)
		OSB	101	99 (98)	94 (93)	87 (86)	78 (77)

Continued

Table 12.6 *Continued*

Gestation (Completed Wks)		Total No. Pregnancies*	No.(%) Equal to or Greater than Cut-off Levels† (Multiples of Normal Median)			
			Specified	Specified +0.5	Specified +1.0	Specified +1.5
			4.0	4.5	5.0	5.5
All samples:	Non–NTD	12,804	61 (0.48)	31 (0.24)	21 (0.16)	14 (0.11)
	Anencephaly	222	218 (98)	218 (98)	217 (98)	216 (97)
	OSB	123	120 (98)	114 (93)	108 (88)	99 (80)

*Excluding unaffected pregnancies ending in miscarriage.
†Excluding unaffected pregnancies with serious fetal abnormalities.

Reprinted with permission from UK Collaborative Study on Alpha-fetoprotein in Relation to Neural Tube Defects. Amniotic fluid alpha-fetoprotein measurement in antenatal diagnosis of anencephaly and open spina bifida in early pregnancy. Lancet 1979; 2:651.

Table 12.7 Odds of Having Fetus with Open Spina Bifida Before and After Positive Amniotic Fluid AFP Test at 16–18 Weeks' Gestation, According to Prevalence of Open Spina Bifida and Reason for Amniocentesis.

Prevalence of Open Spina Bifida	Reason for Amniocentesis	Odds of Having Fetus with Open Spina Bifida:				
		Before Amniotic Fluid AFP Test	After Amniotic Fluid AFP Level at 16–18 wk Gestation Found to Be ≥ Cut-off Level (Multiple of Normal Median)†			
			3.0	3.5	4.0	4.5
1 per 1,000	Serum AFP ≥ 2.5 x median*	1:26	9:1	16:1	17:1	26:1
	Previous infant with an NTD	1:100	2:1	4:1	4:1	7:1
	Other	1:1000	1:4	1:2	1:2	2:3
2 per 1,000	Serum AFP ≥ 2.5 x median*	1:13	18:1	32:1	35:1	52:1
	Previous infant with an NTD	1:50	5:1	8:1	9:1	14:1
	Other	1:500	1:2	1:1	1:1	3:2
3 per 1,000	Serum AFP ≥ 2.5 x median*	1:9	26:1	46:1	50:1	75:1
	Previous infant with an NTD	1:33	7:1	13:1	14:1	20:1
	Other	1:333	2:3	1:1	3:2	2:1

*At 16–18 weeks' gestation based on a single serum AFP test; if patients with raised levels are tested twice and average value used, odds ratios would be increased by about one-third.
†Odds based on practical false-positive and detection rates associated with single tests using data relating to all samples (i.e., including blood-stained ones) are shown in Table 12.6.

Reprinted with permission from UK Collaborative Study on Alpha-fetoprotein in Relation to Neural Tube Defects. Amniotic fluid alpha-fetoprotein measurement in antenatal diagnosis of anencephaly and open spina bifida in early pregnancy. Lancet 1979; 2:651.

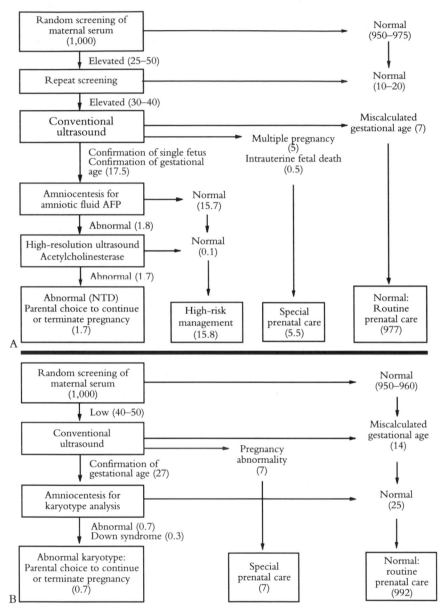

Figure 12.6 Anticipated results of MSAFP screening of 1,000 prenatal patients at 16–18 weeks of gestation. (**A**) Elevated results. (**B**) Low results.

Reproduced with permission from Haddlow JE. New England Regional Genetics Group Prenatal Collaborative Study of Down Syndrome Screening. Combining maternal serum alpha-fetoprotein measurements and age to screen for Down syndrome in pregnant women under age 35. Am J Obstet Gynecol 1989; 160:575–581.

screening in the United States. In 1985, the Department of Professional Liability of the American College of Obstetricians and Gynecologists circulated an opinion to Fellows of the College, advising them of the FDA approval of commercial marketing for MSAFP screening kits and the consequent liabilities of failure to counsel a pregnant patient of the implications and the availability of these kits. At the time, there was insufficient consideration given to the implications of advising screening without accessibility of an appropriate full-service screening program. The American Society of Human Genetics has detailed the complex elements of an adequate program for screening (10).

MSAFP screening should occur at 15–21 weeks (ideally 16–18), in the frame of reference of a complete program of counseling prior to screening and well-established appropriate logistics for follow-up. Each laboratory performing assays should establish normal median values for the population served. This requires a data base of at least 100–200 patients at each gestational week used in screening, followed through delivery to ensure the inclusion of values only from normal pregnancies with normal outcomes in determining normal medians. Commonly, a value above 2.5 MoM indicates further study: repeat sample or ultrasound study to rule out incorrect pregnancy dating, multiple gestation, dead fetus, missed abortion or obvious major anomaly, such as anencephaly (Figure 12.6) (11). If the reason for the abnormal value is not clear, amniocentesis for assay of amniotic fluid AFP (AFAFP) and, if necessary, acetylcholinesterase (AChE) offer more specific testing than just serum screening and are reassuring if the AFAFP level is normal. If the amniotic fluid AFP level is elevated, AChE assessment offers another marker more specific to NTD, and high-resolution ultrasound searching for fetal anomalies will generally reveal the cause of the elevated level of either AFAFP alone or elevated AFAFP and AChE.

If the gestational dating is correct, one can calculate from the MoM a specific risk of neural tube defect or ventral wall defect, such as 1:150, instead of relying on an arbitrary cutoff for the MoM, such as 2.5. This method uses a known prevalence of open spina bifida (OSB) within the population, the distributions of concentrations of MSAFP from both affected and unaffected pregnancies, and Bayes' theorem (12). The advantage is that the patient can compare the risk of abnormal outcome to the risk of a specific intervention, such as amniocentesis, rather than just considering the abstract >2.5 MoM. Whether the reference value is a MoM cutoff or a specific risk calculation, the MoM must be adjusted for maternal weight (volume of distribution); race (13, 14); and diabetes (12). Using the specific risk-based method proposed by Adams and preferred by the American Society of Human Genetics (15) requires application of the resultant adjusted MoM to a population-specific prevalence based on geographic region and race. Using Adams' methods also permits calculation of risks of undiagnosed twins and ventral wall defects (VWD) from the MoM. After combining risks mathematically, one can quote a total risk of either VWD or OSB (14). Table 12.8 is an example of specific risk reporting for the Washington, D.C. area based on Adams' methods. Adams et al. adjusted

Table 12.8 Risk of Open Spina Bifida (OSB) and Combined Risks of OSB and Ventral Wall Defect (VWD) for Various Weight-Adjusted MSAFP MoM After Twins, Anencephaly, and Erroneous Gestational Dates Have Been Detected by Ultrasound*

| | Population and Prevalence | | | |
| | Black, DC Area 3/10,000 | | White, DC Area 6.5/10,000 | |
MoM	OSB (1/Risk)	OSB + VWD (1/Risk)	OSB (1/Risk)	OSB + VWD (1/Risk)
16–18 Weeks				
1.5	5495	2748	2607	1765
2.0	1692	972	782	580
2.1	1245	738	573	436
2.2	985	594	453	349
2.3	815	497	374	291
2.4	695	428	319	249
2.5	606	375	278	218
2.6	469	294	216	170
2.7	383	242	177	140
2.8	323	205	149	119
2.9	280	178	130	103
3.0	247	158	114	91
3.1	199	127	92	73
3.2	167	106	77	61
3.3	144	91	66	53
3.4	126	80	58	46
3.5	112	71	52	41
4.0	56	35	26	20
4.5	29	18	14	11
5.0	16	10	7	6
19–21 Weeks				
1.5	2327	1630	1071	895
2.0	799	561	369	310
2.1	599	424	275	229
2.2	479	341	219	182
2.3	399	285	182	151
2.4	342	245	156	128
2.5	299	214	136	112
2.6	230	163	105	85
2.7	187	132	86	69
2.8	158	110	73	58
2.9	136	95	63	50
3.0	120	83	55	44
3.1	95	65	44	34

Continued

Table 12.8 *Continued*

Population and Prevalence

MoM	Black, DC Area 3/10,000		White, DC Area 6.5/10,000	
	OSB (1/Risk)	OSB + VWD (1/Risk)	OSB (1/Risk)	OSB + VWD (1/Risk)
3.2	79	53	37	28
3.3	67	45	32	24
3.4	58	39	28	21
3.5	52	34	24	18
4.0	24	15	11	8
4.5	12	7	6	4
5.0	6	5	4	3

*Example: Black patient in DC area with MoM = 2.6 at 16 weeks has 1/469 risk of OSB and 1/294 combined risk of OSB and VWD.

Reprinted with permission from Adams MJ Jr, Windham GC, James LM, et al. Risk reporting of maternal serum alpha-fetoprotein (AFP) concentrations. Atlanta: U.S. Department of Health and Human Services, 1985.

these risks in an update to their monograph that accounted for decreased risks of OSB and a slight increase in risk for VWD after ultrasonography had ruled out twin pregnancy, anencephaly, and mistaken gestational age (14).

Early investigators estimated that screening in this way in the United Kingdom should detect nearly 90% of anencephalic fetuses, and nearly 80% of those with OSB, at a cost of identifying about 3% of normal pregnancies incorrectly as at risk (see discussion above). The lower the frequency of NTDs in the population screened (as in the United States), the lower will be the risk of true abnormality with an abnormal test result (12). But the sensitivity of such a program of prospective screening should be just as high in the United States. Table 12.9 summarizes three series of MSAFP screening in the United States (3). Table 12.10 addresses the significance of an elevated AFAFP in the United States in two series (3).

The state of California began a mandatory counseling program requiring that every pregnant woman have an opportunity to participate voluntarily in routine MSAFP screening, followed by the offer of more specific testing when indicated. We hope much data useful for describing risks in the U.S. population will come from this project, which began in April, 1986. Table 12.11 reveals preliminary results from the first year of screening in the California state program (through April 30, 1987) (16).

These results are preliminary and represent the largest single series to date. Over 200,000 women accepted screening (over 60% of all pregnancies in the state), and initial analysis suggests that sensitivity for NTD detection was 70%.

For cases in which the elevated MSAFP remains unexplained, the test may be considered a nonspecific screening tool for "high-risk" pregnancy. Thomas and Blakemore recently provided an extensive review of causes of abnormal MSAFP levels without a fetal NTD or VWD (17). Brock et al. reported an association between premature delivery and small-for-gestational-age infants and unexplained elevated MSAFP (18, 19). Purdie et al. found an association between unexplained elevated MSAFP and both

Table 12.9 Experience in Three Large United States Studies with Maternal Serum AFP Testing

	Macri & Weiss	Burton et al	Milunsky & Alpert
No. women screened	17,703	12,084	21,000
No. open NTD total	22	18	25
No. open NTD detected by screening program	20	15	20*
Women with elevated serum AFP (%)	7.1†	3.7‡	1.2
Women with repeat elevated serum AFP (%)	3.9	2.1	
Women requiring ultrasound (%)	3.7	2.2	
Women requiring amniocentesis (%)	2.1	1.2	0.3
Women with amniocentesis who had fetus with NTD (%)	5.5	10.0	13.2§

*Two diagnosed by ultrasound rather than serum AFP.
†Cut-off used 2 x median for given gestational age.
‡Cut-off used 2.5 x median for given gestational age.
§32% of women undergoing amniocentesis had a fetus with a major malformation or fetal death.

Reprinted with permission from Main DM, Mennuti MT. Neural tube defects: issues in prenatal diagnosis and counselling. Obstet Gynecol 1986;67:1

Table 12.10 Significance of an Elevated Amniotic Fluid AFP Result in Two Large United States Series

	Milunsky	Crandall	Crandall
Total sample size	20,000	34,000	34,000
Cut-off for abnormal	≥3 SD above mean	≥3 SD above mean	≥5 SD above mean
Elevated AFP (%)	1.7	0.7	0.4
No. open NTD diagnosed by AFP alone	136	69	59
No. open NTD missed by AFP alone	0	3	13
No. other abnormalities associated with elevated AFP	90	66	64
No. normal fetuses with elevated AFP	108	90	9
True false positives—no. normal infants aborted after all tests*	11[†]	3[††]	2[††]
No. open NTD missed after all tests	0	0	0

*Additional tests performed in selected cases included amniotic fluid acetylcholinesterase, ultrasonic evaluation of the fetus, and repeat amniocentesis for AFP testing.

[†]Only two of 11 cases would not have been diagnosed by current techniques including acetylcholinesterase testing. Several of the 11 were terminated without further testing because the mother did not want the pregnancy. Others involved errors in tube labeling, AFP measurement, and ultrasonic evaluation.

[††]Grossly normal but microscopic autopsy of kidneys was not performed.

Reprinted with permission from Main DM, Mennuti MT. Neural tube defects: issues in prenatal diagnosis and counselling. Obstet Gynecol 1986; 67:1.

Table 12.11 Preliminary Results from the First Year of the California MSAFP Screening Program

Fetal Abnormality	High MSAFP Value	Low MSAFP Value	History	Total
Anencephaly	63	1	5	69
Spina bifida	32	0	0	32
Encephalocoele	10	0	0	10
Ventral wall defect	40	0	0	40
Other physical defects	NR	NR	NR	35
Trisomy 21	0	17	0	17
Other chromosomal defects	NR	NR	NR	30
Total				223

Note: NR = not reported.

Reprinted with permission from Anderson RL. Maternal serum alpha-fetoprotein: more than a screening test for neural tube defects. In: Parer JT, ed. Antepartum and intrapartum management. Philadelphia: Lea & Febiger, 1989.

MSAFP <2 MoM, 89 with MSAFP between 2 and 4 MoM, and 10 with MSAFP ≥ 4 MoM. The total perinatal mortality increased from 32.6/1,000, to 73.3/1,000, and to 400/1,000, respectively.

Some might ask if amniocentesis is necessary, or if sonography might supplant amniocentesis for evaluation of elevated MSAFP. Table 12.12 outlines results from three series, illustrating the point that "routine" sonography in a low-prevalence population had poor sensitivity (40%)(24). The table also illustrates the value of experience and higher-

Table 12.12 Accuracy of Ultrasound in the Prenatal Diagnosis of Spina Bifida

	n	Prevalence (%)	Sensitivity (%)	Specificity (%)	PPV	NPV
Allen et al.	374	2.1	87	99	87	99
Persson et al.	10.147	0.1	40	100	100	99
Roberts et al.	1261	1.4	30	96	92	99
Roberts et al.	1991	1.7	80	99	80	99

Note: PPV = positive predictive value; NPV = negative predictive value.

Reprinted with permission from Romero R, Pilu G, Jeanty P, et al. Prenatal diagnosis of congenital anomalies. Norwalk CT: Appleton & Lange, 1988.

intrauterine growth retardation and placental abruption (20). Walters et al. related unexplained MSAFP elevation to later development of preeclampsia (21).

Ghosh et al. recommended a cutoff of five multiples of the singleton median for assessment of twin gestations for occurrence of an NTD since all 11 of their patients with twins discordant for NTD had MSAFP levels higher than this (22). Redford and Whitfield reported that with elevations in MSAFP over 2 MoM for singletons, the frequency of occurrence of low birthweight, prematurity, and perinatal mortality in twin gestations correlated with the level of MSAFP elevation (23). They listed 46 twin gestations with

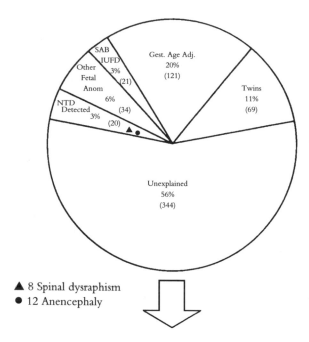

▲ 8 Spinal dysraphism
● 12 Anencephaly

Amniocentesis Offered:

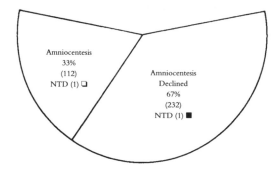

☐ MS-AFP 3.6 MoM (risk 2.8%), Adj. risk 0.28%, elevated
AF-AFP and ACHE, rescan showed L-S open spine defect
■ MS-AFP 7.7 MoM (risk > 10%), Adj. risk > 1%, declined
amnio, Spont Ab at 21 wks gest. Autopsy showed sacral open spine
defect.

Figure 12.7   Results of ultrasound (top) and amniocentesis for
609 patients referred for evaluation because of elevated MSAFP
values. IUFD = intrauterine fetal death; NTD = neural tube
defect; Adj = adjusted; MoM = multiples of the median; AF =
amniotic fluid; ACHE = acetylcholinesterase; L-S = lumbosacral;
Ab = abortion.

resolution equipment, as the two time periods reported by
Roberts (1977–1980 versus 1980–1983) varied greatly in
sensitivity (25). Based partially on assessments of similar
data, Richards et al. counseled their patients with elevated
MSAFP that a normal sonographic evaluation including
"optimal" views of the fetus decreased the risk of NTD by
90% (26). Based on this counseling, two thirds of their 609
high-risk patients declined amniocentesis. Their sensitivity
for anencephaly was 100% and for OSB was 80%, for a
combined sensitivity of 91%. Both the specificity and positive predictive values were 100%. The negative predictive
value was 99.66%. Figure 12.7 graphically depicts the
results of their experience.

The recognition of cranial signs associated with OSB
facilitates a higher detection rate using ultrasound without
amniocentesis. The fetus afflicted with OSB usually has
some or most of the following abnormalities: small BPD;
small head circumference; ventriculomegaly; concave frontal bones ("lemon sign"); obliteration of the cisterna magna;
diminution in size of and abnormal forward–curving of the
cerebellum ("banana sign") (27–31).

Two recent publications have reached differing conclusions on the advisability of omitting amniocentesis when
no abnormality is seen on ultrasound. Nadel et al. (32) used
a malformation surveillance program and a retrospective records search to identify all significant anomalies among 51
fetuses imaged in their facility without resorting to amniocentesis. Platt et al. (33), based on data from the California
MSAFP Program, argue that competent sonographers participating in a rigidly controlled large screening program
can miss OSB in the fetus of a patient with a known high
MSAFP. From January 1988 through June 1990, more than
640,000 pregnancies had MSAFP screening performed.
Approximately 92% of the patients with abnormal values
had follow-up at one of the 20 state-authorized prenatal
diagnostic centers. Within this group, 161 cases of spina
bifida were identified. Ultrasound identified 148 (92%) of
the fetuses with defects, although some also had amniocentesis. There were 13 (8%) cases of spina bifida undetected
by the initial sonogram, although repeat scanning after
detection of elevated amniotic fluid AFP identified 10
lesions. There were three lesions that remained undetected
until after birth. In two of these cases, patients declined

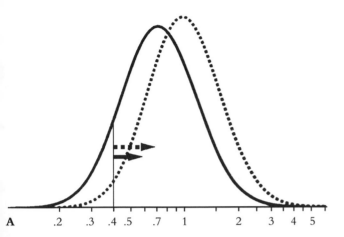

Figure 12.8 Distribution of MSAFP (as MoM) in Down syndrome (solid line) and unaffected pregnancies (dotted line). Arrows indicate the most probable direction of repeat sample with an initial MoM of 0.4 (light vertical line).

Reproduced with permission from Knight GJ, Palomaki GE, Haddow JE. Use of maternal serum alpha-fetoprotein measurements to screen for Down's syndrome. Clin Obstet Gynecol 1988;31:306.

amniocentesis after ultrasound failed to detect anomalies. In the third, redating of the pregnancy based on ultrasound measurements corrected the MSAFP to a normal value for the assumed gestational age.

A recent development in MSAFP screening programs is the discovery of an increased risk of fetal trisomy, especially trisomy 21, among women with low MSAFP values. In 1984, Merkatz et al. reported retrospectively that, in 41 evaluable pregnancies with proven trisomic outcomes, the midtrimester MSAFP MoM had been at or above 1.0 in only five (34). The distribution of MoMs from affected pregnancies was significantly lower than that from a matched control population. Others have reported similar findings from both retrospective and prospective investigations, and many centers use this information for counseling women under the age of 35 of increased risks of trisomy, with the offer of amniocentesis.

Unlike testing for NTDs, a repeated sample is not helpful if the first is low. Figure 12.8 illustrates this principle. To modify a gravida's age-specfic risk of Down syndrome based on a low level of MSAFP, a likelihood ratio is calculated, which is then applied to her age-specific risk

prior to testing (Figure 12.9). To test this concept prospectively, Palomaki, Williams, and Haddow designed, coordinated, analyzed, and reported a collaborative study of Down syndrome screening in women under age 35 (35).

During 1986–1987, the collaborative group screened 77,273 pregnancies from eight cooperating centers, using methodologies previously published (36–38). Based on initial screening, 4.7% of the population qualified for further assessment because of a calculated midtrimester risk of Down syndrome of 1:270, equal to that of an unscreened 35-year-old gravida. Corrections (predominantly sonographic adjustment of estimated gestational age) eliminated 40% from further consideration, and 76% of the remaining 2.7% of the original population consented to amniocentesis. Amniocentesis and karyotype analysis identified 18 cases of Down syndrome, four of trisomy 18, one partial trisomy 7, one mosaic 45,X/46,XX, and one 47,XYY. Among those who declined amniocentesis, three more Down syndrome births resulted. Thus, within the total original population, 25% of the Down syndrome births were identified at a net

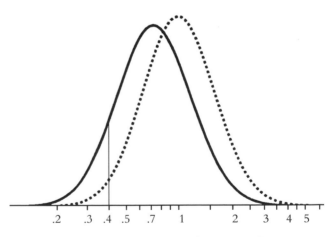

Figure 12.9 Distribution of MSAFP values (MoM) for Down syndrome (solid line) and unaffected pregnancies (dotted line) with light line at 0.4 MoM to demonstrate method of calculating likelihood ratio. Likelihood ratio for 0.4 MoM is vertical distance from the baseline to solid line divided by the vertical distance to the dotted line.

Reproduced with permission from Knight GJ, Palomaki GE, Haddow JE. Use of maternal serum alpha-fetoprotein measurements to screen for Down's syndrome. Clin Obstet Gynecol 1988;31:306.

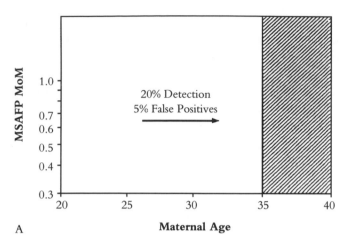

A

Figure 12.10 (**A**) Women at increased risk for carrying a Down syndrome fetus (hatched area) as defined by maternal age > 35 years.

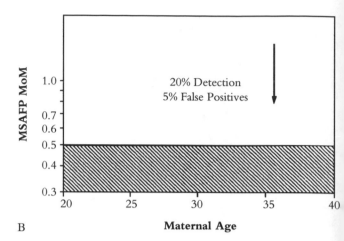

B

Figure 12.10 (**B**) Women at increased risk for carrying a Down syndrome fetus (hatched area) as defined by MSAFP MoM <0.5.

"cost" of proposal of amniocentesis to 2.7% of the gravidas. In other terms, one case of Down syndrome was identified per 89 amniocenteses (95% CI=1:64 to 1:178), or one case of chromosomal aberration per 64 amniocenteses (95% CI=1:48 to 1:110) (38).

General estimates are that amniocentesis among women over 35 (5% of pregnancies historically, but this may be rising) may identify 20% of fetuses with trisomy 21, and MSAFP screening may identify another 20%. (Figures 12.10(*A*), (*B*), and (*C*)) (7). As of early 1993, the American Society of Human Genetics had not completely embraced this concept (15). Part of the significant reluctance to recommend these techniques for wide application is that MSAFP test kits have been optimized and approved for labeling for use only for NTD screening (high values, as opposed to low values). Again, the California experience should be very helpful within a short time.

The realization that the distributions of MSAFP levels differed between aneuploid and euploid pregnancies led to investigations of other serum markers. In 1987, Bogart et al. published their findings of higher mean human chorionic gonadotropin (hCG) levels among Down syndrome pregnancies than among normal control pregnancies (39). In 1988, Canick et al. reported lower-than-normal levels of maternal serum unconjugated estriol in 22 pregnancies of Down syndrome fetuses in the United States, while on the next page of the same issue, Wald et al. reported similar

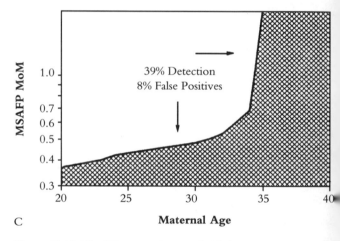

C

Figure 12.10 (**C**) Women at increased risk for carrying a Down syndrome fetus (hatched area) as defined by a combination of MSAFP and maternal age to identify women with risk equal to or greater than that of a 35-year-old woman.

Reproduced with permission from Knight GJ, Palomaki GE, Haddow JE. Use of maternal serum alpha-fetoprotein measurements to screen for Down's syndrome. Clin Obstet Gynecol 1988;31:306.

findings among 77 pregnancies in the United Kingdom (40, 41). Also in 1988, the same two groups combined to describe a statistical algorithm combining maternal age and MoM values for maternal serum α-fetoprotein, hCG, and estriol to predict risk for Down syndrome (42).

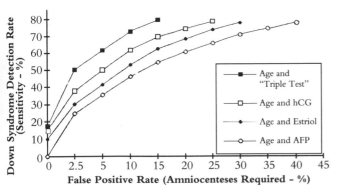

Figure 12.11 Combined age and biochemical screening for Down syndrome (Receiver Operator Characteristic Curves).

This method promised to identify 60% of Down syndrome fetuses at a cost of offering amniocentesis for diagnosis to 5% of pregnant women (Figure 12.11). This figure of 5% false-positive rate is similar to the currently accepted method of offering amniocentesis to all gravidas over 35 years of age at delivery, but should identify two to three times as many Down syndrome fetuses. Estimates of false-positive rates and detection rates for simply using maternal age over 35 as a screening tool range from 5%–7.5% and 20%–35%, respectively, depending upon the demographics of the population (7, 43). Interest in this area is great, and there has been an immediate explosion in related publications (44–50).

Three recent publications have reported prospective trials of triple analyte maternal serum screening in combination with maternal age to predict the risk of Down syndrome in the second trimester (51–53). None of the studies had 100% prospective ascertainment of pregnancy outcome among pregnancies with normal screening values, but all studies reported methods used to ascertain all affected cases "missed" by the screening protocol. The cutoff level that indicates further action is an important consideration in any screening program. The mid-trimester risk of Down syndrome in a 35-year-old is about 1:270. This is the cutoff risk used by Phillips et al. (52) and by the New England Regional Genetics Group Prenatal Collaborative Study of Down Syndrome Screening (35). The mid-trimester risk of Down syndrome in a 37-year-old is about 1:190. This is the cutoff risk used by Cheng et al. (53). Haddow et al.

(51) used 1:270 for patients in Rhode Island, and 1:190 for patients in Maine. They noted that using a cutoff of 1:270 in the Rhode Island patients resulted in a 4% increase in detection rate (one case) at a cost of an additional 192 amniocenteses to find that one case. Table 12.13 reveals important details of the efficacy of these trials. Haddow et al. counted as "detected" three additional cases of Down syndrome discovered only after birth. One mother had refused amniocentesis, and two patients had been reclassified as "low risk" after sonographic evaluation and adjustment of assumed gestational age. Additionally, Haddow's detection rate uses a theoretical calculated birth prevalence as the denominator. In all of the referenced works some methods of estimating the true birth prevalence was used. The marked disparity in birth prevalence among the studies is unexplained as of this writing, one month after Cheng's publication.

Phillips et al. suggested screening might be less effective in a population with a larger proportion of younger patients, as two of their three undetected cases occurred in women age 22 and younger. Cheng et al. (53), supported this concept. The two undetected cases in their study were in women under age 30.

The efficacy of the combination of maternal age and serum screening tests for Down syndrome has not achieved universal acceptance, and Macri specifically decries the inclusion of estriol as a component of what some have termed the "triple test" of serum markers. An informal written debate on the topic appeared in the newsletter of the National Society of Genetic Counselors, Inc. (Summer 1990; Vol. 12, No. 2), with Canick and Knight arguing the pro and Macri stating the con. Macri avers that, in his retrospectively assayed data base of serum samples from mothers carrying Down syndrome fetuses, the median MoM was 0.99 and, further, that some assays may even result in higher-than-expected values in affected pregnancies (54). Canick and Knight retort that the range of published median maternal serum estriol values among affected pregnancies is 0.5 to 0.99, with a consensus median of 0.74 MoM. They note that this is a similar circumstance to the reported range of medians for MSAFP, with one published study also finding no association between MSAFP and Down syndrome. The consensus median for MSAFP is clearly

Table 12.13 Comparison of Prospective Studies of Prenatal Serum Screening for Down Syndrome in the Mid-Trimester

	New England	Haddow	Phillips	Cheng
No. Screened	77,273	25,207	9,530	7,718
Risk Cutoff	1:270	1:190	1:274	1:195
Positive screen (%)	4.7	6.1	7.2	8
Offered amniocentesis (%)	2.7	3.8	3.2	6
Amniocentesis performed (%)	2.1	3.0	*2.2	4.1
Cases of Down syndrome identified	18	20	4	20
No. of amniocenteses per Down syndrome case identified	89	38	54	16
Down syndrome birth prevalence†	9.32	14.28	7.35	28.50
Detection rate (%)	25	56	57	91

*214 samplings: 212 amniocenteses, 2 chorionic villus sampling.
†Based on 10,000 screenings.

low, and they opine that the same will hold true for estriol.

If currently active prospective studies of screening for Down syndrome pregnancies confirm some combination of maternal age and serum markers as effective, some significant cautions remain. Canick and Knight forecast that amniocentesis for only those women over 35 who are high risk by serum markers would identify 85% of Down syndrome fetuses in only 20% of the gravidas in this age group. Thus, a reduction of amniocenteses of 80% among gravidas over age 35 could be realized at a cost of missing only 15% of the Down syndrome-affected pregnancies in this age group. But the patient over age 35 with screening results suggesting low risk for Down syndrome must realize that an amniocentesis will rule out *all* major chromosomal aberrations (not just trisomy 21), while a normal serum screening result will only reduce *her statistical risk of Down syndrome* to that of an unscreened gravida under age 35. Women over 35 are also at increased risk for other significant chromosomal aberrations that would escape detection if the patients were to forego amniocentesis because of a reassuring serum marker test statistically reducing the risk of trisomy 21.

Current protocols recommending consideration for chorionic villus sampling (CVS) or amniocentesis among women over 35 acknowledge the increasing genetic burden for other aneuploidies than just trisomy 21 in association with advancing maternal age. The only aneuploidies thus far found to be associated with abnormal levels of these serum markers have been trisomy 21 and trisomy 18. In fact, the specific case that initiated the Merkatz review was a trisomy 18 (34). In all the studies of serum screening, other karyotypic abnormalities have been observed among the offspring of mothers with both positive and negative screening results. Trisomy 18 is the next most common autosomal trisomy among liveborn. Since the median hCG MoM among Trisomy 18 fetuses is 0.3, they often are not identified if high hCG is included in the Down screening algorithm. But Palomaki et al. (55), have offered a fixed screening protocol for Trisomy 18 that has permitted them to screen 20,000 pregnancies and detect about 3/4 of the Trisomy 18 fetuses (6 detected). Their cutoffs are currently MSAFP $\leq$ 0.75 MoM, Estriol $\leq$ 0.6 MoM, and hCG $\leq$ 0.55 MoM.

For the moment, it is sobering to realize that the median for hCG is low for trisomy 18 pregnancies, versus the higher median for hCG found in trisomy 21 pregnancies. The effect of this difference would be to fail to identify trisomy 18 pregnancies using hCG in the algorithm to screen for trisomy 21 because decreasing the number of amniocenteses for gravidas (of any age) based on a low level of hCG (decreased risk of trisomy 21) would decrease the sensitivity of screening for trisomy 18. A review of published series of aneuploidies associated with low MSAFP finds many have been trisomy 18. Large prospective studies are necessary to validate these concepts, and we hope that important new data will result soon from such studies as the California project.

References

1. Romero R, Pilu G, Jeanty P, et al. Prenatal diagnosis of congenital anomalies. Norwalk, CT: Appleton & Lange, 1988.

2. Greenberg F, James LM, Oakley GP Jr. Estimates of birth prevalence rates of spina bifida in the United States from computer-generated maps. Am J Obstet Gynecol 1983; 145:570.

3. Main DM, Mennuti MT. Neural tube defects: issues in prenatal diagnosis and counselling. Obstet Gynecol 1986; 67:1.

4. Brock DJH, Sutcliffe RG. Alpha-fetoprotein in the antenatal diagnosis of anencephaly and spina bifida. Lancet 1972; 2:197.

5. Habib A. Maternal serum alpha-fetoprotein: its value in antenatal diagnosis of genetic disease and in obstetrical-gynecological care. Acta Obstet Gynecol Scand Suppl 1977;61:14.

6. Report of the U.K. Collaborative Study on alpha-fetoprotein in relation to neural-tube defects. Maternal serum alpha-fetoprotein measurement in antenatal screening for anencephaly and spina bifida in early pregnancy. Lancet 1977; 1:1323.

7. Knight GJ, Palomaki GE, Haddow JE. Use of maternal serum alpha-fetoprotein measurements to screen for Down's syndrome. Clin Obstet Gynecol 1988;31:306.

8. Wald NJ. The interpretation of AFP values and the effect of AFP assay performance on screening efficacy. In: National Center for Health Care Technology. Maternal serum alpha-fetoprotein: issues in the prenatal screening and diagnosis of neural tube defects. Office of Health Research, Statistics, and Technology. Summary of Proceedings, July 1980.

9. Second Report of the U.K. Collaborative Study on alpha-fetoprotein in relation to neural-tube defects. Amniotic fluid alpha-fetoprotein measurement in antenatal diagnosis of anencephaly and open spina bifida in early pregnancy. Lancet 1979;2:651.

10. American Society of Human Genetics. Policy statement for maternal serum alpha-fetoprotein screening programs and quality control for laboratories performing maternal serum and amniotic fluid alpha-fetoprotein assays. Am J Hum Genet 1987;40:75–82.

11. American College of Obstetricians and Gynecologists. Alpha-fetoprotein. Technical Bulletin Number 154. Washington, DC: AGOG, April 1991.

12. Adams MJ, Windham GC, James LM, et al. Clinical interpretation of maternal serum alpha-fetoprotein concentrations. Am J Obstet Gynecol 1984;148:241.

13. Crandall BF, Lebherz TB, Schroth PC, Matsumoto M. Alpha-fetoprotein concentrates in maternal serum: relation to race and body weight. Clin Chem 1983;29:531.

14. Adams MJ Jr, Windham GC, James LM, et al. Risk reporting of maternal serum alpha-fetoprotein (AFP) concentrations. Atlanta: U.S. Department of Health and Human Services, 1985.

15. Garver KL. Update on MSAFP policy statement from the American Society of Human Genetics. Am J Hum Genet 1989;45:332.

16. Anderson RL. Maternal serum alpha-fetoprotein: more than a screening test for neural tube defects. In: Parer JT, ed. Antepartum and intrapartum management. Philadelphia: Lea & Febiger, 1989.

17. Thomas RL, Blakemore KJ. Evaluation of elevations in maternal serum alpha-fetoprotein: a review. Obstet Gynecol Surv 1990;45:269.

18. Brock DJH, Barron L, Raab GM. The potential of mid-trimester maternal plasma alpha-fetoprotein measurement in predicting infants of low birth weight. Br J Obstet Gynaecol 1980;87:582.

19. Brock DJH, Barron L, Watt M, et al. Maternal plasma alpha-fetoprotein and low birthweight: a prospective study throughout pregnancy. Br J Obstet Gynaecol 1982;89:348.

20. Purdie DW, Young JL, Guthrie KA, et al. Fetal growth achievement and elevated maternal serum alpha-fetoprotein. Br J Obstet Gynaecol 1983;90:433.

21. Walters BNJ, Lao T, Smith V. Alpha-fetoprotein elevation and proteinuric pre-eclampsia. Br J Obstet Gynaecol 1985; 92:341.

22. Ghosh A, Woo JSK, Rawlinson HA, Ferguson Smith MA. Prognostic significance of raised serum alphafetoprotein levels in twin pregnancies. Br J Obstet Gynaecol 1982; 89:817.

23. Redford DHA, Whitfield CR. Maternal serum alpha-fetoprotein in twin pregnancies uncomplicated by neural tube defect. Am J Obstet Gynecol 1985;152:550.

24. Persson PH, Kullander S, Gennser G, et al. Screening for fetal malformations using ultrasound and measurements of alpha-fetoprotein in maternal serum. Br Med J 1983;286:747.

25. Roberts CJ, Hibbard BM, Roberts EE, et al. Diagnostic effectiveness of ultrasound in detection of neural tube defect. The South Wales experience of 2509 scans (1977–1982) in high-risk mothers. Lancet 1983;2:1068.

26. Richards DS, Seeds JW, Katz VL. Elevated maternal serum

alpha-fetoprotein with normal ultrasound: is amniocentesis always appropriate? A review of 26,069 screened patients. Obstet Gynecol 1988;71:203.

27. Nicolaides KH, Gabbe SG, Campbell S, Guidetti R. Ultrasound screening for spina bifida: cranial and cerebellar signs. Lancet 1986;ii:72.

28. Campbell J, Gilbert WM, Nicolaides KH, Campbell S. Ultrasound screening for spina bifida: cranial and cerebellar signs in a high-risk population. Obstet Gynecol 1987; 70:247.

29. Thaigarajah S, Henke J, Hogge WA, et al. Early diagnosis of spina bifida: the value of cranial ultrasound markers. Obstet Gynecol 1990;76:54.

30. Pilu G, Romero R, Reece EA, et al. Subnormal cerebellum in fetuses with a spina bifida. Am J Obstet Gynecol 1988; 158:1052.

31. Goldstein RB, Podrasky AE, Filly RA, Callen PW. Effacement of the fetal cisterna magna in association with myelomeningocele. Radiology 1989;172:409.

32. Nadel AS, Green JK, Holmes LB, Frigoletto FD, Benacerraf BR. Absence of need for amniocentesis in patients with elevated levels of maternal serum alpha-fetoprotein and normal ultrasonographic examinations. N Engl J Med 1990;323:557.

33. Platt LD, Feuchtbaum L, Filly R, Lustig L, Simon M, Cunningham GC. The California maternal serum alpha-fetoprotein screening program: the role of ultrasonography in the detection of spina bifida. Am J Obstet Gynecol 1992;166:1328.

34. Merkatz IR, Nitowsky HM, Macri JN, Johnson WE. An association between low maternal serum alpha-fetoprotein and fetal chromosomal abnormalities. Am J Obstet Gynecol 1984; 148:887.

35. New England Regional Genetics Group Prenatal Collaborative Study of Down Syndrome Screening. Combining maternal serum alpha-fetoprotein measurements and age to screen for Down syndrome in pregnant women under age 35. Am J Obstet Gynecol 1989;160:575.

36. Palomaki GE, Knight GJ, Kloza EM, Haddow JE. Maternal weight adjustment and low serum alpha-fetoprotein values. Lancet 1985;1:468.

37. Erratum. Lancet 1985;1:1281.

38. Palomaki GE, Haddow JE. Maternal serum alpha-fetoprotein, age, and Down syndrome risk. Am J Obstet Gynecol 1987; 156:460.

39. Bogart MH, Pandian MR, Jones OW. Abnormal maternal serum chorionic gonadotropin levels in pregnancies with fetal chromosome abnormalities. Prenat Diag 1987; 7:623.

40. Canick JA, Knight GJ, Palomaki GE, et al. Low second trimester maternal serum unconjugated oestriol in pregnancies with Down's syndrome. Br J Obstet Gynaecol 1988; 95:330.

41. Wald NJ, Cuckle HS, Densem JW, et al: Maternal serum unconjugated oestriol as an antenatal screening test for Down's syndrome. Br J Obstet Gynaecol 1988;95:334.

42. Wald NJ, Cuckle HS, Densem JW, et al. Maternal serum screening for Down's syndrome in early pregnancy. Br Med J 1988;297:883.

43. Donnai D, Andrews T. Screening for Down's syndrome. Br Med J 1988;297:887.

44. Bogart MH, Golbus MS, Sorg ND, et al. Human chorionic gonadotropin levels in pregnancies with aneuploid fetuses. Prenat Diagn 1989;9:379.

45. DelJunco D, Greenberg F, Damule A, et al. Statistical analysis of maternal age, maternal serum alpha-fetoprotein, β human chorionic gonadotropin, and unconjugated estriol for Down syndrome screening for midtrimester. Am J Hum Genet 1989;45:A257.

46. Fisher RA, Suppnick CK, Peabody CT, et al. Maternal serum chorionic gonadotropin, unconjugated estriol, and alpha-fetoprotein in Down syndrome pregnancies. Am J Hum Genet 1989;45:A259.

47. Kelly JC, Lee J, Petrocik E, et al. Prenatal Down syndrome screening using a combinational analysis of maternal age, serum alpha fetoprotein and serum human chorionic gonadotropin. Am J Hum Genet 1989;45:A262.

48. Norgaard-Pederson B, Larsen SO, Arends J, et al. Maternal serum markers in screening for Down syndrome. Clin Genet 1990;37:35.

49. Osathanondh R, Canick JA, Abell KB, et al. Second trimester screening for trisomy 21. Lancet 1989;2:52.

50. Suchy SF, Yeager MT. Maternal serum human chorionic gonadotropin screening for Down syndrome in women under 35. Am J Hum Genet 1989;45:A271.

51. Haddow JE, Palomaki GE, Knight GJ, et al. Prenatal screening for Down Syndrome with use of maternal serum markers. N Engl J Med 1992;237:588.

52. Phillips OP, Elias S, Shulman LP, Andersen RN, Morgan CD, Simpson JL. Maternal serum screening for fetal down syndrome in women less than 35 years of age using alpha-fetoprotein, hCG, and unconjugated estriol: a prospective 2-year study. Obstet Gynecol 1992;80:353.

53. Cheng EY, Luthy DA, Zebelman AM, Williams MA, Lieppman RE, Hickok DE. A prospective evaluation of a second-trimester screening test for fetal Down Syndrome using maternal serum alpha-fetoprotein, hCG, and unconjugated estriol. Obstet Gynecol 1993;81:72.

54. Macri JN, Kasturi RV, Krantz DA, et al. Maternal serum Down syndrome screening: unconjugated estriol is not useful. Am J Obstet Gynecol 1990;162:672.

55. Palomaki GE, Knight GJ, Haddow JE, Canick JA, Saller DN, Panizza DS. Prospective intervention trial of a screening protocol to identify fetal Trisomy-18 using maternal serum alpha-fetoprotein, unconjugated oestriol, and human chorionic gonadotropin. Prenat Diag 1992;12:925.

13

Antenatal Diagnosis of Inborn Errors of Metabolism

William L. Nyhan, M.D., Ph.D.

ANTENATAL diagnosis of genetic disease has opened an exciting new chapter in perinatal medicine. This common ground for the obstetrician, geneticist, and biochemist represents one of the most significant advances in pragmatic clinical genetics and is particularly appealing as a vigorous and positive approach to management of genetic disease. The means of making genetic diagnosis in the human fetus, following amniocentesis or chorionic villus sampling, has become established practice.

The more than 3,000 disorders now classified as genetic in origin account for a significant proportion of human morbidity and at least 25% of hospitalizations in children. The possibility of bearing a child with congenital malformation or mental retardation is a prominent fear among pregnant women and even among prospective parents contemplating pregnancy. Probably the most common reaction is to attempt to suppress these fears. Until recently, the physician's only role has been to reassure the patient, but this is changing. It is no longer true that nothing can be done, and it is unrealistic to "reassure" a mother who has previously delivered a child with Down syndrome or cystic fibrosis or Tay-Sachs disease or hemophilia, for example. Most physicians would like to be able to do something more, and, for many genetically determined conditions, this is now possible.

Fortunately, public awareness and interest in genetic disease is at an unprecedented high. Patients and families are less likely to view genetic concerns as "skeletons in the closet" and are seeking counsel. In the past, genetic counseling has been a relatively passive, highly statistical business. Generally, parents known to be at risk have sought a statistical appraisal of their chances of having a child with a particular anomaly. Then, depending on their reaction to the statistics and on how good a listener or how brave a gambler each was, they would decide whether or not to avoid future pregnancy.

This is still a big part of the practice of genetics today, but it represents a passive approach, and geneticists are now finding many ways in which they can undertake more active intervention. These include treating a number of genetic diseases such as galactosemia or agammaglobulinemia, screening newborns for metabolic diseases such as phenylketonuria (PKU), and detecting heterozygotes as in

Tay-Sachs disease. The most active approach to genetic practice and the one that has most caught the imagination of the public is intrauterine diagnosis.

Amniocentesis

Transabdominal amniocentesis for detecting genetic disease is usually carried out between 15 and 18 weeks' gestation. The usual goal is to obtain viable cells to culture the supply needed for a specific diagnosis in time to permit intervention with therapeutic abortion if the diagnosis is positive. It may be carried out earlier when the goal is to obtain fluid for direct chemical examination. We have conducted prenatal diagnosis as early as 12 weeks in this fashion, which makes the procedure competitive in time with chorionic villus sampling, especially if it is necessary to culture the chorionic villus cells.

Amniotic fluid is 98%–99% water. It is the exfoliated fetal cells it contains that we are usually concerned with, and they must be grown in culture prior to analysis; however, an increasing number of conditions can be detected by the direct analysis of a unique metabolite in the amniotic fluid, and techniques of recombinant DNA are sufficiently sensitive that they may be used on uncultured amniocytes. The likelihood that amniotic fluid cells will be viable and will grow in tissue culture is greater early in pregnancy than later, when amniocentesis to detect Rh incompatibility or assess fetal maturity is done. Complications are also fewer. However, it is not advisable to place the patient at risk at a time when the likelihood of obtaining fluid is small; in our experience, failure to obtain fluid is fairly common before 14 weeks. A 5-inch, 22-gauge spinal needle with a stylet is usually employed. Once in place, as determined by a free flow of fluid, the stylet is removed, a plastic syringe is attached, and the fluid is withdrawn. Strict asepsis is required for the protection of both mother and fetus, as well as for protection of the amniotic cells. Cells in culture, especially the few that grow following amniocentesis, are highly susceptible to infection, and aseptic technique should be observed during transfer of the fluid and all procedures it undergoes. Initially, a standard amniocentesis took a 10-mL sample, but it is now routine to withdraw at least 20–30 mL.

We have learned to be very careful about logistics once fluid is obtained. In our center, the specimen is hand-carried to the laboratory by the nurse assigned to the amniocentesis program who has attended the patient throughout the procedure. Once in the laboratory, the sample is centrifuged and the supernatant fluid is removed, tested when indicated, and frozen. The cells are suspended in fetal calf serum, placed in small plastic petri dishes, and covered with microscope cover slips. A nutrient tissue culture medium containing fetal calf serum and antibiotics is added, and the plates are put into incubators in a carbon dioxide-rich atmosphere at 37°C. The cells are fed by changing the medium every other day. It is important to emphasize that this type of farming takes a "green thumb."

Not everyone can successfully grow amniotic cells or even cells from skin or blood. Therefore, it is important in planning for a prenatal diagnosis to arrange to have the cells sent to a laboratory with a high yield of viable cultures. For added assurance, we divide each sample in half and culture each half in a different laboratory, on a different floor, in case of incubator failures or accidents. When a culture does not grow, the alternative is to call the patient back and obtain more fluid, and it is wise to explain these possibilities to the patient ahead of time. It is also advisable to explain to the patient that it will take at least two weeks, and sometimes as long as four, for the cells to multiply enough for testing. Most patients become anxious during this waiting period, and we tell them to call if they would like to obtain a progress report.

Locating the Placenta

Of the problems and potential risks associated with amniocentesis, the major concern is inadvertent puncture of the placenta. The fetus, as a free-floating object, is not readily skewered, and experience bears this out, but the placenta is a highly vascular and fixed organ. Its puncture could lead at least to a bloody tap (which would be useless because cultured cells might be maternal) and at worst to severe hemorrhage. A related potential risk is that of Rh or other isoimmunization of the mother against fetal red cell antigens following disruption of the delicately balanced isolation of the fetal and maternal circulations. Today, the most common technique for locating the placenta is ultrasound.

To date, the percentage of bloody taps has been no greater in a series of patients in whom ultrasound was not employed than in those in whom it was used, but this may well be an index of the real safety of the procedure. Routine use of ultrasound is particularly useful in detecting twins. A major cooperative study undertaken in the United States, funded under contract from the National Institute of Child Health and Human Development, has established the safety of amniocentesis for genetic diagnosis.

Chorionic Villus Sampling

Chorionic villus sampling is discussed in detail in Chapter 7. It provides a method for obtaining fetal tissue for prenatal diagnosis earlier than amniocentesis. Ultrasound visualization is routinely employed in the placing of an aspiration catheter through the cervix to the site of implantation. The method has already been employed for the antenatal diagnosis of both cytogenetic and metabolic disease. It has the advantage that tissue obtained can be analyzed directly. This has been employed particularly in cytogenetic diagnosis and the use of DNA probes. We have found the direct assay to be unreliable for enzymatic diagnosis and now routinely culture the chorionic villus cells when asked to do an antenatal enzymatic diagnosis.

Some of the pitfalls are obvious. There is a somewhat greater risk of complication, especially abortion, than with amniocentesis. There is also a greater risk of obtaining maternal rather than fetal tissue; of course, this is one risk that may be magnified by culture of the cells. In enzymatic diagnosis, one is looking for an absence of enzyme activity for a positive diagnosis of disease. Thus, the assay of nonviable material or even a mixture of viable and nonviable material can yield a false-positive diagnosis and the abortion of an uninvolved fetus. Culturing the cells solves this problem. Other pitfalls are not so obvious. In the assessment of hypoxanthine-guanine phosphoribosyltransferase (HPRT) activity in the diagnosis of the Lesch-Nyhan disease, we measure the incorporation of radioactively labeled hypoxanthine into nucleotides. Most other assays measure incorporation into inosine monophosphate (IMP). In uncultured chorionic villus material, there is sizable and highly variable catabolism of the nucleotide products. This too could lead to a false-positive diagnosis. Cultured cells are less variable and provide enough material to permit parallel study in which a nucleotidase inhibitor is added.

Cytogenetic Analysis

Analysis of amniotic fluid cells for fetal chromosomal study is the basis for most prenatal diagnoses. The fetal karyotype is the simplest information obtainable from amniotic fluid cells; we now routinely karyotype every amniotic fluid cell culture regardless of the indication for amniocentesis today. The most common indication for amniocentesis is advanced maternal age, followed by a previous history of a child with trisomy 21 (Down syndrome). A woman over 40 has a 1:40 chance of having a baby with trisomy 21; most centers doing prenatal diagnosis now offer the procedure to any pregnant woman over 40, and, at many centers, the age range has been extended to those over 34. However, since the overall incidence of chromosomal abnormalities is 1:200 live births, it may one day become practical to offer amniocentesis to all pregnant women. In 234 women over 35 years of age, for example, six fetuses were found to be cytogenetically abnormal. The incidence in women who had had a previous child with trisomy 21 was high (3:182). In all, 19 positive diagnoses were made. The genetic disorder most commonly diagnosed prenatally is Down syndrome. The technique is especially useful in follow-up of a mother who herself has a translocation. Turner's syndrome can also be diagnosed.

The state of the art in diagnosing metabolic disorders was surveyed early; of 119 amniocenteses done in families at risk for 21 different disorders, there were 52 for Tay-Sachs disease, 24 for Pompe's disease, 11 for mucopolysaccharidosis, and six for maple syrup urine disease. Thirty-three affected fetuses were detected in this way, of which 27 were aborted. One error, a false-positive diagnosis of Tay-Sachs disease, was reported. In another extensive tabulation of amniocenteses, nearly 1,700 procedures yielded diagnoses of 127 affected fetuses. On only three occasions were maternal cells seen. The risk of the procedure to mother and infant was minimal. Experience assembled from a number of centers in the United States included 10,431 pregnancies studied by amniocentesis; 598 affected fetuses were found, 466 of which were cytogenetic abnormalities and 132 of which were biochemical defects. Cytogenetic diagnosis is also the predominant reason for chorionic villus sampling.

Enzyme Profiles

Vigorous research in the field of prenatal diagnosis has been devoted to assessment of enzymes in cells in culture. This is the usual method employed for the prenatal diagnosis of inborn errors of metabolism. Occasionally, it is possible to make a diagnosis by assay of enzymes in the fluid directly or of uncultured cells, but the study of cells in culture is more reliable. The cells obtained at amniocentesis are generally large, with irregular borders and very small nuclei, and look like amnion cells or squamous epithelial cells. Occasional cells are round or oval and smooth-bordered but also have small nuclei. They are resistant to mechanical and physical methods of disruption. On cultivation, the cells may be epitheloid or fibroblastic and are readily disrupted by freezing and thawing or sonication for preparation of cell-free extracts. Their fetal origin is supported by a considerable body of evidence, such as the regular demonstration of male karyotypes.

The enzymatic content of these cells and the presence or absence of changes at different stages of development remain to be established for most enzyme systems. A working hypothesis in this field has been that any condition that can be positively diagnosed by studying enzymes of fibroblasts in cell culture can in all probability be diagnosed by assaying enzymes in cells cultured from amniotic fluid. So far, this hypothesis has proved essentially correct. However, in the case of histidase, the result depends on the type of cell studied. When amniotic fluid cells are cultured, epithelial cells and fibroblastic cells may be obtained. Epithelial cells are rich in histidase, but histidase is lacking in fibroblastic cells. Thus, it is obvious that only the former would be useful for prenatal diagnosis of histidinemia. These observations underscore the need for caution and the continued assessment of appropriate controls in any new field.

The genetic diseases that have been diagnosed by enzyme assay of cell cultures derived from amniotic fluid cells are transmitted as autosomal recessive or X-linked recessive traits.

X-linked Disorders

The X-linked disorders were the earliest to be approached by amniocentesis. It was recognized as early as 1956 that the sex of the fetus could be determined by examining desquamated cells in the amniotic fluid for the presence of sex chromatin bodies. In carriers of X-linked conditions, such as hemophilia and pseudohypertrophic muscular dystrophy, in which a specific diagnosis can now be made, recognition that a fetus was male has been considered grounds for interruption of the pregnancy. This is certainly a less-than-satisfactory criterion, for such a male fetus has a 50% chance of being normal. Unfortunately, this approach to prenatal diagnosis remains all that is available in most X-linked disorders. However, cultivation of cells and determination of enzyme contents have put prenatal detection of the X-linked disorders that can be diagnosed at a molecular level on a sound basis. The diseases that should be detected prenatally in this way are cited in Table 13.1.

Lesch-Nyhan Syndrome

The primary expression of the mutant gene determining this disorder is the complete absence of activity of HPRT. Affected patients show increased purine synthesis, hyperuricemia, choreoathetoid cerebral palsy, and aggressive self-mutilating behavior. Mental retardation is severe. The devastating nature of this disorder has certainly qualified it for consideration of control through prenatal diagnosis.

The activity of the enzyme can be assessed quantitatively in cell extracts; it can also be assessed radioautographically, since tritiated guanine must first be converted to guanylic acid (GMP) via HPRT before it is incorporated into RNA. We now routinely employ a whole or intact cell assay in which the assessment is of the incorporation of ^{14}C-hypoxanthine into each of the nucleotide products of the pathway, including guanosine triphosphate (GTP) and adenosine triphosphate (ATP), as well as IMP and intermediates. The method is sensitive enough that small numbers of cells are sufficient. It can be employed with cultured amniocytes or chorionic villus cells. In monitoring a num-

Table 13.1 X-linked Disorders Detectable Prenatally by Assay of Enzymes, Precursors, or Metabolism in Cultured Cells

Disorder	Enzyme System	Prenatal Diagnosis*
Adrenoleukodystrophy	Hexacosanoic acid accumulation	+
Fabry's disease	Ceramide trihexosidase	+
Glucose-6-phosphate dehydrogenase deficiency	Glucose-6-phosphate dehydrogenase	P
Hunter's syndrome	Iduronate sulfate sulfatase	+
Lesch-Nyhan syndrome	Hypoxanthine-guanine phosphoribosyltransferase (HPRT)	+
Partial deficiency of HPRT	HPRT	P
X-linked ichthyosis	Steroid sulfatase	+

*+ = prenatal diagnosis made in one or more proven instances; P = possible.

ber of pregnancies by chorionic villus sampling, we have detected one involved fetus antenatally. The pregnancy was terminated and the diagnosis confirmed. Of four other pregnancies monitored by direct enzymatic assay of chorionic villus material, two fetuses had no activity and the pregnancies were terminated. A third, in which activity was very low, aborted spontaneously, and the fourth was a normal female. This assay detects HPRT deficiency in time to permit therapeutic abortion.

Cloning of fibroblast cultures has shown that the heterozygote for HPRT deficiency carries two populations of cells, one with normal activity of HPRT and the other with complete deficiency. More convenient diagnosis of heterozygosity in cells in culture depends on the ability of selective media containing purine analogues to inhibit the growth of normal cells but not that of HPRT-deficient cells. The most convenient methods of detection of heterozygosity are those employing analysis of the enzyme in singular hair follicles. Unfortunately, it is not possible to detect heterozygous carriers of this gene by analysis of enzymatic activity in blood.

The Lesch-Nyhan syndrome has now been diagnosed prenatally in a sizable number of pregnancies (Table 13.2). No false-positive or false-negative diagnoses have been reported.

Hunter Syndrome

The X-linked form of mucopolysaccharidosis is designated as Hunter syndrome. These patients, like those with the autosomal recessive Hurler syndrome, excrete large amounts of chondroitin sulfate B and heparan sulfate in the urine. The disease is somewhat less severe than Hurler syndrome and is not associated with corneal clouding. These patients store excessive quantities of mucopolysaccharides in the viscera and excessive quantities of gangliosides in the brain.

Specific diagnosis of Hunter syndrome, as well as of the other mucopolysaccharidoses, followed observations reported by Dr. Elizabeth Neufeld and her colleagues who found abnormal kinetics of mucopolysaccharide metabolism in cultured fibroblasts in patients with these diseases. These

Table 13.2 Prenatal Diagnosis of Lesch-Nyhan Syndrome

Method	Fetuses at Risk	Normal HPRT+	Affected HPRT-
Amniocentesis	16	15	1
Chorionic villus sampling	4	3	1
Total	20	18	2

cells incorporate labeled sulfate into mucopolysaccharide in the normal way, but the rates of degradation are very low. It was found that this defect could be corrected by incubating the mutant cells either with normal cells or in medium in which normal cells had grown. Furthermore, the Hunter's defect could be corrected by Hurler's cells, and vice versa. A specific diagnosis can be made on this basis, for a Hunter's cell is one with a defect in kinetics that cannot be corrected by Hunter's cells. This can be done with cells cultured after amniocentesis, and a prenatal diagnosis of Hunter's syndrome has been made in this way.

Cells from individuals with mucopolysaccharidoses accumulate mucopolysaccharides in vitro as well as in vivo. These accumulations can be demonstrated by the presence of metachromatic staining or by chemical analysis, but it is now clear that neither of these methods is sufficiently reliable for accurate prenatal diagnosis. The diagnosis is now made by assay of the enzyme defective in Hunter syndrome: iduronate sulfate sulfatase.

Fabry's Disease

Fabry's disease is also known as angiokeratoma corporis diffusum universale. Affected patients have red, raised angiokeratomatous skin lesions, crises of fever, and excrutiating pain in the extremities. Birefringent lipid deposits occur throughout the body, with particularly high concentrations in the blood vessels, heart, and kidneys. This lipid is a trihexosylceramide (GL$_3$), with the structure galactosyl-galactosyl-glucosyl-ceramide. A defect has been found in an enzyme responsible for hydrolysis of the terminal galactose of this molecule. Accumulation of the GL$_3$ glycolipid has been demonstrated in the fibroblast. A deficiency of α-galactosidase has been demonstrated in leukocytes and fibroblasts from homozygous patients with Fabry's disease as well as from heterozygous carriers. Antenatal diagnosis of Fabry's disease was first undertaken in the fetus of a 22-year-old woman who had been identified as a carrier by fibroblast assay. Enzyme assays of cells cultured from amniotic fluid obtained at 17 weeks' gestation contained a tenth of the activity found in control cell cultures. Diagnosis was confirmed by accumulation of the Fabry's lipid in the fetal tissues.

Other X-linked Disorders

In X-linked ichthyosis the molecular defect is in the enzyme, steroid sulfatase, active in fibroblasts and in amniocytes in culture. The defect was demonstrable in amniocytes from the initial patient discovered to have this enzymatic abnormality. Its relatively benign nature suggests that the demand to monitor pregnancies for this skin disorder might be small

At the other end of the spectrum is adrenoleukodystrophy, a cerebral degenerative disorder in which progressive demyelination is associated with adrenal insufficiency. The disorder has been called bronzed Schilder's disease because of the combination of dark skin pigmentation and a progressive cerebral white matter disease. Onset is in childhood between four and six years of age, and the disease is fatal within one to nine years. Milder and more severe variants have been described. Characteristic cytoplasmic inclusions have been seen in the cerebral white matter and in the adrenal cortex. This suggested that the basic problem was a lipid storage disorder. A specific biochemical abnormality has been documented in the accumulation of unbranched long-chain saturated or monounsaturated fatty acids with a carbon length of 24 to 30. These fatty acids account for up to 40% of the total fatty acids found in cholesterol esters and gangliosides of adrenal cortex and white matter. They are readily detectable in fibroblasts and in the blood plasma. The ratio of C$_{26}$ to C$_{22}$ fatty acids in these materials is employed in diagnosis. This biochemical characteristic has been used in prenatal diagnosis. The ratio in 23 control amniotic fluid cell cultures was 0.17. In seven pregnancies at risk, three were diagnosed as having adrenoleukodystrophy; these pregnancies were terminated, and the diagnosis was confirmed.

Autosomal Recessive Disorders

Autosomal recessive disorders that may be diagnosed by enzymatic reactions in cultured fibroblasts are shown in

Table 13.3 Autosomal Recessive Disorders Detectable by Assay of Enzymes in Cultured Cells

Disorder	Enzyme	Prenatal Diagnosis*
Acatalasemia	Catalase	Pr
Adrenoleukodystrophy, neonatal	Accumulation of very long chain fatty acids; acyl CoA dihydroxyacetone phosphate acyl transferase	+
Alysosomal acid phosphatasia	Lysosomal acid phosphatase	+
Argininemia	Arginase	+
Argininosuccinic aciduria	Argininosuccinase	+
Branched-chain ketoaciduria (maple syrup urine disease)	Branched-chain α-keto acid decarboxylase	+
Citrullinemia	Argininosuccinate synthetase	+
Cystathioninuria	Cystathionase	P
Cystinosis	Cystine accumulation	+
α-Fucosidosis	α-Fucosidase	+
Galactosemia	Galactose-1-phosphate uridyl-transferase	+
Gaucher's disease	Glucocerebrosidase	+
Generalized gangliosidosis (GM$_1$ gangliosidosis)	β-Galactosidases A, B and C	+
Glycogen storage disease (type II Pompe's disease)	α-1,4-Glucosidase	+
GM$_2$ gangliosidosis type 2 (Sandhoff disease)	Hexosaminidases A and B	+
GM$_2$ gangliosidosis type 3	Partial deficiency hexosaminidase A	P
Glutaric aciduria type I	Glutaryl CoA dehydrogenase	+
Glutaric aciduria type II	Multiple acyl CoA dehydrogenase	+
Homocystinuria	Crystathionine synthase	+
Hurler syndrome	α-L-Iduronidase	+
4-Hydroxybutyric aciduria	Succinic semialdehyde dehydrogenase	P
Hyperlysinemia	Lysine-α-ketoglutarate reductase	Pr
Hypervalinemia	Valine transaminase	Pr
I-cell disease	Multilysosomal enzyme deficiency, N-acetylglucosamine-1-phosphotransferase	Pr
Krabbe's disease	Galactocerebroside β-galactosidase	+
Lactosylceramidosis	Lactosylceramide galactosidase	P
Mannosidosis	α-Mannosidase	P
Metachromatic leukodystrophy	Arylsulfatase A	+
Methylmalonic acidemia	Methylmalonyl-CoA mutase	+
Niemann-Pick disease	Sphingomyelinase	+
Orotic aciduria	Orotidylic pyrophosphorylase and decarboxylase	Pr
Propionic acidemia	Propionyl-CoA carboxylase	+
Refsum syndrome	Phytanic acid α-hydroxylase	Pr
Sanfilippo syndrome, type A	Heparan sulfate sulfatase	+
Sanfilippo syndrome, type B	N-acetyl-α-D-glucosaminidase	+
Tay-Sachs disease (GM$_2$ gangliosidosis type 1)	Hexosaminidase A	+
Wolman's disease	Lysosomal acid lipase	+
Xeroderma pigmentosum	DNA repair	
Zellweger syndrome	Accumulation of very long chain fatty acids; acyl CoA dihydroxyacetone phosphate acyl transferase	+

*+ = prenatal diagnosis made in one or more proven instances; P = possible; Pr = presumably possible.

Table 13.3. The following discussion reviews some representative disorders.

Lysosomal Acid Phosphatase Deficiency

Lysosomal orthophosphoric monoester phosphohydrolase (acid phosphatase) deficiency, a metabolic disorder, is a product of research on cultured cells first discovered through studies by Nadler and Egan on fibroblasts from an infant who died at four months. He and two siblings had had histories of vomiting, lethargy, opisthotonos, and terminal bleeding. Acid phosphatase activity was absent from the lysosomal fraction of fibroblasts, as well as from a variety of tissues. Heterozygotes could be distinguished from controls by a failure of stimulation of acid phosphatase activity after addition of phytohemagglutinin to fibroblasts in vitro. In a subsequent pregnancy, an antenatal diagnosis was made by amniocentesis; this pregnancy was interrupted, and the absence of enzyme was confirmed in homogenates of fetal tissues.

Galactosemia

Prenatal diagnosis has been shown to be possible in galactosemia by the assay of galactose-1-phosphate uridyltransferase in cultured cells. In the first approaches to antenatal diagnosis, this enzyme was found to be undetectable in cells derived from amniotic fluid obtained immediately before cesarean section in a woman who had previously delivered a galactosemic infant. The diagnosis was made by assay of the enzyme in cord blood; when the cell culture was ready for assay six weeks later, the enzyme deficiency was documented. Galactosemia is treatable in infants diagnosed at birth. Thus, a prenatal diagnosis of this condition might suggest early treatment rather than therapeutic abortion.

Glycogenosis

Glycogen storage disease type II (Pompe's disease) can also be detected in cultured fibroblasts. The deficient enzyme is a lysosomal hydrolase, (α-1,4-glucosidase, or maltase). Amniocentesis has been reported, with assay of the enzyme in cultured cells, from a woman who had previously delivered a child who died at seven months of Pompe's disease. Enzyme activity in the cells studied was normal, and the infant subsequently delivered was normal. Infants with this disease show a generalized glycogenosis and life-threatening signs associated with deposition in heart and nervous system tissues. They usually die at less than a year of age. Interruption of pregnancy would be a serious consideration in positive antenatal diagnosis.

The α-glucosidase in amniotic fluid is a different enzyme from that found in the cells. Therefore, it is clear that prenatal diagnosis of this condition cannot be based on assay of the free enzyme in amniotic fluid. In an alternative approach to intrauterine diagnosis, Hug et al. have relied on electron microscopic analysis of amniotic cells. Two of four pregnancies at risk were diagnosed to be associated with Pompe's disease in this way, and, in each instance, the diagnosis was confirmed. This approach has a time advantage since it can be used directly on uncultured amniotic fluid cells.

Inborn Errors of Amino Acid Metabolism

A number of disorders of amino acid metabolism can be diagnosed by enzyme studies in cultured cells (Table 13.3). These include argininosuccinic aciduria, maple syrup urine disease, intermittent branched-chain ketonuria, citrullinemia, and homocystinuria. Propionyl-CoA carboxylase deficiency can be detected in the cultured fibroblast directly or by measuring conversion of (^{14}C) propionate to acid-insoluble radioactivity. This latter approach is also useful in methylmalonic acidemia. It may be unreliable in chorionic villus material.

Homocystinuria

Homocystinuria is a disorder of amino acid metabolism that affects multiple systems by producing widespread vascular thrombotic accidents, and many of these patients are mentally retarded. Affected patients usually die of cerebral, pulmonary, renal, or other thromboses. The enzyme cystathionine synthase, which is defective in these patients, can be assayed in tissue culture. Cystathionine synthase has a pyridoxal phosphate prosthetic group. Some patients with this disease respond to large doses of vitamin B_6 with decreased plasma concentrations and urinary excretion of methionine and homocystine.

Prenatal diagnosis has been attempted in homocystinuria. In a known heterozygote for cystathionine synthase deficiency, the fetus was found not to have the disease. A similar result has been obtained in a pregnancy at risk for maple syrup urine disease, in which a healthy infant was born after monitoring. In another instance, a positive prenatal diagnosis of maple syrup urine disease was made; this infant was confirmed at birth as having the disease. A prenatal diagnosis of argininosuccinic aciduria was reported following amniocentesis at 16 weeks in a 31-year-old woman who had had a previous child with the disease. When pregnancy was terminated at 22 weeks, the diagnosis was confirmed by assay of the enzyme in fetal tissues. The argininosuccinic acid concentration in the amniotic fluid around this fetus was appreciable; this amino acid is not normally present in amniotic fluid. Thus, it is presumably possible to diagnose this condition by direct assay of the amniotic fluid. We have diagnosed citrullinuria antenatally on the basis of the citrulline content of amniotic fluid, and the antenatal diagnosis was confirmed by assay of the synthase in cultured amniocytes. In two pregnancies so diagnosed, one affected fetus was aborted. The other was brought to term and treated such that symptomatic hyperammonemia was avoided for a number of years.

Cystinosis

The nephropathic or infantile form of cystinosis is characterized by accumulation of cystine crystals in many tissues. Renal accumulation leads to the Fanconi syndrome of acidosis, growth retardation, glycosuria, phosphaturia, and generalized aminoaciduria. Patients with this condition die in childhood of renal failure. Cystine also accumulates in cultured fibroblasts; both patient and carrier can readily be identified in this way. However, the numbers of cells required for this assay preclude its use for prenatal diagnosis. Therefore, a method has been developed using (^{35}S) cystine that is suitable for use with small numbers of cells in vitro. A number of homozygous fetuses have been detected and the pregnancies terminated.

Mucopolysaccharidoses

The abnormalities in metabolism of the mucopolysaccharidoses and the kinetics of sulfatide degradation that charac-

terize the fibroblasts of these patients, discussed earlier i relation to Hunter syndrome, also apply to the cells from patients with Hurler and Sanfilippo syndromes.

Hurler Syndrome

A prenatal diagnosis of the syndrome has been made in mother who had had two previous affected sons. Amnio centesis at 25 weeks yielded cells that accumulated ^{35}S labeled mucopolysaccharide. The patient elected to com plete the pregnancy and was delivered at 37 weeks of daughter with Hurler syndrome.

The dermatan sulfate and heparan sulfate that accumu late in the tissues of patients with Hurler syndrome are L iduronic acid-containing polysaccharides. Sequential degra dation of dermatan sulfate requires the action of a numbe of enzymes, including α-L-iduronidase, and this enzyme the site of the fundamental defect in Hurler syndrome Cross-correction studies have indicated that the defect i Scheie syndrome occurs in the same enzyme. Prenatal diag nosis of both syndromes can now be done by assay fo iduronidase.

Sanfilippo Syndrome

There are two forms of Sanfilippo syndrome. In Sanfilippo A, the defect is in the sulfatase for heparan sulfate. On th other hand, the Sanfilippo B defect involves an α-glu cosaminidase. Prenatal diagnosis can now be done by assa for these enzymes.

Gangliosidoses

The gangliosidoses are now being very actively explored and their relative frequency and real severity make them major candidates for prenatal study.

Tay-Sachs Disease

Among the important findings in this field was the delin eation by O'Brien and Okada of the defect in Tay-Sach disease, the only ganglioside storage disease known befor 1965. Patients with this disease develop a progressive cere bral degeneration that is invariably fatal by the fourth yea of life. Macular degeneration is evident in the cherry-re spot in the retina. The ganglioside that accumulates in th central nervous system is known as GM_2. The ganglioside is cleaved by an N-acetylhexosaminidase. There are two hexosaminidase components in human tissue, separable by starch gel electrophoresis. One of these, hexosaminidase A, is absent in tissue and fibroblasts of patients with Tay-Sachs disease. In Sandhoff's disease, both the A and B isozymes are missing.

Tay-Sachs disease is the metabolic disorder in which there has been by far the greatest experience with prenatal diagnosis of inherited disease. The number of pregnancies monitored for this condition may well exceed those of all other enzyme deficiency diseases. Many well-documented prenatal diagnoses have been made.

Diagnosis can be made in Tay-Sachs disease using amniotic fluid or uncultured cells, but the most reliable assay is that performed on cells in culture, which yields the greatest difference between affected patient and control. Assays for hexosaminidase A in amniotic fluid or uncultured cells may be unreliable in the presence of contaminating maternal blood. Errors may also be observed in cultured cells contaminated with bacteria, as a bacterial hexosaminidase has a pH optimum, heat lability, and electrophoretic mobility similar to those of hexosaminidase A.

Heterozygotes for the Tay-Sachs gene may be readily detected using a serum fluorometric assay that depends on the thermolability of hexosaminidase A and the stability of hexosaminidase B. This important contribution led the way to mass screening for the gene in high-risk populations of Ashkenazic Jews. These screening programs have increased the demand for prenatal diagnosis in this condition, as well as its effectiveness in control of the disease.

Other Disorders

Xeroderma Pigmentosum

This light-sensitive skin disease, characterized by multiple malignancies and consequent fatality, is inherited as an autosomal recessive trait. Excessive freckling and sunlight sensitivity are sometimes seen in the heterozygote. Some patients with xeroderma pigmentosum have cerebral manifestations, including mental retardation, microcephaly, ataxia, choreoathetosis, and deafness. This group of symptoms is known as the De Sanctis-Cacchione syndrome and appears

to represent a different genetic disease.

An interesting abnormality has been reported in the fibroblasts derived from patients with xeroderma pigmentosum. There appears to be a defective repair mechanism for DNA in these cells. In general, cells in culture incorporate tritiated thymidine into DNA only when they are in the growth phase in which they are synthesizing DNA. However, in response to ultraviolet radiation, lightly labeled cells begin to appear, and labeling of this sort involves 100% of the cells of a culture. This incorporation is interpreted to represent repair of the DNA damaged by irradiation. In cells of patients with the De Sanctis-Cacchione syndrome, this repair response to irradiation is absent. In patients with xeroderma pigmentosum without neurologic abnormalities, there is a very slight degree of repair capability.

Prenatal Diagnosis by Direct Chemical Assay of Metabolites

A new approach to prenatal diagnosis has been developed (Table 13.4) in the study of families at risk for propionic acidemia. Patients with this disorder accumulate a unique metabolite, methylcitrate, and excrete it in the urine. Using techniques of gas chromatography-mass spectrometry, this

Table 13.4 Prenatal Diagnosis by Direct Detection of Metabolites in Amniotic Fluid

Disorder	Metabolite
Adrenogenital syndrome	17 α-hydroxyprogesterone
Argininosuccinic aciduria	Argininosuccinic acid
Citrullinemia	Citrulline
Galactosemia	Galactitol
Glutaric aciduria type I	Glutaric acid
Glutaric aciduria type II	Dicarboxylic acids
4-Hydroxybutyric aciduria	4-Hydroxybutyric acid
Isovaleric acidemia	Isovalerylylglycine
Methylmalonic aciduria	Methylcitric acid, methylmalonic acid
Mevalonic aciduria	Mevalonic acid
Multiple carboxylase deficiency	Methylcitric acid, 3-hydroxy-isovaleric acid
Propionic acidemia	Methylcitric acid
Tyrosinemia, hepatorenal	Succinylacetone

compound was found in the amniotic fluid surrounding a fetus with propionic acidemia. It was absent from amniotic fluid of normal women and from amniotic fluid of a woman at risk for a propionic acidemic fetus when the fetus was normal or heterozygous. This technique permits rapid diagnosis within 24 hours of the amniocentesis. It is also applicable to methylmalonic acidemia, where the fluid can be analyzed directly for methylmalonic acid and for methylcitrate. In methylmalonic acidemia, an involved fetus may be detected by assay of the maternal urine for methylmalonic acid, but this may not be sufficiently elevated until it is much too late to intervene. It is a good marker to monitor intrauterine treatment of B_{12}-responsive methylmalonic acidemia. Direct analysis of the amniotic fluid is generally preferable for antenatal diagnosis.

The sensitivity and accuracy of these procedures have been improved considerably by the use of internal standards labeled with stable isotopes and of selected ion monitoring gas chromatography-mass spectrometry. Deuterium-labeled methylcitric acid has been successfully employed in the prenatal detection of propionic acidemia, methylmalonic acidemia, and multiple carboxylase deficiency. Deuterium-labeled methylmalonic acid is now available as well, permitting assay for methylmalonic acid in the prenatal diagnosis of methylmalonic acidemia. We routinely assay both compounds in pregnancies at risk for methylmalonic acidemia in order to obtain maximum confidence in the antenatal diagnosis. In a recent summary of our experience, there were 43 pregnancies at risk for propionic acidemia, of which 13 were found to be affected. Of 26 at risk for methylmalonic acidemia, five were affected. The total of 18 affected is close to the one-fourth expected for autosomal recessive inheritance. Assay of the amniotic fluid for 3-hydroxyisovaleric acid should be an even better approach than that of methylcitric acid to the prenatal diagnosis of multiple carboxylase deficiency, for the amounts of this metabolite that accumulate in this condition are much greater than those of methylcitric acid.

Argininosuccinic aciduria has been detected prenatally on the basis of the presence of argininosuccinic acid in the amniotic fluid, and citrullinemia has been detected in amniotic fluid of infants with citrullinemia.

Succinylacetone has been found to accumulate i patients with hepatorenal tyrosinemia, and this property ha been successfully employed for prenatal diagnosis. The sit of the molecular defect in that condition is currentl thought to be in fumarylacetoacetic acid hydrolase. Accum ulated fumarylacetoacetic acid would be reduced to suc cinylacetoacetic acid, the precursor of succinylacetone. Th compound is a powerful inhibitor of δ-aminolevulinat hydratase, and this property has been employed in the pre natal assay. A direct chemical method has been develope for the detection of succinylacetone in amniotic fluid afte reaction with hydroxylamine to form an oxime that under goes ring closure to 5-methyl-3-isoxazole propionic aci and formation of the trimethylsilyl derivative. Selected io monitoring permitted the detection in the same sample o 4-hydroxyphenyllactic acid, which should permit the pre natal diagnosis of oculocutaneous tyrosinemia. In one preg nancy at risk, the fetus was normal.

The adrenogenital syndrome that results from a defec in adrenal 21-hydroxylase can be diagnosed prenatally b direct assay of amniotic fluid for 17α-hydroxyprogesteron This is best done at midgestation, when levels are highe and the distinction between affected and normal is mo clearly made. Diagnosis at this time permits a decision as t interruption of the pregnancy. In late pregnancy, after 3 weeks, the concentration of 17α-hydroxyprogesterone i maternal serum rises appreciably, and the diagnosis may b made at this time by assay of the mother's blood. A diagno sis at this time permits the prompt initiation of treatment a birth, which may be life-saving.

Other approaches to the direct chemical assay of ke compounds in amniotic fluid in antenatal diagnosis includ galactitol for galactosemia, glutaric acid for glutaric acide mia, 4-hydroxybutyric acid for 4-hydroxybutyric aciduri and mevalonic acid for the antenatal detection of the new discovered defect in cholesterol biosynthesis, mevalon aciduria. We have developed a stable isotope method fo orotic acid detection in amniotic fluid, which is not usefu in the diagnosis of urea cycle defects such as ornithine tran carbamylase (OTC) deficiency, but should be effective fo the antenatal diagnosis of orotic aciduria, the inborn err of pyrimidine metabolism. Other possibilities for futu development include uracil or thymine for dihydropyrimidine dehydrogenase deficiency, oxalic, glycolic, or glyoxylic acids for oxalic aciduria, and suberylglycine or hexanoylglycine for medium-chain acyl CoA dehydrogenase deficiency.

Direct methods of chemical analysis have considerable advantages in speed over methods that require cell culture. In most instances, an answer is available within two days of the arrival of the sample in the laboratory. Direct chemical assay also avoids the risk, always a worry in cell culture, that maternal cells may contaminate and overgrow the fetal cells. We have encountered just this situation in a pregnancy at risk for propionic acidemia. A prenatal diagnosis was made on the basis of methylcitric acid. When cells became available, the activity of propionyl-CoA carboxylase was normal. The family was not interested in abortion, but the baby was born with propionic acidemia. When cultures were available on mother and infant, it was clear that the mother had a marker chromosome not inherited by the infant, and the cells that had grown following amniocentesis were maternal.

Recombinant DNA Techniques in Prenatal Diagnosis

Techniques generated from the forefront of molecular biology are already being applied in the problem of prenatal diagnosis. The use of restriction endonuclease mapping, polymerase chain reaction, and other elements of recombinant DNA technology in antenatal diagnosis is discussed in detail in Chapter 14. Variation at the molecular DNA level occurs on a wide scale, not only in the coding areas of genes, but also in flanking regions and introns. Research on restriction endonuclease mapping was initially applied to the antenatal diagnosis of thalassemia and sickle cell disease. Syndromes due to gene deletion such as α-thalassemia and hemoglobin H were the first diseases to be detected in this way. More recently, the restriction enzyme DdeI permitted the direct detection of the sickle cell mutation in all cases, but cell culture was necessary to produce enough DNA for analysis. The latest development employs another enzyme, MstII, which is so sensitive that it can be used with uncultured amniocytes.

These techniques have now been applied to a number of inborn errors of metabolism. A probe has been developed for the phenylalanine hydroxylase gene that detects restriction polymorphism. It is utilized to detect heterozygosity and for prenatal diagnosis.

OTC deficiency is the most common of the inherited disorders of the urea cycle. The gene is on the X chromosome, but the disease is expressed in both males and females. Most patients with OTC deficiency have the classic defect in which the disease is uniformly fatal in affected male infants, usually within the first days of life. The syndrome is one of massive hyperammonia and deep coma. In affected females, there is variable expression, due probably to variable inactivation of the X chromosome carrying the normal gene or its counterpart carrying the abnormal gene. The OTC enzyme, like that of phenylalanine hydroxylase, is an exclusively hepatic enzyme. Therefore, prenatal diagnosis has not been possible in the usual ways. Prenatal diagnosis has been carried out by liver biopsy of the fetus and assay of the enzyme in liver tissue, but OTC activity in the liver does not develop until second trimester; therefore, this approach to prenatal diagnosis means delay until 18 to 20 weeks of gestation.

The cloning of the OTC gene has permitted heterozygote detection and prenatal diagnosis of amniocytes and chorionic villus tissue. As in the case of PKU, the cDNA probe does not usually detect the mutation in the gene directly, but, in informative families, restriction fragment length polymorphism (RFLP) linked to the gene permits the diagnosis of the fetus. In two pregnancies at risk, a hemizygous normal male was detected in one and a heterozygous female in the other.

Prenatal diagnosis of the Lesch-Nyhan syndrome, as discussed above, has been available for a number of years by assay of the HPRT enzyme. Cloning of the gene for this enzyme has also made it accessible to diagnosis by recombinant DNA techniques. A few mutations that cause HPRT deficiency are detectable directly because the nature of the defect is directly detected by a restriction site and the cDNA probe. The majority must be looked at for linked RFLP, as in the case of PKU and OTC deficiency.

Heterozygote detection and prenatal diagnosis can be carried out in this way, and a prenatal diagnosis has been reported.

Discussion

The field of antenatal diagnosis is in its infancy. It offers a positive approach to genetic counseling and management of genetic disease, and it can be expected that further research will increase the number of disorders detectable antenatally. Presumably, as techniques improve and become more widely applied, legal, clinical, and moral questions may arise regarding therapeutic abortion, but there are increasing indications that society is now prepared to deal realistically with these controversial issues.

By monitoring pregnancies with amniocentesis or chorionic villus sampling and recommending selective abortion, one can guarantee selection of a child unaffected with the illness monitored, who can then be brought to term. We find that parents seldom come to us seeking to terminate pregnancy. Rather, they come to us wanting children and wondering if a genetic monitoring program can assure them of a chance to have children free of a disease for which they are at risk. Planned parenthood at its best is concerned not only with the quantity of human reproduction but also with its quality.

CASE 13.1   Lesh–Nyhan Syndrome

The first two children of a 33-year-old gravida 8, para 4 had the Lesch–Nyhan syndrome. Both were severely retarded, spastic, and self-mutilative, and had been institutionalized in a state hospital for the mentally retarded.

The third pregnancy was monitored by an amniocentesis at 16 weeks. The fetus was found to be a male with no activity of hypoxanthine-guanine phosphoribosyltransferase (HPRT) in cultured amniotic cells. A therapeutic abortion was performed.

Subsequently, the mother had three monitored pregnancies. In two, the fetuses were found to be female with normal HPRT activity. The pregnancies went to term, and healthy girls were delivered. They are living and well.

In her seventh pregnancy, the fetus was found to be male and involved, and the pregnancy was terminated. The mother had been tested for heterozygosity using the hair root test and confirmed to be a carrier.

In the patient's latest (eighth) pregnancy, a pelvic ultrasound echogram was performed at 15 weeks' gestation and a single intrauterine fetus was identified. Successful amniocentesis was performed. Fetal cells were grown in culture, and, within four weeks, there were sufficient numbers for enzyme assay. The karyotype was that of a normal 46 XY male. Activity of HPRT was undetectable. Therefore, a diagnosis of the Lesch–Nyhan syndrome was made in the fetus, and the mother was admitted to the hospital.

Physical examination revealed a healthy woman at 16 weeks' gestation. The patient's uterus was visualized by ultrasound, and 20 mg prostaglandin $F_{2\alpha}$ and 40 mg urea were instilled intraamniotically. A stillborn male fetus was delivered. Assay of HPRT on homogenates of fetal tissue revealed no evidence of activity, which confirmed the diagnosis of the Lesch–Nyhan syndrome.

Conclusion: This discussion of inborn errors of metabolism clearly demonstrates why tertiary-care centers are necessary. The long list of genetic abnormalities is so complex that the clinician must rely on the expertise available at such centers. The obstetrician and gynecologist must take a careful history of both parents so that these problems may be anticipated and the patient may have the proper examinations.

Suggested Reading

Bakay B, Francke U, Nyhan WL, et al. Experience with detection of heterozygous carriers and prenatal diagnosis of the Lesch-Nyhan disease. In: Muller MM, Kaiser E, Seegmiller JE, eds. Purine metabolism in man. II: Regulation of pathways and enzyme defects. New York: Plenum, 1977:351-8.

Brady RO, Uhlendorf BW, Jacobsen CB. Fabry's disease. Ante

natal detection. Science 1971;172:175.

Buchanan PD, Kahler SG, Sweetman L, et al. Pitfalls in the prenatal diagnosis of propionic acidemia. Clin Genet 1980; 18:177.

Chang JC, Kan YW. A sensitive new prenatal test for sickle-cell anemia. N Engl J Med 1982;307:30.

Fratantoni JC, Neufeld EF, Uhlendorf BW, et al. Intrauterine diagnosis of the Hunter and Hurler syndromes. N Engl J Med 1969;280:686.

Gibbs DA, McFadyen IR, Crawford MD'A, et al. First-trimester diagnosis of Lesch-Nyhan syndrome. Lancet 1984; 2:1180.

Hug G, Schubert WK, Soukup S. Electron microscopy of uncultured amniotic fluid cells. In utero diagnosis of type II glucosidosis. Pediatr Res 1971;5:421.

Jakobs C, Sweetman L, Nyhan WL. Chemical analysis of succinylacetone and 4-hydroxyphenyllactate in amniotic fluid using selective ion monitoring. Prenat Diagn 1984;4:187.

Kaback MM, Brent RL, Crandall BF, et al. Antenatal Diagnosis, NIH Publication No. 79-1973. Bethesda, MD: US Dept. of Health, Education & Welfare, National Institutes of Health, 1979.

Nadler HL, Egan TJ. Lysosomal acid phosphatase deficiency. A new familial metabolic disorder. N Engl J Med 1970; 282:302.

Naylor G, Sweetman L, Nyhan WL, et al. Isotope dilution analysis of methylcitric acid in amniotic fluid for the prenatal diagnosis of propionic and methylmalonic acidemia. Clin Chim Acta 1980;107:175.

Nyhan WL. Prenatal diagnosis of metabolic disease. Yokohama Med Bull 1989;39:219.

Nyhan WL, Sakati NO. Diagnostic recognition of genetic disease. Philadelphia: Lea & Febiger, 1987.

O'Brien JS. San Filippo syndrome. Profound deficiency of alpha-acetylglucosaminidase activity in organs and skin fibroblasts from type B patients. Proc Natl Acad Sci USA 1972; 69: L720.

O'Brien JS, Okada S, Fillerup DL, et al. Tay-Sachs disease. Prenatal diagnosis. Science 1971;172:61.

Orkin SH, Little PFR, Kazazian HH Jr, et al. Improved detection of the sickle mutation by DNA analysis: application to prenatal diagnosis. N Engl J Med 1982;307:32.

Page T, Broock RD. A pitfall in the prenatal diagnosis of Lesch-Nyhan syndrome by chorionic villus sampling. Prenat Diagn 1990;10:153.

Pembrey ME, Old JM, Leonard JV, et al. Prenatal diagnosis or ornithine transcarbamyltransferase deficiency using a gene specific probe. J Med Genet 1985;22:462.

Reed EN, Landing B, Sugarman G, et al. Xeroderma pigmentosum. JAMA 1969;207:2073.

Schneider JA, Veroust FM, Kroll WA, et al. The prenatal diagnosis of cystinosis. N Engl J Med 1974;290:878.

14

Antenatal Diagnosis by DNA Analysis

Jane Chueh, M.D.
Mitchell S. Golbus, M.D.

AS INTEREST in genetic research has shifted recently from the study of animals, particularly *Drosophila*, to the study of humans, investigators have described more than 4,000 distinct mendelian conditions. New techniques in molecular biology have also aided in characterizing these disorders and increasing the possibilities for prenatal diagnosis. Over 200 heritable genetic defects are already isolated and mapped (1). It is clear that prenatal diagnosis will involve more assessment and DNA analysis early in pregnancy.

Initial Assessment

A family history should be part of every new obstetric visit so that the clinician can identify those individuals at risk for heritable disorders. In many cases, risk can be detected only if the clinician knows of a previously affected family member. Such knowledge is especially important in diagnosing recessive disorders.

It's also important to record ethnic origin. For example, Ashkenazi (Eastern European) Jews are at increased risk for Tay-Sachs disease, with a carrier frequency of one in 2 in the Ashkenazi population, compared with one in 150 in the general population. Southeast Asians are at increased risk for α-thalassemia and β-thalassemia mutations. For these diseases, a particular subset of common mutations is present in each ethnic group (2). Knowledge of Chinese ancestry, for example, reduces the number of likely mutations to eight and focuses the diagnostic DNA test required. Similarly, knowledge of Mediterranean ancestry focuses analysis on four specific mutations for β-thalassemia, which account for 79% of β-thalassemia alleles in this population (2).

When to Use DNA Analysis

Once a patient is determined to be at increased risk to deliver a fetus with a particular disorder, the next question often is: Can the condition be diagnosed prenatally? In theory, there's a possibility of diagnosing disorders at the DNA level if they are due to a defect in a single gene. Most mutations are point mutations: changes in one or a few nucleotides. These changes can be substitutions, deletions, or insertions. Only 1%–5% of gene mutations involve such gross gene alterations as insertions or deletions of relatively large pieces of genetic material (3). One exception is the α-globin cluster, where most of the mutations causing α-thalassemia have one or more entire genes missing.

Despite the impressive list of cloned genes, prenatal diagnosis is not yet available for all genetic disorders. Table 14.1 lists diseases for which DNA markers exist within or close to the gene. Sickle cell disease is the only one of these caused by one mutation in all cases. For the other disorders, we must find DNA markers that distinguish the affected (mutant) gene from the normal gene. If we determine the sequence of both the normal and the mutant genes, we can

Table 14.1 Diseases with DNA Markers

Disease	Cloned Gene	Informative (%)
β-thalassemia	β-globin	95
Sickle cell	β-globin	100
α-thalassemia	α-globin	98
Hemophilia A	Factor VIII	94
Hemophilia B	Factor IX	93
Von Willebrand deficiency	Von Willebrand factor	96
Phenylketonuria	Phenylalanine hydroxylase	98
α1-antitrypsin deficiency	α1-antitrypsin	99
Duchenne and Becker Mb	dystrophin	99‡
OTC deficiency	Ornithine transcarbamylase	87†
Lesch-Nyhan	HGPRTase	38
Retinoblastoma	retinoblastoma	95
Her's disease	liver phosphorylase	92
McArdle diaease	muscle phosphorylase	75
Familial hypercholesterolemia	low density lipoprotein receptor	99
X-linked ichthyosis	steroid sulfatase	—
Antithrombin III deficiency	antithrombin III	57
Ehlers-Danlos Type IV	procollagen type III	58
CAT deficiency	ornithine amino transferase	48

*with Hb electrophoresis and blood analysis
**with clotting test
†diagnosis has been made
‡with CPK enzyme test

use precise DNA probes or markers—short sequences of nucleotides (oligonucleotides) synthesized to complement the gene sequence exactly—that will selectively recognize an affected or normal gene.

Unfortunately, use of oligonucleotide probes is limited because we often don't know the exact gene sequence. For a given disease, different families may have different mutations. In some cases, as in β-thalassemia among Chinese, knowledge of the ethnic group defines the likely mutations and therefore certain DNA probes. In other cases, where we don't know the exact molecular defect, we can recognize abnormal genes by using DNA polymorphisms linked to the abnormal gene.

Polymorphisms are differences in DNA base sequences due to normal variability. We can recognize them once the DNA is cut by a restriction endonuclease: an enzyme that recognizes and cleaves DNA at a specific nucleotide sequence. The human genome contains a large number of such DNA polymorphisms: One in 500 nucleotides differs between two randomly selected alleles, and about 5% of this variability can be recognized by a restriction endonuclease (3).

The polymorphism is not the mutation that causes the disorder, but it helps us distinguish the chromosome carrying the mutant gene from the chromosome carrying the normal gene. In a given family, an informative polymorphism occurs when an affected member has identifiable DNA variability closely linked to the affected gene. Using this, we can trace the affected gene and determine its inheritance even if we don't know the precise gene mutation that is causing the disease.

DNA Techniques

The most direct method of detecting gene mutations at the DNA level is through DNA oligonucleotide probes complementary to the gene undergoing study. Human genomic DNA extracted from white blood cells can be cut into small pieces with enzymes (restriction endonucleases) that recognize and cleave specific nucleotide sequences (4). Electrophoresis then separates these DNA fragments according to size on an agarose gel. These are rendered single-stranded, transferred to a filter, and exposed to a radiolabeled DNA probe. After a period of hybridization, while the probe is allowed to find and anneal with its complementary strand, the filter is exposed to photographic film. Bands of radioactivity appear on the film, corresponding to the areas on the filter where the probe attached.

With this method, deletions can be recognized by noting unusual-sized DNA fragments. Point mutations can also be detected because the probe will attach only to a very specific nucleotide sequence. Mutations in this sequence show no hybridization.

Even if the exact nature of the molecular defect of a gene is unknown, indirect methods can be used to identify the affected gene. Thus its inheritance can be traced by using restriction fragment linked polymorphisms (RFLP) (5–7). These RFLPs are found when DNA from different individuals is cut by the same restriction endonuclease. Because of the normal variability among individuals, the enzyme may cut the DNA at a particular site on one chromosome but not on another chromosome. The different sizes of DNA fragments help distinguish the two chromosomes. If this polymorphism lies close to a disease-causing gene, it can be used to identify the chromosome carrying an affected gene. We can trace its inheritance without knowing the precise gene mutation.

An informative polymorphism occurs when an affected member of a family has DNA variability closely linked to the affected gene. This distinguishes the chromosome carrying it from the chromosome carrying the normal allele in this family.

Recently, the polymerase chain reaction (PCR) has contributed another way of detecting genes (8, 9). This new technique allows the use of a small amount of genomic DNA (theoretically, the amount found in a single cell) to make hundreds of thousands of copies of a sequence in a matter of hours. The copies can be used for further DNA analysis.

Human genomic DNA is rendered single-stranded (denatured), and a heat-stable polymerase (Taq polymerase) is used to synthesize the strands complementary to the original single-stranded DNA. Besides free nucleotides, amplification of DNA also requires short starting pieces of DNA: oligonucleotide primers.

The primers (usually around 20 nucleotides long) are

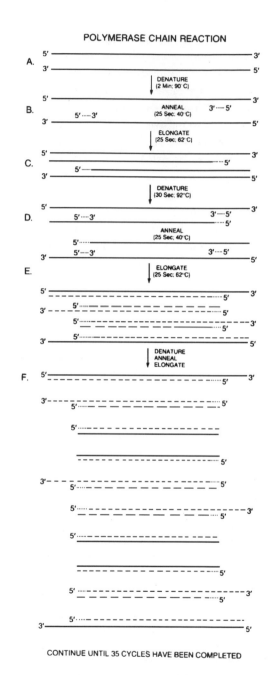

POLYMERASE CHAIN REACTION

CONTINUE UNTIL 35 CYCLES HAVE BEEN COMPLETED

Figure 14.1 Events here are occurring in three cycles of polymerase chain reaction. DNA is denatured at 90°C, oligonucleotide primers complementary to the gene are allowed to attach at 40°C, and elongation is accomplished at 62°C by a heat-stable polymerase. Each cycle doubles the amount of DNA present at the beginning of the cycle. Conditions shown are those for the rapid sex test.

synthesized so that they are complementary to the gene of interest; the sequence of the gene therefore must be known. The primers flank the area of genomic DNA to be studied after amplification. PCR can be used to diagnose the presence or absence of the sickle cell mutation quickly. It is also proving to be a reliable and rapid sex test for prenatal diagnosis because it detects the presence or absence of the Y chromosome. When this technique is used for the rapid sex test, events are described in three cycles of the polymerase chain reaction (Figure 14.1).

Sickle Cell Anemia

One of the first and most important contributions to prenatal diagnosis came with the elucidation of the gene that causes sickle cell disease. Because the genetic mutation is universal, this heritable condition is one of the easiest to diagnose.

Each year, approximately 3,000 pregnancies in the United States are at risk for producing a child with homozygous sickle cell anemia. In the diseased child, an abnormality in the β-globin chain leads to poor solubility of hemoglobin when it is deoxygenated. The responsible mutation lies on the short arm of chromosome 11. In the gene for the β-subunit of hemoglobin, valine is substituted for glutamic acid as the sixth amino acid. Because we know the exact nature of the mutation, we can perform prenatal diagnosis from chorionic villi or amniocytes. Therefore, we don't need DNA information from other members of the family.

Figure 14.2 shows how we diagnose sickle cell anemia using polymerase chain reaction. We extracted DNA from chorionic villi of a fetus of parents known to be carriers of the sickle gene. Then we performed PCR amplification (40 cycles) of 500 ng of genomic DNA. This amplified a 294-base pair fragment of the β-globin gene that traverses the sickle mutation. Oxan I, a restriction endonuclease, digested the resulting DNA, and electrophoresis separated the fragments on an acrylamide gel. Oxan I, which recognizes and cleaves at a particular nucleotide sequence in the normal β-globin gene, produces a 191-base pair and a 103-base pair fragment. A mutation in the gene giving rise to the sickle form abolishes this recognition site. Because Oxan I does not cleave the sequence, only the 294-base pair fragment appears.

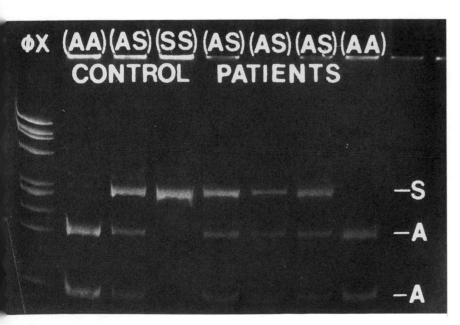

Figure 14.2 Acrylamide gel shows characteristic patterns of DNA fragments from normal patients and patients with heterozygous and homozygous sickle cell disease. Amplification of the β-globin gene in the area of the sickle mutation was accomplished using the polymerase chain reaction method. The resulting 294-base pair fragment of the β-globin gene was digested with Oxan I, which cleaves the normal gene into two fragments (191 bp and 103 bp), but leaves the sickle form intact.

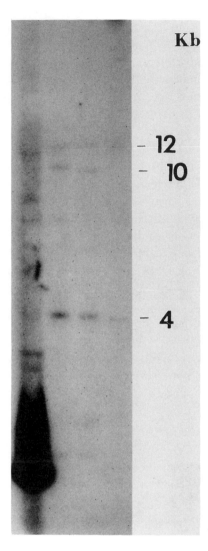

Figure 14.3 This autoradiograph is of two parents with α-thalassemia trait and their fetus. The first lane on the left is the DNA ladder, a marker used to determine what size the DNA fragments are in the samples to the right. The next two lanes are the parents', who have α-thalassemia trait in *cis* configuration. The lane to the far right is that of the fetus, which has only a 12-kb band and therfore must be unaffected.

α-thalassemia

This disorder arises from deletion of one or more genes in the α-globin cluster. The cluster includes two α-globin genes on chromosome 16. Deletion of one or more α-glo-bin genes reduces the amount of α-globin chains, thereby reducing the synthesis of hemoglobin A ($\alpha_2 \beta_2$).

In the homozygous state, all four α genes are absent, no α-chains are produced, and the fetus cannot synthesize hemoglobin F or any of the adult hemoglobins. The predominant hemoglobin made is Hb Bart's (γ^4), which has a high oxygen affinity. Inadequate amounts of oxygen are released at the tissue level, leading to a high-output cardiac failure, hydrops fetalis, and fetal or neonatal death. Deletion of three α genes, called Hb H disease, results in abnormal amounts of Hb H (β_4) and Hb Bart's. Affected individuals will have a moderately severe hemolytic anemia. The detection of the two α genes (α-thalassemia trait) results in a hypochromic, microcytic anemia, with a low mean red cell volume (MCV). The two genes deleted may be from the same chromosome (*cis*), as is frequently seen in an Oriental population, or one gene may be missing from each chromosome (*trans*), as seen in the black population. Deletion of one gene is clinically undetectable (10).

Parents with α-thalassemia trait or Hb H disease are at risk for having offspring with hydrops fetalis or Hb H disease. The presence of a mild hypochromic, microcytic anemia, even though iron study results are normal, indicates parents at risk. Hemoglobin electrophoresis must be used to exclude β-thalassemia, which can also show hypochromic microcytic anemia, and normal iron studies. If the hemoglobin electrophoresis is shown to be normal, the diagnosis of α-thalassemia is made by exclusion.

The normal α-thalassemia gene has cut-sites for restriction endonucleases Bg1 and Asp. Treatment of DNA from an unaffected individual will yield DNA fragments 12 kb long. A deletion of one α gene will eliminate an original cut-site and result in a DNA fragment 15 kb long. A deletion of two α genes from the same chromosome will result in a DNA fragment 10 kb long. Therefore, the DNA from an individual with α-thalassemia trait in *cis* configuration will have both 10- and 12-kb-long DNA fragments after treatment with Bg1 and Asp, whereas the DNA from an individual with α-thalassemia trait in *trans* configuration will have only 15-kb-long fragments. A patient with only one functional α-globin gene will have a 15-kb-long fragment from the chromosome with the gene and a 10-kb-long fragment from the chromosome without any functional α-globin genes. The presence of these DNA fragments is demonstrated by hybridization with α-globin and β-globin probes.

Figure 14.3 is an autoradiograph of two parents with α-thalassemia trait and their fetus. Both parents have 10- and 12-kb bands, indicating that they have two normal α-globin genes on one chromosome and two missing α-globin genes on the other chromosome. The fetus, however, has only a 12-kb band and therefore must have all four normal α genes.

Cooley's Anemia

β-thalassemia results from reduced or absent β-globin chain production. A variety of mutations can cause clinical β-thalassemia (Figure 14.4). Certain mutations segregate within particular ethnic groups. Since there are different intragenic probes for detecting mutations, a knowledge of the ethnic group can reduce the number of probes that must be tried to characterize the mutation. There is an increase in γ-chain (Hb F) production in the fetus, but this protective effect disappears after three months of age. Severe anemia, hepatosplenomegaly, frequent blood transfusions, impaired fertility, myocardial hemosiderosis, and death by the third decade of life usually result (10).

β-thalassemia heterozygotes have high red blood cell counts and moderate microcytosis, resembling iron defi-

ciency. However, their iron studies are normal, and the hemoglobin electrophoresis characteristically shows an increased amount of Hb A_2 (>3.5%).

The technique of polymerase chain reaction has made it easier to detect mutations by selectively amplifying the β-globin gene. Only nanograms of starting DNA are needed. The amplified products are then spotted onto nylon membranes (dot blots) and hybridized with oligonucleotide probes made to detect specific mutations. The probes are labeled with horseradish peroxidase, which turns blue if the mutation is present (11).

In Figure 14.4, which is a dot blot of two families with β-thalassemia, one is due to a mutation at the 41/42 site and the other to a mutation at the β17 site. In the family with the 41/42 mutation, each parent has one mutant gene and one normal gene, whereas the fetus has two copies of the mutant gene and therefore is homozygous for β-thalassemia. In the family with the β17 mutation, both parents are heterozygous for the mutant gene and so is their fetus.

DNA Biology: A Powerful Tool

As recently as 10 years ago, a clinical obstetrician would have found it difficult to imagine the need to study molecular biology and laboratory techniques. Now, however, it has become clear that prenatal diagnosis and therapy will play an increasingly important role in prenatal care, and

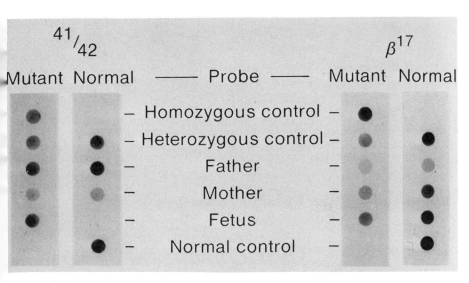

Figure 14.4 In the dot-blot analysis of a family with β-thalassemia, the filled circles represent hybridization with a DNA probe labeled with horseradish peroxidase. The family on the left is at risk for the 41/42 mutation causing β-thalassemia. The parents' dot blots show hybridization with both normal and 41/42 mutant genes. Their fetus shows hybridization with only the mutant gene and therefore will have homozygous β-thalassemia. The family on the right is at risk for the β17 mutation. Both parents and their fetus have one normal and one mutant gene and thus are β-thalassemia carriers.

DNA biology offers powerful tools to achieve these aims. An understanding of the basic theories and techniques of molecular biology available today is helpful in counseling and referring appropriate patients.

References

1. White R, Caskey CT. The human as an experimental system in molecular genetics. Science 1988; 240:1483.

2. Saiki RK, Chang CA, Levenson CH, et al. Diagnosis of sickle cell anemia and beta thalassemia with enzymatically amplified DNA and nonradioactive allele-specific oligonucleotide probes. N Engl J Med 1988; 319:537.

3. Antonarakis SE. Diagnosis of genetic disorders at the DNA level. N Engl J Med 1989; 320:153.

4. Southern EM. Gel electrophoresis of restriction fragments. Methods Enzymol 1979; 68:152.

5. Boehm CD, Antonarakis SE, Phillips JA, et al. Prenatal diagnosis using DNA polymorphisms: report on 95 pregnancies at risk for sickle-cell disease or beta thalassemia. N Engl J Med 1983; 308:1054.

6. Oberle I, Camerino G, Heilig R. Genetic screening for hemophilia A (classic hemophilia) with a polymorphic DNA probe. N Engl J Med 1985; 312:682.

7. Katayama S, Montano M, Slotnick N, et al. Prenatal diagnosis and carrier detection of Duchenne muscular dystrophy by restriction fragment length polymorphism analysis with pERT 87 deoxyribonucleic acid probes. Am J Obstet Gynecol 1988; 158:548.

8. Embury SH, Scharf SJ, Saiki RK, et al. Rapid prenatal diagnosis of sickle cell anemia by a new method of DNA analysis. N Engl J Med 1987; 316:656.

9. Kogan SC, Doherty M, Gitschier J. An improved method for prenatal diagnosis of genetic diseases by analysis of amplified DNA sequences. N Engl J Med 1987; 317:985.

10. Laros RK. The hemoglobinopathies. In: Laros RK, ed. Blood disorders in pregnancy. Philadelphia: Lea & Febiger, 1986: 37–61.

11. Cai SP, Chang CA, Zhang JZ, et al. Rapid prenatal diagnosis of beta thalassemia using DNA amplification and nonradioactive probes. Blood 1989; 73:372.

PART FOUR Monitoring: Biochemical and Biophysical

15

Biochemical Profile of the Fetus

Houchang D. Modanlou, M.D.

HUMAN cellular metabolism occurs in a specific acid-base milieu, and pH values compatible with tissue survival range from 6.8 to 7.7 (1). To maintain proper acid-base balance, the fetus depends on the integrity of the respiratory gas exchanges of the placenta and appropriate oxygen availability. There is a close relationship between maternal and fetal acid-base balance (2–4).

During pregnancy, maternal P_{CO_2} is regulated at a lower physiologic level. Fetal and maternal gradient of P_{CO_2} facilitates exchange. Transport of oxygen from mother to fetus is postulated to occur because gas exchange flow is concurrent (5). Therefore, umbilical cord venous P_{O_2} (highest P_{O_2} in the fetus) depends on and cannot be higher than venous P_{O_2} of the uterine circulation.

Metabolic disturbances of acid–base balance in the mother would cause analogous disturbances in the fetus, although the rate of transmission of such disturbances is not known (2–4). Decreased placental respiratory functions due to maternal factors or uteroplacental factors affect the fetus adversely.

Although the integrity of fetal cellular function depends on the degree and duration of hypoxia, the exact extent of cellular damage cannot be estimated by hypoxia alone. Some have suggested that the placenta provides relatively large amounts of lactate to the fetus and acts as a substrate of fetal metabolism (6). In a normal pregnancy before labor, fetal oxygen extraction from the uteroplacental circulation is adequate to meet all aerobic requirements of the fetus. Further increase in oxygen availability to the fetus, by maternal hyperoxygenation, does not enhance fetal oxygen consumption (7).

Labor and Delivery

Uterine contractions during labor and delivery can impair oxygen transmission to the fetus by reducing uterine and umbilical blood flow. Similarly, cesarean section can decrease fetal oxygen supply since uterine incision and manipulations lessen maternal and fetal-placental blood flow (8).

Although physiologic, normal labor and delivery interfere with uteroplacental gas exchange, resulting in decreased fetal oxygen availability and increased anaerobic glycolytic metabolism and accumulation of excess lactic acid. The exact quantitative relationship between decreased oxygen supply and fetal acidosis is unclear, as is the connection between maternal metabolic and fetal acidosis (9, 10).

During normal labor, the fetus develops some metabolic acidosis (11). This acidosis increases during the second stage, at which time, it is combined with respiratory acidosis caused by interference with CO_2 exchange by frequent, strong uterine contractions.

Intrapartum biochemical assessment of the fetus is associated with decreased perinatal mortality in high-risk pregnancies (12, 13). However, because of the technical difficulty of providing such assessment 24 hours a day, it is far less widespread than biophysical assessment with ultrasound and electronic fetal heart rate (FHR) monitoring. Even in a tertiary perinatal center, equipped with appropriate laboratory facilities and staffed with properly trained personnel, biochemical assessment is used only when the FHR pattern is ominous or equivocal. Scalp blood pH may then provide additional information about fetal status.

Blood Sampling Technique

A fetal blood specimen is obtained from the skin of the presenting part, usually the scalp. A sterile endoscope with a light source is introduced through the cervix by pressing gently against the presenting part. A small area is cleansed of amniotic fluid with a sterile cotton swab, and a thin film of silicone gel applied to assure blood will exude as a drop rather than spread. Ethyl chloride spray may be applied to cause local reflex hyperemia.

A small incision is then made with a specially designed 2-mm-long blade. The specimen is collected in a heparinized glass capillary tube. The Monoject Fetal Blood Sampling Tray (Sherwood Medical, St. Louis, Missouri) is marketed for this technique.

Collected properly and analyzed immediately, a fetal scalp blood specimen yields a fairly reliable pH value between those of arterial and venous blood. Marked hypoxia tends to reflect the venous value more heavily.

Factors that may cause important errors when determining biochemical values are protracted exposure to air with resultant loss of CO_2, prolonged storage in room air, sedimentation of blood, and incorrect calibration, buffering,

temperature regulation, or reading. Other factors affecting accuracy of pH and lactate measurements are timing of sampling in relation to uterine contractions, caput succedaneum, maternal fever or hypertension, pH and lactate, and positioning during collection.

Interpreting Intrapartum pH

Fetal blood during normal labor has a higher hydrogen ion concentration than adult blood. The normal arterial pH range in adults is 7.35–7.45, whereas in the fetus average range is 7.30–7.40, with values above 7.25 considered normal.

In 1961, Oliver and co-workers suggested that delivery, whether vaginally or by cesarean section, is invariably asphyxiating for the fetus (14). Other groups subsequently confirmed this view, using such clinical indicators as lack of apparent fetal distress, spontaneity of delivery, and vigor of the newborn infant (15–17).

My co-workers and I analyzed intrapartum serial biochemical values, selecting infants by Apgar score (11). Comparing second-stage labor values with umbilical cord values in normal fetuses, we documented a rise in PCO_2, a sharp drop in pH, and an increase in base deficit (Table 15.1). Although second-stage fetal biochemical changes were more evident, changes were also found, to a lesser degree, from 5 cm of dilation to the beginning of the second stage. Thus, umbilical cord blood biochemistry reflects stresses, not only of delivery, but also of labor.

Equiluz and co-workers have reported similar alterations in fetal scalp blood pH, PCO_2, PO_2, and base deficit (18). They also showed a gradual rise of intrapartum fetal blood lactate from early labor to the second stage in normal pregnancy. This latter change was greater in fetuses of high-risk pregnancy, who were more depressed and acidotic at birth.

The normal fetus generally shows a tendency toward acidosis. Such acidosis is both respiratory and metabolic, with metabolic acidosis prevalent during the first and early second stages of labor. The fetal base deficit has been found to follow closely the pattern of fetal pH. Respiratory acidosis, with increasing PCO_2, may predominate during the end of the second stage.

Table 15.1 Changes in Fetal Blood Acid-Base Balance Intrapartum and during First 64 Minutes of Neonatal Life

	Early Labor*	Mid-labor†	Full Cervical Dilation	Before Delivery	Umbilical Artery	Umbilical Vein	4 min‡	8 min	16 min	32 min	64 min
					At Birth						
pH	7.30	7.30	7.28	7.26	7.24	7.32	7.20	7.24	7.30	7.32	7.36
PO_2	19.7	21.1	19.1	17.3	17.6	27.8	53.3	62.4	68.0	69.6	70.3
PCO_2	45.5	45.1	47.8	50.4	48.7	38.9	46.1	39.7	35.4	34.8	34.4
Base deficit	6.4	5.4	6.1	7.3	8.8	6.6	10.5	9.3	7.9	6.4	4.2

All findings cited ± SD.
*Cervical dilation less than or equal to 4 cm.
†Cervical dilation 5 cm.
‡All times cited are for arterial blood.

Such second-stage changes have been interpreted as evidence of reduced placental oxygen-carbon exchange during the final phase of delivery and of a brief period of fetal asphyxia (19). Because biochemical surveillance generally is restricted to measurement of pH alone, we cannot directly measure metabolic against respiratory acidosis. Making this comparison is important because changes in partial CO_2 pressures disappear rapidly once acute asphyxia is past. However, the separate values can be calculated by using pHqu40 (pH units measured after equilibration of the fetal blood sample with CO_2 at a tension of 40 mm Hg), which measures the metabolic component of acidosis. The actual pH value also includes the respiratory component.

The fetus's increasing metabolic acidosis during normal labor is due in part to increasing maternal metabolic acidosis. Saling and Schneider have objected to calling this particular fetal acidosis "physiologic," rather than simply calling it "increased," since the term acidosis used clinically refers to a pathologic entity (12).

In the first few minutes after delivery, a further fall in blood pH and increase in base deficit occur, although there is a simultaneous decrease in PCO_2 and increase in PO_2, presumably because of a delayed influx of hydrogen ions from the tissues (19). In a normal newborn, major correction of this metabolic acidosis occurs in the first 10 minutes after respiration begins.

Findings in High-Risk Pregnancies

In a study comparing intrapartum fetal acid-base status in pregnancies associated with such conditions as preeclampsia, Rh isoimmunization, and diabetes mellitus with that in apparently normal pregnancies, we found no difference during early first-stage labor between high-risk fetuses and normal fetuses (20). (Hypoxic acidosis usually develops slowly during labor.) However, with progression of labor, high-risk fetuses showed more marked changes in acid-base status. Particularly notable, in both umbilical arterial and venous blood, were significantly lower pH and higher base deficits at the end of the first stage, during the second stage, and at birth. Significant differences in CO_2 tension were noted only at birth. Equiluz and co-workers have corroborated our findings (18).

These pathophysiologic changes were associated with decreased tolerance of the stress of labor in the high-risk fetuses. The cesarean section rate was higher, as were the number of infants requiring resuscitation at birth because of depression and because of significantly lower Apgar scores at one and five minutes. Postnatally, these infants were more acidotic, and correction of their metabolic acidosis occurred at a much slower pace.

What degree of fetal acidosis can be considered pathologic? Saling proposed that a pH of 7.20 or less be considered significant acidosis and that immediate intervention be undertaken if a value determined 10 minutes later falls more than 0.1 unit (12, 21). Subsequently, several studies have advocated similar values for the lower pH limit, which is considered an indication for immediate intervention (Table 15.2) (22, 23). Since a "preacidotic" fetal pH of 7.20–7.24 is a warning of impending fetal distress, repeat sampling should be done to confirm such distress before taking measures to interrupt pregnancy. Simultaneous measurements of maternal and fetal pH and lactate may be more useful than fetal measurements alone in confirming fetal hypoxic acidosis.

Minimizing Asphyxia

Normal labor and especially delivery cause frank partial asphyxiation. In situations such as complete placental abruption and uterine perforation, this asphyxia can suddenly become total.

Episodes of partial asphyxia in utero are frequently due to mechanisms that reduce maternal blood flow through the placenta, diminishing the net exchange of respiratory gases to produce hypoxia, hypercarbia, and acidosis (24). Term monkey fetuses experiencing such episodes of partial asphyxia show injury to structures in the cerebral hemispheres. Eventual long-term static lesions are very similar to those seen in human perinatal injury or cerebral palsy.

Uterine contractions of labor act as intermittent stressful stimuli. Each contraction temporarily reduces the flow of oxygenated blood through the intervillous space. If placental function is impaired before onset of labor—as may occur in high-risk pregnancies—or contractions are too frequent, the fetus will become vulnerable to asphyxia. Although the intrapartum period is most susceptible, fetal neurologic damage may occur much earlier. A recent study by Goetzman and co-workers showed long-standing neurologic lesions in newborns who died during the first few days of life (25).

Fetal pH measured at different labor stages does not always correlate well with the infant's condition at birth (23, 26–30). Depending on timing of sampling, false normal or abnormal laboratory values can result from umbilical cord blood cholesterol, stage of labor, maternal acidosis or alkalosis, anesthetics or analgesics, or—most important—an ominous FHR pattern.

However, once these factors are considered, the value of fetal blood sampling for biochemical analysis becomes clear. Most fetuses that develop intrapartum hypoxia have a normal blood pH at the beginning of labor (11, 26). Thus, pH determination on a single specimen, particularly early in the first stage, may not correlate well with fetal acid-base balance at birth. Serial measurement during labor is required to identify the fetus at risk of asphyxia and hypoxic acidosis. Continuous intrapartum pH monitoring, now experimental, may avoid the rare complications encountered with intermittent sampling (31).

As we become more confident of our ability to diagnose fetal distress and hypoxia using FHR patterns, the need for determining pH and lactate values from fetal scalp blood should lessen. We may reserve intrapartum biochemical determinations to clarify implications of such ambiguous FHR patterns as intermittent late decelerations with good baseline variability or decreased variability without late decelerations.

Umbilical arterial and venous blood pH, lactate, and blood gas determinations are useful for aiding objective assessment of the newborn and confirming the presence or absence of intrapartum hypoxic acidosis. It is easier to obtain blood from the cord than from the fetal scalp: the cord should be double-clamped at delivery and arterial and venous blood collected in a heparinized plastic syringe. It is

Table 15.2 Lower Limits of Normal Intrapartum Fetal pH Values

Authors	First Stage	Second Stage
Bretscher and Saling (15)	7.20	7.20
Beard and Morris (16)	7.20	7.17
Kubli (17)	7.21*	7.23*
Modanlou, et al. (11)	7.22†	7.18†
Paterson, et al. (22)	7.23	7.17
Paul, et al. (23)	7.20	7.20

pH 2 SD below mean.
*Lower limit of pH range.
†Value of pH 1 SD below the mean.

not necessary to preserve the filled syringe in ice slush before determining pH, lactate, and blood gas values, as room temperature will not significantly alter values if determinations are done within a reasonable time (32).

If cord blood acid-base values are normal, it becomes difficult to infer that perinatal depression resulted from intrapartum events, regardless of Apgar scores (33). Gilstrap and co-workers reported that a normal baseline FHR with beat-to-beat variability correlated 97% with no neonatal acidemia, defined as cord blood pH of less than 7.20 (34).

Cord blood values appear not only to reflect fetal status more accurately than Apgar scores, but also may help determine the mechanism responsible for fetal acidosis, providing information for immediate appropriate management of the newborn (35, 36). Values of more than 7.20 will rule out intrapartum asphyxia/hypoxia, even in the presence of low Apgar scores (37–39).

Determination of cord blood pH is of even greater value in preterm infants because they tend to be given lower Apgar scores, and acidosis correlates more positively with neonatal respiratory distress syndrome and mortality (40). Umbilical artery metabolic values in preterm infants do not correlate closely with Apgar scores except when acidosis is severe (pH < 7.05) (41). Since low umbilical arterial pH reflects the actual physiologic result of placental compromise in gas exchange and oxygen deprivation, leading to anaerobic glycolysis and metabolic acidosis, it should remain our standard for determining intrapartum asphyxia (42).

REFERENCES

1. Parer JT. The current role of intrapartum fetal blood sampling. Clin Obstet Gynecol 1980;23:565.
2. Seeds AE. Maternal-fetal acid-base relationships and fetal scalp blood analysis. Clin Obstet Gynecol 1978;21:579.
3. Roversi GD, Canussio V, Spennocchio M. Recognition and significance of maternogenic fetal acidosis during intensive monitoring of labor. J Perinat Med 1975;3:53.
4. Rooth G, Jacobson L, Heinrich J, et al. The acid-base status of the fetus during normal labor. Testing a model of maternal fetal acid-base exchange on two different series of patients. In: Longo LD, Bartels H, eds. Respiratory gas ex-change and blood flow in the placenta. Bethesda, MD: HEW Publications, 1972.
5. Meschia G. Placental respiratory gas exchange and fetal oxygenation. In: Creasy RK, Resnik R, eds. Maternal-fetal medicine: principles and practice. Philadelphia: WB Saunders, 1984;274.
6. Battaglia FC, Meschia G. Principal substrates of fetal metabolism. Physiol Rev 1978;58:499.
7. Battaglia FC, Meschia G, Makowski FL, et al. The effect of maternal oxygen inhalation upon fetal oxygenation. J Clin Invest 1968;47:548.
8. Datta S, Ostheimer GW, Weiss JB, et al. Neonatal effect of prolonged anesthetic induction for cesarean section. Obstet Gynecol 1981;58:331.
9. Kubli FW, Hon EH, Khazin AF, et al. Observations on heart rate and pH in the human fetus during labor. Am J Obstet Gynecol 1969;104:1190.
10. Low JA, Pancham SR, Worthington D, et al. The acid-base and biochemical characteristics of intrapartum fetal asphyxia. Am J Obstet Gynecol 1975;121:446.
11. Modanlou HD, Yeh S-Y, Hon EH, et al. Fetal and neonatal biochemistry and Apgar scores. Am J Obstet Gynecol 1973;117:942.
12. Saling E, Schneider D. Biochemical supervision of the fetus during labor. J Obstet Gynaecol Br Commonw 1967;74:799.
13. Rey H, Bowe ET, James LS. Impact of fetal heart rate monitoring and blood sampling on infant mortality and morbidity—ongoing study. Pediatr Res 1974;8:450/176.
14. Oliver TK Jr, Demis JA, Bates GD. Serial blood-gas tensions and acid-base balance during the first hour of life in human infants. Acta Paediatr UPPS 1961;50:346.
15. Bretscher J, Saling E. pH values in the fetus during labor. Am J Obstet Gynecol 1967;97:906.
16. Beard RW, Morris ED. Foetal and maternal acid-base balance during normal labour. J Obstet Gynaecol Br Commonw 1965;72:496.
17. Kubli FW. Influence of labor on fetal acid-base balance. Clin Obstet Gynecol 1968;11:168.
18. Equiluz A, Lopez Bernal A, McPherson K, et al. The use of intrapartum fetal blood lactate measurements for the early diagnosis of fetal distress. Am J Obstet Gynecol 1983;147:949.
19. Daniel SS, Adamsons K Jr, James LS. Lactate and pyruvate as an index of prenatal oxygen deprivation. Pediatrics 1966;37:942.
20. Modanlou HD, Yeh S-Y, Hon EH. Fetal and neonatal acid-

base balance in normal and high-risk pregnancies during the first hour of life. Obstet Gynecol 1074;43:347.

21. Saling E. A new method for examination of the child during labor: introduction, technique, and principles. Arch Gynaek 1962;197:108.

22. Paterson PJ, Dunstan MK, Trickey NR, et al. A biochemical comparison of the mature and postmature foetus and newborn infant. J Obstet Gynaecol Br Commonw 1970;77:390.

23. Paul WM, Gare DH, Whetham CJ. Assessment of fetal scalp sampling in labor. Am J Obstet Gynecol 1967;99:745.

24. Myers RE: Two patterns of perinatal brain damage and their conditions of occurrence. Am J Obstet Gynecol 1972; 112:246.

25. Goetzman BW, DiNello C, Lindenberg HA, et al. Brain injury of prenatal origin documented in term and preterm infants. Clin Res 1984;32:123A.

26. Beard RW, Morris ED, Clayton SG. pH of foetal capillary blood as an indicator of the condition of the foetus. J Obstet Gynaecol Br Commonw 1967;74:812.

27. Bowe ET. Assessment of fetal acid-base status during labor. Bull Sloane Hosp Women 1967;13:6.

28. Hon EH, Khazin AF, Paul RH. Biochemical studies of the fetus. II. Fetal pH and Apgar scores. Obstet Gynecol 1969; 33:237.

29. Khazin AF, Hon EH, Yeh S-Y. Biochemical studies of the fetus. V. Fetal PCO_2 and Apgar scores. Obstet Gynecol 1971;38:535.

30. Khazin AF, Hon EH, Quilligan EJ. Biochemical studies of the fetus. III. Fetal base and Apgar scores. Obstet Gynecol 1969;34:592.

31. Modanlou HD, Smith E, Paul RH, et al. Complications of fetal blood sampling during labor. Clin Pediatr 1973; 12:603.

32. Strickland DM, Gilstrap LC III, Hauth JC, et al. Umbilical cord pH and PCO_2: effect of interval from delivery to determination. Am J Obstet Gynecol 1984;148:191.

33. Yeomaus ER, Hauth JC, Gilstrap LC. Umbilical cord pH, PCO_2, and bicarbonate following uncomplicated term vaginal deliveries. Am J Obstet Gynecol 1985;151:798.

34. Gilstrap LC, Hauth JC, Toussaint S. Second-stage fetal heart rate abnormalities and neonatal acidosis. Obstet Gynecol 1984;62:209.

35. Gordon A, Johnson JWC. Value of umbilical blood acid-base studies in fetal assessment. J Reprod Med 1985;30:329.

36. Wible JL, Petrie RH, Koons A, et al. The clinical use of umbilical cord acid-base determinations in perinatal surveillance and management. Clin Perinatol 1982;9:387.

37. Thorp JA, Sampson JE, Parisi VM, et al: Routine umbilical blood gas determinations? Am J Obstet Gynecol 1989; 161:600.

38. Sykes GS, Johnson P, Ashworth F, et al. Do Apgar scores indicate hypoxia? Lancet 1982;1:494.

39. Josten BE, Johnson TRB, Nelson JP. Umbilical cord blood pH and Apgar scores as an index of neonatal health. Am J Obstet Gynecol 1987;157:843.

40. Tejani N, Verma UL. Correlation of Apgar scores and umbilical artery acid-base status to mortality and morbidity in the low birth weight neonate. Obstet Gynecol 1989;73:597.

41. Silverman F, Suidan J, Wasserman J, et al. The Apgar score: is it enough? Obstet Gynecol 1985;66:331.

42. Marrin M, Paes BA. Birth asphyxia: does the Apgar score have diagnostic value? Obstet Gynecol 1988;72:120.

C A S E   1 5 . 1   Primigravida with Elevated Blood Pressure

A 25-year-old primigravida with blood type O, Rh positive, was admitted in early labor at 40 weeks' gestation. Her problems during pregnancy included mild anemia that responded to iron therapy.

Two weeks before admission, she was noted to have an elevated blood pressure, with the diastolic value ranging between 90 and 100 mm Hg, as well as mild pitting edema and 2+ proteinuria. She was treated with phenobarbital and bed rest, but without achieving effective control of her blood pressure.

A week before admission, stress testing (oxytocin challenge) was done and showed mild uterine contractions with normal and reactive FHR.

On admission, external fetal monitoring was applied and showed uterine contractions three to four minutes apart, associated with occasional late FHR decelerations but with average baseline beat-to-beat variability. Because of increased blood pressure and deep tendon reflexes, she was also started on magnesium sulfate by titrated IV infusion.

At 2-cm cervical dilation and 40% fetal effacement,

fetal membranes were ruptured artificially and direct FHR monitoring applied. As labor progressed, baseline FHR increased slightly and was associated with more frequent late decelerations. Beat-to-beat variability decreased significantly. Since late decelerations and decreased FHR variability persisted despite changing the maternal position and administration of oxygen, fetal scalp blood was sampled when the cervix was dilated 6–7 cm. At that time, pH was 7.32, P_{O_2} 25 torr, and P_{CO_2} 45 torr.

A repeat fetal scalp blood sample half an hour later was at pH 7.29. At this point, cervical dilation was complete. Twenty-five minutes later, the patient was delivered of a 3,020 g baby girl with Apgar scores of 7 at one minute and 9 at 5 minutes. The infant's hospital course was uneventful except for mild ABO incompatibility. ∎

C A S E   1 5 . 2   Multigravida with Previous Abortion

A 30-year-old, moderately obese, black gravida 3, para 1, who had had one spontaneous abortion, was admitted in early labor at 42–43 weeks' gestation. She had been followed in the clinic since early in her first trimester. Her pregnancy was uncomplicated.

On admission, the cervix was 2 cm dilated and 50% effaced. Artificial rupture of membranes was done for the purpose of applying an internal FHR and inserting a uterine catheter. The amniotic fluid was stained with thick meconium. Baseline FHR rate was 160 beats per minute (bpm) with decreased beat-to-beat variability. There was no FHR reactivity on vaginal examination and catheter insertion. No periodic FHR changes were observed. Uterine contractions were 5 to 6 minutes apart and of moderate intensity.

At about 3-cm cervical dilation, fetal scalp blood was sampled and showed a pH of 7.19, a P_{CO_2} of 60 torr, and a P_{O_2} of 18 torr. Blood sampling was repeated soon after, resulting in a pH of 7.18.

As labor progressed, baseline FHR variability decreased

Table 15.3 Postmature Infant's Recovery from Acidosis

Minutes	pH	Base Deficit (mEq)	P_{CO_2} (torr)	P_{O_2} (torr)
5	7.04	16.0	55	56
8	7.12	16.2	43	55
16	7.20	16.2	26	53
32	7.28	16.0	21	69
64	7.35	13.5	17	81

further, and occasional late decelerations appeared. Maternal position was changed and oxygen administered. During a vaginal examination, persistent fetal bradycardia as slow as 70 beats per minute was noted, lasting about 90 seconds with very slow recovery.

Preparations were made for cesarean section. A third scalp blood sample, taken within 15 minutes of the second one, showed pH to be 7.08, P_{CO_2} 61 torr, and P_{O_2} 11 torr.

At cesarean section, under general anesthesia, a 3,680-g boy was delivered. He was flaccid and heavily meconium stained, and showed other signs of postmaturity. Heart rate at birth was less than 50 bpm.

He was intubated immediately for direct tracheal suctioning, which yielded copious thick meconium. Intermittent positive pressure ventilation with 100% oxygen, alternated with suctioning, was continued. The infant responded relatively well, with increased heart rate and improvement in color.

By three minutes, he was breathing spontaneously, and, by five minutes, he was extubated but was receiving free-flow oxygen. Umbilical arterial blood, obtained after double clamping of the cord at delivery, showed pH to be 7.01, P_{CO_2} 69 torr, P_{O_2} 11 torr, hematocrit 50%, and base deficit 16 mEq. An umbilical arterial catheter was inserted, and neonatal heart rate was continuously monitored. Mean blood pressure at eight minutes was 49 torr. Heart rate was 60 bpm at one minute, 165 bpm at four minutes, and 140 bpm at 32 and 64 minutes, respectively, but still showed decreased baseline variability (Table 15.3).

The infant had moderate respiratory difficulty because of meconium aspiration syndrome, but recovered within three days. He was discharged home on the seventh day of life, apparently in good condition. ∎

16

Fetal Lung Maturity

Steven G. Gabbe, M.D.

WITHIN the past decade, investigators have developed a second generation of methods for evaluating fetal pulmonary maturation. These tests appear to be more specific than assessments of lung surfactant synthesis (lecithin/sphingomyelin or L/S ratio). They should reduce the number of false-immature predictions. As screening tests, these assays have the advantage of being fast, yet accurate. Like the L/S ratio, such tests are performed on amniotic fluid.

Measuring Saturated Phosphatidylcholine

The major component of pulmonary surface-active phospholipid, saturated phosphatidylcholine (SPC), may be separated from unsaturated lecithin using osmium tetroxide. This assay requires two hours to complete and is unaffected by the presence of blood or meconium.

Torday and colleagues have found SPC concentration and the L/S ratio of equal predictive value in uncomplicated pregnancies (1). However, in contaminated specimens or in those from high-risk patients, the SPC assay is significantly better than the L/S ratio in decreasing false-immature results. Whether SPC concentrations could, in fact, be altered by changes in amniotic fluid volume has not been determined.

Lung Profile

Gluck, the developer of the L/S ratio, now emphasizes that complete assessment of fetal lung maturity requires determination of the L/S ratio, the percent of acetone precipitable lecithin, and the acidic phospholipids phosphatidylinositol (PI) and phosphatidylglycerol (PG) (2). The complete analysis is performed by two-dimensional, thin-layer chromatography and takes 2.5 to 3 hours.

Recognizing the presence of PG, a marker of completed pulmonary maturation, may be useful for timing elective delivery of diabetic patients. The lung profile will also reduce the number of false-immature predictions, as some infants with L/S ratios below 2.0 do show PG. This observation has been made in so-called stress pregnancies complicated by severe hypertension, prolonged premature rupture of membranes, or diabetes with vascular involvement.

Slide Agglutination Test for PG

An immunologic semiquantitative agglutination test that takes only 10 minutes to perform can now detect phosphatidylglycerol at a concentration greater than 0.5 µg/mL of amniotic fluid. This method correlates well with discovery of PG by thin-layer chromatography and is highly predictive of fetal lung maturation (3).

Using the Microviscosimeter

The relative lipid content of amniotic fluid may be determined by fluorescence depolarization analysis (4). Analysis is performed by incubating a lipid-soluble dye with the amniotic fluid specimen for 30 minutes and assessing the amount of dye absorbed into phospholipid membrane structures by measuring the fluorescence of polarized light. The fluorescence polarization (FP) value falls as the L/S ratio rises and correlates with the presence of PG.

This rapid screening technique gives few false-positive results but has a false-negative rate of approximately 70%. In pregnancies complicated by diabetes, the FP value and L/S ratio show the same sensitivity and false-mature prediction rate (5). PG determination has proven to be the most sensitive method.

The foam stability index (FSI) is derived from the shake test, an assay of surfactant function that evaluates the ability of pulmonary surfactant to generate stable foam in the presence of ethanol. The commercially prepared test kit contains wells with a predispensed volume of ethanol. Adding amniotic fluid to each test well produces final ethanol concentrations ranging from 44% to 50%.

After shaking the amniotic fluid-ethanol mixture, one reads the FSI as the highest well in which a rim of stable foam persists. Respiratory distress syndrome (RDS) has been reported unlikely with an FSI of 47 or higher. The FSI cannot be derived from an amniotic fluid specimen contaminated by blood or meconium (6).

Interpreting Amniotic Fluid Optical Density

Determining the optical density (OD) of fresh amniotic fluid at 650 nm permits a quick assessment of fetal lung maturity. The fluid must be uncontaminated by meconium, blood, or bilirubin and should not be refrigerated. Cetrulo and associates found that only four of more than 300 infants with mature OD values of 0.15 or greater developed RDS (7).

Although few false-positive results have been noted, only 20% of infants with immature OD readings will manifest RDS after delivery. Therefore, amniotic fluid specimens with immature OD readings at 650 nm and those with immature FP determinations must be evaluated further with an L/S ratio and lung profile.

Placental Morphology and Fetal Cephalometry

Several investigators have examined the correlation of placental morphology and fetal cephalometry with pulmonary maturation. The term placenta that exhibits uniform grade III changes is highly predictive of fetal pulmonary maturation in an uncomplicated pregnancy.

A fetal biparietal diameter (BPD) of 9.0 or 9.2 cm at 38 weeks' gestation can be used to predict fetal pulmonary maturation. However, the BPD cannot be relied on in pregnancies complicated by diabetes mellitus (8, 9).

Less Need for Testing

Recent changes in clinical practice have, in many cases, reduced the need for determining fetal lung maturity. More obstetricians are scheduling ultrasound examinations early in pregnancy, thereby establishing gestational age more accurately. The result is that elective deliveries at term can be scheduled without determining fetal lung maturation. Also, more patients who have had a previous cesarean section are being allowed to have a vaginal delivery after entering spontaneous labor. This change has also decreased the need for measuring fetal lung maturity before cesarean section.

Similarly, in pregnancies complicated by diabetes mellitus, excellent maternal glucose control through self-monitoring of blood-glucose levels and carefully planned insulin regimens, combined with intensive antepartum fetal surveillance, has reduced the fear of unexpected intrauterine death late in the third trimester. More patients with insulin-dependent diabetes mellitus are being allowed to enter spontaneous labor at term, making amniocentesis to establish fetal lung maturity unnecessary

When fetal lung maturation is determined, it may be best to begin with a simple screening test (10, 11). For example, in many cases, if the FSI, OD at 650 nm, FP, or slide agglutination test for PG were positive, one would not need to determine the L/S ratio. This approach reduces the time, as well as the cost, required to determine fetal lung maturation.

References

1. Torday J, Carson L, Lawson EE. Saturated phosphatidylcholine in amniotic fluid and prediction of the respiratory-distress syndrome. N Engl J Med 1979; 301:1013.
2. Kulovich MV, Hallman MB, Gluck L. The lung profile. I. Normal pregnancy. Am J Obstet Gynecol 1979; 135:57.
3. Towers CV, Garite TJ. Evaluation of the new Amniostat-FLM test for the detection of phosphatidylglycerol in contaminated fluids. Am J Obstet Gynecol 1989; 160:298.
4. Golde SH, Mosley GH. A blind comparison study of the lung phospholipid profile, fluorescence microviscosimetry, and the lecithin/sphingomyelin ratio. Am J Obstet Gynecol 1980; 136:222.
5. Simon NV, Levisky JS, Lenko PM. The prediction of fetal lung maturity by amniotic fluid fluorescence polarization in diabetic pregnancy. Am J Perinatol 1987; 4:171.
6. Lipshitz J, Whybrew W, Anderson G. Comparison of the Lumadex-foam stability test, lecithin:sphingomyelin ratio, and simple shake test for fetal lung maturity. Obstet Gynecol 1984; 63:349.
7. Cetrulo CL, Sbarra AJ, Selvaraj RJ, et al. Amniotic fluid optical density and neonatal respiratory outcome. Obstet Gynecol 1980; 55:262.
8. Kazzi G, Gross T, Sokol R, et al. Noninvasive prediction of hyaline membrane disease: an optimized classification of sonographic placental maturation. Am J Obstet Gynecol 1985; 152:213.
9. Golde SH, Tahilramaney MP, Platt LD. Use of ultrasound to predict fetal lung maturity in 247 consecutive elective cesarean deliveries. J Reprod Med 1984; 29:9.
10. Garite TJ, Freeman RK, Nageotte MP. Fetal maturity cascade: a rapid cost-effective method for fetal lung maturity testing. Obstet Gynecol 1986; 67:619.
11. Herbert WNP, Chapman JF. Clinical and economic considerations associated with testing for fetal lung maturity. Am J Obstet Gynecol 1986; 155:820.

17

Antepartum Fetal Monitoring

Barry S. Schifrin, M.D.
Daniel Clement, M.D.

TECHNOLOGIC innovations in perinatal care over the past two decades have enlarged our understanding of fetal physiology and anatomy. As a result, clinicians are far better able than before to diagnose potential abnormalities and are more confident about pronouncing a fetus normal. Clinicians have also reached a better understanding of the limitations of the designations "high" and "low" in categorizing risks of pregnancy. As a consequence, obstetricians are using tests of fetal well-being more extensively throughout the obstetrical population.

As such tests have become more specific, their number has decreased. For the most part, we have abandoned the indirect biochemical tests so prevalent 20 years ago and now concentrate on direct biophysical testing of the fetus. The most popular tests of fetal well-being during the third trimester include the nonstress test (NST) and biophysical profile (BPP). Use of the contraction stress test (CST) has waned. The trend away from the CST has parallelled the evolving emphasis in fetal heart pattern interpretation from contraction-related events to an analysis of the epochal responses to various intrinsic and extrinsic provocations: fetal behavior patterns.

Although these tests remain popular and widely applicable, details of interpretation, testing schemes, and management strategies vary, sometimes considerably. In most institutions, the NST acts as a primary screening test. If the result is nonreactive, the test is followed by either the CST or, more commonly, the BPP. The latter consists of an assessment of fetal breathing movements, body movements, tone, and amniotic fluid volume (AFV) (1).

Anticipation, prevention, and timely intervention in the distressed fetus are the basis of monitoring. Yet the greatest virtue of testing is to provide reassurance that fetal milestones of growth and maturity, oxygen availability, and neurologic function have been reached and that no intervention is necessary. Because no single test provides sufficient information about all these measurements, several may be required.

The Nonstress Test

The NST is predicated on the cardioaccelerative response

to the provocation, arguably stress, of fetal movement or activity patterns (2, 3). It has been appreciated for several decades that fetal cardiac accelerations to fetal movement reliably indicate fetal well-being. Various names have been applied to tests using fetal accelerations as the end point. The most widely used term, the NST, is probably the least appropriate. The designation has been retained even though a host of external provocations (stresses) have been invoked to elicit the pattern and the test duration has been extended, all without compromising the predictive value of the test (4, 5). These diversions only underscore the concept that, regardless of the effort, time, or stimulus used to elicit the reactive pattern, once obtained, it is a sign of fetal well-being. The response cannot be counterfeited.

The NST is the most widely used screening test of fetal well-being. Depending on the end point, the reactive NST is the best predictor of fetal well-being yet devised. A nonreactive test result is far less accurate in predicting outcome, though it does show significant risk (4).

Debates over the value of the NST relate in part to the lack of specificity of the abnormal pattern. Depending on what criteria are used, the false abnormal rate inconveniently ranges from 50% to 80%. Moreover, the dichotomous division of test results (reactive/nonreactive or normal/abnormal), which has doubtless contributed to its acceptability, now serves more as an impediment than as a facilitator of proper interpretation. While most would agree that it is unreasonable to wait until the NST becomes flat before intervening, there has been little understanding of the pattern of deterioration from reactive to nonreactive (Figure 17.1). Today, we realize that analysis of the overall fetal heart rate (FHR) patterns is more useful than relying on the frequency of accelerations (4, 6, 7). These benefits, in turn, emerge from a better understanding of fetal behavioral cycles and the cardiac responses to them.

As gestation advances, the baseline heart rate falls, variability and the amplitude and frequency of accelerations and decelerations increase, and patterns become grouped into epochs of rest and activity (state changes) (8–10). These activity patterns reflect the increasingly complex organization of the fetal central nervous system (Figure 17.2). The normal range of the baseline heart rate is 110–150 beats per minute (bpm). The individual fetus, however, attempts to maintain a unique, stable baseline heart rate. Heart rates above 150 bpm, especially in the postdate fetus, are suspect. On the other hand, heart rates as low as 90 bpm, especially in postdate pregnancy, are of little consequence if reactivity continues to be normal. A rise in baseline heart rate over sequential testing (rarely higher than 160 bpm) carries an increased risk of adverse outcome.

Accelerations associated with fetal movement are angular; those associated with contractions are usually smoother. In a normal reactive pattern, accelerations appear in epochs (sleep/wake cycles) of about 40 minutes, with considerable variation. Constant activity may sometimes be seen in the fetuses of mothers addicted to cocaine or narcotics. Within these cycles, the baseline between accelerations shows variability; some accelerations invariably coalesce. Formerly, variability was generally discounted as part of the NST, partly because variability was artifactually increased by older cardiotachometers. Newer external transducers permit better registration of variability and easier perception of fetal state changes.

Preliminary studies suggest that changes of state and variability precede the loss of accelerations. As the fetus deteriorates, rest cycles lengthen, accelerations become more uniform, the interval between accelerations increases (accelerations do not coalesce), variability between accelerations disappears, and the baseline rate may rise. Only then do accelerations disappear. This process parallels the disappearance of accelerations with asphyxial stress during labor (11).

Conspicuously, the definition of the reactive NST applies to the mature infant. Fetal heart rate patterns can be used to infer maturity, not only of the mechanism controlling the heart, but also that of the lung. At comparable gestational ages, the risk of respiratory distress syndrome is less in fetuses with normal reactivity (variability) than in those without it (12). By 28 weeks, mature reactivity is present in more than 65% of infants; by 34 weeks, about 95% of infants are reactive (13). Before 28 weeks of gestation, the relatively higher heart rate and the diminished variability, the smaller, more isolated accelerations, and the less obvious epochs of sleep/wake cycles, though present, make the diagnosis of reactivity more elusive (14). In addition, in the preterm fetus, movement may be accompanied by transient decelerations rather than accelerations (7).

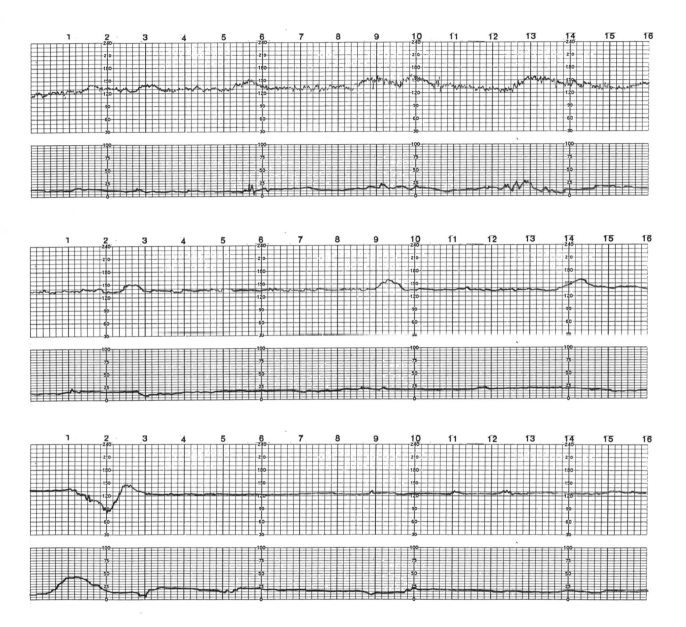

Figure 17.1 Evolution of reactivity in a healthy fetus. (**A**) Three distinct fetal heart rate (FHR) patterns. Accelerations are isolated and variability is decreased. (**B**) This pattern evolves into coalesced accelerations and normal variability. From 12 to 16 minutes, the tracing becomes reactive, with normal variability, obvious accelerations, and (presumably) fetal movement. (**C**) Coalesced accelerations undershoot the baseline (lambda pattern). This is a benign occurrence.

Monitoring Procedure

The nonstress test and the CST are usually performed during the postprandial period, with the patient in semi-Fowler's or left lateral decubitus position. Fetal heart rate, uterine contractions, and fetal movement are obtained with an ultrasound transducer and external tocotransducer, as combined in a standard fetal monitor. If a reactive NST is

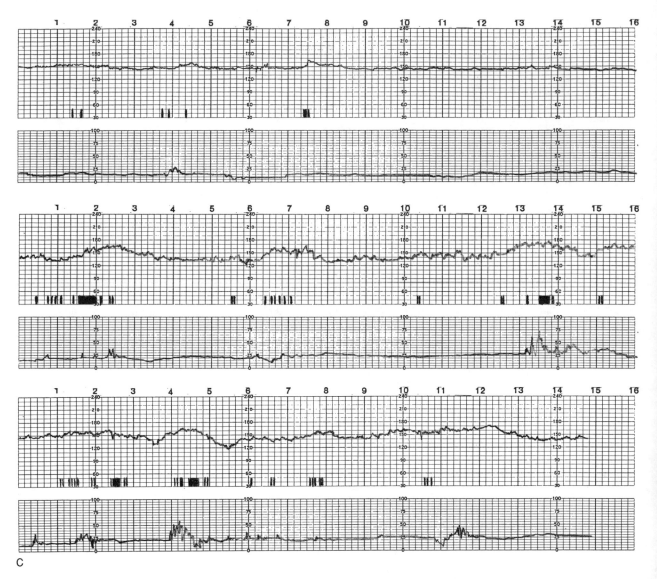

C

Figure 17.2 Schematic tracing of nonstress test (NST) deterioration. (**A**) Reactive NST. Frequent accelerations arise from average variability and coalesce. (**B**) Intermediate NST. Accelerations are less variable and spaced further apart. (**C**) Nonreactive NST. Variability is absent and there are occasional variable decelerations with overshoot ("atypical variable decelerations").

not found within 20 minutes, one should stimulate the fetus either by abdominal palpation or by giving a glucose-containing beverage to the mother. Recently, a number of investigators have applied a vibroacoustic stimulus to the maternal abdomen (5).

Regardless of the stimulus or provocation used, all cri-

teria of the NST must be elicited. Stimulation of a single acceleration does not constitute an appropriate response. If sufficient accelerations are not seen within 40 minutes of the onset of testing, the pattern is deemed nonreactive. Originally, we performed a CST if the NST was nonreactive. Now we perform a biophysical profile to evaluate the nonreactive test. Both schemes will be described (3, 15).

The Contraction Stress Test

The search for late decelerations during the antepartum period is an extrapolation of fetal cardiac surveillance during labor. The earliest signs of placental respiratory distress in the fetus are elicited in this way. But, unlike the situation with the reactive NST, late decelerations can be induced in any fetus when sufficiently provoked by excessive contractions or maternal hypotension. "Late decelerations" occasionally accompany fetal breathing movements in the normal fetus and probably account for a substantial number of false-positive stress tests. Fetal breathing movements may be easily seen with ultrasound scanners, but can also be appreciated on the uterine contraction channel if the tocotransducer is appropriately positioned over a palpable fetal extremity.

Braxton Hicks contractions apparently do not influence fetal state; fetal state is not influenced by contractions. Contractions normally increase the amount of variability and may induce transient flurries of movement at the beginning of a contraction and clustered fetal breathing movement at the end of it (16). During antepartum testing, late decelerations with an otherwise reactive pattern are invariably false positive, while those without reactivity usually, but not invariably, represent fetal deterioration (17).

Both during labor and before, variable decelerations are the most commonly seen deceleration pattern. They increase in frequency with advancing gestation. Early in pregnancy, variable decelerations may normally accompany fetal movement (7). Later in pregnancy, variable decelerations may accompany spontaneous contractions or fetal movements especially if oligohydramnios is present.

With normal variability, accelerations may appear both before the downslope and after the upslope of variable decelerations. In this context, they are referred to as "shoulders" and carry no adverse connotation about the condition of the infant. When variability is persistently absent and a smooth acceleration appears after the return of the variable deceleration, it is termed "overshoot" or "atypical variable decelerations," and the prognosis is guarded (18–20). Occasionally, the acceleration component is larger than the

deceleration. This "overshoot" feature represents autonomic imbalance with compromised parasympathetic (vagal) tone and, in addition to significantly asphyxiated fetuses, may be seen in very immature fetuses, those given atropine, and those with chronic neurologic handicap or congenital anomaly (20).

Oligohydramnios, pathologic conditions, and encumbrances of the umbilical cord increase the likelihood of variable or prolonged decelerations during antepartum and intrapartum testing (15, 21). Oligohydramnios may also produce broad, shallow, intermittent decelerations, out of proportion to the uterine contraction, which must not be confused with late decelerations. In a study by Eden and co-workers, more than 40% of postdate pregnancies with decreased AFV demonstrated FHR decelerations during the NST (15). Yet over 90% of patients whose fetuses had FHR decelerations during the NST had decreased AFV.

The high frequency of FHR decelerations associated with decreased AFV suggests that the umbilical cord is vulnerable to compression and may be the mechanism of deterioration in the babies allowed to remain in utero. With adequate AFV, infants rarely, if ever, demonstrate postmaturity syndrome as neonates. Abnormalities of AFV and FHR decelerations during antepartum testing should also raise the suspicion of fetal anomaly. About 10%–20% of abnormal antepartum tests are found in anomalous babies (22).

Transient decelerations below the previous baseline ("undershoot," or lambda pattern) are a frequent but benign commentary on the return of acceleration to the baseline and also should not be confused with late decelerations (23).

If the frequency of contractions is less than three per 10 minutes, contractions are induced either with oxytocin or by breast stimulation, according to preference. Oxytocin is administered by means of a constant infusion pump beginning at 0.5 mU/minute and increasing the rate of infusion by 0.5 mU/minute every 15 minutes until three contractions are palpable within a 10-minute period. Breast stimulation is done with any number of techniques. Whatever technique is used to begin contractions, no more than three contractions per 10 minutes should be permitted.

Uterine activity under the NST or CST is always monitored. If spontaneous uterine contractions take place, the NST strip is evaluated for the fetal response to contractions as well.

Biophysical Profile

The biophysical profile consists of a general survey of intrauterine contents, including fetal presentation, position, biparietal diameter, and FHR. The placenta is localized, and the AFV is determined. During this survey and for 10 to 30 minutes thereafter, fetal body movements and fetal breathing movements are counted, and fetal tone is determined. There seems little to choose among the dynamic features of the biophysical profile and breathing movements, trunk movements, tone, and cardiac accelerations, if the pattern of any of these is normal (14). The one possible exception is that of tone (15). Multiple dynamic indicators of normality do not improve accuracy for predicting normal outcome. Only when all are abnormal are babies invariably affected. The organized, epochal flurries of movement are the best predictors of fetal well-being, whether those movements are of the eyes, of breathing, or otherwise (8, 10, 24). Isolated single movements that suggest fetal malaise represent either an effect of medication or deterioration. Within reason, the frequency and amplitude of accelerations or movements do not critically define fetal well-being. It is the pattern and sequence of movements and the responses to them that best define fetal reactivity and normal neurologic function.

Amniotic fluid volume may diminish acutely or reflect an underlying congenital anomaly of the central nervous system (CNS), gastrointestinal (GI), or genitourinary (GU) system. As part of the biophysical profile, it seems to provide the measure of nutritional placental function (25-27). It does not appear to be a function of fetal hypoxia, either chronic or acute. Abundant evidence suggests that the loss of amniotic fluid is part of a generalized depletion of water from the fetal compartment, from the skin, the cord, and the blood volume (28). Similarly, nutritional deficiency and respiratory deficiency of the placenta need not develop simultaneously.

As paradoxical as it may seem, the fetus may not flourish nutritionally despite adequate oxygenation. The clinical model here is the postdates infant, who, though dysmature, usually shows no respiratory placental insufficiency in the form of late decelerations. Similarly, experimental animals maintained under chronic hypoxia do not develop oligohydramnios.

Antepartum Testing and Results

The published criteria for a reactive NST—that is, the number of accelerations with fetal movement in a given time—vary considerably and have created some confusion about the use and interpretation of the NST. These differences doubtless influence the duration of testing and to some extent the prevalence of a reactive pattern. They appear to have little clinical importance, although standardization is desirable.

In general, the various tests predict normal outcome well, but are much less accurate in predicting poor outcome (3, 29). Each test shows a relatively high false-positive rate (40% to 80%) but low false-negative rate (around 1%). Such findings have resulted in a well-known aphorism in perinatal medicine: It's easy to make a "good" baby look "bad," but hard to make a "bad" baby look "good." The diagnostic failures in patients with normal antepartum test results (false normal) are most often due to factors such as congenital fetal anomaly or a later acute problem that are unrelated to or unamenable to diagnosis by such surveillance. Nevertheless, a small portion of these unexpectedly poor outcomes may be related to failure to intervene when fetal variable decelerations are associated with an otherwise normal test.

Despite widespread utilization of the NST, there are no controlled studies validating the interval between tests. One week was chosen arbitrarily, but is probably inappropriate under certain conditions. Patients with oligohydramnios, postdate pregnancy, suspected intrauterine growth retardation (IUGR), or diabetes and those who have been hospitalized for other reasons are monitored at least twice weekly (15, 30). Otherwise, weekly testing seems reasonable. No test interval guarantees a normal outcome (3, 29, 30).

The results of studies designed to elucidate the benefit of antepartum testing are so diverse that one or another can be offered as the revealed word of medical evangelists of any persuasion. The reproducibility of these test results ha been questioned repeatedly, but the disastrous results of neglecting abnormal patterns have also been noted (31, 32). The studies also reveal a number of apparent paradoxes. Fetal death has occurred after a reactive NST, for example, but this is rare and usually related to a factor other than that for which testing was undertaken (33).

If stress testing is used to validate the reactive NST, however, babies with reactive positive test results do better than those with reactive results alone. In explanation, the reactive NST is such a good predictor of fetal well-being that, if an indication such as a false-positive CST is used to terminate the pregnancy, the baby will invariably do well. Similarly, whatever the test or management scheme, the more frequently testing is carried out or the greater the number of measurements required for the definition of normal, the better the results (15).

Ultimately, however, we must increase the breadth of our analysis to include, not only oxygenation, but also neurologic integrity and maturity. For these purposes, the NST seems optimal, but it does not predict abnormal outcome, anomaly, or IUGR well. Most growth-retarded fetuses have normal NST or CST results. Heart rate testing is inappropriate for the diagnosis—as opposed to the management—of fetuses with this condition (34). While decelerations on the NST or CST may provide a clue to the possibility of growth failure, the diagnosis is more reliable if supported by the determination of AFV and fetal mensuration with ultrasound (26).

Controversy remains concerning the best way to manage the uncomplicated prolonged pregnancy (15, 35, 36). Those advocating conservative management rely on the NST, CST, or BPP. Others believe that the hazards of continuing pregnancy after the 42nd week are so great they routinely intervene at that time (35). The issue of which management strategy and testing scheme is superior remains unresolved because no controlled study has yet compared the various tests in postdate pregnancy. In addition, differences in methodology, test criteria, and intervention strategy make comparisons of published data less than ideal (15).

Given the rapidity with which AFV may diminish, both semiweekly testing and liberalized criteria for intervention are recommended in postdate pregnancies, whatever test scheme is used (6). In fact, the test chosen is probably not important. The data support the concept that any of them sufficiently evaluates fetal well-being in postdate pregnancies. That is, when delivery is effected immediately after a normal test result, there is virtually no serious morbidity, even if AFV is diminished or FHR decelerations are present.

When conservative management is chosen, results are best when the clinician pays attention to FHR decelerations, as well as the AFV. When any antepartum test shows FHR decelerations or decreased AFV, the postdate patient should be hospitalized and the pregnancy terminated, irrespective of the underlying FHR pattern. If AFV is decreased, anticipate postmaturity syndrome (actually chronic nutritional placental insufficiency related to advanced gestational age).

The benefits of routine NST testing in late pregnancy have been widely debated. In a previous study, we found that about 20% of low-risk patients became high risk under care (33). We also found that NST results correlated better with outcome than did maternal risk classification. About 90% of high-risk patients and 95% of low-risk patients had reactive NST results. But low-risk patients with nonreactive NSTs fared worse than high-risk patients with reactive NSTs. Furthermore, perinatal deaths and anomalies were equally divided among low- and high-risk patients and among reactive and nonreactive NST results. We continue to believe that a program of care that includes fetal evaluation in the assessment of risk improves outcome of both high- and low-risk pregnancies. These and abundant other data support the concept that risk status of the fetus must be tested directly before the mother is designated to be at low risk. Which specific test is used is probably a less important consideration. Positions to the contrary have also been presented.

The issue of routine testing has usually been deliberated as the value of the search for abnormality. This seems to be the wrong perspective. Testing of the individual fetus is necessary to define its own risk status (33). Either the NST with an evaluation of AFV or the BPP seems to perform this function more accurately than any historical assessment of maternal risk or programs based solely on fetal mensuration with ultrasound.

Both from the concept of the definition of the well

fetus or the elucidation of the need to intervene in the potentially growth-retarded infant, a routine NST and measurement of AFV or determining the BPP seems a more rational screening strategy than does the intermittent ultrasonic mensuration of fetal growth.

References

1. Manning FA, Baskett TF, Morrison I, et al. Fetal biophysical profile scoring: a prospective study in 1,184 high-risk patients. Am J Obstet Gynecol 1981;140:289.

2. Evertson LR, Gauthier RJ, Schifrin BS, et al. Antepartum fetal heart rate testing. I. Evolution of the nonstress test. Am J Obstet Gynecol 1979;133:29.

3. Schifrin BS. The rationale for antepartum fetal heart rate monitoring. J Reprod Med 1979;23:213.

4. Devoe LD, McKenzie J, Searle NS, et al. Clinical sequelae of the extended nonstress test. Am J Obstet Gynecol 1985; 151:1074.

5. Brubaker K, Garite T. The lambda fetal heart rate pattern: an assessment of its significance in the intrapartum period. Obstet Gynecol 1988;72(6):881–5.

6. Brioschi PA, Extermann P, Terracina D, et al. Antepartum nonstress fetal heart rate monitoring: systematic analysis of baseline patterns and decelerations as an adjunct to reactivity. Am J Obstet Gynecol 1985;153:633.

7. Timor-Tritsch IE, Dierker LJ, Zadan J, et al. Fetal movements associated with fetal heart rate accelerations and decelerations. Am J Obstet Gynecol 1978;131:276.

8. De Vries JIP, Visser GHA, Prechtl HFR. The emergence of fetal behavior. I. Qualitative aspects. Early Hum Dev 1982; 7:301.

9. Nijhuis JG, Prechtl HFR, Martin CB Jr, et al. Are there behavioral states in the human fetus? Early Hum Dev 1982; 6:177.

10. Patrick J, Carmichael L, Chess L, et al. The distribution of accelerations of the human fetal heart rate at 38 to 40 weeks' gestational age. Am J Obstet Gynecol 1985;151:283.

11. Murata Y, Martin CB, Ikenoue T, et al. Fetal heart rate accelerations and late decelerations during the course of intrauterine death in chronically catheterized rhesus monkeys. Am J Obstet Gynecol 1982;144:218.

12. Rochard F, Schifrin BS, Goupil F, et al. Nonstressed fetal heart rate monitoring in the antepartum period. Am J Obstet Gynecol 1976;126:699.

13. Lavin JP Jr, Miodovnik M, Barden TP. Relationship of nonstress test reactivity and gestational age. Obstet Gynecol 1984;63:338.

14. Vintzileos AM, Campbell WA, Nochimson DJ, et al. The use and misuse of the fetal biophysical profile. Am J Obstet Gynecol 1987;156:527.

15. Eden RD, Gergely RZ, Schifrin BS, et al. Comparison of antepartum testing schemes for the management of the postdate pregnancy. Am J Obstet Gynecol 1982; 144:683.

16. Mulder EJH, Visser GHA. Braxton Hicks contractions and motor behavior in the near-term human fetus. Am J Obstet Gynecol 1987;156:543.

17. Braly P, Freeman RK. The significance of fetal heart rate reactivity with a positive oxytocin challenge test. Am J Obstet Gynecol 1977;50:689.

18. Baskett TF, Sandy EA. The oxytocin challenge test: an ominous pattern associated with severe fetal growth retardation. Am J Obstet Gynecol 1979;54:365.

19. Freeman RK, James J. Clinical experience with the oxytocin challenge test. II. An ominous atypical pattern. Obstet Gynecol 1977;46:255.

20 Shields JR, Schifrin BS. Perinatal antecedents of cerebral palsy. Obstet Gynecol 1988;71:899.

21. Druzin ML, Gratacos J, Keegan KA, et al. Antepartum fetal heart rate testing. VII. The significance of fetal bradycardia. Am J Obstet Gynecol 1981;139:194.

22. Garite TJ, Linzey EM, Freeman RK: Fetal heart rate patterns and fetal distress in fetuses with congenital anomalies. Obstet Gynecol 1979;53:716.

23. Spencer JAD, Deans A, Nicolaidis P, Arulkumaran S. Fetal heart rate response to vibroacoustic stimulation during low and high heart rate variability episodes in late pregnancy 1991;165(1):86–90.

24. Birnholz JC, Stephens JC, Faria M. Fetal movement patterns: a possible means of defining neurologic developmental milestones in utero. Am J Roentgenol 1978;130:537.

25. Clement D, Schifrin BS, Kates RB. Acute oligohydramnios in postdate pregnancy. Am J Obstet Gynecol 1987;157:884.

26. Manning FA, Hill LM, Platt LD. Quantitative amniotic fluid volume determination by ultrasound: antepartum detection of intrauterine growth retardation. Am J Obstet Gynecol 1981;139:254.

27. Mercer LJ, Brown LG, Petres RE, et al. A survey of pregnancies complicated by decreased amniotic fluid. Am J Obstet Gynecol 1984;149:355.

28. Paterson PJ, Dunstan MK, Trickey NRA, et al. A biochemical

comparison of the mature and postmature fetus and new-born infant. J Obstet Gynaecol Br Commonw 1970; 77: 390.

29. Druzin ML, Gratacos J, Paul RH. Antepartum fetal heart rate testing. VI. Predictive reliability of "normal" tests in the prevention of antepartum death. Am J Obstet Gynecol 1980;137:746.

30. Barrett JM, Salyer SL, Boehm FH. The nonstress test: an evaluation of 1,000 patients. Am J Obstet Gynecol 1981; 141: 153.

31. Bobitt JR. Abnormal antepartum fetal heart rate tracings, failure to intervene, and fetal death: review of five cases reveals potential pitfalls of antepartum monitoring programs. Am J Obstet Gynecol 1979;133:415.

32. Borgatta L, Shrout PE, Divon MY. Reliability and reproducibility of nonstress test readings. Am J Obstet Gynecol 1988;159:554.

33. Schifrin BS, Foye G, Amato J, et al: Routine fetal heart rate monitoring in the antepartum period. Obstet Gynecol 1979;54:21.

34. Schifrin BS, Lapidus M, Doctor GS, et al. Contraction stress test for antepartum fetal evaluation. Obstet Gynecol 1975; 45:433.

35. Dyson DC, Miller PD, Armstrong MA. Management of prolonged pregnancy: induction of labor versus antepartum fetal testing. Am J Obstet Gynecol 1987;156:928.

36. Freeman RK, Garite TJ, Modanlou H, et al. Postdate pregnancy: utilization of contraction stress testing for primary fetal surveillance. Am J Obstet Gynecol 1981;140:128.

37. Schifrin BS. Exercises in fetal monitoring. Los Angeles: BPM, Inc., 1988:(2)2–41.

18

Interpreting Fetal Heart Tracings

Thomas J. Garite, M.D.
Richard A. Pircon, M.D.

FETAL heart rate (FHR) monitoring has great potential for avoiding antepartum and intrapartum fetal asphyxia and death. It is also useful in monitoring uterine contractions, observing fetal response to anesthesia, and observing fetal response to changes in the maternal medical condition. Additionally, FHR monitoring is an aid in determining the best time and route of delivery. Unfortunately, interpretation of FHR tracings is difficult, imprecise, and often controversial. It is a matter of pattern recognition and hence depends on past observation of similar patterns and knowledge of their cause and significance with respect to fetal and neonatal outcome.

Prior to presenting case examples, it is necessary to review the basic principles of fetal heart rate interpretation. The fetal heart rate tracing is composed of a continuous recording of not only the fetal heart rate but also uterine contraction activity. Uterine activity is described by 1) baseline tonus, 2) contraction amplitude, 3) contraction duration, and 4) contraction interval. Contractions are monitored using an external tocodynamometer or an internal pressure catheter. Baseline tonus and amplitude can be measured accurately only by using the internal pressure catheter. Contraction duration is often underestimated using an external monitor. Adequate contractions for labor are defined as those contractions of sufficient amplitude, duration, and interval to cause progressive cervical dilatation.

The fetal heart rate is described by 1) baseline rate, 2) variability, and 3) periodic changes. The baseline rate is the fetal heart rate that predominates over a given time interval (usually more than 15 minutes). Normal baseline rate is 120–160 beats per minute (bpm). However, a normal fetus can have a rate that is less than this value. Baseline rate greater than 160 bpm can be a sign of fetal hypoxia or possibly a normal response to maternal fever or maternal drugs (i.e., terbutaline). The normal fetal heart rate response to maternal fever is approximately a 10 bpm rise for every one degree of temperature elevation.

Variability is an important fetal heart rate characteristic which predicts the status of the fetus at any given point in time. Variability reflects normal neurologic modulation of the heart rate. The variability can be described as either short-term or long-term. The short-term variability is the beat-to-beat irregularity. If one considers the FHR to be a series of electrocardiograph QRS complexes, the short-term variability is the difference in R-R interval from one heart beat to the next. Therefore, short-term variability can only be determined using direct internal scalp electrode fetal heart rate monitoring. Doppler external fetal heart rate monitoring can artifactually increase short-term variability. Recently, this artifact has been minimized with modern Doppler units using autocorrelation technology.

Long-term variability is the cyclic waviness of the fetal heart rate tracing. This can be assessed using either internal electrode or external Doppler monitoring. With early hypoxia, increased variability is often seen. Progressive hypoxia and acidosis are associated with decreasing variability.

In patients with decreased variability, as with any non-reassuring FHR pattern, the fetus can be further evaluated by a scalp blood pH. A complete discussion of fetal scalp blood sampling is discussed elsewhere. Fetal scalp stimulation can also be used to assess the fetal status. Fetuses that respond to scalp stimulation with an acceleration of the heart rate (15 bpm for at least 15 seconds) have been shown to have a scalp pH greater than 7.20 (1). This technique has been proposed as an alternative to fetal scalp blood sampling in patients with worrisome intrapartum fetal heart rate tracings.

Periodic changes are fetal heart rate decelerations that occur with uterine activity. There are four principle types of decelerations described: early, late, variable, and prolonged. A complete discussion of fetal heart rate changes and heart rate regulation has been described by Martin (2). An early deceleration is a symmetric U-shaped drop in the fetal heart rate which begins with the onset of the uterine contraction and ends with the uterine contraction. It is not associated with fetal hypoxia, acidosis, or low Apgar scores.

Late decelerations, like early decelerations, are symmetrical and U-shaped. However, the onset of the deceleration is delayed and occurs after the onset of the uterine contraction. Late decelerations are associated with inadequate oxygen delivery, exchange, or uptake. This is classically described as uteroplacental insufficiency.

Uteroplacental insufficiency can result from uterine hypoperfusion from causes such as maternal hypotension or drug-induced vasospasm (i.e., maternal cocaine use). Other causes of uteroplacental insufficiency include placental pathology resulting in decreased oxygen diffusion. This can result from chronic medical disorders (i.e., diabetes mellitus, chronic hypertension) or acute processes such as abruptio placentae.

Late decelerations can also result from acute maternal and fetal medical conditions. These include maternal anemia, maternal diabetic ketoacidosis, and fetal anemia. Finally, late decelerations can result from uterine hyperstimulation occurring naturally or secondary to labor induction or augmentation (i.e., use of prostaglandin or oxytocin).

When late decelerations are recognized, management should include several basic steps: 1) placement of the patient in the lateral recumbent position, 2) intravenous fluid infusion, 3) maternal oxygen administration, and 4) evaluation of the patient to identify a possible treatable cause of late decelerations. Patient positioning and intravenous fluid infusion improve uterine blood flow. Placing the patient in the right or left recumbent position displaces the uterus laterally and reduces compression of the inferior vena cava. This results in an increased venous cardiac return, with improved maternal cardiac output. The left and right lateral positions are equally effective in improving cardiac output (3).

There are several treatable causes of late decelerations. In these patients, therapy is directed at the specific medical condition. Late decelerations secondary to uterine hyperstimulation can be treated with subcutaneous terbutaline, intravenous beta sympathomimetics, and intravenous magnesium sulfate (4–7).

Variable decelerations are the most frequently seen fetal heart rate deceleration. The drop in the fetal heart rate is variable in duration, intensity, and timing relative to uterine contractions. The cause of variable decelerations is compression of the umbilical cord. Repetitive variable decelerations can result in significant fetal hypoxia and acidosis. As variable decelerations become more severe (deeper and longer lasting), the patient can be repositioned in an effort to relieve cord compression. Recent studies have demonstrated that intrapartum variable decelerations that develop before the second stage of labor can be treated with saline amnioinfusion. The technique was originally described by Miyazaki et al. (8, 9). Prophylactic use in preterm premature rupture of membranes has also been shown to be effective (10).

Prolonged decelerations may result from any number of causes. Profound and sudden hypoxia, as with any form of uteroplacental insufficiency, or prolonged umbilical cord compression can result in prolonged decelerations. Rapid descent of the fetus can also result in a prolonged deceleration.

With this background, one of the best ways to teach and reinforce knowledge of FHR monitoring is by presenting case examples. It is hoped that reviewing this collection of clinical cases will be a useful and educational experience.

Fetal Monitoring Patterns

CASE 18.1 Variable Decelerations

A 34-year-old primigravida was admitted at 43 weeks' gestation, three hours following spontaneous premature rupture of the membrane (PROM), with complaints of irregular uterine contractions every two to five minutes. A fetal scalp electrode and external tocodynamometer were placed with subsequent continuous monitoring of the fetal heart rate and uterine contractions. The irregular contractions continued three hours after admission, and labor was augmented with oxytocin. An internal pressure catheter was then placed to more accurately monitor uterine activity. The patient made adequate progress in labor and had intermittent mild variable decelerations during that time. The tracing shown in Figure 18.1 was recorded during the second stage of labor and revealed the following data:

Uterine activity
Baseline tonus: 10–15 mm Hg
Amplitude: >100 mm Hg with pushing
Duration: 40–60 seconds
Interval: 1.25–1.5 minutes, regular

Fetal heart rate
Baseline rate: 150 bpm, rising to 170 bpm
Variability: decreased
Periodic changes: variable decelerations

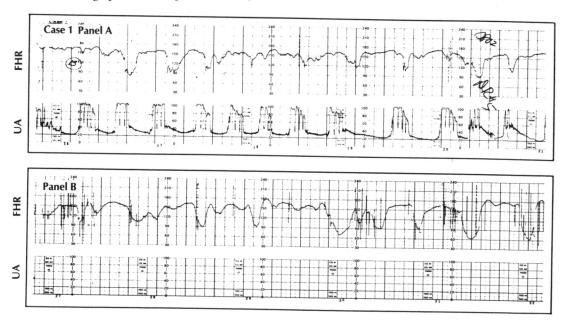

Figure 18.1   Monitor: Hewlett-Packard model 8030A. Paper speed: 3 cm/min. Vertical scale: 30 bpm/cm. Method: Direct (fetal scalp spiral electrode and intrauterine pressure catheter). Note that the pressure catheter has been removed in panel B.

INTERPRETATION

In panel A (Figure 18.1), there are a few mild variable decelerations, down to a maximum of 90 bpm, lasting up to 30 seconds. These are associated with a mild fetal tachycardia of 150–160 bpm and average-to-slightly decreased FHR variability. This patient should be treated initially with position change. If such a pattern persists in the second stage of labor, then close observation is required. This pattern at this time is not an indication for operative delivery. However, approximately 45 minutes later, in panel B, the variable decelerations go down to 70 bpm and last up to 45 seconds. More importantly, they are associated with a gradually rising FHR baseline, up to 170 bpm, with a further reduction in FHR variability. Also note that, after several of the decelerations, accelerations are rather blunted. In fact, there is a general blunting of the response of the heart rate changes (slow and not abrupt). These signs suggest a progressive fall in the fetal pH. In the presence of developing tachycardia and loss of variability in the second stage, intervention is probably indicated.

MANAGEMENT AND OUTCOME

The physician managing this patient decided that the more ominous variable decelerations, loss of variability, and tachycardia indicated intervention. The patient was delivered by vacuum extraction of a 6-lb, 9-oz girl with Apgar scores of 4 at one minute and 8 at five minutes. The baby has done well. There was no apparent cord entanglement to explain the variable decelerations. However, postdate patients with oligohydramnios often have this type of FHR pattern.

This case illustrates the difficulty in managing second-stage variable decelerations. Usually, the variable decelerations look rather profound but are associated with a normal FHR and normal variability. The most important parameters to monitor are 1) rising baseline and 2) loss of variability. One can be more tolerant of abnormal FHR changes in the second stage; delivery is expected shortly, and, if intervention is required, it can be performed quickly and easily. ∎

CASE 18.2 Persistent Late Decelerations

The patient was a 27-year-old primigravida, admitted in early labor at 42 weeks' gestation with intact membranes. On admission, the cervix was 1 cm dilated and 50% effaced, with the vertex presenting at -3 station. About four hours after commencement of labor, the patient's contractions were regular. Artificial rupture of membranes revealed a scant amount of amniotic fluid lightly tinged with meconium. An internal electrode was inserted, and contractions were monitored with an external tocodynamometer. Several hours later, the patient's temperature and physical examination suggested early amnionitis.

Uterine activity
Baseline tonus: not interpretable on external monitor
Amplitude: not interpretable on external monitor
Frequency: every 2–3.5 minutes
Duration: 60–80 seconds

Fetal heart rate
Baseline rate: 135 bpm
Variability: normal
Periodic changes: intermittent variable decelerations and intermittent late decelerations

INTERPRETATION

The panels in Figure 18.2 were recorded about one hour apart. In panels B and C, the patient was having persistent late decelerations with each contraction, as well as several mild variable decelerations. It should be noted that some contractions were not being recorded well. The sometimes more obvious, but mild, variable decelerations should not prevent the observer from noticing the coincident late decelerations. Furthermore, in panel C, there appears to be a further rise in the baseline heart rate to 150 bpm and some decrease in FHR variability. The combination of late decelerations and variable decelerations can appear as a variable deceleration, with slow return to baseline. This is

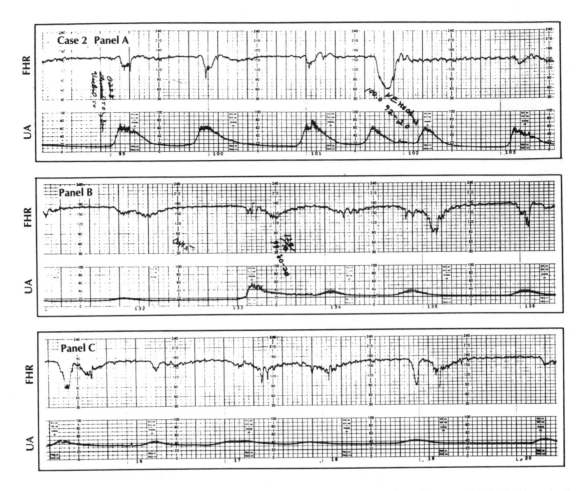

Figure 18.2 Monitor: Hewlett-Packard model 8030A. Paper speed: 3 cm/min. Vertical scale: 30 bpm/cm. Method: Direct (scalp spiral electrode) and external tocodynamometer.

common in the postdate pregnancy associated with postmature fetus. The variable decelerations occur because amniotic fluid, which is scant, normally protects the umbilical cord from compression during labor. The persistent late decelerations are a result of placental insufficiency.

MANAGEMENT AND OUTCOME

Between panels A and B, the patient was placed on her side and given fluids and oxygen; however, the late decelerations persisted. Additionally, the patient's temperature

declined to 99°F, but the fetal tachycardia persisted. Apparently, this pattern was not appreciated for several hour Three hours after the beginning of Figure 18.2B, becaus of irreversible late decelerations, a primary cesarean sectio was performed for fetal distress. A 6-lb, 3-oz boy was deliv ered, with Apgar scores of 6 at one minute and 9 at fiv minutes. Thick meconium was present at delivery.

Persistent late decelerations, not uncommon in pos date pregnancy, require some form of action. If late dece erations remain unrecognized and persist during labor, fet acidosis can result. This must be regarded as an ominou pattern. If repositioning, oxygen, and fluids do not change the pattern, then the clinician needs to assess the patient's stage and progress of labor. If a vaginal delivery is expected within a short period of time, then fetal scalp stimulation or repeated measurements of scalp blood pH are recommended. Saline amnioinfusion may also be beneficial in this situation. The variable decelerations may be relieved with amnioinfusion. Additionally, amnioinfusion has been shown to dilute thick meconium and can improve neonatal outcome (11). If the scalp pHs are abnormal, or if delivery is not imminent, an immediate cesarean section is appropriate.

This baby had stigmata of postmaturity, including loss of subcutaneous fat. While in the newborn nursery, the infant had transient hypoglycemia and hyperbilirubinemia. The baby was discharged with the mother five days after birth. There were no apparent further sequelae. ■

CASE 18.3 Prolonged Decelerations

This patient was a 33-year-old gravida 5, para 3 admitted in early labor at term. On admission, her cervix was dilated to 3 cm, and she was having contractions every five minutes. She was placed on external fetal heart rate and uterine contraction monitors. The baseline FHR was 150 bpm, with accelerations and no decelerations. Approximately six hours after admission, the pattern on the external monitoring was as follows:

Uterine activity
Baseline tonus: not interpretable
Amplitude: not interpretable
Duration: 1.5–2 minutes
Interval: 3–5 minutes

Fetal heart rate
Baseline rate: 150 bpm
Variability: apparently normal
Periodic changes: prolonged decelerations

INTERPRETATION

A prolonged deceleration is seen in Figure 18.3A, going down to 90 bpm, with the deceleration lasting 10 minutes. The patient was placed on her side and given oxygen, and her attending physician was notified. Shortly after the FHR had returned to the previous baseline, another prolonged deceleration occurred, again down to 90 bpm, lasting eight minutes. Vaginal examination revealed no umbilical cord prolapse or sudden descent of the presenting part. Nor was there any predisposing cause of the prolonged decelerations.

It is appropriate to term these decelerations "prolonged" rather than severe variable decelerations or bradycardia. Bradycardia refers to the baseline FHR, and this is clearly not a change in the baseline. This is indeed a periodic change. Variable decelerations are caused by umbilical cord compression and generally are characterized by abrupt onset of the deceleration and abrupt return to the baseline FHR. Frequently, they are associated with accelerations that precede the deceleration or follow the deceleration or both.

Prolonged decelerations may have a number of causes: uterine hyperstimulation, umbilical cord prolapse, hypotension, paracervical anesthesia, or rapid descent through the birth canal. Maternal hypotension can be caused by conduction anesthesia, supine position, or maternal hemorrhage. Maternal hypoxia can result from seizures, pulmonary edema, pulmonary embolus, or respiratory depression secondary to drug overdose (i.e., magnesium sulfate, narcotics). Occasionally, such decelerations (usually of shorter duration) may be seen during pelvic examination, application of a scalp electrode, or sustained maternal Valsalva's maneuver.

When a patient develops such prolonged decelerations, an immediate vaginal examination should be done to rule out cord prolapse or rapid descent of the fetus. The patient should have a complete set of vital signs taken, looking for hypotension, tachypnea, apnea, or bradycardia. If an abnormality is found, then the previously listed conditions should be sought and treated, if possible. If uterine hyperstimulation is diagnosed, then the patient can be treated with subcutaneous or intravenous terbutaline (4–6). In the absence of such apparent causes, one must conclude that prolonged umbilical cord compression is the cause. Repositioning, infusing intravenous fluids, and providing oxygen can often be corrective. Saline amnioinfusion may also be helpful.

Recurring prolonged decelerations to less than 70–80 bpm when delivery is not expected soon is one of the most difficult FHR patterns to manage. Whenever possible, the FHR should be allowed to return to the previous baseline, waiting for "placental resuscitation" as the baby recovers. Still, it is often difficult to know exactly when such a pattern will go down and not return. Cesarean section may be justified when decelerations go below 80 bpm, lasting

longer than three or four minutes, and recurring three or four times during early labor.

An equally difficult situation is when the fetal heart rate drops without return to baseline for four to five minutes. If the preceding segment of the fetal heart rate tracing is reassuring, then the fetal heart rate will most probably return to baseline. However, the patient needs to be transferred to the operating room in the event that the fetal heart rate doesn't return. Prior to performing an operative delivery, the fetal heart rate should be remonitored. If the fetal heart rate has returned, then an operative delivery can be avoided.

MANAGEMENT AND OUTCOME

This pattern recurred twice within the next hour; there was no response to position change. No apparent cause could be identified. Therefore, the patient was taken for cesarean section where, under epidural anesthesia, a 9-lb, 11.5-o boy was delivered, with Apgar scores of 7 at one minute

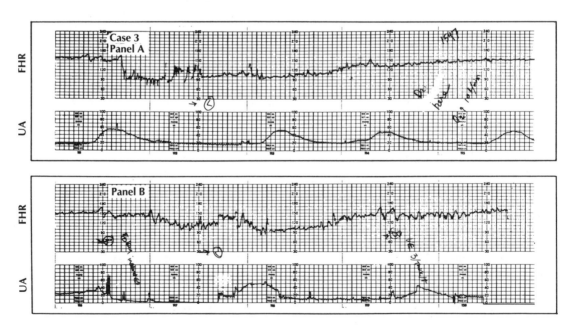

Figure 18.3   Monitor: Hewlett-Packard model 8030A. Paper speed: 3 cm/min. Vertical scale: 30 bpm/cm. Method: External (Doppler FHR monitor and external tocodynamometer).

and 9 at five minutes. There was a loop of umbilical cord adjacent to the baby's head. Compression of the cord in the lower segment may have been the cause of these prolonged decelerations.   ▄

CASE 18.4   Increased Variability

The patient was a 19-year-old primigravida admitted at 37 weeks' gestation in active labor with mild preeclampsia. On admission, the patient was having regular contractions, and, on examination, the cervix was noted to be 5 cm dilated, 50% effaced, and the vertex presenting at -1 station. Amniotomy was performed after the patient was externally monitored for two hours. She had progressed to 7 cm and 0 station. An internal electrode and pressure catheter were placed at that time and revealed the following pattern:

Uterine activity
Frequency: irregular, every 2–5 minutes
Duration: 60–70 seconds
Baseline tonus: 20–25 mm Hg
Amplitude: 60–80 mm Hg

Fetal heart rate
Baseline rate: 130 bpm
Variability: decreased
Periodic changes: increased variability in period immediately following the contractions

INTERPRETATION

The significance of a repetitive pattern of increased variability in the period immediately following the contractions was not appreciated. The decreased FHR variability was recognized, but, in the absence of periodic decelerations, no further evaluation or intervention was pursued. In Figure 18.4A, there is a period of increased long-term variability that can be seen immediately following each contraction. There is no substantial change in the baseline. Also, the increased variability is seen with the stronger contractions and, in one instance, is not apparent with the weaker contraction. The timing and relationship of the contractions make the pattern remarkably similar to late decelerations. This persisted for approximately an hour. Then, in panel B, while this pattern persists with several of the contractions, the backbone of a late deceleration can also be noted. A short time later, in panel C, obvious and typical late decelerations became apparent. While not typical, occasionally the onset of late decelerations is herald by increased variability following contractions (where late decelerations would normally appear). Therefore, increased variability late in timing should be considered to be as important as persistent late decelerations and warrants further assessment.

MANAGEMENT AND OUTCOME

The FHR pattern was appreciated only in Figure 18.4C. At this time, the patient had made no further progress in labor, and the persistent late decelerations did not respond to oxygen, intravenous fluids, and position change. The patient was taken for emergent cesarean section. A 5-lb, 10-oz girl was delivered, with Apgar scores of 6 at one minute and 7 at five minutes. Umbilical cord pHs were taken: the arterial pH was 7.17, and the venous pH was 7.19. At delivery, thick meconium, which had not been detected earlier, was also noted. There was no apparent explanation for the uteroplacental insufficiency other than the mild preeclampsia. Subsequently, the baby did well in the newborn nursery and had no particular complications.

Optimal management for this patient should have included scalp stimulation or determination of fetal scalp pH as soon as the internal electrode was placed, revealing the pattern of decreased variability in the period immediately following the late decelerations (Figure 18.4C). An ideal use for fetal scalp sampling is in the instance of a confusing pattern, especially if the pattern is associated with such non-reassuring signs as decreased variability.   ▄

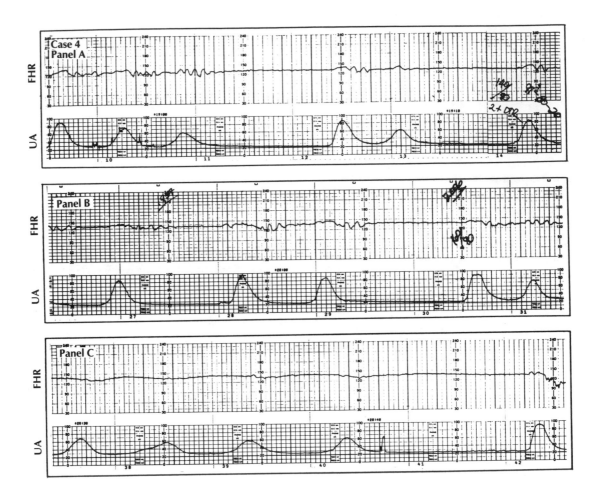

Figure 18.4   Monitor: Hewlett-Packard model 8030A. Paper speed: 3 cm/min. Vertical scale: 30 bpm/cm. Method: Direct (fetal scalp

C A S E   1 8 . 5   Decreased Variability

This 32-year-old gravida 3, para 0 was admitted in early labor at 42-1/2 weeks' gestation with spontaneously ruptured membranes, but no apparent meconium staining. Three hours after admission, the patient's cervix was 2 cm dilated, 80% effaced, and the presenting vertex was floating.

The external monitor tracing revealed the following data in Figure 18.5A:

Uterine activity
Baseline tonus: not interpretable on external monitor
Amplitude: not interpretable on external monitor

Duration: 1.5–2 minutes
Interval: 5–8 minutes, irregular

Fetal heart rate
Baseline rate: 160 bpm
Variability: decreased
Periodic changes: none

INTERPRETATION

Shortly after the end of the tracing in panel A, because the unexplained baseline tachycardia and the flattened he rate, an internal scalp electrode was inserted, and the patie was placed on her side and given oxygen. These measu

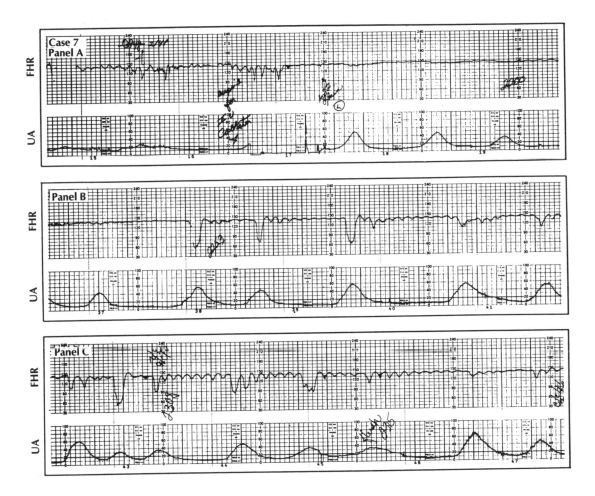

Figure 18.5   Monitor: Hewlett-Packard model 8030A. Paper speed: 3 cm/min. Vertical scale: 30 bpm/cm. Method: Initially, external FHR by Doppler; subsequently, internal scalp spiral electrode. Contractions were monitored by external tocodynamometer.

were taken immediately before the beginning of panel B. In panels B and C, the variability, especially the long-term, is markedly decreased. There is persistent tachycardia of 165 bpm, and there are persistent, subtle late decelerations occurring with each contraction. These decelerations were recognized only after placement of the internal monitor.

A fetus with apparent decreased short-term variability and absent accelerations, especially in the presence of tachycardia, requires very careful monitoring. Whenever possible, an internal scalp electrode should be placed. Persistent late decelerations, particularly in the postterm pregnancy, may go unrecognized for hours because of their subtle nature. Their depth generally correlates with the degree of

hypoxia; however, when the fetus becomes acidemic, the decelerations that were initially reflexive may subsequently be caused by direct myocardial depression and consequently become shallower in character. When the pregnancy is prolonged, late decelerations may be especially shallow and subtle. Such patients should be monitored with particular care to detect fetal distress. Occasionally, one may encounter a fetal heart rate tracing where there is decreased variability without apparent periodic changes. This can occasionally result from severe hypoxia. Other causes in the nonhypoxic fetus include maternal drug abuse, fetal central nervous system (CNS) anomaly, or CNS damage from a previous episode of hypoxia that has since resolved. A fetal scalp pH is very helpful in such a clinical situation.

MANAGEMENT AND OUTCOME

Despite oxygen and lateral positioning, the late decelerations persisted (even though uterine activity was relatively infrequent) and were present with each contraction. It was impossible to obtain a scalp pH to confirm fetal hypoxia because the cervix was undilated. Thus, given the gestational age and FHR pattern, a cesarean section was done.

The patient delivered an 8-lb, 6 oz–girl, with Apgar scores of 2 at one minute and 6 at five minutes and stigmata of postmaturity. The infant was treated for hyperbilirubinemia and polycythemia, but otherwise did well and was in apparently good condition at time of discharge. The mother's postoperative course was uneventful. ■

C A S E   1 8 . 6   Baseline Bradycardia

A 22-year-old primigravida at 37 weeks' gestation was admitted in active labor. One hour after admission, an amniotomy was performed, and an internal electrode was placed. The amniotic fluid was clear at the time of rupture. Her contractions were monitored with an external tocodynamometer. Several hours later, the labor was progressing normally, and the fetal monitor revealed the following data:

Uterine activity
Baseline tonus: not interpretable on external monitor
Amplitude: not interpretable
Durations: 50–90 seconds
Interval: 1–3 minutes

Fetal heart rate
Baseline rate: 90 bpm, rising to 110 bpm
Variability: normal
Periodic changes: accelerations initially and second-stage variable decelerations

INTERPRETATION

Initially, a fetal bradycardia of about 90 bpm was noted. This was not associated with any loss of variability, and accelerations above this baseline were present. In Figure 18.6A, there were no other significant periodic changes, except for some minimal variable decelerations. Approximately an hour later, in panel B, the patient had progressed into the second stage of labor. More typical second-stage variable decelerations were noted. These returned to baseline and were associated with normal FHR variability. When the patient was admitted, the baseline FHR was 130 bpm. As labor progressed, the rate gradually drifted down to 90 bpm, as seen in Figure 18.6A. Before that, there were no significant periodic changes.

MANAGEMENT AND OUTCOME

Whenever a fetus has baseline bradycardia, one should determine whether this is a baseline change or possibly a prolonged deceleration. Baseline changes persist and are associated with accelerations and decelerations. Additionally, with bradycardia, it is important to assess the baseline FHR variability. A bradycardia that is not a deceleration and is associated with normal beat-to-beat variability is usually a benign pattern. Bradycardia may represent a pathologic condition such as fetal heart block. This can result from blocked premature atrial contractions or complete heart block. With complete heart block, a baseline FHR is 60–70 bpm, and there are minimal variability and no periodic changes. Such a pattern can be associated with significant fetal cardiac anomalies or maternal systemic lupus erythematosus (12). However, baseline bradycardia with normal variability in the 80–110 bpm range is generally associated with normal outcome and has no apparent explanation.

Approximately half an hour after the end of panel B, the patient spontaneously delivered a 6-lb girl, with Apgar scores of 9 at one minute and 9 at five minutes. The baby did well in the newborn nursery and had a normal heart rate. Both baby and mother were discharged two days later.

This case illustrates the importance of proper terminology in assessing the FHR. Prolonged decelerations down to 90 bpm may be an indication of fetal hypoxia. Baseline bradycardia with normal variability is usually benign. ■

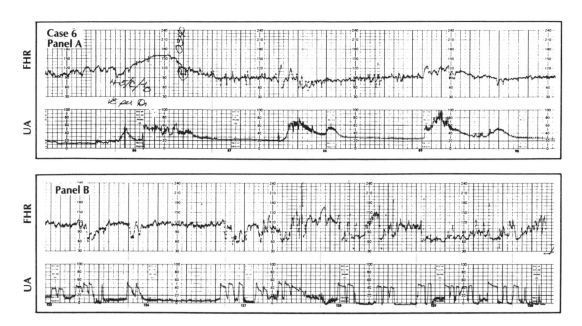

Figure 18.6   Monitor: Hewlett-Packard model 8030A. Paper speed: 3 cm/min. Vertical scale: 30 bpm/cm. Method: Direct (fetal scalp spiral electrode) and external tocodynamometer.

C A S E 1 8 . 7   Sinusoidal Pattern

A 27-year-old gravida 2, para 1, admitted at 39 weeks' gestation in active labor, had an uncomplicated prenatal course and no apparent problems. On admission, her cervix was found to be 4–5 cm dilated, 80% effaced, and the presenting vertex was at -1 station. Vital signs were normal. Because of difficulty in obtaining an adequate tracing from the external monitor, an amniotomy was performed 45 minutes after admission, and an internal electrode and pressure catheter were placed. At amniotomy, moderately thick meconium was noted. The initial monitoring period in Figure 18.7A revealed the following:

Uterine activity
Frequency: 2.5–3 minutes
Duration: 60 seconds
Baseline tonus: 5 mm Hg
Amplitude: 35–50 mm Hg

Fetal heart rate
Baseline rate: 140 bpm

Variability: initially normal, followed by a period of decreased variability
Periodic changes: initially, there are several small variable appearing decelerations, followed by an early deceleration

INTERPRETATION

Approximately an hour later, in panels B and C the FHR became unusual and somewhat bizarre. Several large, deep, variable decelerations occurred. However, these were relatively short in duration, with a rapid return to baseline. In and of themselves, they suggested mild umbilical cord compression, but the baseline heart rate met all the criteria necessary to describe a sinusoidal pattern. These included stable baseline heart rate of 120–160 bpm with regular oscillations. The amplitude of the oscillation was 5–15 bpm, and rarely greater. The frequency of the oscillation was 2–5 cycles per minute (as long-term variability) with fixed or flat short-term variability and no areas of normal FHR variability or reactivity. Such patterns have been associated with severe fetal anemia, severe hypoxia, or following maternal injection of alphaprodine hydrochloride. Recent-

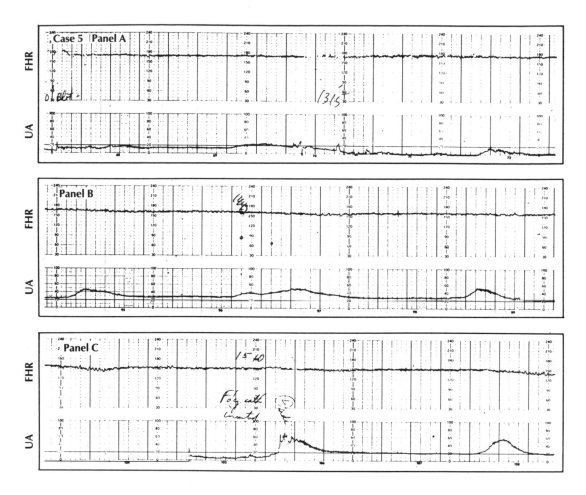

Figure 18.7   Monitor: Hewlett-Packard model 8030A. Paper speed: 3 cm/min. Vertical scale: 30 bpm/cm. Method: Direct (fetal scalp spiral electrode and intrauterine pressure catheter).

ly, an intermittent sinusoidal pattern has been described (13). This pattern was seen in less anemic fetuses where segments of the fetal heart rate tracing (less than 10 minutes) met criteria of true sinusoidal pattern. Yet, in the same tracing, there were areas of normal fetal heart rate reactivity.

Sinusoidal patterns are extremely rare. More commonly, other patterns are often confused with the truly sinusoidal pattern. These are usually normal patterns with either increased variability or frequent small accelerations above the baseline. Unfortunately, such patterns, when mistaken for sinusoidal, have led to inappropriate intervention. Therefore, when there is any question, a fetal scalp sam-

pling for pH and fetal hematocrit are indicated.

MANAGEMENT AND OUTCOME

The physician managing this case did not appreciate the significance of this FHR pattern. A spontaneous vaginal delivery occurred shortly after the end of panel C. Before delivery of the shoulders, the oronasal pharynx was suctioned. Following delivery, the baby was intubated, and meconium was suctioned from below the vocal cords. Apgar scores were 4 at one minute and 6 at five minutes. The baby was a 3,200-g girl, that was appropriate for gestational age. The umbilical cord venous pH was 7.33. A central hematocrit on the neonate was 22%. The apparent explanation for this severe anemia was found when a Kleihauer-Betke test on maternal blood detected a fetomaternal transfusion. The estimated volume of fetal blood loss was 200–300 mL. This anemia may have caused the sinusoidal pattern. The newborn had seizures and renal failure, but responded to medical management. There was no evidence of intracranial hemorrhage. The baby was discharged on the 15th day of life, doing fairly well.   ■

CASE 18.8 Low-Risk Patient

A 19-year-old nullipara was admitted in early labor at 37 weeks' gestation with premature ruptured membranes. The patient's cervix was 1 cm dilated and uneffaced, and the presenting vertex was floating. The patient was monitored using external Doppler and external tocodynomonitor. Fifteen minutes after her admission to the hospital, the tracing (Figure 18.8) was interpreted as follows:

Uterine activity
Baseline tonus: not interpretable
Amplitude: not interpretable
Duration: 60–90 seconds
Interval: 1.25–4 minutes, irregular

Fetal heart rate
Baseline rate: 140–150 bpm
Variability: apparently normal
Periodic changes: one small variable deceleration and
    one prolonged deceleration

INTERPRETATION

This patient was not considered high-risk, but was monitored electively. After 45 minutes of monitoring, a sponta-

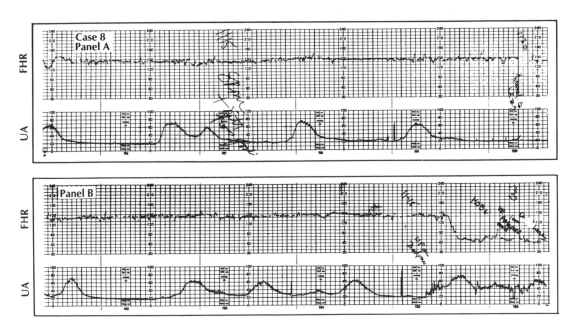

Figure 18.8   Monitor: Hewlett-Packard model 8030A. Paper speed: 3 cm/min. Vertical scale: 30 bpm/cm. Method: External (Doppler FHR monitor and external tocodynamometer).

neous prolonged deceleration began when the patient was sitting up on the bedpan. As previously noted, prolonged decelerations can result from uterine hyperstimulation, umbilical cord prolapse, hypotension, paracervical anesthesia, maternal hypoxia, or rapid descent through the birth canal. A vaginal examination should be done immediately because umbilical cord prolapse or rapid descent with impending delivery must be recognized and addressed quickly. In this case, the cord prolapse was detected within 90 seconds of the onset of the deceleration.

MANAGEMENT AND OUTCOME

The examiner kept her hand in the patient's vagina to keep the pressure of the presenting part off the cord. The patient was taken to the operating room, where an emergency cesarean section was performed under general anesthesia. Eleven minutes after detection of the prolapsed cord, a 6-lb, 9-oz boy was delivered, with Apgar scores of 9 at one minute and 9 at five minutes. Umbilical cord prolapse is relatively rare, occurring in approximately 0.5% of vertex presentations. It is much more common with nonvertex presentations and preterm pregnancies. The routine use of intrapartum FHR monitoring obviously benefited this patient. Intermittent auscultation might have detected this deceleration, but probably not as quickly. Continuous FHR monitoring allowed prompt recognition of a serious problem in a patient who was considered low-risk. Swift intervention resulted in a baby with normal Apgar scores. ∎

CASE 18.9 Abruptio Placentae

A 28-year-old gravida 3, para 1 at 39 weeks' gestation complained of frequent uterine contractions. She denied vaginal bleeding but reported unusual discomfort. On admission, the cervix was 2 cm dilated, 50% effaced, with the vertex presenting and membranes bulging. Vital signs were normal.

External monitors were placed for uterine contractions and FHR. The tracing in Figure 18.9A showed the following:

Uterine activity
Baseline tonus: not interpretable on external monitor
Amplitude: not interpretable on external monitor
Duration: 1 minute
Interval: 1.5–2 minutes

Fetal heart rate
Baseline rate: 140 bpm
Variability: decreased long-term variability on external monitor
Periodic changes: none apparent on admission

INTERPRETATION

What is striking about this patient's monitor tracing is the degree of uterine hyperactivity. The contraction pattern is tachysystolic, with little or no apparent relaxation between contractions. Several contractions appear to run into each other. Even with external monitoring, this labor pattern is abnormal.

About two hours after admission, at the beginning of panel B, it became apparent that late decelerations were developing. With this degree of uterine hyperactivity, it is often difficult to detect subtle late decelerations. Shortly after the onset of the late decelerations, the patient began having increased vaginal bleeding. Such a pattern of frequent uterine contractions, little relaxation between contractions, late decelerations, and vaginal bleeding, all in the absence of oxytocin, is most consistent with an abruption. Other maternal conditions associated with spontaneous uterine hyperactivity include polyhydramnios, preeclampsia, chorioamnionitis, and maternal drug use (i.e., cocaine). Drugs such as oxytocin or prostaglandin can cause uterine hyperactivity, but this patient had not been given these drugs.

MANAGEMENT AND OUTCOME

The decelerations were noticed almost immediately. The patient was placed on her left side and given oxygen by mask, and IV fluids were started. When the late decelera-

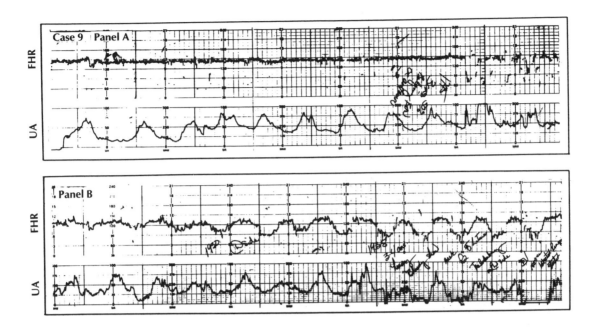

Figure 18-9   Monitor: Corometrics model 911. Paper speed: 3 cm/min. Vertical scale: 30 bpm/cm. Method: External (Doppler FHR monitor and external tocodynamometer).

tions persisted despite these resuscitative measures, the patient was taken for immediate cesarean section. A complete abruptio placentae was found. A 5-lb, 11-oz girl was delivered, with Apgar scores of 2 at one minute and 7 at five minutes. The baby did well in the newborn nursery.

Rupturing the membranes and placing an internal electrode might have confirmed fetal distress. However, the physician felt that the patient's clinical condition was consistent with abruption, and an immediate cesarean section seemed appropriate. The early recognition of fetal distress and prompt intervention probably prevented asphyxial complications or even fetal death. The mother, who had neither coagulopathy nor substantial problems with blood loss, did well in the immediate postpartum period. ∎

CASE 18.10   Cord Prolapse

A 21-year-old gravida 2, para 2 at 34 weeks' gestation was transferred from an outlying hospital because of preeclampsia. Evaluation included an amniocentesis for fetal pulmonary maturity. Fetal lung maturity was documented, and the patient was subsequently given magnesium sulfate, and oxytocin induction was started. Membranes were artificially ruptured, and an internal scalp electrode and pressure catheters were inserted. Several hours after amniotomy, Figure 18.10A revealed the following data:

Uterine activity
Baseline tonus: registering at 0
Amplitude: 60–75 mm Hg
Duration: 60 seconds
Interval: 2–4 minutes

Fetal heart rate
Baseline rate: 135 bpm
Variability: average
Periodic changes: variable decelerations with associated
    accelerations

INTERPRETATION

The monitor pattern in panel A was interpreted as mild, variable decelerations, consistent with mild umbilical cord compression. This pattern was considered reassuring. Intervention did not appear necessary because there was not a sharp decrease in variability nor a rise in the baseline FHR.

MANAGEMENT AND OUTCOME

While panel A was being recorded, the patient was examined. The cervix was 2 cm dilated, 50% effaced, and the vertex was presenting at -2 station. Approximately two hours later, variable decelerations were somewhat more prolonged, but there did not seem to be any substantial change in baseline FHR nor FHR variability.

When the patient was examined, several loops of umbilical cord were prolapsed through the cervix into the vagina, with the cervix 4 cm dilated and the vertex at -1 station. The vertex was elevated, and the patient was taken immediately to the operating room, where a primary cesarean section was performed. A 2,140-g boy was delivered, with Apgar scores of 4 at one minute and 7 at five minutes.

Generally, a prolapsed cord is associated with more profound variable or prolonged decelerations. However, since the presenting part had not descended, the variable decelerations appeared mild. Without the diagnosis of frank umbilical cord prolapse, these decelerations would not have warranted immediate intervention. But it is clear that a pelvic examination is needed in order to rule out an umbilical cord prolapse whenever the FHR pattern suggests cord compression.

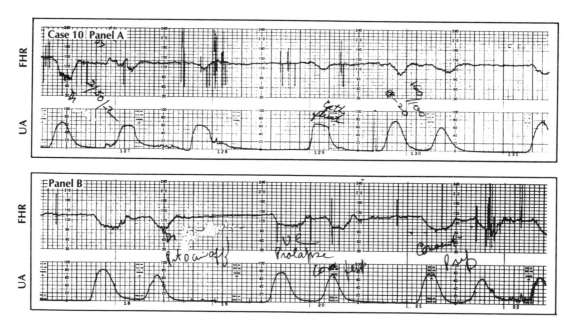

Figure 18.10   Monitor: Hewlett Packard model 8030A. Paper speed: 3 cm/min. Vertical scale: 30 bpm/cm. Method: Direct (fetal scalp spiral electrode and intrauterine pressure catheter).

CASE 18.11 Uterine Hyperstimulation

The patient was a 19-year-old nullipara with severe pre-eclampsia at 34 weeks' gestation. Labor induction with oxytocin began six hours before the start of Figure 18.11A. Examination just before the beginning of this tracing found the patient to be 1–2 cm dilated, 80% effaced, and the vertex presenting at 0 station. The oxytocin was increased per induction protocol. The infusion rate eventually reached 22 MU/min. In panel A, the external tocodynamometer did not pick up uterine activity. However, when the internal electrode and pressure catheters were placed, the monitor record in panel B yielded the following information:

Uterine activity
Baseline tonus: 15–20 mm Hg
Amplitude: 85–100 mm Hg
Duration: 60–80 seconds
Interval: every 2 minutes

Fetal heart rate
Baseline rate: 140–150 bpm
Variability: normal
Periodic changes: late decelerations

INTERPRETATION

Figure 18.11A shows persistent, repetitive, smooth, symmetric decelerations to 90 bpm. Dips of this type generally are either early or late decelerations. A look at the uterine contractions is necessary to time and describe them accurately. Since the tocodynamometer was not adequately recording uterine contractions, the exact diagnosis could not be made in this case. Furthermore, a common cause of late decelerations is uterine hyperstimulation. External monitoring cannot determine with certainty whether or not this is the case. Therefore, amniotomy was performed, and an internal electrode and a pressure catheter were inserted. After the internal monitors were placed, it was evident that these were indeed late decelerations. The oxytocin was immediately stopped when it became apparent that uterine activity was over-

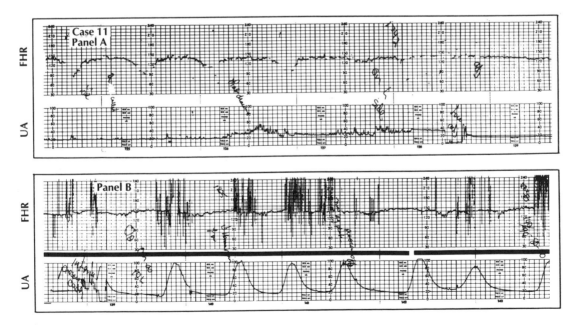

Figure 18.11 Monitor: Hewlett-Packard model 8030A. Paper speed: 3 cm/min. Vertical scale: 30 bpm/cm. Method: In panel A, external (tocodynamometer and Doppler); in panel B, direct (scalp electrode and internal pressure catheter).

stimulated. Additionally, the patient was placed on her side and given oxygen by mask.

MANAGEMENT AND OUTCOME

After the end of panel B, when the uterine activity had substantially decreased, the late decelerations disappeared and did not reappear. Four hours later, the patient had a spontaneous vaginal delivery of a 1,660-g boy, with Apgar scores of 8 at one minute and 9 at five minutes. He did well in the newborn nursery.

This case illustrates problems of oxytocin induction in a patient at risk for uteroplacental insufficiency. Frequently, placental perfusion is marginal, and overstimulation of uterine activity may cause fetal hypoxia. Thus, it is important to use the uterine pressure catheter when uterine activity cannot be adequately monitored externally. This case also illustrates that relative uterine hyperstimulation can be recognized by the appearance of late decelerations. For this patient, decreasing the oxytocin improved fetal oxygenation. Another therapy that has demonstrated benefit in situations of uterine hyperstimulation is the use of beta sympathomimetics such as terbutaline. As noted previously, this can be administered either by subcutaneous or intravenous injection. ▪

CASE 18.12 Conduction Anesthesia Hypotension

A primigravida at term was admitted in active labor, with the cervix dilated 3–4 cm and the membranes ruptured. Oxytocin augmentation was begun because of lack of progress and inadequate uterine activity. An internal electrode was placed at the time. The first dose of bupivacaine hydrochloride (Marcaine) for continuous epidural anesthesia was administered at the beginning of Figure 18.12A. Dilation was 5 cm, and blood pressure was 110/70. An internal uterine pressure catheter was placed in Figure 18.12C.

Interpretation of panel A is as follows:

Uterine activity
Baseline tonus: not interpretable
Amplitude: not interpretable
Duration: 40–60 seconds
Interval: 1.5–2.5 minutes

Fetal heart rate
Baseline rate: 130 bpm, rising to 150 bpm
Variability: average
Periodic changes: one variable deceleration and recurrent late decelerations

INTERPRETATION

The variable deceleration at the beginning of panel A seems to be associated with a long contraction. We cannot be certain whether this represents a real four-minute contraction or if it represents an increase in the intraabdominal pressure caused by having the mother sit up during administration of the epidural.

Persistent late decelerations begin approximately 16 minutes after the anesthetic and are associated with a drop in maternal blood pressure to a minimum of 90/60. Appropriate actions to counteract these late decelerations begin near the end of panel B. The patient was placed on her side, given oxygen by face mask, and had the oxytocin discontinued. A very important therapy for this patient was the administration of intravenous fluids. An internal pressure catheter was placed at the beginning of Figure 18.12C because of some difficulty in timing the decelerations; however, it did not appear to function well. In the middle of panel C, the late decelerations disappear. While the late decelerations were occurring, the FHR baseline rose from 130 bpm to a maximum of 150 bpm. Eventually, there was a return to the original baseline. A slight decrease in the variability was also associated with the late decelerations.

MANAGEMENT AND OUTCOME

Following the correction of this hypotension, the patient's labor progressed rapidly, and the late decelerations did not recur. Several hours later, she had a spontaneous vaginal

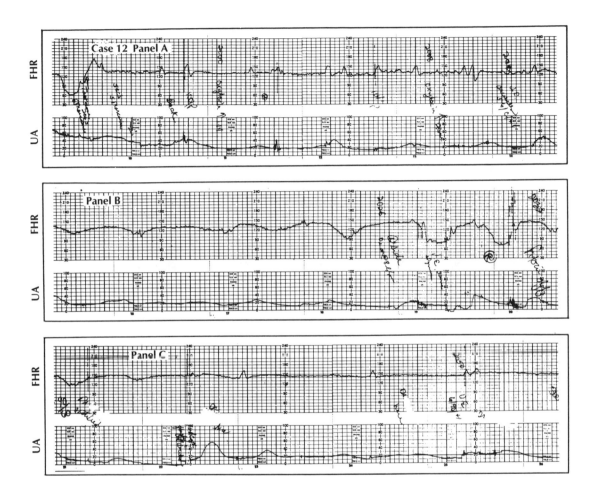

Figure 18.12   Monitor: Hewlett-Packard model 8030A. Paper speed: 3 cm/min. Vertical scale: 30 bpm/cm. Method: FHR was measured directly by scalp electrode. Uterine contractions were initially measured indirectly with an external tocodynamometer. In panel C, they were measured directly by intrauterine pressure catheter.

delivery of a 7-lb, 8-oz boy, with Apgar scores of 9 and 9. The baby did well in the newborn nursery.

Relative hypotension is a common complication of conduction anesthesia. Giving the patient an adequate fluid load before administering the epidural usually, but not always, averts this problem. When hypotension occurs, the late decelerations are most probably caused by a decrease in uterine blood flow. It this occurs, the patient should be placed on her side and given oxygen and a large volume of IV crystalloid. If oxytocin is being given, it should be discontinued. If these measures fail to elevate blood pressure, a medication such as ephedrine may be indicated.

In most cases, repositioning and hydration correct the hypotension. Usually, the FHR baseline rises, and there may be some loss of variability associated with the late decelerations. Some time after the late decelerations resolve, the FHR usually returns to the normal baseline, and the variability returns.

Every effort should be made to reverse the persistent late decelerations rather than intervene for the baby. Once such a condition has been resolved, the placenta can resuscitate the baby. In this case, intrauterine resuscitation was successful. The baby was vigorous at birth.

CASE 18.13 Loss of Fetal Movement

A 25-year-old primigravida with no risk factors at 32 weeks' gestation called her physician because she had felt no fetal movement since awakening that morning. Brought in for immediate fetal evaluation, she was placed on external fetal monitors that revealed the following:

Uterine activity
Only one contraction during the entire monitoring period

Fetal heart rate
Baseline heart rate: 135 bpm
Apparent variability: markedly decreased

Periodic changes: no accelerations and two late decelerations

INTERPRETATION

Variability cannot always be determined on an external monitor, since such monitoring can increase variability artifactually. Therefore, when a marked decrease in variability appears on the external monitor, the real variability is no greater than what is seen and is possibly even less. Two smooth, symmetrical decelerations were noted during the monitoring period. The first followed the contraction in Figure 18.13A and was associated with loss of signal; the second was shallow and not associated with an apparent contraction. Both were probably late decelerations. Such a nonreactive antepartum tracing associated with loss of fetal movement and spontaneous late decelerations requires immediate evaluation.

MANAGEMENT AND OUTCOME

Upon noticing the ominous antepartum monitoring strip, the physician requested an immediate ultrasound exam.

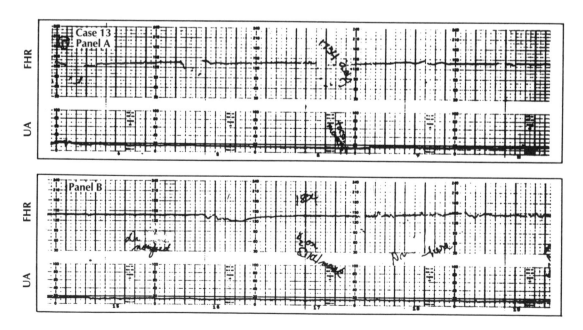

Figure 18.13   Monitor: Hewlett-Packard model 8030A. Paper speed: 3 cm/min. Vertical scale: 30 bpm/cm. Method: External.

The purpose of the scan was to obtain a fetal biophysical profile (BPP) and to rule out gross congenital anomalies. Congenital anomalies have been reported to be more likely with ominous FHR patterns (14). Another consideration in this clinical situation is possible illicit drug use. Cocaine, in particular, can cause arterial vasospasm with resultant late decelerations and loss of variability.

On real-time ultrasound, the fetus appeared grossly normal without apparent congenital anomalies. Measurements of biparietal diameter, abdominal diameters, and femur length were normal for gestational age. Amniotic fluid volume was also reported to be normal. With regard to the biophysical profile, the fetus had no spontaneous respiratory movements during a 30-minute period. There were no gross fetal body movements. Basing a decision on the above information, the managing physician elected for an operative delivery. The patient was taken for emergency cesarean section under epidural anesthesia, where a 1,380-g girl was delivered. She was appropriate for gestational age, with Apgar scores of 2 at one minute and 7 at five minutes. The umbilical venous pH was 7.15, and the umbilical arterial pH was 7.00. The baby had no congenital anomalies and no evidence of congenital infection. Both grossly and histologically, the placenta was unremarkable. There was no apparent cause for the antepartum fetal distress. The baby had mild respiratory distress, hyperbilirubinemia, and some feeding difficulties; otherwise, she did remarkably well. She was discharged from the hospital on the 33rd day of life.

Antepartum fetal testing contraction stress test (CST), nonstress test (NST), (BPP) of the high-risk patient has been very successful in lowering the incidence of unexpected stillbirth in that population. The result is that most stillbirths now occur in low-risk patients. Applying antepartum fetal testing to all patients would be costly and impractical. However, encouraging methods such as patients' perception of fetal movement might be useful. Formal counting of the fetal movements may be unnecessary, but a general awareness of overall fetal movement should be taught to all patients. If fetal movements substantially decrease, it is appropriate to begin other antepartum evaluation of the fetus. Approximately 7% of these patients will have a non-reactive NST, and 6% will demonstrate fetal heart rate decelerations (15). These patients also have a significant risk

of decreased amniotic fluid.

This patient had no antepartum risk factors until she perceived decreased fetal movement. Judging by the Apgar scores and umbilical pH values, the institution of fetal monitoring probably saved this baby's life. ∎

CASE 18.14 Intermittent Complete Heart Block

A 26-year-old primigravida, with no past problems, was admitted at 40 weeks' gestation, seven hours after spontaneous rupture of membranes. The patient was not in labor at the time of admission. Internal electrode and external contraction monitors (Figure 18.14) were placed, and labor was induced with IV oxytocin by continuous infusion pump.

Fetal heart rate
Baseline rate: apparently dropping from 130–70 bpm
Variability: normal at the higher heart rate and decreased at the lower rate
Periodic changes: accelerations only

INTERPRETATION

This is an unusual case of intermittent fetal atrioventricular dissociation (intermittent complete heart block). Those involved had several theories to explain this FHR pattern. One possibility was "halving," a characteristic only of Doppler external monitors. It cannot happen with direct electrodes unless heart rates of 240 bpm or greater are achieved. Another guess was intermittent tracing of the fetal heart rate and occasional recording of maternal heart rate. Recording of the maternal heart rate with an internal monitor does not occur with a live fetus. When the fetus is dead, however, maternal heart rate may be conducted and recorded. A third possibility was profound decelerations to 70 bpm from a baseline of 130 bpm. This was not a reason-

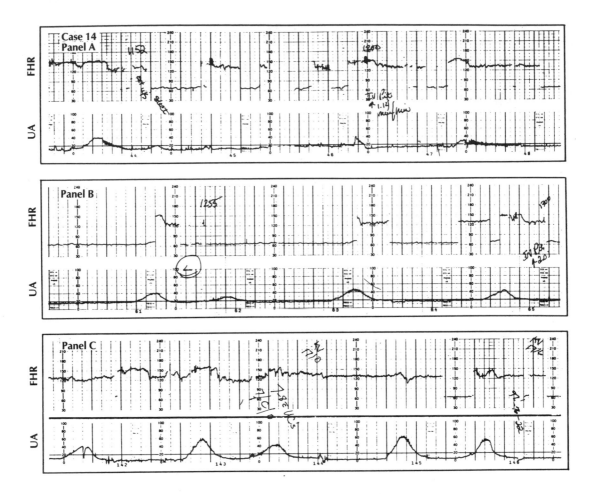

Figure 18.14 Monitor: Hewlett-Packard model 8030A. Paper speed: 3 cm/min. Vertical scale: 30 bpm/cm. Method: Direct FHR monitor (scalp spiral electrode) and external contraction monitor (tocodynamometer).

able explanation because transition from the higher to the lower heart rate was immediate.

Another explanation is an intermittent fetal heart block. There are several techniques for confirming the diagnosis of intermittent heart block. An electrocardiogram (ECG) machine may be connected to the fetal monitor, and a fetal ECG can be recorded or observed using an oscilloscope. Real-time/M-mode echocardiography is an effective means to study this arrhythmia. The atrial and ventricular rates are counted simultaneously with M-mode echocardiography. Asynchrony between atrial and ventricular contractions would be seen during periods of dissociation. These techniques are also useful in diagnosing complete heart block when FHRs of 60–80 bpm are seen.

MANAGEMENT AND OUTCOME

The patient was allowed to labor without intervention. The FHR between episodes of heart block were without apparent decelerations, and there was good fetal heart rate variability with FHR accelerations. The patient progressed normally in labor, and a 7-lb, 12-oz boy was delivered spontaneously, with Apgar scores of 9 at one minute and 9 at five minutes. In the first hour of life, the infant had periods of intermittent atrioventricular dissociation. These became less frequent and lasted a shorter period of time. The dysrhythmia eventually resolved completely. Echocardiography was normal, and the baby had no apparent clinical problems in the newborn period.

Complete fetal heart block may be associated with serious congenital heart disease or with maternal systemic lupus erythematosus. Those patients with anti Ro antibody (SSA) have a high risk of fetal congenital heart block. The fetuses of these patients can also have bundle branch block or intermittent complete heart block. A review of fetal dysrhythmias in pregnancy has been published (12). ■

branes. The patient was afebrile and not having contractions. The speculum examination confirmed membrane rupture. Ultrasound revealed a single fetus in vertex presentation whose biparietal diameter and other fetal biometric measurements were consistent with dates.

Management was expectant until later that evening when the patient began having regular contractions. After several hours, she had progressed to 5-cm cervical dilation. Decelerations were noted on the external monitor. These decelerations were not tracing well, so an internal scalp electrode was inserted. Reviewing the tracing revealed the following data:

Uterine activity
Baseline tonus: not interpretable on external monitor
Amplitude: not interpretable on external monitor
Duration: 40–60 seconds
Interval: every 4–8 minutes

Fetal heart rate
Baseline rate: 140 bpm, rising to 170 bpm
Variability: normal
Periodic changes: severe variable decelerations

CASE 18.15 Premature Rupture of Membranes

A 23-year-old gravida 1, para 0 was admitted at 28 weeks' gestation, several hours after apparent rupture of mem-

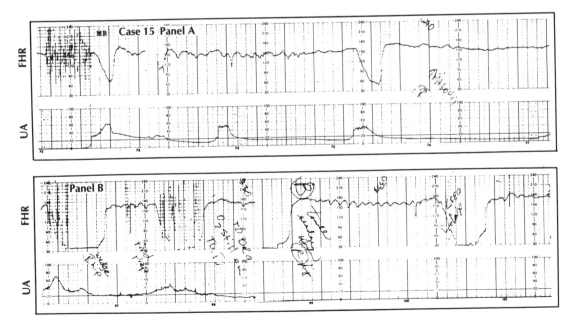

Figure 18.15 Monitor: Hewlett-Packard model 8030A. Paper speed: 3 cm/min. Vertical scale: 30 bpm/cm. Method: Direct FHR monitor (fetal scalp spiral electrode) and external tocodynamometer.

INTERPRETATION

Severe variable decelerations were occurring even though the contractions were infrequent and somewhat irregular. Such decelerations are common with oligohydramnios. Amniotic fluid seems to protect the umbilical cord from compression during contractions or fetal movement. When the amniotic fluid is decreased or absent, cord compression and thus variable decelerations are much more common. Some of the most severe variable decelerations occur in very small, premature fetuses with premature rupture of membranes (16).

MANAGEMENT AND OUTCOME

Placing the patient on her side and in Trendelenburg position failed to relieve the variable decelerations. The increased depth and duration of the decelerations and the associated tachycardia (Figure 18.15B), suggested that the fetus was hypoxemic between contractions. Because of these fetal heart rate changes, the early gestational age, and a vaginal delivery not being eminent, a cesarean section was performed.

A 860-g boy with Apgar scores at 1 at one minute and 4 at five minutes was delivered and responded well to resuscitation. The infant had an extremely rocky four months in the nursery, with many complications of prematurity. The only evidence of any permanent sequelae at this time is some hearing impairment. ∎

CASE 18.16   Maternal Cocaine Use

The following is a recently published report illustrating the effect of cocaine on the fetal heart rate (17). The patient was a 23-year-old multigravida female presenting at term with regular uterine contractions. She was examined and found to be 2 cm dilated and 50% effaced. The admission fetal heart rate tracing can be seen in Figure 18.16A. The pattern was reassuring, with no periodic changes and good long-term variability. Several hours following the admission, a significant change was noted in the fetal heart rate tracing. Rupture of membranes was performed, and a scalp electrode was placed. The subsequent tracing can be seen in Figure 18.16B:

Uterine activity
Baseline tonus: not interpretable on external monitor
Amplitude: not interpretable on external monitor
Frequency: every 6 minutes
Duration: 60–90 seconds

Fetal heart rate
Baseline rate: 165 bpm
Variability: decreased
Periodic changes: persistent late decelerations

INTERPRETATION

There was a significant loss of variability from panel A to panel B, with a rise in the baseline from 155 to 165. Additionally, there were persistent late decelerations noted. This was a worrisome tracing, necessitating further evaluation. At that time, the patient informed the staff that she had been supplied with cocaine by a visitor and that she had used it intranasally while in the labor room. She felt that this would lessen the pain associated with labor.

Psychoactive drugs such as cocaine can effect the fetal heart tracing most notably by decreasing variability. In addition to this effect on the central nervous system, cocaine is an active vasoconstrictor. Animal studies have shown that this results in maternal hypertension, decreased uterine blood flow, and a reduction of fetal P_{O_2} without a significant effect on the fetal pH.

MANAGEMENT AND OUTCOME

Due to the nonreassuring pattern, a fetal scalp pH was performed, with a resultant value of 7.35. The pattern remained worrisome, and a second pH was obtained, with a value of 7.38. Subsequently, the pattern improved, with return of good variability and abatement of late decelerations. The patient's labor progressed, with eventual vaginal

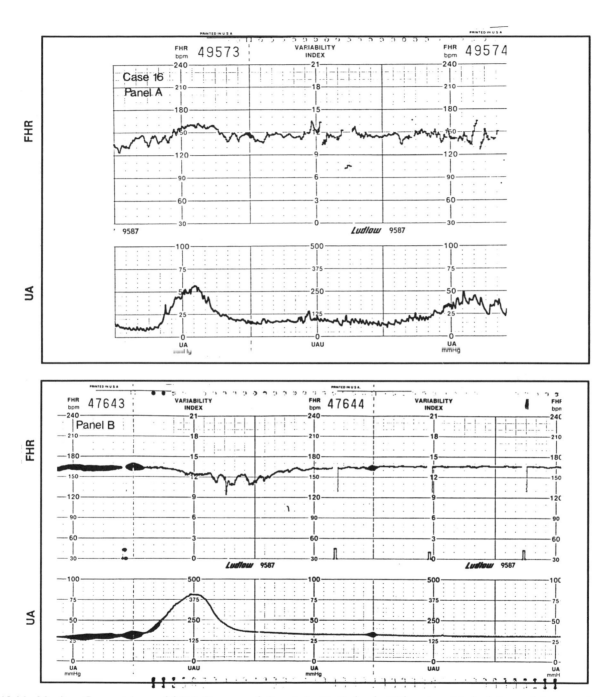

Figure 18.16 Monitor: Corometrics model 911. Paper speed: 3 cm/min. Vertical scale: 30 bpm/cm. Method: In panel A, external Doppler FHR monitor and tocodynamometer). In panel B, direct (fetal scalp spiral electrode) and external tocodynamometer.

delivery of a female infant with Apgar scores of 9 and 9 at one minute and five minutes, respectively.

It is important to confirm fetal well-being with a scalp pH when faced with an abnormal fetal heart rate tracing and with continuing labor. This patient was not delivered by cesarean section since this is a potentially reversible condition. The pH needs to be repeated every 20–30 minutes until the patient is delivered or the tracing improves. ■

Antepartum CST

CASE 18.17 Nipple Stimulation

The monitor strip (Figure 18.17) represents an antepartum contraction stress test of a 36-year-old gravida 5, para 4 at 39 weeks' gestation. The test was done because of her history of a previous stillbirth. She had no other known complications of pregnancy. This test was a repeat because the CST the day before had been equivocal. The monitor tracing shown in Figure 18.17 revealed the following data:

Uterine activity
Initially, only one contraction is seen; after nipple stimulation, more frequent uterine contractions appear, until a contraction frequency of three in 10 minutes is reached

Fetal heart rate
Baseline rate: 140–150 bpm
Variability: possibly increased variability on external monitor
Periodic changes: frequent accelerations

INTERPRETATION

This is a reactive nonstress test, followed by a negative CST achieved with nipple stimulation. Particularly interesting are the areas of increased FHR variability, or possibly small and frequent FHR accelerations, seen on the middle of panel A and most of panel B. Such a pattern might be misinterpreted as sinusoidal because of the relatively regular, undulating appearance and frequency. Sinusoidal-like patterns are often seen in fetuses who subsequently have normal outcomes. There has been much debate about the importance of such patterns. However, this particular pattern does not fit the strict definition of sinusoidal uniform

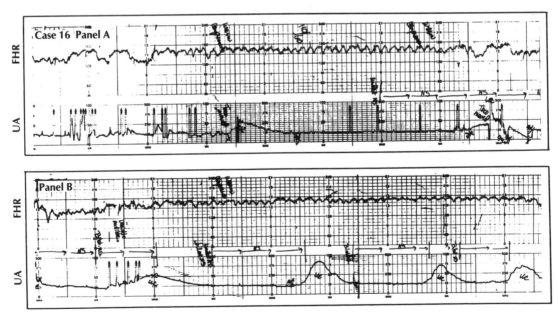

Figure 18.17   Monitor: Corometrics model 911. Paper speed: 3 cm/min. Vertical scale : 30 bpm/cm. Method: External (Doppler FHR monitor and external tocodynamometer).

long-term variability: generally at three to five cycles per minute, no short-term variability, no acceleration or reactivity, and often associated with other ominous patterns such as late decelerations. When considering whether a FHR pattern might indeed be sinusoidal, it is important to look at enough of the monitor strip to be sure that it is uniform and persistent. This patient's FHR baseline was 140–150 bpm. What looks like a sinusoidal pattern are actually accelerations above that baseline. Additionally, there were no associated decelerations. In fact, there were obvious FHR accelerations associated with fetal movements.

Nipple stimulation achieved adequate uterine contractions for the CST. In fact, most patients can have an adequate CST without oxytocin. Its efficacy and reliability has been tested and is similar to the oxytocin contraction stress test (18, 19).

MANAGEMENT AND OUTCOME

This test was appropriately read as reactive and negative. A repeat test was scheduled in a week, but, before it was done, the patient had an uneventful monitored labor with a spontaneous vaginal delivery. The term-size newborn had normal Apgar scores and did well in the nursery. The FHR during labor was normal. The pattern of increased long-term variability seen on the antepartum test did not recur. ∎

CASE 18.18 False-Positive CST

This patient was a 27-year-old gravida 3, para 2, was transferred to a tertiary-care center because her CST was positive. The patient was at 31 weeks' gestation and was tested because of two previous unexplained antepartum stillbirths. The first stillbirth occurred at 8.5 months and the second at 7.5 months.

INTERPRETATION

The test in Figure 18.18A represents the first effort at antepartum fetal surveillance. Nipple stimulation, started at the beginning of the panel, was used to stimulate contractions. The patient began having contractions every two minutes that apparently lasted 40–50 seconds. Amplitude was uninterpretable on the external monitor. Reactivity (accelerations) was absent, and there were persistent late decelerations with each contraction.

MANAGEMENT AND OUTCOME

Suspicion that the test results in Figure 18.18A may have represented uterine hyperstimulation was raised by the fact that the tocodynamometer was set at 0 for a baseline rather than at 10–20 mm Hg where the instrument tends to work best. If the recorded contractions represented only the "top of the hump," they may really have lasted longer. After transfer to the tertiary-care center, another CST (not shown) was performed after the baseline monitoring revealed some reactivity. The patient immediately began having contractions after the oxytocin was started at 0.5 mU/minute.

Uterine hyperstimulation was absent (Figure 18.18B and C) when the tocodynamometer was set at 20 mm Hg baseline. The result was an adequate test, with three contractions in 10 minutes. The test became reactive, with obvious accelerations visible. There were no late decelerations.

When this test was repeated the next day, the result was again negative. The patient was subsequently followed with weekly CSTs that, except for an occasional equivocal result, were reactive and negative. At 38 weeks' gestation, the patient's cervix was found to be favorable for induction. Amniocentesis revealed a mature lecithin/sphingomyelin (L/S) ratio. Seven hours after labor was induced, the patient had a spontaneous vaginal delivery of a 5-lb, 7-oz girl, with Apgar scores of 8 at one minute and 9 at five minutes. There was apparently no fetal distress during labor. Mother and baby both did well, and they were discharged from the hospital on the second postpartum day.

Figure 18.18A represents one of the pitfalls of contrac-

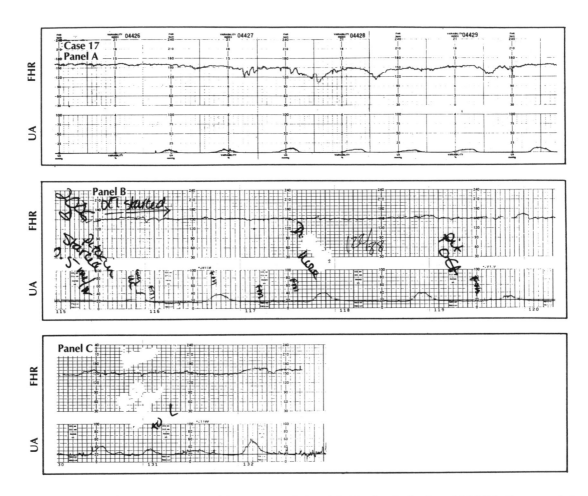

Figure 18.18   Monitor: In panel A, Corometrics model 112. In panels B and C, Hewlett-Packard model 8040A. Paper speed: 3 cm/min. Vertical scale: 30 bpm/cm. Method: External (Doppler FHR monitor and tocodynamometer).

tion stress testing. It has been said that any fetus can be shown to have a false-positive CST when sufficiently excessive uterine activity is created. Certainly, failure to monitor contractions adequately by correct placement of the tocodynamometer and by having a nurse at bedside to observe the contractions can lead to such a problem. Whenever one considers the possibility of intervention, it is important to be absolutely sure that there is no hyperstimulation.

Additional tests of fetal well-being such as the biophysical profile can be considered to corroborate fetal distress before intervention. For this patient, such a step was unnecessary because the repeat CST was reassuring. Data on nipple-stimulated CSTs do not suggest that they are more prone to hyperstimulation than oxytocin-induced tests. Reliability of the nipple stimulation contraction stress test is comparable to the oxytocin contraction stress test. This patient had sufficient contractions induced with minimal amounts of oxytocin; therefore, her uterus was quite sensitive to such stimulation. Excessive stimulation can be caused by nipple stimulation or oxytocin if care is not taken.

References

1. Clark SL, Gimorsky ML, Miller FC. Fetal heart rate response to scalp blood flow sampling. Am J Obstet Gynecol 198 144:706.

2. Martin CB. Regulation of the fetalheart rate and genesis of FHR patterns. Semin Perinatol 1978;2:131.

3. Clark SL, Cotton DB, Lee W, et al. Central hemodynamic assessment of normal third trimester pregnancy: a simultaneous comparison of Fick principle, thermodilution, continuous wave doppler, pulsed doppler and electrial impedance measurements of cardiac output, and effects of position changes in hemodynamics and oxygen delivery. Society of Perinatal Obstetricians, 1989.

4. Patriarco MS, Viechnicki BM, Hutchinson TA, et al. A study on intrauterine fetal resuscitation with terbutaline. Am J Obstet Gynecol 1987;157:384.

5. Mendea-Bauer C, Sherkarloo A, Cook V, et al. Treatment of acute intrapartum fetal distress by B_2-sympathomimetics. Am J Obstet Gynecol 1987;156:638.

6. Sherkarloo A, Mendez-Bauer C, Cook V, et al. Terbutaline (intravenous bolus) for the treatment of acute intrapartum fetal distress. Am J Obstet Gynecol 1989;160:615.

7. Reece EA, Chervenak FA, Romero R, et al. Magnesium sulfate in the management of acute intrapartum fetal distress. Am J Obstet Gynecol 1984;148:104.

8. Miyazaki FS, Taylor NA. Saline amnioinfusion for relief of variable or prolonged decelerations: a preliminary report. Am J Obstet Gynecol 1983;146:670.

9. Miyazaki FS, Nevarez F. Saline amnioinfusion for relief of repetitive variable decelerations: a prospective randomized study. Am J Obstet Gynecol 1985;153:301.

10. Nageotte MP, Freeman RK, Garite TJ. Prophylactic intrapartum amnioinfusion in patients with preterm premature rupture of membranes. Am J Obstet Gynecol 1985;153:557.

11. Wenstrom KD, Parson MT. The prevention of meconium aspiration in labor using amnioinfusion. Obstet Gynecol 1989;73:647.

12. Reed KL. Fetal arrhythmias: etiology, diagnosis, pathophysiology, and treatment. Semin Perinatol 1989;13:294.

13. Porto M, Murata Y, Keegan KA, Ray DA, Garite TJ. Intermittent sinusoidal fetal heart rate: a sign of moderate fetal anemia. Am J Obstet Gynecol (in press).

14. Garite TJ, Linzey EM, Freeman RK, et al. Fetal heart rate patterns and fetal distress in fetuses with congenital anomalies. Obstet Gynecol 1979;53:716.

15. Ahn MO, Phelan JP, Smith CV, et al. Antepartum fetal surveillance in the patient with decreased fetal movement. Am J Obstet Gynecol 1987;157:860.

16. Moberg LJ, Garite TJ, Freeman RK. Fetal heart rate patterns and fetal distress in patients with preterm premature rupture of membranes. Obstet Gynecol 1989;64:60.

17. Perlow JH, Schlossberg DL, Strassner HT. Intrapartum cocaine use: a case report. J Reprod Med (in press).

18. Huddleston JF, Sutliff G, Robinson D. Contraction stress test by intermittent nipple stimulation. Obstet Gynecol 1984;63:669.

19. Lenke RR, Nemes JM. Use of nipple stimulation to obtain contraction stress test. Obstet Gynecol 1984;63:345.

19

Fetal Movements

Eliahu Sadovsky, M.D.

FETAL monitoring in high- as well as low-risk pregnancies is aimed at detecting possible signs of chronic fetal distress and impending fetal death. Antenatal fetal heart rate (FHR) recording, contraction stress test (CST), and biophysical profile (BPP) have been used for this purpose, as has maternal assessment of fetal movement (1, 2). Using these tests, fetal death and, with experience, neonatal morbidity can be prevented by prompt delivery, provided that the fetus is viable. It is accepted today that fetal activity expresses fetal condition in utero, and daily monitoring of fetal movements provides a good way of assessing fetal well-being (1, 3, 4).

Fetal movement monitoring first started in 1971 when a pregnant diabetic woman with a previous cesarean section was admitted to the department for an elective cesarean section that was scheduled for three days later. The woman complained that the fetal movements had decreased and become weaker. The fetal heart beats were audible, and she was reassured that everything was in order. During the following day, she did not feel any fetal movements although again the fetal heart beats were heard. One day later, when she persistently complained of not feeling fetal movements, the fetal heart beats were no longer heard.

It was obvious that her complaints were not taken seriously, but since then attention has been paid to the onset of decreased fetal movements, and of course there have been additional similar cases. The main object is how to avoid such an event. This chapter will deal with this problem.

Nature of Fetal Movements

From the fifth month of pregnancy, and sometimes even earlier, women feel fetal movements. Although at first infrequent, weak, and indistinguishable from other abdominal movements such as those in the intestine, fetal movements gradually become stronger and more frequent as pregnancy progresses.

In my own study of 127 pregnant women with normal outcome, I found that the mean daily fetal movement recording (DFMR) rises from about 200 in the 20th week to a maximum of 500 in the 32d week of gestation. Then it gradually decreases to a mean of 282 at delivery (2). It was suggested that the decreased activity at term may be related to fetal sleep states, which increase with maturity (5). The number of daily fetal movements ranged from 50 to 956. As expected, the mean DFMR is significantly higher in twin gestations and even higher in triplets (6).

The daily fluctuation in a given woman may range from 200 to 700 fetal movements. Except for very low DFMRs, and especially where there is a definite trend toward decreasing motion, the clinical value of the absolute number of fetal movements has not been established; the only exception is when fetal movements cease entirely for a period of 12 hours (2).

Our cases of postmaturity were associated with very low DFMR values (3), a finding confirmed by Edwards and Edwards (7). Our mean DFMR (2) was higher than that found by Pearson and Weaver (4), who reported a daily count of 60–70 movements, but lower than that reported by Spellacy's group (8), who obtained 30 movements in 10 minutes, a DFMR of about 2,000 spread over 12 hours. Pearson and Weaver (4) may have detected fewer movements because they recorded for longer periods, as well as during meals, work, and rest, when the women may have been less alert. The high DFMR reported by Spellacy and associates (8) is probably explained by their patients' short assessment time.

Interpretation is complicated because every pregnancy has its own rhythm; moreover, a woman's reports are subjective, influenced by character, occupation, and readiness to cooperate. Gestational age is also a factor (9), and a change in the mother's position may vary the frequency of fetal activity. The frequency of movements may alter during the day, becoming higher while the woman rests and lower after exercise. But there is no significant difference in fetal movements before or after meals, or in the morning, afternoon, or evening. Drugs such as barbiturates and tranquilizers probably reduce fetal movement (10). These tentative conclusions, however, rest purely on observations from mothers' daily records and need confirmation by electromagnetic or electronic devices.

We have shown that fetal movements did not vary with the sex of the fetus (2). Wood et al. (11) found reduction of fetal movements among mothers who smoke. Edwards and Edwards (7) pointed out that there did not appear to be any systemic relationship between the moth-

er's activity and changes in daily rates of fetal movements. But intrauterine anoxia caused by diminished uteroplacental blood flow, as in preeclampsia, may be important.

Pattern of Movements

Timor-Tritsch and associates (12), using a pressure transducer (tokodynamometer), distinguished four types of motion: rolling, simple, high-frequency (isolated and repetitive), and respiratory. In our study (13), we had 120 women who were in the 20th–41st week of gestation record fetal movements and also class the movements as weak, strong, or rolling. There was good correlation between the types of movement described by the women and recordings with a piezoelectric recorder. Weak movements appeared as single spikes of short duration (one second) and low amplitude above and below the baseline; strong movements showed as spikes of short duration (one second) and higher amplitude. Rolling movements were recorded by the device as biphasic, N- or W-shaped, and of longer duration (3–10 seconds). At about 20 weeks' gestation, weak movements predominated; then their percentage in the total count decreased until the 36th to 37th week, when they increased slightly until term. The strong and rolling movements, which appeared in the 22d to 23d week, increased proportionally until the 36th to 37th week, then decreased slightly until term.

Assessment of Movements

Many women reported that fetal activity during the day is not constant; they distinguished periods of 10–30 minutes or more of pronounced decreased fetal movements ("fetal sleep"), not dependent on the time of day or on the habits of the mothers. It would therefore be incorrect to evaluate fetal movements only once a day for a short period of time.

The patient was instructed to assess and record each movement for 30 minutes, two to three times daily. If there were fewer than four movements per hour, the assessment was continued for 1–4 hours/day. By prorating the movement totals over 12 hours, it is possible to obtain the DFMR.

We recorded movements with an electromagnetic device (10) and found that patients could sense about 87%

of the motions it recorded. We also used a new, simpler instrument (14), composed of two piezoelectric sensors. Highly sensitive to rapid straining forces such as fetal movements and relatively insensitive to steady or slowly changing movements such as uterine contractions or maternal respiratory movements, this device gave results that correlated well with maternal assessment. The 20 women checked by this instrument recorded 80% of the movements that the device picked up.

Fetal Movements Assessment by Real-time Ultrasound

Due to developments of good resolution in real-time ultrasound, fetal activity, felt or not felt by the mother, can now be studied in detail, quantitatively and qualitatively. With the real-time ultrasound, a larger portion of the fetus can be observed, and the complexities of individual fetal movements can be described more accurately. In addition, the image produced on the oscilloscope can be recorded by a videotape recording system (5).

Hertogs et al. (15), using real-time ultrasound, confirmed the occurrence of many movements that the mothers did not perceive. Most of their subjects were sensitive to major fetal movements. Maternal awareness of fetal movements correlated with the number of fetal parts contributing to the movement, but the duration of the movement, maternal age, and parity were unimportant. Gettinger et al. (16) measured fetal movements by real-time ultrasound and found that the real-time ultrasound recorded about twice as much fetal movement as the mother sensed within the same period. Birnholz et al. (17) used phased-array ultrasound in 37 patients between 6 and 40 weeks of gestation; they identified 11 separate movement patterns in normal pregnant women. Several groups of patterns appear to correlate with gestational age. They suggested that there are primitive responses that are lost with further development of the fetus and that it is possible that identification of a movement pattern inappropriate to gestational stage may add further sensitivity to movement observation as a possible monitor of fetal status for diagnosis of distress (17). Tajani et al. (18) studied 1,200 pregnancies between 6 and 42 weeks of gestation with real-time ultrasound and recognized six patterns of fetal movement, or motor behavior, which were ordered by gestational age. This pattern analysis was presented as an effective method for developmental diagnosis and prognosis.

Sudden, Increased Movements

High DFMR is normal if it is constant, but a pattern of sudden, strong, vigorous movements of increased frequency followed by cessation is almost invariably a sign of acute fetal distress and death. A cord complication, such as compression, may be the cause. If the fetus is able to release the cord, the woman continues to feel normal movement. If not, the fetus usually dies. A similar sequence of events characterizes sudden abruptio placentae. In these cases, recording the DFMR is of little clinical use.

Decreased Movements

First Half of Pregnancy

Ultrasound studies convinced Reinold (19) that, when spontaneous movements are absent, the fetus is at risk. Haller and co-workers (20) stated that, although evaluating type of movement is more difficult than detecting its presence or absence, the data are more useful. They established the normal range and pattern of movement in early pregnancy and also demonstrated the prognostic value of abnormal frequencies, duration, and patterns of movements associated with impending fetal death.

Second Half of Pregnancy

In cases of preeclampsia, and before intrauterine death, patients have complained of reduced or absent fetal movements, although fetal heartbeats were still audible (1). Reduction or cessation of activity may signify fetal distress caused by anoxia or other factors. Bernstine (21) pointed out that decreased activity in a previously active fetus may reflect disturbance of placental function and may be a clue to impending demise.

Patients have reported that, before fetal movement ceased, there was a change in type of fetal activity, with the weaker movements predominating (13). I suspect that the change in pattern toward an increase in weak movements may be an additional sign of fetal distress and may help distinguish between a mere fluctuation and a real decrease in movement.

Movement Alarm Signal

It has been shown (1, 4, 9, 22) that, in high-risk pregnancies, the decrease to cessation of fetal movement (FM) occurred before fetal death in utero. The reduction in FM to three or fewer or their cessation for at least 12 hours while fetal heart beats were still audible was referred to by us (1, 23) as a movement alarm signal (MAS). This signal points to a severely distressed fetus and indicates impending fetal death. Such a development, when verified, is an indication for immediate delivery of the fetus, provided that it is viable.

Short time of absence of FM does not indicate fetal jeopardy, as was shown by Patrick et al. (24); complete absence of gross fetal body movements for 75 min has been recorded by ultrasound in normal pregnancy. Only much longer periods of absence of FM should be regarded as fetal jeopardy.

We studied daily fetal movements in 164 women with normal pregnancies and with complications such as preeclampsia, diabetes, and postmaturity (9). Fifty patients had MAS, and death in utero occurred in 22. Twenty-eight fetuses were delivered alive, vaginally or by cesarean section, as soon as MAS was observed. Four of the 28 died several hours after delivery from respiratory distress syndrome. Of the 22 stillborn babies that had shown MAS, eight were of low birthweight (<1,500 g). For the other 14, whose weights were 1,500 g or more, estriol determinations had not clearly shown fetal jeopardy, and an expectant approach had been followed. Probably, these fetuses could have been saved if they had been delivered promptly. The duration of MAS ranged from 12 hours to three days; in one case, movements were absent for 12 days. In our series, there were only a few instances of fetal death not preceded by MAS: for example, a case of acute fetal distress caused by sudden abruptio placentae.

We had four diabetic cases with MAS; two of them died in utero 10–11 hours after the cessation of fetal movements. It seems that, in cases of diabetic pregnancy, MAS should be defined as cessation of fetal movements for at

least 6–8 hours, not 12 hours as in all other cases.

Decreased Fetal Movements Not Indicating Intervention

In some cases of a malformed or severely damaged fetus, decreased fetal movements are not an indication for prompt delivery. Of 822 cases of high-risk pregnancy, 55 had decreased fetal movements, nine of which (16%) had congenital malformations. Among the remaining 767 patients, eight (1%) had malformations. If decreased movement occurs, especially in cases of polyhydramnios, every effort—e.g., ultrasonography—should be made to exclude malformations before a preterm termination of pregnancy, especially by cesarean section (25).

In another group of patients, those with severe Rh isoimmunization, the routine monitoring of fetal activity has been reported by Queenan to be very worthwhile (26). Rayburn (27) has found these recordings to be particularly useful following intrauterine transfusion or when other antepartum fetal tests (nonstress test) are limited in interpretation in this condition.

We have found in these cases that decreasing FM until cessation warns of a severely distressed fetus and impending death. This situation may point to the diagnosis of hydrops fetalis. We studied 17 cases with Rh isoimmunization: seven were mild, and 10 were severe. In the mild cases, fetal activity was within normal range. MAS was manifested in three of the 10 severe cases. All of them died in utero. Two of these were associated with hydrops fetalis. As to the controversy regarding intrauterine transfusion or preterm delivery in the later weeks of gestation when hydrops fetalis is already present, it seems to us that the existence of MAS points to a very poor prognosis and that any treatment is futile.

The MAS, which is based on no fetal movement for at least 12 hours with the possibility of impending fetal death, explains why fetal movement should be recorded two–three times in 12 hours and not once in 24 hours, as suggested by Pearson and Rayburn (27). In every case of chronic fetal distress with intrauterine death, there was a period of cessation of FM which could be detected and acted upon; there were a few cases of antenatal fetal death, however, in the acute distress group because of cord complications and abruptio placentae with sudden increase in fetal movement without the manifestations of MAS. The presence of normal fetal movement is a good predictor of a good outcome in the low- or high-risk pregnancies (HRP).

As regards false-positive results, in a study (28) of 616 cases of HRP in which 97 patients had MAS, the outcome was evaluated by perinatal death, intrauterine growth retardation (IUGR), Apgar score of ≤6, meconium in labor, and fetal distress in labor. It was shown that, in 76 cases (78.4%), there was a poor outcome, and, in 21 cases (21.6%) with MAS, the outcome was favorable, according to the above-mentioned criteria. Of these, some patients complained of cessation of movements for some time, but, when a nonstress test (NST) was performed, fetal movements were then felt by the mother. These are presumably false-positive cases. We suggest that the MAS be verified by other biophysical tests for fetal distress such as oxytocin challenge test (OCT) or FHR monitoring. Proven cases of false-positive MAS may be detected by these means.

We have evaluated the rate of MAS in 662 cases of high-risk pregnancy from 1976 to May 1984 (29). The rate of MAS was 6.5%. An especially high incidence of MAS was found in cases with fetal malformations, oligohydramnios, polyhydramnios, Rh isoimmunization, asymmetrical growth retardation, and systemic lupus erythematosus.

Correlating Fetal Heart Rate and Movements

Sporadic increases in fetal heart rate variability, which are often seen in association with fetal movements, are an indication of fetal well-being. Lee and associates (30) suggested that this fact can be used to monitor the fetus in high-risk pregnancies.

We have studied the relationship of fetal movements as felt by the mother and as observed by real-time ultrasound to simultaneous continuous fetal heart rate recording (31). It was shown that all the movements that were both felt by the mother and seen by ultrasound were associated with large (>15 beats per minute (bpm), >15 seconds' duration), or small fetal heart rate accelerations. All of the large accelerations were accompanied by fetal movements seen by ultrasound, and, of these, 78% were associated with

fetal movements felt by the mother. We therefore suggest that fetal movements can be verified by counting the number of large accelerations on fetal heart tracing.

FHR Monitoring during Reduced Fetal Movements

We studied FHR changes during pregnancy in cases of known fetal distress not related to delivery (32). We selected five uncomplicated pregnancies with MAS and 25 high-risk cases with MAS. An external cardiograph recorded the fetal heartbeats for 20–30 minutes, once or twice daily. They were evaluated according to Simmons's method (33).

The FHR recordings were obtained from 12 to 48 hours after decrease of fetal movements until cessation. Of the 30 cases, nine showed normal FHR patterns. The remaining 21 showed loss of long-term variability (LLTV), variable deceleration, and other changes. Of the nine cases with normal FHR for the first 48 hours, four eventually developed abnormal FHR during the next 48 hours. The remaining five were born before any changes were recorded.

In 15 patients, the FHR monitoring was done one to four days before MAS appeared. In nine, FHR was normal and, in six, there was a LLTV; in one of the latter, tachycardia was also present.

There was only one stillbirth; 29 fetuses were delivered alive, but three premature newborns died several hours after delivery. It has been shown that, before fetal death occurs, pathologic changes in FHR will appear (34, 35). In 25 of our 30 cases with MAS, pathologic FHR change appeared. This further supports the view that MAS is an indication that termination of pregnancy is necessary to avoid death in utero. The FHR changes in cases of MAS are only additional evidence that the fetus is in severe distress. LLTV may be the earliest FHR change that appears spontaneously in chronic fetal distress.

Fetal Movement and Fetal Breathing

Dawes et al. (36) were able to demonstrate an association between fetal breathing movements and gross body movements. Fetal movements and fetal breathing movements show some coincidence in time of occurrence but do not show any statistically significant consistent relationship.

Fetal Movements as a Response to Various Stimuli

Sound

Grimwade and co-workers (37) placed sound stimuli near the abdomens of 14 women in the 38th to 42d week of pregnancy and caused changes in FHR in half the cases (94% tachycardia and 6% bradycardia); in 83%, these were associated with fetal movements. The mean noise level used by the Grimwade group was 85 dB (38). The finding that the fetus responds to external sound suggests that intra-uterine noises related to maternal cardiovascular dynamics might also stimulate the fetus and cause it to move.

We studied the ability of the fetus to respond to vibroacoustic stimulation, generated by an electrolarynx, in 28 normal pregnant women in the 27th to 41st week of gestation (39). The fetal movement response until habituation was achieved was evaluated by real-time ultrasound in the form of startle movement of the body, head, or both. The results showed fetal ability to respond and habituate to vibroacoustic stimuli. The number of stimuli required for habituation of the normal fetus decreased with gestational age.

It was shown by Ohel, et al. (40) that vibroacoustic stimulation of the fetus in a period of low activity and low heart rate variability which resembles quiet sleep can cause fetal movement that can be appreciated by the mother or by real-time ultrasound (RTUS). In this way, a distinction between fetal distress with the same low activity and low heart rate variability can be diagnosed. In cases of fetal distress, no fetal response to vibroacoustic stimulation will result. According to Read and Miller (41), positive response to acoustic stimulation obviates the need for OCT. Jensen, in 1984 (42), showed that there was a good outcome in cases when the response was positive. The evoked fetal activity after an acoustic stimulation may indicate fetal well-being, and it is well correlated with good fetal outcome. If fetal activity is not evoked, fetal well-being should be verified by other means.

Light

We studied fetal reaction to external light in 110 normal and 33 pathologic pregnancies (preeclampsia, diabetes, and placental insufficiency) between the 26th and 42d week (43). A 250-W bulb lit for 20 minutes provided the stimulus.

There was an increase in fetal movement in 66% of the normal women, but in only 50% of those with pathologic pregnancy. Measures of reaction to light stimulation may not yet be clinically useful, but, with further refinement, such techniques may be promising.

Amniocentesis

FHR monitoring during 107 amniocenteses (44) suggested that an accelerated FHR response immediately following the insertion of the needle into the amniotic sac indicated fetal well-being (82%). Of those with acceleration, 97% were delivered as healthy babies with a good Apgar score; of the fetuses that did not show this response (18%), 42% had a significantly higher rate of later fetal distress. In 11 high-risk pregnancies, where MAS indicated fetal distress, FHR monitoring during amniocentesis revealed abnormal FHR response, manifested by absence of acceleration. The response of FHR during amniocentesis may be an additional tool for evaluating the severity of fetal distress. This test can be performed only in cases of MAS where the FHR is still normal.

Doppler Ultrasound

David, et al. (45) showed that, in normal pregnancies in which the fetal outcome was satisfactory, there was a 90% increase in fetal activity during the 15-minute exposure to Doppler ultrasound. In mothers who reported absence of fetal movements for at least 12 hours before the fetal heart rate became inaudible, the external Doppler ultrasound cardiotocograph did not elicit a fetal response. However, these findings were not confirmed by Rosen, et al. (46) who reported that a continuous ultrasound signal in a controlled series of 13 patients did not increase fetal activity. Weinstein, et al. (47) showed that external cardiotocography with Doppler ultrasound did not result in an increase in fetal movements in either low-risk or in mild high-risk pregnancy. On the other hand, in the severe high-risk pregnancy and in four patients who felt few fetal movements per day, the ultrasound provoked a significant increase in fetal movements. The disparity in results between these studies may relate to differences in the growth of signal energy reaching the fetus and to differences in experimental design.

Oxytocin Challenge Test and MAS

We have observed pathologic FHRs in a number of cases of MAS when delivery was induced by oxytocin infusion. In cases of decreased fetal movements or MAS with normal FHR, the OCT may be used—with great caution—to seek additional evidence of fetal distress. If MAS appears, cesarean would be preferable to vaginal delivery.

Fetal Movement and Tests of Respiratory Failure

We suggest that the sequence of appearance of abnormal signs in the deteriorating fetus before fetal death is as follows: 1) positive contraction stress test, followed by 2) nonreactive fetal nonstress test, then 3) decreased fetal movements usually, until cessation (MAS), and eventually 4) pronounced FHR changes. If we accept the above sequence of tests in cases of fetal distress before fetal death, we can accept the possibility of one test revealing pathology with another test still being normal. This does not contradict the value of the normal test, but merely indicates that the impairment of health is not severe. With impending fetal death, the tests invariably become positive. It should be pointed out that there is overlap among the tests and that some tests, those that are mildly abnormal, are sometimes reversible.

Management of High- and Low-Risk Pregnancy Employing Fetal Movements and FHR Monitoring

In addition to clinical data, FHR monitoring and ultrasonic methods, the subjective assessment of fetal movements should be the principal screening test for chronic fetal distress in ambulant women. It is simple, universally available, applicable to large numbers of patients, and does not interfere with daily routines. When obstetricians and nurses are positively oriented to the importance of fetal movements, self-monitoring can be a powerful, as well as inexpensive, diagnostic test.

Among other instructions given in the antenatal clinic, the clinician should stress to the patient how important fetal movements are and introduce our protocol of FM assessment (48) (Figure 19.1). From the 25th week until term, we ask patients to report to the hospital whenever fetal movements are reduced to several a day or cease altogether for four hours. Some ambulant patients who notice a reduction or cessation of fetal movements will feel normal fetal activity if they lie down for several hours and concentrate on the assessment.

Indeed, Neldam (49) has shown the value of maternal monitoring of FM in 2,250 pregnant women. Half of the women were instructed to count the FM methodically and contact the hospital if they felt less than 3 FM per hour. The controls were not given any specific indications about counting FM. There were eight intrauterine deaths in fetuses weighing more than 1,500 g without malformations in the control group and no deaths in the group with maternal monitoring of FM. These results demonstrated the value of subjective counting of fetal movements by ambulant pregnant women.

For hospitalized high-risk women, especially those with intrauterine growth retardation, we devised the scoring system outlined below (50) and shown in Table 19.1 to help us decide what to do when there is chronic fetal distress. It combines daily fetal movement recording, stress and nonstress tests, FHR monitoring, and lung maturity tests. When the score is 5 or higher, the pregnancy should be terminated, if the fetus is viable. We don't intervene when the contraction stress test is positive and nonstress test (NST) is nonreactive but the lungs are immature (score of 4). This check is important because, before 33 weeks' gestation, the NST test is nonreactive in about 30% of normal cases (51).

If the lungs are mature, the risk of delivery is not great. The scoring system will confirm fetal distress when the fetal movements are severely decreased or cease altogether, and there is an additional pathologic test (NST or CST) (score of 5 or 6).

Low-risk patients
1. Pay attention to fetal movements two to three times a day.
2. If fetal movements are markedly reduced, treat as high-risk patients.

High-risk patients

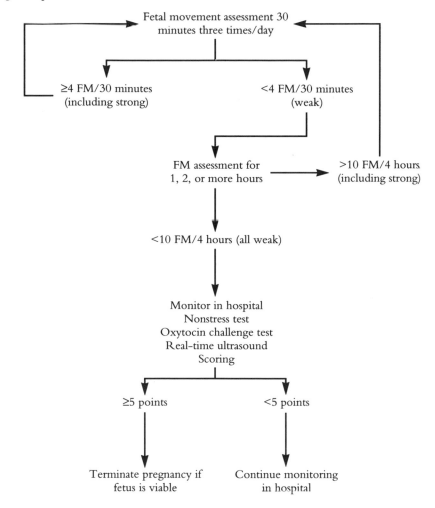

Figure 19.1   Protocol for fetal movement (FM) assessment.

Reproduced with permission from Sadovsky E. A scoring system using fetal movements. Contemp Ob/Gyn 1982;19:142.

Delivery is not indicated when only one test is patho-logic (score of 3), but is indicated when at least two tests show severe fetal distress and impending death: fewer than three movements in 12 hours—the movements alarm signal (MAS)—or persistent severe FHR changes (score of 6), although the lungs are not mature. Note that two different types of abnormality within the severe FHR category will give a score of 6. This is an important indication in cases of severe *acute* fetal distress. The fetal movements may be decreased for a short time, but not enough to establish MAS, and the CST is contraindicated.

The decision to deliver should be established by CST, NST, and fetal movement assessment, not by the severe FHR changes considered diagnostic of the more severely compromised fetus close to death, who may already have cerebral damage. In this way, we approach the most impor-

Table 19.1 Elements of the Scoring System

Parameter	Definiton	Score*
Contraction stress test (CST): *positive*	Three contractions followed by late decelerations (10-minute period)	2
Non stress test (NST) *nonreactive*	Fewer than two accelerations associated with FM (20-minute period)	2
Daily fetal movements recording (DFMR): *pathologic*	Fewer than 10 movements (12-hour period) (DFM)	2
	Fewer than three or no movements (12-hour period) (MAS)	3
Fetal heart rate (FHR): *pathologic changes*	Base level: <100 bpm, >180 bpm (3)	
	Repeated severe variable or late decelerations (3)	
	Loss of long-term variability (amplitude <5, frequency <2) (3)	3
	Constant sinusoidal pattern (3)	
Lung maturity	Lecithin/sphingomyelin (L/S) ratio ≥2	1

*If score is 5 or more, terminate pregnancy if fetus is viable.

tant challenge facing the obstetrician today: the reduction of the perinatal mortality rate, as well as of neonatal morbidity, that has its origin in the antenatal period.

CASE 19.1

A 33-year-old G1P0 with a history of chronic hypertension, was hospitalized at 30 1/2 weeks gestation for superimposed PIH with BP of 160/95, 3+ protein, and 10 lb weight gain over the last 4 days.

Admitting evaluation identified the fetus at the 15th % for gestational age with AFI 5.9 and reactive NST. The patient was placed at bedrest with 30 min fetal movement assessments TID and biweekly NSTs.

Forty-eight hours following admission, DFMR were found to be <5 over last 24 hours. NST remained reactive. An amniocentesis for maturity revealed L/S 1.9 PG 0%. Over the next 24 hours <3 movements were noted (MAS). BPP demonstrated AFI to 3.8, and questionable fetal breathing. NST was now nonreactive (Sadovsky score = 5 with BPP = 4).

A C/S was carried out secondary to noninducible cervix and fetal distress. A 1200 g female with Apgar scores of 5 and 8 was delivered. ∎

Conclusion

Fetal movement monitoring has made an enormous contribution to perinatal medicine. It must be emphasized that this type of monitoring detects, qualitatively, a different sort of fetal movement from what is seen with real-time ultrasound. One has only to observe the fetus with real-time ultrasound to realize that the mother perceives only 20%–80% of fetal movements. A real-time ultrasound scanner reveals many types of fetal movements, which are more frequent than movements perceived by the mother (for instance, she often does not feel movements of the fetal hand and forearm).

This work has been shown to reduce perinatal mortality when used as a clinical protocol. The simplicity of this test makes it extremely valuable in clinical medicine. A classic example of this sort of monitoring is seen in a patient with severe erythroblastosis fetalis: The fetus almost always becomes inactive for one to three days before dying in utero.

The deteriorating or chronically distressed fetus has a change in the number and pattern of fetal movements. First, the number of fetal movements is decreased. The patient no longer feels strong or rolling movements, but perceives only what she describes as weak movements

After some hours or days, no movements at all are felt for at least 12 hours. This is what is described as the movements alarm signal.

Certainly, fetal activity as seen with real-time ultrasound can be correlated with fetal well-being or fetal jeopardy. But many variables, such as fetal resting state and maternal glucose load, medications, or exercise, make the interpretation of fetal movement patterns difficult. Vigorous fetal activity indicates well-being, but decreased fetal movements are difficult to interpret. Much research remains to be done before routine clinical application will be practical.

Manning, Platt, and colleagues developed a fetal biophysical profile for antenatal fetal evaluation. They evaluated five biophysical parameters: fetal breathing, fetal movement, fetal tone, amniotic fluid volume, and fetal reactivity (nonstress test). Combining these parameters gives a much more accurate indication of fetal condition then observing a single parameter (see Chapter 15).

References

1. Sadovsky E, Yaffe H. Daily fetal movement recording and fetal prognosis. Obstet Gynecol 1973;41:845.
2. Sadovsky E. Fetal movements and fetal health. Semin Perinatol 1981;5:131.
3. Sadovsky E, Weinstein D, Polishuk WZ. Timing of delivery in high risk pregnancy by monitoring of fetal movement. J Perinat Med 1978;6:160.
4. Pearson JF, Weaver JB. Fetal activity and fetal well being: an evaluation. Br Med J 1976;1:1305.
5. Timor-Tritsch IE, Dierker LJ, Hertz RH, et al. Fetal movements: a brief review. Clin Obstet Gynecol 1979;22:583.
6. Samueloff A, Evron S, Sadovsky E. Fetal movements in multiple pregnancy. Am J Obstet Gynecol 1983;146:789.
7. Edwards DA, Edwards JS. Fetal movements: development and time course. Science 1970;169:95.
8. Spellacy WN, Cruz AC, Gelman SR, et al. Fetal movements and placental lactogen levels for fetal-placental evaluation. Obstet Gynecol 1977;49:113.
9. Sadovsky E, Polishuk WZ. Fetal movements in utero. Obstet Gynecol 1977;50:49.
10. Sadovsky E, Polishuk WZ, Mahler Y, et al. Correlation between electromagnetic recording and maternal assessment of fetal movement. Lancet 1973;1:1141.
11. Wood C, Gilbert M, O'Connor A, et al. Subjective recording of fetal movements. Br J Obstet Gynaecol 1979;86:836.
12. Timor-Tritsch I, Zador I, Hertz RH, et al. Classification of human fetal movement. Am J Obstet Gynecol 1976;126:70.
13. Sadovsky E, Laufer N, Allen JW. The incidence of different types of fetal movement during pregnancy. Br J Obstet Gynaecol 1979;86:10.
14. Sadovsky E, Polishuk WZ, Yaffe H, et al. Fetal movements recorder, use, and indications. Int J Gynaecol Obstet 1977;15:20.
15. Hertogs K, Roberts AB, Cooper D, et al. Maternal perception of fetal motor activity. Br Med J 1979;2:1183.
16. Gettinger A, Roberts AB, Campbell S. Comparison between subjective and ultrasound assessments of fetal movements. Br Med J 1978;2:88.
17. Birnholz JC, Stephens JC, Faria M. Fetal movement patterns: a possible means of defining neurologic developmental milestones in utero. AJR 1978;130:537.
18. Tajani E, Ianniruberto A, Iancarrino M, et al. Motoscopic examination of the fetus. Presented at the International Symposium on Fetal Medicine, Venice, June 1979.
19. Reinold E. Clinical value of fetal spontaneous movements in early pregnancy. J Perinat Med 1973;1:65.
20. Haller H, Wille HD, Henner H, et al. Quantification of active fetal movements in the first half of pregnancy. Presented at Eighth World Congress of Gynecology and Obstetrics, Mexico, Oct 1976.
21. Bernstine RL. Placental capacity and its relationship to fetal death. Clin Obstet Gynecol 1960;3:852.
22. Ehrstrom C. Fetal movement monitoring in normal and high risk pregnancy. Acta Obstet Gynecol Scand (Suppl) 1979;80:1.
23. Sadovsky E, Yaffe H, Polishuk WZ. Fetal movement monitoring in normal and pathological pregnancy. Int J Gynaecol Obstet 1974;12:75.
24. Patrick J, Campbell K, Carmichael L, et al. Patterns of gross fetal body movements (GFBM) over 24 hours observation intervals during the last 10 weeks of pregnancy. Am J Obstet Gynecol 1982;142:363.
25. Sadovsky E, Rabinowitz R, Yaffe H. Decreased fetal movements and fetal malformations. J Foet Med 1981;1:62.
26. Queenan JT. Modern management of Rh problem. 2nd ed. New York: Harper and Row, 1977.
27. Rayburn WF. Antepartum fetal assessment clinics. Perinatol 1982;9:231.
28. Sadovsky E, Ohel G, Havazeleth H, et al. The definition and

the significance of decreased fetal movements. Acta Obstet Gynecol Scand 1983;62:409.

29. Sadovsky E. Fetal movements in complication of pregnancy. Israel J Obstet Gynecol 1992;3:121.

30. Lee CY, Di Loreto PC, O'Lane JM. A study of fetal heart rate acceleration patterns. Obstet Gynecol 1975;45:142.

31. Rabinowitz R, Persitz E, Sadovsky E. The relation between fetal heart rate accelerations and fetal movements. Obstet Gynecol 1983;61:16.

32. Sadovsky H, Polishuk WZ. FHR monitoring in cases of decreased fetal movements. Int J Gynaecol Obstet 1976; 14:285.

33. Simmon SC. Organization of fetal intensive care. Clin Obstet Gynecol 1974;1:217.

34. Emment L, Huisjes HJ, Aaronson JG, et al. Antepartum diagnosis of the "terminal" fetal state by cardiotocography. Br J Obstet Gynaecol 1973;82:353.

35. Tushuizon PB, Stood JE, Ubachs JMH. Fetal heart rate monitoring of the dying fetus. Am J Obstet Gynecol 1974; 120:922.

36. Dawes GS, Visser GHA, Goodman IDA, et al. Numerical analysis of the human fetal heart rate: modulation by breathing and movement. Am J Obstet Gynecol 1981; 140:535.

37. Grimwade JC, Walker DW, Bartlett M, et al. Human fetal heart rate change and movement in response to sound and vibration. Am J Obstet Gynecol 1971;109:86.

38. Walker D, Grimwade J, Wood C. Intrauterine noise: a component of the fetal environment. Am J Obstet Gynecol 1971;109:93.

39. Rabinowitz R, Yarkoni S, Sacks B, et al. The prognostic and diagnostic value of the auditory habituation reflex of the fetus. Presented at the Second Internatioal Workshop on the At-Risk Infant. Jerusalem, May 1983.

40. Ohel G, Birkenfeld A, Rabinowitz R, Sadovsky E. Fetal response to vibratory acoustic stimulation in periods of low heart rate reactivity and low activity. Am J Obstet Gynecol 1986;154:619–21.

41. Read JA, Miller FC. Fetal heart rate acceleration in response to acoustic stimulation as a measure of fetal well-being. Am J Obstet Gynecol 1977;129:512–17.

42. Jensen OH. Fetal heart rate response to a controlled sound stimulus as a measure of fetal well-being. Acta Obstet Gynecol Scand 1984;63:97–101.

43. Polishuk WZ, Laufer N, Sadovsky E. Fetal response to external light stimulus. Harefuah 1975;89:395.

44. Ron M, Yaffe H, Sadovsky E. Fetal heart response to amniocentesis in cases of decreased fetal movements. Obstet Gynecol 1976;48:456.

45. David H, Weaver JB, Pearson JP. Doppler ultrasound and fetal activity. Br Med J 1975;2:62.

46. Rosen MG, Hertz RH, Dierker LJ, et al. Monitoring fetal movement. Clin Obstet Gynaecol 1979;6:325.

47. Weinstein D, Navot D, Sadovsky E. Antepartum ultrasound fetal heart rate monitoring and fetal movements. J Obstet Gynaecol 1981;2:85.

48. Sadovsky E. Monitoring fetal movements: a useful screening test. Contemp Ob/Gyn 1985;25:123.

49. Neldam S. Fetal movements as an indicator of fetal wellbeing. Lancet 1980;1:1222.

50. Sadovsky E. A scoring system using fetal movements. Contemp Ob/Gyn 1982;19:142.

51. Sadovsky E, Navot D, Yaffe H. Antenatal evaluation of FHR accelerations associated with fetal movements. Int J Gynaecol Obstet 1981;19:441.

PART FIVE Maternal Disease

20

Sickle Cell Anemia

Edgar O. Horger III, M.D.

SICKLE cell (S/S) anemia is an inherited chronic hemolytic anemia characterized clinically by symptoms of anemia, arthralgia, and recurrent painful crises. The disease occurs almost exclusively in blacks. Many afflicted individuals die within the first decade of life; few survive to age 40. Since there is no known cure, treatment is only palliative at present

The disorder, which is associated with a physical appearance and clinical course that are both quite distinctive, affects most organ systems. Patients with sickle cell disease generally appear to be undernourished and have a short trunk, narrow hips and shoulders, and long, spindly extremities. The skin around the ankles has a marked tendency to chronic ulceration. Splenomegaly is frequently noted in children, but seldom found in adults. Cardiomegaly and heart murmurs may lead to an erroneous diagnosis of rheumatic heart disease. A mild-to-moderate hyperbilirubinemia, causing a peculiar muddy yellow color in the sclerae, is commonly seen. Most patients with sickle cell anemia adapt remarkably well to their anemia. They are able to tolerate a hemoglobin concentration as low as 7 or 8 g/dL, without a great deal of difficulty, although they often tire easily.

The condition is characterized by crises with a sudden onset of pain in the extremities or abdomen. An attack may last for several days and can lead to unnecessary surgery unless S/S anemia is suspected.

Pathogenesis

In sickle cell anemia, the pathogenic mechanism lies in the synthesis of the hemoglobin molecule. Investigators have identified a single structural anomaly in the β chain of the globin molecule that differentiates sickle cell hemoglobin (HbS) from normal adult hemoglobin (HbA): specifically, the amino acid valine replaces glutamic acid in position 6.

Under conditions of decreased oxygenation, this abnormal molecule undergoes reversible aggregation. This results in a semisolid gel with sufficient rigidity to distort the erythrocyte into a characteristic sickle shape. The abnormal morphology of these erythrocytes causes them to flow poorly through the capillary lumina, thereby leading to obstruction within the microvasculature and tissue hypoxia. A cycle results in which blood stasis, tissue acidosis, and continued oxygen deficit combine to increase the number of sickled cells and thus augment the stasis. Microinfarction of ischemic tissue then occurs. This is most likely the cause of the pain accompanying a crisis. Additionally, the sickled red cells are more susceptible to hemolysis and phagocytosis than are normal erythrocytes.

Sickle cell hemoglobin is inherited in dominant fashion. Although variable among blacks in different parts of the United States, the incidence of sickle cell trait averages 8% (1). One out of 400 American blacks is homozygous for HbS and has full-blown sickle cell anemia.

When an individual inherits both HbS and HbA alleles, the resulting heterozygote usually remains asymptomatic throughout life. However, sickling can occur under conditions of severe hypoxia, such as that imposed by high altitudes. In addition, studies have shown that those patients heterozygous for both HbS and HbA have an increased incidence of asymptomatic bacteriuria and clinical pyelonephritis, particularly during pregnancy. The heterozygous combination of HbS and other abnormal hemoglobins, such as HbC or beta thalassemia, may lead to a clinical course closely resembling that of sickle cell anemia. These heterozygous combinations are included in the all-encompassing term "sickle cell disease."

Pregnancy

For many years, practitioners believed that S/S anemia markedly decreased fertility in women. In fact, as late as 1971, pregnancy had been reported in only 236 patients with S/S anemia (2). This decreased fertility rate apparently results from both the chronic illness and the fact that these patients often die before reaching childbearing age. However, pregnancy certainly is a possibility among adults. Recent studies show that the incidence of S/S anemia in the pregnant population is no smaller than that in the general population.

Sickle cell anemia has profound effects on maternal morbidity and on both perinatal and maternal mortality (3, 4). These patients are particularly susceptible to infection; pneumonia, urinary tract infection, and puerperal endometritis head the list. Anemia is a universal finding and almost invariably becomes more severe as pregnancy pro-

gresses. Approximately one-third of these patients develop preeclampsia. Acute sickle cell crisis commonly occurs during pregnancy and may, in fact, appear for the first time after a patient becomes pregnant. Congestive heart failure and pulmonary infarction are not infrequent. These complications necessitate frequent hospitalizations and greatly prolong the patients' confinements.

Despite these potential problems, the gestational course for most patients with S/S anemia reflects their history prior to pregnancy. That is, patients with uncomplicated past histories usually will have relatively uncomplicated pregnancies and deliveries. Unfortunately, this is not universally true. Previously asymptomatic patients may experience serious—even fatal—complications during pregnancy.

Most reports since 1970 show significant improvements in both maternal and perinatal outcomes. Although maternal mortality rates as high as 25% were once reported in patients with sickle cell anemia, reviews since 1970 have shown maternal death rates to be much less than 1% (4). Similarly, perinatal mortality rates have decreased from as high as 50% to as low as 2.4% (Table 20.1). These improvements probably reflect earlier entry into the health care system, better antepartum monitoring, and new management techniques.

Most perinatal deaths occur in utero. Low birthweight deliveries are common, resulting both from preterm birth and intrauterine growth retardation. Intrauterine hypoxia caused by the sluggish circulation of sickled erythrocytes in uterine and decidual arterioles may be at least partially responsible for both the rise in the rate of stillbirths and the greater incidence of low birthweight infants. However,

Table 20.1 Pregnancy Outcome in Patients with S/S Anemia (Data from 309 Pregnancies in Seven Reports Since 1976 (5–11))

	Range	Mean
Spontaneous abortion (%)	11–16	12.4
Stillbirth (%)	2–8	4.2
Neonatal death (%)	0–9	2.0
Low birthweight (%)	7–33	21.3
Perinatal mortality	24.4–121.1/1,000	61.5/1,000

such factors as chronic anemia, maternal debility, and the high rate of preeclampsia must also be considered.

Management

The appropriate management of pregnant patients with S/S anemia requires close observation and frequent office visits throughout the antenatal course. As sudden drops in hemoglobin concentration and hematocrit may occur with alarming abruptness, blood counts should be obtained at frequent intervals. Folic acid supplements are necessary throughout pregnancy because of the increased utilization of folate through rapid erythrocyte turnover. Iron therapy is controversial and may contribute to iron storage disease. Iron deficiency should be documented before implementing supplemental iron.

While intermittent transfusions of packed erythrocytes may be necessary to correct severe anemia (hematocrit (Hct) <20%), most patients tolerate their anemia with little difficulty. Nevertheless, less anemic patients generally appear to have fewer painful crises, infections, and other complications. A collaborative project involving blood transfusion in pregnant patients with sickle cell anemia found fewer painful crises in patients managed with prophylactic transfusions than in the group transfused only on indications. However, no other benefits were noted in complication rates or outcome (11).

Recent studies advocate partial exchange transfusions for managing these patients. This procedure increases red blood cell volume and the blood's oxygen-carrying capacity, decreases the number of circulating erythrocytes capable of sickling, and suppresses the production of erythrocytes containing HbS. However, these benefits must be weighed against the risks of transfusion reaction, hepatitis, AIDS, and blood group isoimmunization (12). Although several reports have demonstrated reduced maternal morbidity and perinatal mortality rates following prophylactic partial exchange transfusion (5, 7), others have implied that the statistics reflect a general improvement in obstetrical care rather than the procedure's therapeutic efficacy (8). Partial exchange transfusion is of unquestioned value in the treatment of crisis and infection.

Hospitalization becomes mandatory when such complications as preeclampsia, infection, or crisis occur. Diuretics must be avoided, as any degree of dehydration can precipitate sickling. Fever also has been implicated as a potential sickling inducer and must be treated promptly.

Specific therapy for S/S anemia is essentially nonexistent (13). Corticosteroids, vasodilators, anticoagulants, cobaltous chloride, acetazolamide, dextran, urea, magnesium salts, and phenothiazines all have had therapeutic trials, with results ranging from questionable to disappointing. Current research efforts are directed toward conversion of hemoglobin synthesis from HbS to HbF, identification and repression of a sickling cofactor (possibly prostaglandin E_2), and preventing or reversing intravascular sickling. Extra-corporeal cyanate carbamylation currently is being tested in nonpregnant patients.

Available treatment modalities are aimed at preventing or relieving painful crisis. The most useful options are bed rest, increased atmospheric oxygen, intravenous hydration, analgesics, and blood transfusion. Although hyperbaric oxygen may be effective, this approach is extremely cumbersome and not readily available.

Some practitioners advocate preterm induction of labor or cesarean section to prevent death in utero because of placental insufficiency. There seems to be little merit for this policy. Fetuses lost in utero generally die too early in the pregnancy to survive elective delivery. Nonetheless, there may be some justification for elective delivery in certain cases when a patient's condition remains relatively stable. As with other high-risk pregnancies, antepartum fetal heart rate testing is indicated. If these tests remain reassuring, it is generally safe to await spontaneous labor. The route of delivery should be based solely on obstetric considerations, bearing in mind that prolonged labor increases the risks of maternal acidosis, dehydration, and infection, all of which predispose to sickling. Anesthesia must be administered with extreme caution to avoid hypoxia and hypotension, and blood loss must be held to a minimum.

Genetic Counseling

Patients with S/S anemia require careful counseling concerning potential pregnancy-related hazards. For example, there is a strong likelihood of serious morbidity and an increased incidence of maternal mortality in this group. These patients also must realize that they face increased risks of stillbirth and neonatal death. In view of these concerns, it is understandable that many consider S/S disease an indication for sterilization, whether or not previous pregnancies have been attempted.

Ideally, patients should be so advised before marriage. However, many S/S patients don't receive adequate counseling and are already pregnant when seen by a physician. Because of the myriad maternal complications closely related to the duration of pregnancy, therapeutic abortion may be considered. No patient with sickle cell anemia should be required to continue a potentially threatening pregnancy. The patient should be apprised fully of these potential problems and offered the option of early abortion.

Theoretically, a mass screening program to detect heterozygotes, coupled with effective genetic counseling, could abolish all S/S anemia in the United States. In fact, such detection programs are currently in progress in many areas to screen black children and adolescents for HbS. However, extraordinarily persuasive counseling would be necessary to discourage childbearing by heterozygotes.

The prenatal diagnosis of fetal S/S disease represents a further refinement in genetic counseling. Recent techniques demonstrate reliable prediction and exclusion of fetal sickle hemoglobinopathies through restriction endonuclease analysis of the DNA present in uncultured amniotic fluid cells (14). Similar analysis of trophoblastic DNA, obtained by chorionic villus sampling, has led to the diagnosis of fetal hemoglobinopathies as early as seven to 13 weeks of gestation.

Patients with S/S anemia face formidable complications during pregnancy, with marked increase in maternal morbidity and perinatal mortality rates. These patients—and their obstetricians—must recognize these facts to ensure meticulous care during the prenatal period, labor, and the puerperium. All medical facts considered, a liberal approach to therapeutic abortion and sterilization seems to be warranted for these patients.

CASE 20.1

A 23-year-old primigravida with S/S disease reported for prenatal care at nine weeks' gestation. Her past history revealed two hospitalizations for painful sickle cell crises, most recently at 16 years of age. Her initial hemoglobin was 8.4 g/dL, hematocrit 25%, and urine culture showed more than 100,000 *Escherichia coli* bacteria/mL, for which she was treated with oral ampicillin for 14 days.

At 25 weeks' gestation, she was found to have right lower lobe pneumonia. She was hospitalized for 19 days and treated with penicillin. Her hemoglobin fell as low as 6.5 g/dL and hematocrit 19.5%, but no blood transfusions were given.

At 31 weeks' gestation, preeclampsia was diagnosed. She was hospitalized and put on complete bed rest. Hemoglobin was 7.2 g/dL and hematocrit 20.5%. Approximately 48 hours after hospital admission, no fetal activity was observed, and no fetal heartbeat could be detected. Forty-eight hours later, labor was induced with oxytocin. She delivered a 1,220-g macerated stillborn infant.

The patient developed postpartum endometritis. She was treated initially with ampicillin, but, after no response in 72 hours, clindamycin and gentamicin were added to her regimen. On the fourth postpartum day, her hemoglobin was 6.1 g/dL and hematocrit 17%. Transfusion of two units of packed erythrocytes raised the hemoglobin to 8.4 g/dL and hematocrit to 25%. She became afebrile on the sixth postpartum day and was discharged home three days later.

This patient's pregnancy and puerperium were complicated by three different infections, preeclampsia, fetal death, and severe anemia requiring blood transfusions. She was hospitalized for 33 days during and after her pregnancy. ∎

CASE 20.2

A 15-year-old primigravida with S/S disease was referred for management at 28 weeks' gestation. She had been hospitalized elsewhere for sickle cell crisis several times, including three admissions during the first 26 weeks. On each occasion, she had been treated with IV fluids, oxygen, and analgesics.

Partial exchange transfusion was performed at 29 weeks' gestation. Prior to exchange, her electrophoretic pattern revealed 89% HbS, 2% HbA$_2$, and 9% HbF, while her hemoglobin concentration was 8.5 g/dL and hematocrit 24.6%. After exchange, she had 56% HbS, 42% HbA, and 2% HbF. Her postexchange hemoglobin was 11.2 g/dL and hematocrit 32%. Weekly evaluations over the next 10 weeks revealed a slowly progressive fall in HbA to 33% and rise in HbS to 65%. The hematocrit decreased only to 28%.

She experienced no further complications or crises during pregnancy. Weekly oxytocin challenge tests begun at 34 weeks' gestation were negative. Spontaneous labor began at 39 weeks. A 3,008-g healthy male infant was delivered. The patient and her infant were discharged three days later. ∎

References

1. Motulsky AG. Frequency of sickling disorders in U.S. Blacks. N Engl J Med 1973;288:31.
2. Perkins RP. Inherited disorders of hemoglobin synthesis and pregnancy. Am J Obstet Gynecol 1971;111:120.
3. Horger EO III. Hemoglobinopathies in pregnancy. Clin Obstet Gynecol 1974;17:127.
4. Morrison JC. Hemoglobinopathies and pregnancy. Clin Obstet Gynecol 1979;22:819.
5. Morrison JC, Wiser WL. The effect of maternal partial exchange transfusion on the infants of patients with sickle cell anemia. J Pediatr 1976;89:286.
6. Charache S, Scott J, Niebyl J, et al. Management of sickle cell disease in pregnant patients. Obstet Gynecol 1980;55:407.
7. Morrison JC, Schneider JM, Whybrew WD, et al. Prophylactic transfusions in pregnant patients with sickle cell hemoglobinopathies: benefit versus risk. Obstet Gynecol 1980;56:274.
8. Miller JM Jr, Horger EO III, Key TC, et al. Management of sickle hemoglobinopathies in pregnant patients. Am J Obstet Gynecol 1981;141:237.
9. Cunningham FG, Pritchard JA, Mason R. Pregnancy and sickle cell hemoglobinopathies: results with and without prophylactic transfusions. Obstet Gynecol 1983;62:419.
10. Powars DR, Sandhu M, Niland-Weiss J, et al. Pregnancy in sickle cell disease. Obstet Gynecol 1986;67:217.
11. Koshy M, Burd L, Wallace D, et al. Prophylactic red-cell transfusions in pregnant patients with sickle cell disease. N Engl J Med 1988;319:1447.
12. Orlina AR, Sosler SD, Koshy M. Problems of chronic transfusion in sickle cell disease. J Clin Apheresis 1991;6:234.
13. Rodgers GP. Recent approaches to the treatment of sickle cell anemia. JAMA 1991;265:2097.
14. Chang JC, Kan YW. A sensitive new prenatal test for sickle-cell anemia. N Engl J Med 1982;307:30.

21

Thrombocytopenia: The ITP and TTP Syndromes

David Z. Kitay, M.D.

DIAGNOSIS of thrombocytopenia in pregnancy is no longer rare as a result of increased awareness of the platelet in maternal disease and routine automation of the complete blood count. Clinically significant thrombocytopenia in pregnancy remains unusual and is almost always caused by a coincidental medical problem, the latter possibly aggravated or precipitated by gestation. The major conditions associated with occasionally profound thrombocytopenia include immunologic (idiopathic) thrombocytopenic purpura (ITP), the microangiopathic hemolysis (HELLP syndrome) of toxemia, and thrombotic thrombocytopenic purpura (TTP). These are separate clinical entities that have certain hematologic features in common but are not related in etiology.

The laboratory diagnosis of thrombocytopenia is of prime importance because spuriously low platelet counts may lead to erroneous diagnosis and unnecessarily zealous therapy. This is especially important in a pregnant woman without purpura, hemorrhage, or bleeding diathesis because chronic ITP is most frequently seen in young women, and the disease may first appear during pregnancy. Although there are a number of causes of spurious thrombocytopenia, EDTA-induced platelet clumping and improper blood withdrawal and anticoagulation appear most frequently. The diagnosis should always be verified either by finger-stick blood collection with phase microscopy counting or by a sodium citrate-anticoagulated venous blood sample. Examination of a peripheral smear for platelet morphology and clumping is essential. Newer instruments for automated counting with histograms have been of some assistance (1, 2).

The behavior of the platelet count in otherwise normal pregnancy has been well studied. There is a significant drop with gestational progression. This fall in platelet count is most pronounced after 32 weeks, does not affect hemostasis, and almost always remains in the normal range of $150,000–450,000/mm^3$. The mean platelet volume, a measure of platelet size (normal: 8.5–9.0 femtoliters), rises dramatically in the late third trimester. Young platelets or macrothrombocytes are large and become progressively smaller with age. These findings are compatible with increased platelet destruction, similar to what occurs in ITP, where a fall in count and increase in volume are characteristic. It has been suggested that pregnancy is a state of chronic intravascular coagulation, and normal platelet behavior supports this concept. It is important to remember that iron deficiency, so prevalent in pregnancy with or without iron deficiency anemia, may either raise or lower the platelet count (3).

Chronic ITP is an immunologic problem. Peripheral platelet destruction occurs in the presence of a normal or hyperplastic megakaryocyte population in bone marrow. In toxemia, platelet destruction may be mechanical, presenting as a heightened response to endothelial injury. During pregnancy, ITP is usually a benign chronic disease affecting both mother and newborn; in contrast, TTP in the past was almost universally fatal when associated with pregnancy. Treating ITP can yield satisfactory results with little or no maternal or perinatal mortality; until recently, therapy for TTP has been empiric. ITP is not associated with preeclampsia; the TTP syndrome, however, can be clinically indistinguishable from severe toxemia, with many of the same hematologic and organ system features.

Immunologic Thrombocytopenic Purpura

Immunologic thrombocytopenic purpura is an autoimmune disorder in which an antibody is produced to a platelet-associated antigen. Binding of the antibody to the platelet results in platelet destruction in the spleen, liver, and bone marrow. The two forms of ITP, acute and chronic, differ in clinical course and probably in pathogenesis. The acute form is most common in children, and both sexes are equally affected.

Chronic ITP has a female-to-male incidence of 3:1, and the peak age affected is between 20 and 40 years. It is not surprising to find ITP associated with pregnancy, the incidence being about 1–2 in 10,000 pregnancies. Most cases have an insidious onset, with easy bruising or bleeding localized to one site, such as epistaxis or menorrhagia. Thrombocytopenia is often not severe. The disease lasts for months to years, with a course that is fluctuating, and spontaneous remissions are uncommon. ITP seems to be a disorder of immune regulation in which lymphocytes produce antibody to a platelet-associated antigen. It is of particular concern during pregnancy because the placenta has receptors for the Fc portion of the IgG molecule and actively transports IgG antibodies from maternal to fetal circulation. This may or may not cause thrombocytopenia in the fetus, as well as the major risk of central nervous system hemorrhage during vaginal delivery. Many aspects of the pathogenesis and treatment of ITP, as well as management of labor in the presence of this disease, remain unknown or controversial, although methods for determining level of antiplatelet antibody, intravenous gamma globulin therapy, and fetal scalp or cord blood sampling for platelet counts before or during labor are among advances that may assist the clinician (Table 21.1) (4).

Megakaryocyte number in the bone marrow of patients with ITP averages three times normal. The megakaryocyte volume averages 1.6 times normal. Megakaryocyte mass increases 4.8 times, indicating that the marrow is able to increase platelet production about fivefold. Platelet turnover, which reflects both platelet delivery from the marrow and platelet disappearance from the blood, has been shown to increase to 2.25–4.9 times normal. Since platelets and megakaryocytes share common antigens, the antibody present in ITP may be affecting the megakaryocytes as well. Evidence of antibody bound to megakaryocytes has been shown with immunofluorescent antiglobulin antiserum and with radioautographs. Large platelets or megathrombocytes are found in the peripheral blood of patients with ITP. The number of these "stress" platelets parallels the increased number of megakaryocytes in the bone marrow. Megathrombocyte diameter is inversely proportional to platelet survival. About 50% of ITP patients in clinical remission have increased megathrombocytes, indicating increased platelet turnover, despite normal platelet counts. Paradoxically, the bleeding time in patients with ITP is often normal. This is due to the increased hemostatic competence of large, young platelets. However, a qualitative or functional platelet defect has been described in a few patients with ITP. These patients were symptomatic despite platelet counts greater than 50,000/mm^3. Abnormal platelet aggregation and arachidonate metabolism were demonstrated. In addition, patients with an "easy bruising syndrome" and a normal platelet count have been described, in which the thrombopathia, an aspirinlike platelet aggregation defect, is associated with an antiplatelet antibody. It has been suggested that the antiplatelet antibody may be responsible for a qualitative, as well as a quantitative, defect. The immune system may respond to platelet antigen by producing antibody or by activating cell-mediated immunity. Humoral immunity seems to play the central role in ITP.

Presenting symptoms in ITP vary, and the onset is usually insidious. Manifestations include petechiae, purpura, ecchymoses, gingival bleeding, epistaxis, menometrorrhagia, hematuria, melena, hematemesis, intracranial hemorrhage, and excessive bleeding following trauma or surgery. Bleeding into joints or the retina is unusual. Hemorrhagic bullae in the oral mucosa indicate that platelet levels are very low, usually $<5,000/mm^3$ and that aggressive treatment is needed. Episodes of bleeding may last days or weeks. Not infrequently, the course is surprisingly benign. Spontaneous remissions are uncommon and likely to be incomplete. The spleen is palpable in less than 10% of cases. Splenomegaly argues strongly against the diagnosis of ITP.

Thrombocytopenia is defined as a platelet count of $<100,000/mm^3$. An initially low platelet count must be verified since falsely low values may occur with automated counters, ineffective anticoagulant, or faulty blood-drawing technique, and examination of the peripheral smear is indicated.

The platelet count may fluctuate widely but usually is in the $10–75,000/mm^3$ range. Bizarre, giant platelets are commonly seen. The white cell count and differential are normal except for neutrophilia associated with acute bleeding. Lymphocytosis with atypical cells has been reported. Anemia secondary to blood loss is not infrequent and is usually normocytic unless iron deficiency is present. If an autoimmune hemolytic anemia and ITP occur together, the Coombs' test will be positive. Serum acid phosphatase may be elevated because of increased platelet turnover. The bleeding time may be prolonged but less than would be expected by the platelet count. Clot retraction, tourniquet test, and prothrombin consumption vary with the severity of the thrombocytopenia. Prothrombin time, partial thromboplastin time (PTT) and coagulation time are normal. The bone marrow shows normal or increased megakaryocytes, but they are less granular, more basophilic, and smoother in contour. These findings all suggest that ITP is a quantitative platelet problem, and, although qualitative defects are occasionally described, maternal and fetal thrombocytopenia are the most important considerations in therapy.

ITP is a diagnosis of exclusion. The first consideration should be exposure to drugs or chemicals; the second, sys-

Table 21.1 Brief History of ITP in Pregnancy

Year	Finding
1929	First successful splenectomy for ITP during pregnancy
1950	Suggestion that maternal mortality is no higher than general population; fetal mortality 15%
1953	Demonstration of humoral thrombocytopenia-producing factor in peripheral blood of patients with ITP
1954	Maternal mortality 2.1%, fetal mortality 15%
1957	Maternal mortality 1.6%, fetal mortality 1.9%
1973	Cesarean section to prevent fetal intracranial hemorrhage if maternal platelet count less than 100,000 mm³
1975	Assay for platelet-associated IgG
1978	Scalp platelet counts to determine route of delivery
1982	Prediction of neonatal thrombocytopenia by measurement of maternal antiplatelet antibody level
1987	Only one maternal death with ITP reported since 1960; perinatal mortality 6.2%
	Prenatal cordocentesis for diagnosis

temic lupus erythematosus. Indeed, ITP may occur as a precursor to lupus and precede this disease by years. Hereditary thrombocytopenia can be excluded by family history, laboratory studies of platelet function, and examination of family members. Splenomegaly from any cause may result in secondary thrombocytopenia, although this finding argues against the diagnosis. Underlying hematologic disorders such as leukemia, myeloma, aplastic anemia, lymphoma, and myelophthisic processes are usually associated with anemia, changes in leukocytes, or bone marrow abnormalities. Infectious causes such as septicemia, infectious mononucleosis, and cytomegalovirus merit consideration. In addition, diffuse intravascular coagulation, thrombotic thrombocytopenic purpura, and posttransfusion purpura should be ruled out.

The course of ITP is so varied that treatment is difficult to evaluate. Because the rarity of the disease has prohibited controlled studies, personal bias sometimes enters management with excellent results. It must be emphasized that *the goal of therapy is a hematologically asymptomatic patient, not a normal platelet count* (5). Steroids followed by splenectomy has withstood the test of time; there is fair, but not complete, agreement on this approach. Asymptomatic patients with profound thrombocytopenia (4,000+/mm^3) have been closely followed throughout pregnancy, labor, and delivery by cesarean section that produced healthy unaffected infants with minimal operative blood loss, a totally benign puerperal course, and none of the side effects of drug therapy. Attainment of a platelet count of 30,000/mm^3 is usually sufficient to prohibit serious bleeding, and 50,000/mm^3 is sufficient to assure safety. With current therapy, death from ITP is very unusual. Heroic therapy should be reserved for life-threatening situations. Factors that will aggravate the bleeding tendency and should be avoided include antiplatelet drugs such as aspirin and alcohol, infection, trauma, azotemia, hypermetabolism, and vaccinations.

A corticosteroid, usually prednisone, in doses of 1–1.5 mg/kg/day is the first drug used. The platelet count usually increases in 70%–80% of patients within 1–2 weeks. The dose is continued for 2–3 weeks and then tapered to a low-dose, alternate-day regimen sufficient to maintain the platelet count at greater than 50,000/mm^3. If the platelet count in symptomatic patients does not increase to greater than 50,000/mm^3 or can be maintained only with massive doses of steroids, the spleen should be removed. A sustained remission with steroids occurs in from 15%–60% of patients, and only an occasional case will have a sustained remission after steroids are discontinued. The mechanism of action of corticosteroids in ITP is to decrease antibody production, inhibit phagocytosis of sensitized platelets, and decrease capillary fragility. Rarely, steroid therapy may actually perpetuate thrombocytopenia, and remission occurs when the drug is discontinued. When the choice between increased or decreased dosage has to be made in refractory patients, an initial large increase of prednisone for one week should be tried (6).

Splenectomy removes the major site of platelet destruction and a significant source of antibody synthesis. The overall permanent remission rate is in the range of 70%–80%, and mortality is less than 1%. The prednisone dosage should be increased prior to surgery in an attempt to raise the platelet count. Platelet transfusions may be used in the presence of severe thrombocytopenia but are usually not required and should be reserved, if possible, for life-threatening situations. Lessening of any bleeding is commonly noted as soon as the splenic pedicle is clamped, and the platelet count rises within a few hours to two weeks. Following splenectomy, steroids should be withdrawn gradually over a three-week period. Even with complete remission, evidence of increased platelet production and decreased platelet survival may persist as evidence of a "compensated" state where production can keep up with destruction. Because of its rapid effect, emergency splenectomy, along with platelet transfusions and steroids, are recommended for treatment of intracranial bleeding.

There is no foolproof way to predict who will respond to splenectomy. An accessory spleen was formerly considered to be a common cause of relapse after splenectomy. Autopsy studies have shown patients dying with accessory spleens without recurrence of their thrombocytopenia, and patients who relapse rarely have accessory spleens. Recurrence usually represents an exacerbation of the underlying immune disorder. A simple method to detect persistent splenic activity is to examine peripheral blood for Howell-Jolly and Heinz bodies, both of which should be present after splenectomy.

The major remote complication of splenectomy is fulminant sepsis and death, usually due to encapsulated organisms such as the pneumococcus. This risk is 2–3 times that in the general population.

A variety of immunosuppressant agents have been used in patients refractory to steroids and splenectomy. However, because the fate of treatment failures is not too bad and because there are troublesome side effects with immunosuppressant therapy, including a predisposition to malignancy, it is often prudent to accept an incomplete response. The most commonly used agents are azathioprine, cyclophosphamide, and the vinca alkaloids.

The mitotic spindle poisons, vincristine and vinblastine, are unique in that they are cytolytic for macrophages but also induce thrombocytosis. Vincristine is given in a dosage of 0.025 mg/kg intravenously (maximum dose 2 mg). Vinblastine is given at 0.125 mg/kg (maximum dose 10 mg) intravenously. Injections are repeated every 7–10 days. A rise in platelets is usually observed within 5–7 days. This early response is an advantage in life-threatening situations. If there is no response after three doses, the likelihood of a response is lessened. Response rates approximate 55%. Once remission is obtained, no maintenance therapy is given. The two agents appear to be about equally effective, although duration of remission may be longer with vincristine. The main side effects of vincristine are troublesome peripheral neuropathy and temporary jaw pain. Vinblastine may also produce the neuropathy, but leukopenia is the major dose-limiting toxicity. Other side effects reported with both agents include autonomic dysfunction, producing obstipation and urinary retention, fever, alopecia, gastrointestinal symptoms, inappropriate ADH secretion, and skin sloughing if the agent is extravasated. The vinca alkaloids have been used to "load" platelets which are then given intravenously; macrophages ingest the platelets and are themselves destroyed. Although response rates of 70% have been obtained, the remission is not sustained. Anaphylactic reactions have occurred, and in vitro studies have shown that the drug is eluted from platelets within two hours.

Plasmapheresis has been useful in a number of diseases with an immunologic pathogenesis such as Goodpasture's syndrome, myasthenia gravis, and multiple sclerosis. The goal of plasmapheresis in ITP is to remove antiplatelet antibody. Plasmapheresis may be effective in patients with acute ITP, but it does not benefit patients with long-standing disease. It may decrease the need for splenectomy in acute disease.

Another treatment modality is the use of high-dose intravenous gamma globulin. This therapy was discovered by chance when two children receiving intravenous gamma globulin for congenital agammaglobulinemia and thrombocytopenia had an unexpected rise in platelet counts. In the original series of 13 children with ITP, the platelet count rose sharply within five days of therapy in all patients, but the peak and duration of the response were variable. Some patients with acute ITP and with intermittent ITP had sustained responses. No untoward side effects were observed (7, 8).

This work has been confirmed by others using the same dosage of gamma globulin, 400 mg/kg/day for five days. Intravenous gamma globulin is marketed in the United States and has met with variable response in pregnancy. Both in vitro and in vivo studies show platelet function to be unaffected with treatment, and, to date, a number of reported cases have had at least an initial response.

Indications for IgG infusion are unclear, but the rapid initial response makes it attractive for the control of acute hemorrhage and for preparing the steroid-resistant patient for splenectomy and other surgical procedures. The most effective and economical dose has yet to be determined. Because of expense, long-term maintenance requiring weekly infusions is a problem.

Danazol, the synthetic androgen initially formulated for use in endometriosis, has been employed in treatment of ITP. The duration of remission has ranged from 2–13 months. The drug is well-tolerated and is thought to have a synergistic action with steroids. The mechanism of action is unknown. Its use in pregnancy is contraindicated. Colchicine has also been used, although the place of both danazol and colchicine in the long-term management of ITP has yet to be determined.

Pregnancy seems to have no effect on the course of ITP. On the other hand, ITP has a marked effect on pregnancy. Increased maternal and fetal mortality from thrombocytopenia has been variously confirmed and denied. Perinatal deaths are most commonly caused by prematurity, intracranial hemorrhage, or maternal hemorrhage and shock. The neonate requires close observation but usually does not require treatment. The nadir in the platelet count may not occur until 2–4 days after birth, and thrombocytopenia is self-limited, lasting 3–4 weeks. If petechiae or purpura develop, platelet transfusion and steroids are given. Exchange transfusion may be used in life-threatening situations. Splenectomy is not indicated. Breast-feeding is controversial because minute amounts of antiplatelet antibody are present in breast milk. Circumcision is deferred.

The incidence of antepartum hemorrhage is not increased in ITP, but there is an increased frequency of postpartum hemorrhage from lacerations and episiotomies. Spontaneous abortion rates may be increased, ranging from 5%–53%.

Corticosteroids are used if the platelet count is <50,000 /mm³, as described previously, although this is not a hard-and-fast rule since a number of patients without a bleeding diathesis have been managed with counts lower than 10,000. If the count is >50,000/mm³, close follow-up without therapy is advised. Side effects peculiar to pregnancy include fetal adrenal suppression and questionable increases in preeclampsia and postpartum psychosis. Cleft palate and other congenital malformations are probably not increased by steroid therapy. Antenatal steroid administration for a few weeks prior to anticipated delivery has been proposed to enhance neonatal platelet counts. Significantly higher counts were found in infants of mothers given prednisone versus controls. These findings may well have been serendipitous, since 87% of a prednisone dose is inactivated by a placental dehydrogenase. Several authors have cited cases in which steroids did not prevent neonatal thrombocytopenia. Betamethasone and dexamethasone have been proposed as substitutes for prednisone since their maternal/fetal partition coefficients are 3:1 instead of 10:1, although cases of dexamethasone use with no effect on fetal platelets are reported.

Splenectomy, when necessary, is best performed in the second trimester because of technical difficulties later in pregnancy. There is a risk of abortion, premature labor, and intrauterine fetal demise. The older literature reports a 9%–10% maternal mortality rate and a 25% perinatal mortality rate. Current operative mortality should be comparable to that achieved in the nonpregnant patient. Concomitant cesarean and splenectomy at term have been done, but some advise against this because of an increased complication rate.

Immunosuppressants should be avoided, although experience with azathioprine in pregnant renal transplant patients has shown surprisingly few congenital anomalies. The main problems encountered were growth retardation and prematurity. In such patients, it is impossible to separate the effect of the drug from the effect of the underlying disease.

The most controversial aspect in the management of ITP in pregnancy is the mode of delivery of a potentially thrombocytopenic infant. There are currently six reasonable approaches to management, which are outlined in Table 21.2.

The single greatest factor in neonatal loss is intracranial hemorrhage secondary to birth trauma, favoring cesarean delivery. The 27% incidence of thrombocytopenia in infants of mothers whose platelet counts are greater than 100,000/mm³ is not an acceptable risk. Platelet transfusions should prevent excessive bleeding at cesarean section. This approach has much support. Without the experience and equipment to do fetal scalp sampling (which technique may in itself be flawed because of coagulation), cordocentesis for platelet counts prior to or during labor, or measurement of maternal antiplatelet antibodies, cesarean section may be the most practical approach.

The fourth alternative is to determine fetal platelet counts via scalp sampling. The platelet count is measured after the membranes are ruptured and the cervix is 2–3 cm dilated. This is done early in labor or, in some cases, before labor. If the count is <50,000/mm³, cesarean section is performed; otherwise, vaginal delivery is permitted. It is usually necessary to have some labor to dilate the cervix sufficiently to allow scalp sampling. This may be sufficient trauma to cause intracranial bleeding. There is some worry about excessive bleeding after scalp sampling of the thrombocytopenic fetus, especially if station is lost after the sampling procedure and the bleeding goes undetected. Finally, there is reported concern about clotting leading to falsely

Table 21.2 Management Alternatives in ITP in Pregnancy

1. If the platelet count is >100,000 and there has been no prior splenectomy, perform vaginal delivery. If the platelet count is <100,000 or there has been a prior splenectomy, perform a cesarean section.

2. Deliver all patients vaginally, irrespective of the maternal platelet count, reserving cesarean section for obstetric indications only.

3. Cesarean section for all patients.

4. Perform fetal scalp platelet count early in labor. If the count is >50,000, deliver vaginally. If the count is < 50,000, deliver by cesarean section.

5. Assay maternal blood for platelet-bound IgG antibody or circulating antiplatelet antibody. Women with high antibody levels should be delivered by cesarean section.

6. Perform cordocentesis (funicentesis, percutaneous umbilical blood sampling) at term or prior to delivery, with the extent of neonatal thrombocytopenia, if present, guiding management.

low platelet counts (9, 10).

There have been recent studies using maternal antiplatelet antibody levels to predict fetal platelet count, the fifth alternative. Maternal PAIgG has been predictive of infant thrombocytopenia but not of its severity. This may be because severity is related to a number of factors, including the quantity and characteristics of the IgG antibody, activity of the fetal reticuloendothelial system, steroid therapy, and the capacity of the infant's marrow to produce platelets. Maternal PAIgG does not correlate with maternal platelet counts and is not absolutely predictive.

The sixth and final alternative involves direct determination of fetal hematology prior to delivery. This is the preferred approach when available. A number of studies have now demonstrated the accuracy and feasibility of cordocentesis to determine the fetal platelet count directly prior to labor. The maternal platelet count may vary tremendously without a bleeding diathesis, and the goal in maternal therapy (or expectant therapy) is a hematologically stable patient, regardless of the platelet count. However, in the fetus, there seems to be a general consensus that thrombocytopenia (<100,000/mm^3) greatly increases the chances of intracranial hemorrhage. Although this value may be somewhat arbitrary in that many infants have been delivered by the abdominal or vaginal route with profound thrombocytopenia and absence of gross neonatal sequelae, at present, this seems a prudent laboratory parameter. Below a fetal count of 100,000 mm^3, cesarean section is performed; above this value, operative delivery is undertaken only for obstetric reasons (11).

It is emphasized that, even when cesarean section is done in the presence of thrombocytopenia, fetal intracranial hemorrhage may still occur.

The advantages of cordocentesis in ITP are obvious, the most important being a logical approach to delivery. There are no other antepartum or maternal laboratory antecedents reliable enough to predict fetal thrombocytopenia. Cordocentesis can be performed after 37 weeks, with elective induction, spontaneous labor, or cesarean section planned. Some have suggested that the cord platelet count may be reliable up to three weeks prior to delivery. Maternal-fetal antibody transfer and fetal platelet destruction should be evident by the 37th week.

The greatest disadvantage of cordocentesis is its limited availability to centers with appropriate ultrasound equipment and physicians trained in umbilical cord blood sampling, although, following cord platelet count determination, the patient may be returned to her primary center for delivery. Associated risks are sporadic and include fetal heart rate decelerations, cord bleeding, thrombosis or hematoma, fetal or placental trauma, infection, and failure to obtain a sample. Blood obtained may be confirmed as fetal in origin by an elevated mean corpuscular volume (fetal value >100 microns^3), the Kleihauer-Betke stain (fetal red cells), or hemoglobin electrophoresis (hemoglobin F). In addition to diagnosis, direct transfusion of platelet packs has been performed, with success in raising fetal counts, although this rise will be extremely transient because of destruction, and imminent delivery should be planned.

Thrombotic Thrombocytopenic Purpura

Thrombotic thrombocytopenic purpura was first described in 1924. It is now recognized as an acute illness (syndrome), characterized by fever, thrombocytopenia, microangiopathic hemolytic anemia, slowly progressing or dramatic renal failure, and variable neurologic signs. The pathologic hallmark is hyaline thrombosis of small blood vessels throughout the body. The disorder is uncommon, with females affected more frequently than males, in a ratio of 3:2; the highest incidence is in childbearing years (ages 10–40). The literature regarding TTP and pregnancy consists primarily of case reports and small series of patients, primarily because the disease is uncommon, and mortality in the past has been prohibitive. The etiology remains unknown and strict management is uncertain, although much progress has been made in the past 10 years. When left untreated, the syndrome follows an almost invariably fatal course. The mortality rate within three months of diagnosis is at least 80%, and long-term survival has been about 10% (12).

The characteristic pentad of clinical findings in TTP includes thrombocytopenia, anemia, neurologic abnormalities, fever, and renal dysfunction. Clinical illness usually begins with sudden onset of neurologic symptoms such as headache, visual difficulty, aphasia, paresis, or convulsion. Other common initial presentations may be petechiae, eccymoses, and other hemorrhagic manifestations. The patient may present with simple epistaxis, a common problem in otherwise normal pregnancy, then proceed to the devastating full-blown syndrome. Fever is invariably present. Severe thrombocytopenia and anemia are almost always present. Schistocytes, helmet cells, and other distorted, fragmented erythrocytes are seen in the peripheral blood smear and are the hallmark of a microangiopathic hemolytic phenomenon. Reticulocytosis, hemosiderinuria, and increased plasma hemoglobin levels are additional evidence of hemolysis. Leukocytosis is very common. Platelet survival is decreased, but normal fibrinogen turnover and plasma fibrinogen levels are present unless there is a coexisting consumption coagulopathy such as abruptio placentae. Fibrin split products are occasionally elevated. The Coombs' test and other immuno-logic studies are characteristically negative; abnormal results suggest other underlying disease.

Initial renal manifestations include hematuria and albuminuria. Progressive impairment, with oliguria, azotemia, and complete renal failure, are common. Microangiopathic hemolysis and rapid occurrence of renal failure are the most important findings for the obstetrician because, together, they represent significant diagnostic tools and suggest immediate therapeutic goals.

Although TTP formerly was thought to be a distinct disease entity, it is more appropriately classified as a syndrome associated with a number of etiologic antecedents. Almost any condition that affects the microcirculation may lead to TTP; it has been found in association with infections, autoimmune diseases, drug allergies, oral contraceptives, HIV-positivity, and pregnancy. TTP has been reported in two sisters, with sudden onset in late pregnancy (13). Whatever the associated clinical problem, the basic defect in TTP appears to be increased platelet aggregation (14). For this reason, considerable research has been conducted by many investigators to identify a platelet aggregating factor. Characterization of such a factor could lead to subsequent identification of a medication or a plasma factor that could neutralize its action in the syndrome.

Following vascular endothelial injury, platelets adhere to collagen fibrils in the damaged tissue. Subsequent platelet degranulation results in release of adenosine diphosphate, serotonin, thromboxane, and other compounds that promote further platelet aggregation. Under normal circumstances, this phenomenon is a physiologic response to vessel injury and is self-limited. Release of a platelet aggregation inhibitor (e.g., prostacyclin) from the vessel wall normally limits thrombus formation. Loss of this equilibrium in TTP favors platelet aggregation and leads ultimately to the pathognomonic histologic feature of widespread hyaline thrombi occluding terminal arterioles and capillaries. Microangiopathic hemolytic anemia results from damage to and lysis of erythrocytes by collision with intraluminal thrombi which partially occlude smaller vessels. More complete vascular occlusion leads to ischemia and the characteristic neurologic and renal abnormalities.

The factor initiating this abnormal platelet aggregation in TTP is unknown. Three major processes have been proposed: 1) disseminated intravascular coagulation (DIC), 2) vascular damage by an infectious or toxic agent, and 3) immune-mediated vascular damage. Coagulation studies fail to confirm DIC. Although TTP may accompany some infectious diseases, no specific microbiologic or toxic etiology of the syndrome can be confirmed. The frequent association of TTP with immune diseases, the increased platelet-associated immunoglobulin G, presence of unusually large von Willebrand factor multimers, and the complement-dependent endothelial cell lysis caused by sera from patients with TTP suggest that the increased platelet aggregation may have an immunologic basis. A fourth proposal is that plasma from patients with TTP lacks a naturally occurring inhibitor of platelet aggregation (for whatever reason), which could be prostacyclin, the most potent inhibitor known. Lack of synthesis or increased destruction of the inhibitor might occur. The latter observations, now more than ten years old, form the basis of TTP therapy with plasma infusion and plasma exchange.

The diagnosis of TTP is based most often on a complex of clinical symptoms and laboratory findings, as previously described. Gingival biopsy for histologic confirmation has been recommended but shows characteristic microvascular hyaline thrombi composed of platelets and fibrin in only half of TTP cases diagnosed clinically and is poorly tolerated (15). Although TTP occurs most commonly in women of childbearing age, its association with pregnancy is sufficiently frequent to suggest the latter as a possible predisposing factor. Maternal outcome of these pregnancies has traditionally been poor, although, since 1976, survival of both mothers and infants has improved significantly.

Intrauterine growth retardation (IUGR) has been described with TTP. Both IUGR and perinatal death may be caused by placental dysfunction secondary to hyaline thrombi in endometrial and decidual arterioles. However, pregnancy does not appear to influence the course of the disorder, and TTP is similarly devastating to pregnant and nonpregnant women.

The clinical picture of the TTP syndrome in pregnancy may be indistinguishable from that of severe preeclampsia–eclampsia. The vascular spasm of severe preeclampsia may cause endothelial damage with subsequent platelet aggregation, leading to thrombocytopenia and microangiopathic hemolytic anemia. A decrease in the number of circulating platelets has been reported to be one of the first detectable abnormalities in women who develop preeclampsia. The diagnosis is confused further by albuminuria and convulsions. It seems very likely that the TTP syndrome represents an extension or variation of the pathophysiology operative in severe preeclampsia, and these events may be a final common pathway leading to death in eclampsia. Clinically, however, there appear to be two extremely significant differences: timing and severity of the hemolysis and renal failure.

Microangiopathic hemolytic anemia manifestations in toxemia and the TTP syndrome are the same in peripheral blood. In the presence of preeclampsia or eclampsia, these findings variably appear with a rough incidence of 30%. This figure is highly dependent on the obstetrician's willingness to examine peripheral blood and familiarity with the significance of these characteristic findings if they are reported by laboratory technicians. Virtually 100% of TTP patients have schistocytes, burr cells, helmet cells, polychromasia and nucleated red cells, or some combination of this peripheral smear evidence of increased erythrocyte destruction. The extent of these findings in TTP is profound and will always assist in diagnosis, whereas, in toxemia, signs of red cell fragmentation may be mild to absent, and nucleated erythrocytes on peripheral smear are not common. These differences probably reflect the degree and extent of small vessel damage rather than a difference in pathogenesis, but this very difference may assist in distinguishing the two syndromes. Red cell transfusion is necessary quite early in the development of the TTP syndrome because of a rapidly falling packed cell volume.

Development of renal dysfunction in TTP is also rapid in comparison to toxemia and may be so profound that preparations for dialysis must be considered almost simultaneously with diagnosis. This observation comes from a number of patients with TTP in association with pregnancy and is easily confirmed by obtaining a serum creatinine every 6–12 hours. The rise more often than not is dramatic as the syndrome progresses and renal function rapidly deteriorates.

Suggested serial laboratory tests (q 6–12 hours) when TTP is suspected in association with pregnancy:

Hematocrit/hemoglobin (fall)

Peripheral smear description (rising number of nucleated red blood cells/100 white blood cells, erythrocyte fragmentation)

Serum creatinine (rise)

Lactic dehydrogenase (rise)

Plasma hemoglobin (rise)

Reticulocyte count (rise)

Until recently, therapy of TTP has been empirical and multifarious. Many different regimens, including corticosteroids, heparin, urokinase, dextran, antiplatelet agents, hemodialysis, and splenectomy produced only occasional remissions, alone or in combination. However, several reports in the last decade have described encouraging responses to whole blood exchange transfusion, plasma exchange, and plasma infusion. It appears that TTP in association with pregnancy can be treated successfully while rational decisions on delivery are contemplated. Remissions following exchange transfusion and plasma exchange suggest that removal of a toxin or platelet-aggregating factor is important. The effectiveness of simple plasma infusion indicates that patients with TTP may be deficient in a plasma factor needed to inhibit aggregation. The nature of this plasma factor has not yet been defined, but prostacyclin, or a factor stimulating prostacyclin activity, seems likely. In addition, the effectiveness of antiplatelet agents, such as aspirin, dipyridamole, and sulfinpyrazone, may be potentiated by treatment with plasma. The latter drugs alone have not been promising.

A combination of plasma and corticosteroids offers the most recently described effective therapy. Plasma infusion or plasma exchange should be performed on a schedule and as volume infusion permits until the platelet count returns to normal and the neurologic abnormalities resolve. Dramatic symptomatic improvement has been noted within hours after plasma infusion. A significant rise in platelet count is usually apparent within a few days, and total resolution of neurologic symptoms within 3–7 days has been reported. Recent reports describe the effectiveness of periodic infusions of the high-molecular-weight fraction of

plasma and higher rates of platelet response to plasma exchange than simple plasma infusion (16–19).

The equivalent of prednisone 1–2 mg/kg/day is begun after diagnosis. Dipyridamole, 400–600 mg, and aspirin, 600–1200 mg daily, have been suggested as maintenance therapy for 6–12 months to prevent relapse.

Management of TTP is not altered by pregnancy, and remissions have been reported following plasmapheresis or plasma infusion therapy during pregnancy. Since the fetus is not involved in the pathogenesis of TTP and is not directly affected by the disorder, a conservative approach regarding delivery seems warranted. However, because of the difficulty encountered in differentiating TTP from severe pre-eclampsia and eclampsia and the excellent response of the latter problems to delivery, prompt delivery has also been recommended. Individualization of pregnancy management based on the time of diagnosis is always prudent. When manifestations of TTP are apparent early in pregnancy, treatment with plasma infusions, plasma exchange, and corticosteroids seems appropriate. However, when renal dysfunction, rapidly developing anemia, and hypertension herald the onset late in pregnancy, prompt delivery is recommended.

References

1. Payne BA, Pierre RV. Pseudothrombocytopenia: a laboratory artifact with potentially serious consequences. Mayo Clin Proc 1984;59:123–5.

2. Rappaport ES, Helbert B, Beissner RS, Trowbridge A. Automated hematology: where we stand. South Med J 1988; 81:365–70.

3. Tygart S, McRoyan D, Kitay D, et al. Longitudinal study of platelet indices during normal pregnancy. Am J Obstet Gynecol 1986;154:883–9.

4. McCrae KR, Samuels P, Schreiber AD. Pregnancy-associated thrombocytopenia: pathogenesis and management. Blood 1992;80:2697–714.

5. Cook RL, Miller RC, Katz VL, Cephalo RC. Immune thrombocytopenic purpura in pregnancy: a reappraisal of management. Obstet Gynecol 1991;78:578.

6. Gernsheimer T, Stratton J, Ballem PJ, Slichter SJ. Mechanisms of response to treatment in autoimmune thrombocytopenic purpura. N Eng J Med 1989;320:974–80.

7. Bussel JB, Kimberly RP, Inman RD, et al. Intravenous gamma globulin treatment in chronic idiopathic thrombocytopenic purpura. Blood 1983;62:480–6.

8. Tomiyama Y, Mizutani H, Tsubakio T, Kurata Y, Yonezawa T, Tarui S. High-dose intravenous IgG before delivery for idiopathic thrombocytopenic purpura: transplacental treatment of the fetus. Acta Haemat JPN 1987;50:890–4.

9. Burrows RF, Kelton JG. Thrombocytopenia at delivery: a prospective survey of 6715 deliveries. Am J Obstet Gynecol 1990;162:731.

10. Moise KJ, Patton DE, Cano LE. Misdiagnosis of a normal fetal platelet count after coagulation of intrapartum scalp samples in autoimmune thrombocytopenic purpura. Am J Perinatol 1991;5:295–6.

11. Scioscia AL, Grannum PAT, Copel JA, Hobbins JC. The use of percutaneous umbilical blood sampling in immune thrombocytopenic purpura. Am J Obstet Gynecol 1988; 159: 1066–8.

12. Horger EO. Thrombotic thrombocytopenic purpura. In: Kitay DZ, ed. Hematologic problems in pregnancy. Oradell, NJ: Medical Economics Books, 1987;353–9.

13. Wiznitzer A, Mazor M, Leiberman JR, Bar-Levie Y, Gurman G, Glezerman M. Familial occurrence of thrombotic thrombocytopenic purpura in two sisters during pregnancy. Am J Obstet Gynecol 1992;166:20–21.

14. Kelton JG, Moore JC, Murphy WG. The platelet aggregating factor(s) of thrombotic thrombocytopenic purpura. Prog Clin Biol Res 1990;337:141–9.

15. Miller JM, Pastorek JG. Thrombotic thrombocytopenic purpura and hemolytic uremic syndrome in pregnancy. Clinical Obstet Gynecol 1991;34:64–71.

16. Koyama T, Suehiro A, Kakishita E, Taira S, Isojima S, Norioka M, Ito K. Efficacy of the high molecular weight fraction of plasma for the maintenance of pregnancy associated with thrombotic thrombocytopenic purpura. Am J Hematol 1990;35:179–83.

17. Shepard KV, Fishleder A, Lucas FV, Goormastic M, Bukowski RM. Thrombotic thrombocytopenic purpura treated with plasma exchange or exchange transfusion. West J Med 1991;154:410–13.

18. Rock GA, Shumack KH, Buskard NA, Blanchette VS, Kelton JG, Nair RC, et al. Comparison of plasma exchange with plasma infusion in the treatment of thrombotic thrombocytopenic purpura. N Engl J Med 1991;325:393–7.

19. Bell WR, Braine HG, Ness PM, Kickler TS. Improved survival in thrombotic thrombocytopenic purpura—hemolytic uremic syndrome. N Engl J Med 1991;325:398–403.

22

The Cardiac Patient

Kent Ueland, M.D.

A DEFINITE pattern of cardiovascular changes accompanies normal pregnancy and parturition. Clinicians should be aware of and evaluate the hemodynamic burden that pregnancy places on patients with acquired or congenital heart disease. These patients may require special management because their disorder puts them or their fetuses at greater risk. As pregnancy becomes more common among women with fully or partially corrected heart defects, obstetricians should also be prepared to care for more patients who have had cardiac surgery or who require continued medication.

The burden of pregnancy on the woman with heart disease is only temporary. There is no evidence that pregnancy affects the natural history of the disease. This chapter describes the hemodynamic changes to be expected during normal pregnancies and indicates problems that various cardiovascular conditions may cause mother, fetus, and newborn.

Cardiovascular Changes of Pregnancy

Cardiac output rises early in pregnancy (a significant elevation has been demonstrated at 12 weeks' gestation), continues to rise until 28–32 weeks' gestation, and then remains at a relatively high level until term. Late in pregnancy, it drops significantly only if patients are measured when supine.

A serial study has shown the increasing influence of posture on maternal hemodynamics as pregnancy advances (1). A change from supine to lateral produced a rise in cardiac output of 8% at 20–24 weeks' gestation, 14% at 28–32 weeks' gestation, and 29% at term. Radiography has demonstrated that uterine compression of the vena cava produces the hemodynamic changes related to posture (2). This compression markedly reduces the venous return to the heart.

The heart rate increases by approximately 10 to 15 beats per minute during pregnancy; the peak change occurs near term. Stoke volume, however, appears to be highest in early to midpregnancy; it then declines progressively to term, when it reaches levels at or below those of the nonpregnant person.

Blood pressure declines near the end of the first trimester and generally throughout the second trimester. The diastolic fall is greater than the systolic and results in a rise in pulse pressure. The supine position accentuates the change.

The increment in blood volume during gestation varies considerably in different people. The percentage of increase ranges from 20 to 100, rising most rapidly during the first 20–30 weeks' gestation and continuing gradually to term. Frequently, the increase in plasma volume exceeds that of the red cell mass, and there is a decline in hemoglobin values. This phenomenon, however, appears to depend entirely on the availability and utilization of iron. Patients receiving oral iron do have a slight decline in hemoglobin concentrations late in pregnancy, but it is not significant.

Changes of Parturition

Table 22.1 shows the cardiovascular changes that normally occur during pregnancy and parturition. The changes in cardiac output, heart rate, and stroke volume during labor and delivery are greater than those of pregnancy. Because labor and delivery impose an added burden on the heart, women who suffer from serious heart disease most often die of pulmonary congestion or heart failure during parturition and the early puerperium.

Both anesthesia and method of delivery can modify the maternal hemodynamic response to labor and provide a relatively stress-free delivery. Because each contraction has a significant hemodynamic effect, systemic analgesia and sedation should be used early to modify these changes. Conduction anesthesia (i.e., segmental epidural) should be administered for active labor and delivery in order to circumvent the hemodynamic response to pain and anxiety.

Hypotension is best avoided by using a narcotic epidural and by giving the least amount of local anesthesia needed to relieve pain, omitting epinephrine from the local anesthetic solution, turning the patient from side to side while the anesthetic takes effect, and allowing her to labor only in lateral recumbency. To avoid bearing-down efforts in the second stage of labor, delivery by forceps is indicated as soon as it is deemed safe.

Careful monitoring of the mother and fetus is mandatory. Cesarean section may increase the risk of some pregnant cardiac patients, and fetal monitoring may prevent unnecessary abdominal delivery.

Because of the potential for bacteremia and bacterial endocarditis, all patients with cardiovascular disease should be placed on antibiotic prophylaxis at delivery. Broad-spectrum antibiotics are recommended by the American Heart Association (3). Even though bacterial endocarditis is rare following normal delivery and routine antibiotic prophylaxis cannot be justified statistically, the disease is so devastating when it occurs that the use of antibiotics seems reasonable.

Heart Disease Problems during Pregnancy

Table 22.2 lists the eight most common causes of maternal mortality in the United States between 1980 and 1985. Cardiovascular disease is listed fourth. However, embolism and hypertensive disease, both cardiovascular problems, are numbers one and two, respectively. This emphasizes the importance of the problem. The incidence of heart disease

Table 22.1 Cardiovascular Changes of Normal Pregnancy and Parturition

	Pregnancy (%)	Delivery* (%)
Cardiac output	+30 to 50	+60 to 80
Heart rate	+10 to 15	-15 to 20
Stroke volume	+20 to 40	+60 to 80
Blood volume	+20 to 100	-5 to 15

*Maximum changes from supine prelabor values to early puerperium (delivery changes not superimposed on those of pregnancy).

Table 22.2 Maternal Mortality, 1980–1985

1. Embolism (102)
2. Hypertensive disease (74)
3. Ectopic Pregnancy (60)
4. Cardiovascular (56)
5. Hemorrhage (55)
6. Cerebrovascular accidents (51)
7. Anesthesia complications (42)
8. Infectious conditions (34)

Modified from Obstet Gynecol 1988;72:91.

in pregnancy varies widely but has declined from a high of 2.3%–3.7% between 1940 and 1950 (4, 5) to 0.5%–1.5% between 1960 and 1970 (6, 7) and to a low of 0.3% between 1977–1986 (8). A significant change in the type of heart disease encountered has accompanied this trend. In the past, rheumatic heart disease was by far the most prevalent cardiac problem in pregnancy, occurring 20 times more often than congenital cardiovascular lesions (4, 5). Lately, however, an increased incidence of congenital cardiovascular disease has reduced the ratio to 3:1 (6) and more recently to 10:1 (8). The overall decline in this country is attributable largely to a decline in active rheumatic fever.

Surgical advances have produced yet another major change. An increasing number of women who have had palliative or corrective cardiovascular surgery are undertaking pregnancy. It is important to understand, not only the anatomic and functional characteristics of the original lesion, but also the altered hemodynamics resulting from surgery. This knowledge must be integrated with an understanding of the normal hemodynamic changes accompanying pregnancy and parturition.

Frequently, the lesion is completely corrected by surgery, as in most instances of atrial septal defect, patent ductus arteriosus, and simple coarctation of the aorta. Pregnancy for such patients is not an added risk. But when surgery is only palliative, as in mitral valvotomy, or partially corrective, as in the repair of certain cyanotic lesions (tetralogy of Fallot, for example), pregnancy remains an added risk. Prior cardiac surgery may produce additional problems for the pregnant patient. For example, certain types of prosthetic valves achieve significant functional improvement, but require long-term treatment with oral anticoagulants.

Some cardiovascular lesions place the pregnant woman at a high risk of major disability and death, and pregnancy is contraindicated. Table 22.3 lists the most common cardiovascular diseases that are particularly dangerous to pregnant women (7, 9–16). Some are dangerous because they present a specific anatomic deformity (Marfan's syndrome, complicated coarctation of the aorta). Others are dangerous because of the specific hemodynamic impairment (primary pulmonary hypertension, Eisenmenger's syndrome). In the latter group, the degree of pulmonary hypertension is most important in determining outcome. In the author's opin-

ion, pregnancy is contraindicated in any woman with documented pulmonary hypertension (regardless of etiology), peripartum cardiomyopathy, mitral stenosis with atrial fibrillation, and Marfan's syndrome with aortic root dilation. Maternal mortality rates for these lesions ranges between 15% and 60% (Table 22.3).

In general, the outcome of pregnancy in mothers with acquired heart disease depends on overall functional impairment, as expressed by the New York Heart Association classification (class I, asymptomatic; class II, symptomatic with heavy exercise; class III, symptomatic with light exercise; and class IV, symptomatic at rest) (17). Patients classified as III and IV logically make up the highest-risk group, especially when their dysfunction is associated with an anatomic lesion such as mitral stenosis.

The mainstay of medical management for the cardiac patient is limitation of physical activity: bed rest and, if necessary, prolonged hospitalization. For patients with severe mitral stenosis who develop pulmonary edema that is unresponsive to strict medical management, a closed mitral valvotomy may be necessary. The need for such surgical

Table 22.3 Maternal Mortality Rates for High-risk Cardiovascular Diseases

Lesion	Maternal Mortality (%)
Coarctation of the aorta	
All	9*
Complicated (7)	(doubled)
Marfan's syndrome	50
(with aortic dilatation)	(estimated)
Tetralogy of Fallot (9)	12
Eisenmenger syndrome (10, 11)	33
Primary pulmonary hypertension (12)	53
Mitral stenosis	
All classes (12–14)	1
Classes III, IV (9, 14)†	4–5
With atrial fibrillation (9, 15)	14–17
Closed valvotomy (15)	4–6*
Peripartum cardiomyopathy (7)	15–60
Prosthetic heart valves (all) (16)	2

*Expressed with respect to patients, not pregnancies.
†New York Heart Association functional classification.

intervention is now becoming rare, however, probably because of the changing pattern of rheumatic heart disease. In patients with rheumatic heart disease, the incidence of major complications such as pulmonary edema, right-sided heart failure, and atrial fibrillation has greatly diminished (7).

Cardiovascular Drugs and Their Effects on the Fetus

The following are some of the drugs commonly used in the management of patients with cardiovascular disease. Some of these potent drugs have potential harmful effects on the developing embryo and fetus. The data in the literature will be reviewed briefly in the following paragraphs. Analyzing the data is hazardous because it is frequently difficult to determine accurately whether or not one is seeing the result of the interaction of specific drugs with pregnancy or with the underlying cardiovascular disease, or both.

Anticoagulant Drugs

Oral anticoagulants not only have potential teratogenic effects when given in the first trimester, but may also cause a multitude of subtle physical deformities in the fetus from repetitive small hemorrhages when given during the second and third trimesters of pregnancy (18). At least 12 cases of fatal hemorrhages in the fetus have been reported in the literature from the use of oral anticoagulants during pregnancy. Most of the cases were associated with poor control of the anticoagulant therapy. Control of oral anticoagulation can be difficult during pregnancy. In view of the data, I believe the use of oral anticoagulants at any time during pregnancy is contraindicated. Subcutaneous heparin is the anticoagulant of choice during pregnancy. Its successful long-term use has been documented (19, 20). Because of its large molecular size, it does not cross the placenta and poses no threat to the fetus.

Antiarrhythmic Drugs

There are no reports of harmful effects to the fetus from the use of quinidine during pregnancy. Although quinidine shares many of the pharmacological actions of quinine and is its D isomer, it does not appear to have any significant oxytocic action. Therefore, quinidine appears safe to use during pregnancy. Other choices of therapy for arrhythmia of recent onset include intravenous procainamide or lidocaine. Electroshock therapy may also be tried. This form of treatment has been used successfully during pregnancy in several instances without causing harm to the fetus.

Propranolol is a β-adrenergic blocking agent that works directly on the heart through the β-receptors. Propranolol also has a direct quinidinelike action on the heart. In addition to its usefulness in the treatment of certain cardiac arrhythmias, it is effective in treating angina pectoris and hypertension. This drug should be used with caution during pregnancy because it has the potential of initiating premature labor through its β-blocking action on the uterus. The chronic increase in uterine tone induced by this drug could potentially lead to a small and infarcted placenta and low-birthweight infant, as suggested by some. The fact that this β-adrenergic blocker enhances uterine contraction is demonstrated by its successful use in the treatment of dysfunctional labor. Its reported effects on the neonate include respiratory depression, hypoglycemia, and bradycardia.

Another antiarrhythmic agent, disopyramide, has been reported to have an oxytociclike effect. This drug has electrophysiologic properties similar to quinidine's and is effective in suppressing ventricular and supraventricular tachyarrhythmias. In a recent case report, this drug was used to treat cardiac arrhythmias due to mitral valve prolapse in a pregnant woman at 32 weeks' gestation; therapy resulted in the initiation of hypertonic uterine contractions. When the drug was stopped, the contractions subsided. Because of the potential uterine-stimulating effect of many of the antiarrhythmic agents, they must be used with caution during pregnancy and with careful monitoring of uterine activity and fetal response.

Cardiac Glycosides

There is no report in the literature suggesting that the digitalis glycosides are teratogenic in animals or humans. Nor is there any evidence that the digitalis compounds have any deleterious effect on the fetus later in pregnancy. A recent report, however, suggests that digitalis may have a myometrial-stimulating effect, as it appears to influence the time of onset of labor and the duration of labor in women with heart disease. Spontaneous labor occurred more than a week earlier and lasted about half as long in cardiac patients taking digitalis as compared with a control group of cardiac patients not taking digitalis. This interesting observation may have some merit because digitalis has been shown to increase uterine muscle tone in vitro. Other indirect evidence of the potential effects of digitalis on the uterus may be inferred from the similarity of its chemical structure to that of estrogen. An estrogen surge has been shown to occur in some animals (possibly the human as well) just prior to the initiation of labor. These theoretical considerations are of interest, but they should not preclude the use of digitalis when it is therapeutically indicated during pregnancy.

Diuretics (Thiazides)

These drugs were used extensively two decades ago to treat edema of pregnancy and for prophylaxis against preeclampsia. The current understanding that dependent edema is a physiologic accompaniment of pregnancy and requires no therapy and the documentation that diuretics and sodium restriction do not prevent preeclampsia have led to a marked and appropriate reduction in the use of these potentially harmful drugs. There is little doubt that the thiazide diuretics can reduce plasma volume during pregnancy, but there are no data to show whether or not this reduced volume is maintained by prolonged therapy.

Sporadic reports of harmful effects to the fetus as a result of prolonged use of oral diuretics, especially late in pregnancy, include severe electrolyte imbalance, neonatal jaundice, thrombocytopenia, liver damage, and death. The use of thiazide diuretics during pregnancy should therefore be limited to very specific clinical indications. The most common cardiovascular indication would be in the prevention or treatment of pulmonary edema. When using diuretic therapy, it is important to administer potassium supplementation, especially if digitalis is also being given.

Effect of Maternal Heart Disease on the Fetus and Newborn

Acquired Heart Disease

The babies of women who are asymptomatic or mildly symptomatic show only an insignificant increase in perinatal mortality. But when the mother has class III dysfunction, perinatal mortality reaches 12%; class IV patients show a mortality of perhaps 31%. However, the latter figure includes therapeutic abortion. The surviving offspring of symptomatic patients with acquired heart disease demonstrate no increased incidence of congenital deformity.

There appear to be subtle effects on fetal growth and development even when the mother is asymptomatic or mildly symptomatic. In a group of 21 women of classes I and II, my co-workers and I found an increased number of premature deliveries and small infants at term (21). Niswander and associates (22) in retrospective analysis of over 300 charts of pregnant women with heart disease, found a prematurity rate of 18%, which was significantly higher than in a control group. Our work suggests a mechanism by which maternal heart disease may affect fetal health. The oxygen concentration in mixed venous blood decreases during pregnancy in, for example, patients with mitral stenosis. This decrease is attributed to the low cardiac output of these women compared with what is normal during pregnancy.

Congenital Heart Disease

The fetus whose mother has congenital heart disease may suffer, not only from environmental handicaps, but also from genetic problems. Congenital heart disease occurred in 1.8% of children born to parents of whom one has congenital heart disease, according to a study of more than 500 patients by Neill and Swanson (23). This is six times the incidence in the normal population. More recent data have shown a much higher hereditary risk of 10.4% and 16.1% (24, 25). The data also show that the risk of heart disease in the child is much greater if the mother has congenital heart disease rather than the father. Of interest is the fact that the child is likely to have the same abnormality as the parent. Additionally, corrective surgery prior to undertaking a pregnancy substantially reduces the hereditary risk. Mothers with cyanotic heart disease have a high incidence of spontaneous abortion, and their liveborn children are small compared with those of cyanotic fathers. This finding suggests that a reduced supply of oxygen to the fetus is also a causative factor; hypoxia is a known teratogen. Genetic counselling is important for both parents, to assist them in better understanding the complex hereditary pattern of congenital heart disease (26).

In cyanotic heart disease, outcome of pregnancy correlates with hematocrit (27). The higher the hematocrit, the higher the incidence of abortion and prematurity. This clearly demonstrates the importance of early diagnosis and surgical correction of cyanotic congenital heart disease, preferably before childbearing age.

Conclusion

In managing the pregnant cardiac patient, the clinician must exercise especially careful judgment. Most of the medications necessary for the maternal problem have a direct effect on the fetus. Proper selection of drugs will make a major difference in the outcome of the pregnancy. For instance, the coumarins are known to be teratogenic, and therefore anticoagulation should be managed with heparin, even though it can be difficult to administer during pregnancy. However, with proper instruction and encouragement, this medication may be administered at home. Similar judgments must be made concerning other cardiac medications throughout pregnancy.

CASE 22.1

A 24-year-old primigravida with probable congenital mitral stenosis had at age five undergone open heart surgery and had her deformed mitral valve replaced with a porcine heterograft. Because of restenosis and functional deterioration, she required a second operation at age 16, with the reinsertion of another porcine heterograft valve. She was first seen in the first trimester of pregnancy, complaining of fatigue and dyspnea on mild exertion. Cardiac evaluation showed right ventricular hypertrophy, an enlarged left atrium at 6 cm, severe mitral stenosis with a valve area of 0.8 cm^2, and minimal mitral regurgitation. Multiple PACs were also noted. Initial therapy consisted of digoxin, lasix, and marked limitation of physical activity. At approximately 28 weeks' gestation, she experienced her first bout of hemoptysis at rest, necessitating several days of hospitalization. During the remainder of her pregnancy, she experienced recurrent hemoptysis, and, at 37 weeks, she was hospitalized until delivery. With bed rest and aggressive diuresis, her dyspnea and hemoptysis abated and induction of labor was decided upon at 38 weeks' gestation. Because of an unfavorable cervix (Bishop score of 3), priming was undertaken with 0.5 mg intracervical PGE2 gel. The following morning, in anticipation of induction of labor with oxytocin, central hemodynamic monitoring was begun. At the start of her induction, a narcotic epidural was initiated which kept the patient free of pain in early labor. As labor progressed and with increasing intensity of contractions, a mixture of narcotic and local anesthetic solution was utilized for epidural analgesia. She delivered spontaneously 10 hours after the start of the induction. Hemodynamically, she remained stable throughout. Her postpartum hospital course was uneventful. Four weeks following delivery she underwent her third open heart procedure, this time with the insertion of a ball valve prosthesis.

This patient had severe mitral stenosis with recurrent hemoptysis at rest, placing her in functional class IV. In women seriously ill with heart disease, the author recommends induction of labor at or near term. A carefully timed induction and delivery with hemodynamic monitoring and adequate analgesia is preferred when all consultants are readily available, as opposed to allowing the patient to go into spontaneous labor when all of these conditions may not pertain.

CASE 22.2

A 17-year-old white female was transferred to our hospital at 35 weeks' gestation with her first pregnancy. She was in moderate respiratory distress and looked acutely ill. On physical examination, positive findings included a palpable liver edge 5 cm below the right costal margin, 3+ pitting edema of the legs, jugular venous distention with prominent V waves, a left parasternal lift and a grade 4/6 systolic ejection murmur along the lower left sternal border. On chest x-ray, right ventricular and right atrial enlargement were noted, along with dilatation of the main pulmonary artery. An electrocardiogram (EKG) showed right ventricular hypertrophy. Right heart catheterization showed a right ventricular pressure of 90/30, pulmonary artery pressure of 80/68 with a wedge pressure of 26 mm Hg. These findings supported the diagnosis of primary pulmonary hypertension. The high pulmonary wedge pressure was attributed to hypervolemia secondary to excessive fluid administration at the referring institution.

Within 24 hours of admission, the patient was noted to be in preterm labor. She was also noted to be hypotensive and with a tachycardia of up to 130 beats per minute. After appropriate consultation, a cesarean section was decided upon, feeling that the patient would not tolerate labor. Swan Ganz hemodynamic monitoring was instituted and preparation immediately made for surgery in the cardiac surgery operating suite. The cesarean section was performed under deep cardiovascular anesthesia in order to attempt to optimize the patient's unstable cardiovascular status.

A sleepy, anesthetized, but healthy 5-pound, 2-ounce infant was delivered and successfully resuscitated by the neonatal team in attendance. The mother's course, however, was one of steady deterioration, with a falling cardiac output and progressive hypotension. She died of a cardiac arrest eight hours following delivery in spite of intense cardiorespiratory support, oxygen, and dopamine.

This tragic ending has been encountered by the author on several occasions in women with pulmonary hypertension with or without intracardiac or extracardiac shunts. Pregnancy is contraindicated in these women, and, if a patient is seen early, therapeutic abortion should be offered as the safest therapeutic alternative. Unfortunately, symptomology is not a clear predictor of right ventricular failure or sudden death. Although a disaster can occur at any time during pregnancy, it is much more common surrounding delivery and in the early puerperium, as represented by this case. At the time of delivery and the early puerperium,

continuous hemodynamic monitoring is imperative, as is avoiding or treating hemodynamic collapse and avoiding venous pooling.

Maintaining venous return is critical. ∎

References

1. Ueland K, Novy MJ, Peterson EN, et al. Maternal cardiovascular dynamics. IV. The influence of gestational age on the maternal cardiovascular response to posture and exercise. Am J Obstet Gynecol 1969;104:856.
2. Kerr MG. The mechanical effects of the gravid uterus in late pregnancy. J Obstet Gynaecol Br Commonw 1965;72:513.
3. Dajani AS, Bisno AL, Chung KJ, et al. Prevention of bacterial endocarditis—recommendations by the American Heart Association. JAMA 1990;264:2919.
4. Demakis JG, Rhimtoola SH. Peripartum cardiomyopathy. Circulation 1971;44:964.
5. Mortensen JD, Ellsworth HS. Pregnancy and cardiac surgery. Circulation 1963;28:773.
6. Bloomfield DK. Fetal deaths and malformations associated with the use of coumarin derivatives in pregnancy. A critical review. Am J Obstet Gynecol 1970;107:883.
7. Szekely P, Snaith L. Heart disease and pregnancy. London: Churchill, 1974.
8. Bitsch M, Johansen C, Wennevold A, et al. Maternal heart disease. A survey of a decade in a Danish university hospital. Acta Obstet Gynecol Scand 1989;68:119.
9. Mendelson CL. Cardiac disease in pregnancy. Philadelphia: Davis, 1960.
10. Jones AM, Howitt G. Eisenmenger syndrome in pregnancy. Br Med J 1965;1:1627.
11. Neilson G, Galea EG, Blunt A. Eisenmenger's syndrome and pregnancy. Med J Aust 1971;1:431.
12. Dawkins K, Burke CM, Billingham M, et al. Primary pulmonary hypertension and pregnancy. Chest 1986;89:383.
13. Gilchrist AR. Cardiological problems in younger women, including those of pregnancy and puerperium. Br Med J 1963;1:209.
14. Deal K, Wooley CF. Coarctation of the aorta and pregnancy. Ann Intern Med 1973;78:706.
15. Wallace WA, Harken DE, Ellis LB. Pregnancy following closed mitral valvuloplasty: a long-term study with remarks concerning the necessity for careful cardiac management. J Am Med Assoc 1971;217:297.
16. Buxbaum A, Aygen MM, Shahin W, et al. Pregnancy in

patients with prosthetic heart valves. Chest 1971; 59:639.

17. Metcalfe J, McAnulty JH, Ueland K. Heart disease and pregnancy: physiology and management. 2nd ed. Boston: Little, Brown, 1986.

18. Stevenson RE, Burton M, Frelanto GH, et al. Hazards of oral anticoagulants during pregnancy. JAMA 1985;243:1549.

19. Hellgren M, Nygards EB. Long-term therapy with subcutaneous heparin during pregnancy. Gynecol Obstet Invest 1982; 13:76.

20. Ginsbert JS, Kowalchuk G, Hirsh J, et al. Heparin therapy during pregnancy. Arch Intern Med 1989;149:2233.

21. Ueland K, Novy MJ, Metcalfe J. Hemodynamic responses of patients with heart disease to pregnancy and exercise. Am J Obstet Gynecol 1972;113:47.

22. Niswander KR, Berendes H, Deutschberger J, et al. Fetal morbidity following potentially anoxigenic obstetric conditions. V. Organic heart disease. Am J Obstet Gynecol 1967; 98:871.

23. Neill CA, Swanson S. Outcome of pregnancy in congenital heart disease. Circulation 1961;24:1003.

24. Rose V, Gold RJM, Lindsay G, et al. A possible increase in the incidence of congenital heart defects among offspring of affected parents. J Am Coll Cardiol 1985;63:376.

25. Whittemore R, Wells JA, Castellsaque-Piqne X, et al. Congenital heart defects in the second generation—a comparative study. Am J Cardiol 1991;66:524.

26. Callan NA, Blakemore KJ, Kan JS. Counselling in congenital heart defects. Obstet Gynecol Survey 1991;46:651.

27. Cannell DE, Vernon CP. Congenital heart disease and pregnancy. Am J Obstet Gynecol 1963;85:744.

23

Renal Disease

Marshall D. Lindheimer, M.D.
Adrian I. Katz, M.D.

FORMERLY, obstetricians often considered preexisting renal disease alarming enough to justify interrupting pregnancy and advising contraception. However, results from recent studies suggest that many women with known renal parenchymal disease can give birth successfully if carefully managed.

Urinary Tract Changes

During pregnancy, the kidneys increase in size, probably because of increments in renal interstitial volume and blood flow. For example, researchers noted that kidney size in the immediate puerperium was greater than predicted by standard height-weight nomograms, but that x-ray examinations six months later showed it had decreased an average of 1 cm (1, 2).

Calyceal, pelvic, and ureteral dilation accompanied by hypertrophy and hyperplasia of the ureteral smooth muscle occur as early as the second trimester (2–4). Hormonal alterations of pregnancy, such as increased progesterone, may cause these changes. Later, assumption of a supine or upright posture can create partial ureteral obstruction, since the enlarged uterus may entrap the ureters at the pelvic brim (5).

One observer concluded that ureteral dilation terminates at the level of the true bony pelvic brim where the ureter crosses the iliac artery (6). The same author noted that IV pyelography reveals a filling defect, which he terms "the iliac sign." However, termination of dilation at the level of the bony pelvis is not absolute proof of obstruction. Waldeyer's sheath, which hypertrophies during pregnancy, could prevent hormone-mediated dilation of the ureter within the pelvis.

The right ureter tends to dilate more than the left. Perhaps this difference is caused by its more exposed course at the pelvic brim and protection of the left ureter by the colon and possibly by torsion of the uterus. Finally, dilation of the ureters has been ascribed by some—but not by others—to the increased diameter of the ovarian vein (4).

Although pathogenesis may be controversial, ureteral dilation has practical consequences. The dilated urinary collecting system may contain volumes of urine so large as to cause significant errors in measurements requiring timed urine output, such as quantitative determinations of protein or creatinine excretion rates. For example, if a hydropenic patient whose 24-hour urine output is less than 1 L voids in the morning and 100 mL remains in the bladder and dilated ureters, the total collection will be underestimated by more than 10%. There is also a timing error involved, since the urine remaining in the urinary tract may have been formed several hours before collection. One may minimize such errors by giving the pregnant woman a water load and telling her to stay in bed in a lateral recumbent position for one hour before starting and one hour before terminating collection.

The tendency of asymptomatic bacteriuria to progress to pyelonephritis during pregnancy may arise from ureteral obstruction, dilation, and stasis. It is unclear whether this predisposition is owing simply to obstruction, reflux, or characteristics of the pregnant woman's urine, such as physiologic glucosuria, that favor bacterial growth. Pregnant patients having chronic pyelonephritis experience frequent relapses. They may benefit from a high fluid intake combined with frequent rest periods in a lateral recumbent position.

Finally, there is a complication of late gestation, the distension syndrome, characterized by abdominal pain associated with marked hydronephrosis and often slight increments in serum creatinine (7). Whether this syndrome, which is managed by ureteral stents, is an extreme case of the dilation occurring in normal pregnancy or reflects underlying pathology is unclear.

The most remarkable changes affecting the kidney during pregnancy are the striking increases in glomerular filtration rate (GFR) and renal plasma flow (RPF) to approximately 50% above prepregnancy levels (2, 4, 8, 9). Significant increments in creatinine clearance are apparent four weeks after the last menstrual period and reach a peak 9–11 weeks later. They are sustained to gestational week 36, after which a modest decrease may occur (8, 10).

Because of the increased GFR, greater quantities of plasma solute pass through the glomerulus per unit of time. These increments in filtered load may partly explain certain phenomena seen in normal pregnancy, such as physiologic glucosuria and aminoaciduria. However, such findings may also relate to decrements in fractional tubular reabsorption.

Since GFR increases without major alterations in the production of creatinine and urea, serum concentrations of these solutes decrease. Investigators observed that values of serum urea nitrogen (SUN) and creatinine decreased from 13 ± 3(SD) mg/dL and 0.67 ± 0.14 mg/dL, respectively, in normal nonpregnant women, to 8.7 ± 1.5 mg/dL and 0.46 ± 0.13 mg/dL, respectively, in pregnant women (11). Therefore, values considered normal in nonpregnant women may reflect decreased renal function during pregnancy. Concentrations of SUN in excess of 13.0 mg/dL or of serum creatinine exceeding 0.8 mg/dL call for further evaluation of renal function.

Volume Homeostasis

The kidney regulates the body's excretion of salt and water and is the effector organ for regulation of volume homeostasis. The best measurements of total body water (using deuterium oxide) indicate increments during pregnancy of 7–8 L (4, 9, 12). Data on extracellular volume suggest gains of 4–6 L, including an increase in plasma volume of approximately 1,200 mL.

Normally, there is a cumulative retention of approximately 950 mEq of sodium, distributed between products of conception and maternal extracellular fluid. Thus, retained sodium represents not only fetal needs but maternal physiologic hypervolemia of pregnancy.

Plasma levels of aldosterone, desoxycorticosterone, estradiol, progesterone, prolactin, angiotensin II, and probably several vasodilating prostaglandins all increase during normal pregnancy (4, 9, 12, 13). The effects of these hormones on sodium homeostasis during pregnancy are not yet fully understood by researchers. For example, in preeclampsia, in which interstitial volume increases while intravascular volume decreases, both serum renin activity and aldosterone excretion may decrease (4, 9, 12–14).

Various changes occurring during pregnancy may affect sodium excretion (Table 23.1). Of note is a rise in filtered sodium estimated to exceed 10,000 mEq daily and one in concentration of progesterone of tenfold to one hundredfold. These increases argue strongly against regarding pregnant women as potential sodium retainers. Most tolerate diets high in sodium and should be given consider-

Table 23.1 Factors that May Influence Renal Sodium Handling

Increase Excretion

1. 50% increment in glomerular filtration rate.
2. Increased progesterone production.
3. Physical factors.
   a. Decreased plasma albumin (reduced postglomerular oncotic pressure).
   b. Decreased vascular resistance.
4. Possible increment in natriuretic factors and hormones, including atrial peptides and endogenous digitalis-like factors.

Decrease Excretion

1. Plasma aldosterone concentration increased.
2. Increased conversion of progesterone to desoxycorticosterone.
3. Increased levels of other hormones (estrogen, prolactin, angiotensin, cortisol, and placental lactogen).
4. Physical factors.
   a. Placenta mimics arteriovenous shunt.
   b. Upright and supine posture.
   c. Increased ureteral pressure.

able latitude in food choice.

Ankle edema, found in up to 80% of normal pregnancies, and weight gain in excess of accepted norms need not cause alarm or be taken as indications for severe sodium restriction or administration of diuretics (9, 12). Except for patients with symptomatic heart disease, diuretics appear unnecessary in management of pregnancy. Besides occasioning side effects in both mother and fetus, they may cause excessive volume depletion, decrease placental perfusion, and interfere with using hyperuricemia in diagnosing preeclampsia.

Renal Function Tests

Except for GFR and RPF, few controlled studies have tested the validity of applying values generally considered normal to pregnant women (Table 23.2). Even for urinary sediment, very few data are available to determine if quantitative excretion of casts and cells is similar in pregnant and nonpregnant subjects.

Measurement of urinary protein excretion, essential for uncovering preeclampsia, is also valuable in detecting renal disease. Nonpregnant women rarely excrete more than 150 mg of protein daily, whereas during normal pregnancy excretion doubles. Some authorities accept 500 mg daily as a normal upper limit (12, 15). Reasons for the increment are obscure but may reflect increased glomerular blood supply and the tendency to assume a lordotic position as pregnancy progresses.

Excessive proteinuria is either functional or pathologic. In functional proteinuria, such as after exercise, exposure to heat or cold, or assumption of an upright posture (especially exaggerated lordosis), both renal parenchyma and vasculature are intact. Pathologic proteinuria occurs with most—but not all—diseases of the renal parenchyma and vasculature, including preeclampsia (4, 9, 12).

Urinary Tract Infection

Belief that incidence of asymptomatic bacteriuria increases during pregnancy has proved incorrect. Matching of pregnant and nonpregnant populations by socioeconomic status shows frequency of infected urine to be similar (4, 16, 17).

Because asymptomatic bacteriuria left untreated during pregnancy often progresses to overt pyelonephritis, *all pregnant women with confirmed positive urine cultures should be treated with appropriate antibiotics* (whose sensitivities should be verified by culture). Currently used, if sensitivities are verified by culture, are two-week courses of short-acting sulfa drugs or nitrofurantoin derivatives (although research in progress and results of preliminary studies indicate that single doses or three- to five-day courses may suffice).

Sulfa drugs should not be used near term since they displace bilirubin from albumin and aggravate kernicterus in newborns. Also, the clinician should be aware of other relative contraindications, such as glucose-6-phosphate dehydrogenase deficiency. Ampicillin and cephalexin are other agents used frequently, especially in symptomatic infections. After initial therapy, each patient requires reculture and careful clinical scrutiny.

All women should be screened serially for urinary tract infection (UTI) during pregnancy. Use of relatively inexpensive procedures that detect bacterial growth rather than changes in chemical indicators (such as the older filter paper, dip slide, and streak plate methods) is recommended. However, other clinicians would screen only women

Table 23.2 Renal Function Tests in Pregnancy

Function	Specific Tests	Clinical Tests	Use in Pregnancy
Glomerular filtration	Inulin clearance	Creatinine clearance	Should average 30%–50% above normal nonpregnant means.
		Serum creatinine	Values above 0.8 mg/dL suspicious.
		Serum urea nitrogen	Values above 13mg/dL suspicious.
Renal plasma flow	PAH clearance Diodrast clearance	PSP excretion	PSP test invalid since it back-diffuses in the dilated ureters.
Proximal tubular transport	Tm glucose (reabsorptive) TmPAH or Tm Diodrast (secretory)	PSP excretion	PSP test invalid since it back-diffuses in the dilated ureters.
Distal tubular transport	Concentration and dilution Tc_{H_2O}, C_{H_2O}	Concentration and dilution	Normal values have not been established by critical testing but appear to be similar to those published for nonpregnant populations.
	Maximal and minimal U/P osmolality	Maximal and minimal specific gravity or osmolality	Women should be in bed, laterally recumbent, when dilution is tested.
		U/P osmolality	
Acid-base metabolism	Tm bicarbonate	Minimal urine pH after acid loading	Gravidas' urines are frequently above pH 5.5 even when serum bicarbonate is in the range of 22–24 mmol/L; NH_4Cl loading test rarely indicated in pregnancy.
	Ammonia and titratable acid excretion after NH_4Cl loading		

Specific tests are those generally available in specialized laboratories and used primarily in research. Clinical tests are those available in most hospital laboratories.

PAH: p-aminohippurate; PSP: phenosulphthalein; Tm: tubular maximum; Tc_{H_2O}: free water reabsorption; C_{H_2O}: free water excretion; U/P: urine to plasma ratio

whose history suggests previous urinary tract infection and question the cost effectiveness and sensitivity of routine screening (18).

Some advise further evaluating patients who had bacteriuria detected during pregnancy after the routine postpartum checkup because this group has shown an increased incidence of urinary tract abnormalities (4). Finally, whether asymptomatic bacteriuria predisposes to premature delivery or preeclampsia remains controversial.

The approach to the pregnant woman with symptomatic UTI differs markedly from that for one with asymptomatic bacteriuria. Acute pyelonephritis in pregnancy, which occasionally led to maternal death in the preantibiotic era, is even now associated with hypotension and decreased renal function. Furthermore, it has been implicated in intrauterine growth retardation, prematurity, and fetal death.

Symptomatic UTI should be treated aggressively.

While most patients respond quickly and their fever disappears in 24 to 48 hours, pregnant women are likely to relapse or become reinfected. Such patients should therefore receive antibiotics for 3–5 weeks and thereafter have their urine screened frequently.

Pregnancy Complications Affecting Kidneys

GFR and RPF both decrease during preeclampsia, the former more than the latter, with a resulting decrease in filtration fraction. Reduction in renal hemodynamics is frequently around 25% (9, 19). Thus, GFR in the preeclamptic patient often equals, and may even exceed, prepregnancy levels (again illustrating how early detection of a disease can be missed if one accepts nonpregnancy norms).

When severe, preeclampsia may be accompanied by acute renal failure or even renal cortical necrosis. The latter may occur with a disseminated intravascular coagulation

(DIC) syndrome that usually remits with delivery (4, 9, 14, 19).

Preeclampsia occasionally manifests as the nephrotic syndrome, and at our institution is the most common cause of this syndrome in pregnancy (20). Clinicians often fail to consider preeclampsia in making a differential diagnosis because diastolic blood pressures frequently range only between 80 and 95 mm Hg. However, even such values are high for pregnancy, where average diastolic pressure is usually 15 mm Hg lower than prepregnancy measurements. On occasion, the clinician suspects the true diagnosis only when larger blood pressure increments occur after infusion of albumin for restoration of plasma volume.

Placental abruption may lead to both acute renal failure and renal cortical necrosis (21). One report suggests that abruption may be accompanied by light and electron microscopic patterns in the kidney similar to those seen in preeclampsia (22). Although preeclampsia may have been present, hypertension remained undetected because of the heavy bleeding accompanying abruption.

In addition, acute renal failure has been reported in association with pernicious vomiting of pregnancy (23). It may also accompany acute yellow atrophy of pregnancy, whose etiology is uncertain. In this condition, marked by rapid appearance of jaundice and clinical evidence of severe hepatic dysfunction, immediate evacuation of the uterus may reverse the pathologic process (24).

An important cause of acute tubular necrosis and rarely cortical necrosis early in pregnancy is septic instrumentation of the uterus in an attempt to end an unwanted pregnancy. This possibility should be considered in young women with infection and decreasing renal function (21, 24). Evacuation of the uterus—and perhaps hysterectomy in selected cases—may be lifesaving.

A syndrome related to gestation reported by various names but best called idiopathic postpartum renal failure was first described in 1968 (21, 24–26). In it, the patient, who often has experienced little trouble with gestation or delivery, displays uremia and severe hypertension 3–6 weeks into the puerperium.

Etiology is obscure, and viral agents, ergot compounds, oral contraceptives, and retained placental fragments have all been implicated. Pathophysiology has been likened to diseases characterized by DIC and to scleroderma. Most women affected have either died or survived with severely reduced renal function. Some physicians claim to have reversed or arrested the disease with heparin or antithrombin III concentrates, and one may try these agents, as well as dilation and curettage, when faced with the syndrome.

Influence of Pregnancy on Renal Disease

Preexisting Mild Impairment

In general, pregnancy should not affect disease course adversely, and the gestation will be successful in women with preserved or mildly decreased renal function and normal blood pressure at conception. However, certain conditions, such as lupus and membranoproliferative glomerulonephritis, appear more sensitive to gestation, and pregnancy should not be undertaken in the presence of renal scleroderma and periarteritis (Table 23.3). Also, authorities disagree as to whether pregnancy adversely influences IgA or reflux nephropathy or focal glomerulosclerosis (27–32).

Preexisting Moderate Impairment

Prognosis is poorer if serum creatinine is 1.5 mg/dL or more and/or hypertension is present before conception. About one third of these patients will experience either renal function deterioration, labile hypertension, or both during pregnancy, and some will have accelerated progression of underlying disease after delivery.

Preexisting Severe Impairment

Women with serum creatinine of 3 mg/dL or more are often infertile. In their rare conceptions, the likelihood of successful outcome is low and maternal morbidity high: two compelling reasons to discourage pregnancy in these patients.

General Clinical Observations

Approximately 50% of pregnant women with renal disease and mild dysfunction exhibit increments in proteinuria, often to the nephrotic range (33). However, appearance of heavy proteinuria in such patients does not usually mean that the disease has worsened but may merely reflect nor-

Table 23.3 Chronic Renal Disease and Pregnancy Interactions

Disease	Effects of and on Pregnancy
Chronic glomerulonephritis and focal glomerular sclerosis (FGS)	Increased incidence of high blood pressure late in gestation, but usually no adverse effect if renal function preserved and hypertension absent before pregnancy. Some disagree, believing that coagulation changes in pregnancy exacerbate disease, especially IgA nephropathy, membranoproliferative glomerulonephritis, and FGS.
Systemic lupus erythematosus	Controversial: Prognosis most favorable if disease in remission 6 or more months before conception. Some increase steroid dosage in the immediate puerperium. Presence of lupus anticoagulant or anticardiolipin antibodies imparts a poor fetal prognosis.
Periarteritis nodosa and scleroderma	Fetal prognosis is poor. Disease associated with maternal deaths. Reactivation of quiescent scleroderma can occur during pregnancy and postpartum. Consider therapeutic abortion.
Diabetic nephropathy	No adverse effect on renal lesion. Increased frequency of hypertension, infections, edema, nephrotic syndrome, and preeclampsia.
Chronic pyelonephritis (infectious tubulointerstitial disease)	Bacteriuria in pregnancy may lead to exacerbation.
Polycystic disease	Functional impairment and hypertension usually minimal in childbearing years and not affected by pregnancy. Increased incidence of preeclampsia.
Urolithiasis	Ureteral dilation and stasis do not seem to affect natural history, but infections can be more frequent. Stents have been successfully placed during gestation.
Reflux nephropathy	Controversial: Some believe pregnancy accelerates functional loss; others note course similar to most other diseases.
Permanent urinary diversion	Depending on original reason for surgery, there may be other malformations of the urogenital tract. Urinary tract infection common during pregnancy, and renal function may undergo reversible decrease. No significant obstructive problem, but cesarean section might be necessary for abnormal presentation.
After nephrectomy, solitary and pelvic kidneys	Pregnancy well tolerated. Might be associated with other malformations of the urogenital tract. Dystocia rarely occurs with a pelvic kidney.

mal urinary protein excretion increases of pregnancy.

Preexisting hypertension imparts a poorer prognosis, even when GFR is well preserved, but strict control of blood pressure markedly improves outcome (34). Late pregnancy hypertension or superimposed preeclampsia may be more likely in women with glomerular, compared to tubular, disease, while the latter are more likely to have accompanying UTI (33) (see Case 23.1). Finally, although one should avoid diuretics during pregnancy, they may be needed for severely nephrotic women, especially those displaying diabetic nephropathy (35).

Renal Biopsy Indications

Although pregnancy does not entail increased risks for renal biopsy, many clinical investigators disagree about indications. For example, Packham and Fairley believe in performing percutaneous needle biopsies often to detect those glomerular disorders that they think worsen during pregnancy and might benefit from therapy with antiplatelet or other specific agents (36). Therefore, they endorse biopsy for most pregnant women seen with undiagnosed hematuria or increased proteinuria.

However, some consider these indications too broad and advise continuing to perform renal biopsy infrequently during pregnancy. Current recommendations include considering biopsy when renal function suddenly deteriorates without obvious cause any time before 32 weeks' gestation (37). When diagnosed early, certain forms of rapidly progressive glomerulonephritis may respond to aggressive treatment with steroid pulses and perhaps plasma exchange.

Another appropriate occasion for biopsy is symptomatic nephrotic syndrome noted before 32 weeks. Although some might consider a therapeutic trial of steroids first, it is preferable to determine beforehand whether the lesion is likely to respond to steroids, pregnancy being in itself a hypercoagulable state prone to worsening by such treatment.

However, proteinuria alone in a normotensive woman who has neither marked hypoalbuminemia nor intolerable edema requires only conducting examinations more frequently, while deferring biopsy to the postpartum period. In this situation, we believe that the prognosis is determined primarily by renal function and presence or absence of hypertension rather than the type of renal lesion. We view similarly pregnancies with asymptomatic microscopic hematuria alone, when ultrasonography suggests neither stone nor tumor.

A gray area is a finding of urinary red and white blood cells and casts with proteinuria and borderline renal function in a patient not previously evaluated. In this case, one could argue that diagnosis of a collagen disorder, such as scleroderma or periarteritis, would be grounds for terminating the pregnancy or that the class of lesion caused by systemic lupus erythematosus (SLE) would determine type and intensity of therapy.

However, scleroderma and periarteritis are only infrequently diagnosed by renal biopsy. Rather than intervening, it is important to closely watch normotensive women having stable renal function and neither systemic involvement nor laboratory evidence of these collagen disorders. By contrast, biopsy may be indicated in selected patients with SLE and lupus nephropathy of uncertain histopathology (see Case 23.2). Finally, biopsy during gestation may uncover unusual causes of acute renal failure (38).

In brief, there are few indications for renal biopsy in pregnancy. It should be resorted to only in cases of sudden renal insufficiency or massive nephrotic syndrome of unknown origin occurring before the final two months. Antenatal progress of normotensive women with mild or moderate proteinuria or asymptomatic microscopic hematuria but well-preserved renal function should be monitored frequently and their disease evaluated more completely postpartum.

Transplantation Problems

The number of pregnancies in renal allograft recipients presently exceeds 3,000 (12, 39–41). While most succeed, complications occasionally include irreversible declines in GFR. Other problems are steroid-induced hyperglycemia, severe hypertension, septicemia, uterine rupture, ectopic pregnancy, prematurity, respiratory distress syndrome, growth retardation, congenital anomalies, hypoadrenalism, hepatic insufficiency, thrombocytopenia, and serious fetal infection.

Patients with a homograft from a living donor fare better than those who have received cadaver transplants. The former are counselled to wait one and the latter two years before attempting pregnancy and then to do so only if renal function is adequate and hypertension absent.

Most studies are of women treated with azathioprine and steroids alone (39–41). It is preferable that allograft recipients planning to conceive discontinue or substantially reduce dosage of cyclosporine until more is known concerning its effects in pregnancy.

Dialysis

Many of the pregnant women who conceive while undergoing dialytic therapy for end-stage renal disease do so because they mistakenly believe that they are infertile (40, 42, 43). These women do ovulate, the prevalence being greatest among those undergoing chronic ambulatory peritoneal dialysis. Unfortunately, most such pregnancies fail.

Both peritoneal and hemodialysis have been used in

obstetric patients. The former is preferred because it is less frequently associated with precipitous hypotension and premature contractions. To minimize these problems when using hemodialysis, we suggest daily treatment for shorter periods and avoidance of high-flux technology.

What to Tell Patients

Some clinicians advise against pregnancy if serum creatinine exceeds 1.5 mg/dL. Others allow it in women with preconception levels up to 2 mg/dL, especially those with a single kidney, transplant recipients with stable function (preferably for two years), and women with primary interstitial disease. Diastolic blood pressure before conception should be 90 mm Hg or less, and one must rigidly control levels in women with mild or moderate hypertension who conceive. Failure to control blood pressure early in gestation is reason to consider termination.

Management Steps

All pregnant women with renal disease are best managed at a tertiary care center under the coordinated care of a maternal-fetal specialist and a nephrologist. Initial laboratory tests should include a data base, which aids in early detection of renal functional loss, as well as of superimposed preeclampsia. Besides the usual prenatal screening tests, the following renal parameters should be sought:

- Serum creatinine and its timed clearance
- SUN, albumin, and cholesterol concentrations
- Electrolytes, urinalysis, screening bacterial culture, and 24-hour protein excretion
- Uric acid levels, oxaloacetic and pyruvate transaminases, lactic dehydrogenase, prothrombin time, partial thromboplastin time, and platelet count (superimposed preeclampsia screening tests)

Biweekly prenatal visits should be scheduled until week 32 and weekly ones thereafter. Unless more frequent evaluations become necessary, renal parameters should be tested every 4–6 weeks. Fetal assessment, in particular electronic monitoring, is best started between 30 and 32 weeks,

especially in nephrotic patients with hypoalbuminemia.

Diuretics should be avoided, as nephrotic gravidas are often oligemic, and further intravascular volume depletion may impair uteroplacental perfusion. In addition, since blood pressure normally declines during pregnancy, saliuretic therapy could conceivably precipitate circulatory collapse or thromboembolic episodes. However, some patients have been documented whose kidneys were retaining salt so avidly that cautious use of diuretics was necessary.

Nephrotic gravidas should not be prophylactically anticoagulated because the known risk outweighs alleged benefits. Finally, protein restriction—advocated in management of nonpregnant patients with renal insufficiency—should not be attempted until more is known about effects on fetal development.

CASE 23.1 Late-Pregnancy Hypertension with Decreasing Renal Function

A 25-year-old multipara with known hypertension was hospitalized at 31 weeks' gestation with a blood pressure of 200/140 mm Hg. Treatment included a single 20-mg dose of hydralazine, 2 mg of trichlormethiazide daily for three days, lateral recumbent bed rest, and restriction of dietary sodium.

After two weeks, weight had decreased 10 lb, and diastolic blood pressure averaged 90 to 100 mm Hg. Unfortunately, urine volumes declined to 2.3 mL per minute by hospital day 16, and creatinine clearance decreased from 106 mL per minute on day 6 to 82 mL per minute on day 16. Simultaneously, blood urea nitrogen increased from 8 to 25 mg/dL.

Physicians considered interrupting pregnancy, since deteriorating renal function was regarded as a sign of superimposed and progressing preeclampsia. However, a diagnosis of salt depletion was also entertained.

A trial period in which sodium intake was increased to 206 mEq daily followed. After sodium intake was liberalized, weight increased 3 lb, but diastolic blood pressures remained between 90 and 100 mm Hg and creatinine clearance increased to 118 mL/minute by day 26. Serum creatinine (1.1 mg/dL on day 6 and 1.3 mg/dL on day 16) and urea nitrogen decreased to 0.9 and 16 mg/dL, respectively. Urine volume increased to 8.7 mL per minute. The pregnancy was allowed to continue until the patient went into spontaneous labor.

In this case alterations in serum creatinine mirrored changes in its clearance. The GFR was slightly decreased for pregnancy, and the serum creatinine values of 0.9 to 1.3 (hospital days 26 and 16) were abnormal during gestation. On the other hand, the patient had a normal urea nitrogen on admission, perhaps reflecting poor nutrition. With dehydration and oliguria, concentration of urea increased threefold, while serum creatinine clearance decreased only 23%. However, when GFR increased above admission values, urea nitrogen was still 16 mg/dL, probably reflecting a good hospital diet (44). ∎

CASE 23.2 A Case of Lupus

A 19-year-old woman developed fever, arthritis, pleuritic chest pains, and a malar skin rash two weeks after a miscarriage during her first pregnancy. Positive lupus erythematosus (LE) test results and the presence in her serum of antinuclear and anti-DNA antibodies led to a diagnosis of systemic lupus erythematosus.

Her blood pressure was 115/75 mm Hg. Laboratory examination revealed anemia and leukopenia. Serum creatinine and urea nitrogen were 1.0 and 15 mg/dL, respectively. Qualitative protein excretion was negative, and creatinine clearance was 110 mL per minute. A renal biopsy revealed diffuse glomerulonephritis. She was treated initially with 100 mg of prednisone daily, which was slowly tapered to 30 mg daily. Therapy was complicated by development of a gastric ulcer.

She became pregnant for the second time one year later, while in remission and after her prednisone dose had been further tapered to 15 mg daily. Her prenatal course was uneventful, and during gestation her serum creatinine and urea nitrogen decreased to 0.8 and 11 mg/dL, respectively. Her diastolic blood pressures ranged between 70 and 80 mm Hg. The patient discontinued using prednisone during her fifth gestational month, at a time when all clinical and serologic parameters were normal.

Labor was induced at 40 weeks' gestation, resulting in delivery of a healthy 3,420-g baby. The patient received 100 mg of hydrocortisone during labor and 50 to 75 mg every 6–8 hours for the next two days. During the third postpartum day, she developed transient hypotension, which apparently responded to hydration and an additional 150 mg of hydrocortisone. Oral prednisone was then restarted and was maintained at 20 mg daily.

One year after delivery, the patient was operated on for acute appendicitis. At that time, her serum creatinine was 0.9 mg/dL and her blood pressure was 136/70 mm Hg.

Her third pregnancy occurred at age 23, four years after the initial diagnosis of lupus. At that time, she was in clinical remission, and her prednisone dose was decreased to 15 mg daily. During gestation, her blood pressure was approximately 125/80 mm Hg, and serum creatinine, urea nitrogen, and uric acid were 0.8, 7, and 4.6 mg/dL, respectively. Qualitative urinary protein excretion were negative or trace. Insulin and p-aminohippurate clearances during the seventh gestational month were 157 and 678 mL per minute, respectively.

Her prenatal course continued uneventfully until her 37th gestational week, when decrements in her hemolytic complement and a rise in her antinuclear factor titer led physicians to increase the prednisone dose to 30 mg daily. The complement activity then increased to low normal values.

Delivery was induced at 39 weeks and resulted in a healthy 3,675-g baby. Again, she received IV hydrocortisone during labor and in the immediate puerperium, after which oral prednisone was restarted.

Three months postpartum, her blood pressure was

100/65 mm Hg. Serum creatinine and urea nitrogen were 0.9 and 17 mg/dL, respectively, and urinary protein excretion was 350 mg every 24 hours. Repeat insulin and p-aminohippurate clearances were 93.5 and 405 mL per minute, respectively. Her steroid therapy had been tapered to 5 mg daily.

This case illustrates several points concerning renal disease and pregnancy. This woman's initial manifestations of lupus erythematosus appeared to be related to gestation, and her renal biopsy revealed a lesion that had a guarded prognosis. However, because functional parameters and blood pressure were normal, she was permitted to become pregnant and both gestations succeeded.

During her second pregnancy, steroid therapy was tapered perhaps too quickly. However, it was wisely initiated in the puerperium. The patient's third pregnancy was characterized by close scrutiny of serologic factors, and these factors suggested the possibility that an exacerbation occurred shortly before term. Again, steroid therapy was judiciously increased. It is noteworthy that, in spite of a diffuse kidney lesion, the patient experienced physiologic increments in renal hemodynamics during pregnancy. ■

References

1. Bailey RR, Rolleston GL. Kidney length and ureteric dilatation in the puerperium. J Obstet Gynaecol Br Commonw 1971;78:55.

2. Conrad KP. Renal changes in pregnancy. Urology Annual 1992; 6:313.

3. Rasmussen PE, Nielsen FR. Hydronephrosis during pregnancy. Eur J Obstet Gynecol Reprod Biol 1988;27:249.

4. Lindheimer MD, Katz AI. Kidney function and disease in pregnancy. Philadelphia; Lea & Febiger, 1977.

5. Rubi RA, Sala NL. Ureteral function in pregnant women. Effect of different positions and of fetal delivery upon ureteral tonus. Am J Obstet Gynecol 1968;101:230.

6. Dure-Smith P. Pregnancy dilatation of the urinary tract. The iliac sign and its significance. Radiology 1970;96:545.

7. Nielsen FR, Rasmussen PE. Hydronephrosis causing symptoms during pregnancy. Eur J Obstet Gynecol Reprod Biol 1988; 27:245.

8. Dunlop W, Davison JM. Renal haemodynamics and tubular function in human pregnancy. Baillières Clin Obstet Gynaecol 1987;1:769.

9. Chesley LC. Hypertensive disorders in pregnancy. New York: Appleton-Century-Crofts, 1977.

10. Davison JM, Noble MCB. Serial changes in 24 hour creatinine clearance during normal menstrual cycles and the first trimester of pregnancy. Br J Obstet Gynaecol 1981;88:10.

11. Sims EAH, Kranz KE. Serial studies of renal function during pregnancy and the puerperium in normal women. J Clin Invest 1958;37:1764.

12. Lindheimer MD, Katz AI. Renal physiology in pregnancy. In: Seldin DW, Giebisch G, eds. The kidney: physiology and pathophysiology. New York: Raven Press, 1986:2017.

13. August P, Sealy JE. The renin-angiotensin system in normal and hypertensive pregnancy. In: Laragh JH, Brenner BM, eds. Hypertension: pathophysiology, diagnosis and management. New York: Raven Press, 1990:1761-78.

14. Lindheimer MD, Katz AI. Preeclampsia: pathophysiology, diagnosis and management. Annu Rev Med 1989;40:233.

15. Davison JM. The effect of pregnancy on kidney function in renal allograft recipients. Kidney Int 1985;27:74.

16. McFadyen IR, Eykyn SJ, Gardner NH, et al. Bacteriuria in pregnancy. J Obstet Gynaecol Br Commonw 1973;80:385.

17. Cunningham FC. Urinary tract infections complicating pregnancy. Baillière's Clin Obstet Gynaecol 1987;1:891.

18. Campell-Brown M, McFadyen IR, Seal DV, et al. Is screening for bacteriuria worthwhile? Br Med J 1987;294:1579.

19. Chesley LC, Lindheimer MD. Renal hemodynamics and intravascular volume in normal and hypertensive pregnancy. In: Rubin PC, ed. Handbook of hypertension. Amsterdam: Elsevier, 1988:38.

20. Fisher KA, Luger A, Spargo BH, et al. Hypertension in pregnancy: clinical pathological correlations and late prognosis. Medicine 1981;60:267.

21. Pertuiset N, Grünfeld J-P. Acute renal failure in pregnancy. Baillières Clin Obstet Gynaecol 1987;1:873.

22. Thompson D, Patterson WG, Smart GE, et al. The renal lesions of toxaemia and abruptio placentae studied by light and electron microscopy. J Obstet Gynaecol Br Commonw 1972;79:311.

23. Soyannwo MAO, Armstrong MJ, McGeown MG. Survival of the fetus in a patient in acute renal failure. Lancet 1966; 2:1009.

24. Lindheimer MD, Katz AI, Ganeval D, et al. Acute renal failure in pregnancy. In: Brenner BM, Lazarus JM, eds. Acute renal failure, 3rd ed. New York: Churchill Livingstone, 1993:417.

25. Robson JS, Martin AM, Ruckley VA, et al. Irreversible post-partum renal failure: a new syndrome. Q J Med 1968; 37:423.

26. Wagoner RD, Holley KE, Johnson WJ. Accelerated nephro-sclerosis and postpartum acute renal failure in normotensive patients. Ann Intern Med 1968;69:237.

27. Lindheimer MD, Katz AI. The kidney and hypertension in pregnancy. In: Brenner BM, Rector FC Jr, eds. The kidney, 4th ed. Philadelphia: Saunders, 1991:1551.

28. Lindheimer MD, Katz AI. Gestation in women with kidney disease: prognosis and management. Baillière's Clin Obstet Gynaecol 1987;1:939.

29. Imbasciati E, Ponticelli C. Pregnancy and renal disease. Predictors for fetal and maternal outcome. Am J Nephrol 1991; 11:353.

30. Abe S. An overview of pregnancy in women with underlying renal disease. Am J Kidney Dis 1991;17:112.

31. Jungers P, Houillier P, Forget D, et al. Specific controversies concerning the natural history of renal disease in pregnancy. Am J Kidney Dis 1991,17.116.

32. Abe S. Pregnancy in IgA nephropathy. Kidney Int 1991; 40:1098.

33. Katz AI, Davison JM, Hayslett JP et al. Pregnancy in women with kidney disease. Kidney Int 1980;19:192.

34. Packham DK, Fairley KF, Ihle BV, et al. Comparison of pregnancy outcome between normotensive and hypertensive women with primary glomerulonephritis. Clin Exp Hypertens [A] 1987–1988;B6:387.

35. Reece EA, Coustan DR, Hayslett JP, et al. Diabetic nephropathy, pregnancy performance and fetal-maternal outcome. Am J Obstet Gynecol 1988;159:56.

36. Packham D, Fairley KF. Renal biopsy: indications and complications in pregnancy. Br J Obstet Gynaecol 1989;94:935.

37. Lindheimer MD, Davison JM. Renal biopsy during pregnancy. "To . . .or not to . . ." Br J Obstet Gynaecol 1987; 94:932.

38. Warren V, Sprague SM, Corwin HC. Sarcoidosis presenting as acute renal failure in pregnancy. Am J Kidney Dis 1988; 12:161.

39. Hou S. Pregnancy in organ transplant recipients. Med Clin North Am 1989;73:667.

40. Davison JM. Dialysis, transplantation and pregnancy. Am J Kidney Dis 1991;17:127.

41. Lindheimer MD, Katz AI. Pregnancy in the renal transplant patient. Am J Kidney Dis 1992;19:173.

42. Hou S. Peritoneal dialysis and haemodialysis in pregnancy. Baillière's Clin Obstet Gynaecol 1987;1:1009.

43. Hou SH, Grossman SD. Pregnancy in chronic dialysis patients. Semin Dial 1990;3:224.

44. Polomaki J, Lindheimer MD. Sodium depletion simulating deterioration in a toxemic pregnancy. N Engl J Med 1977; 282:88.

24

The Renal Transplant Recipient

Joseph V. Collea, M.D.
Mohammad R. Alijani, M.D.
Irwin R. Merkatz, M.D.

Introduction

Chronic renal failure or end-stage renal disease (ESRD) requiring either dialysis or transplantation for survival is a major health problem in the world today. Defined as a creatinine clearance of 5 mL/min or less and a serum creatinine of 12 mg/dL or more (1), ESRD may result from a myriad of disorders of the renal-urologic system (Table 24.1) (2), which, according to The National Kidney Foundation, affects as many as 20 million men, women, and children in the United States alone, resulting in over 120,000 cases of ESRD and over 80,000 deaths annually (3).

The Canadian Renal Failure Registry in 1985 estimated the incidence of ESRD in North America as 60 patients per million population (pmp) (4). Other recent publications (Table 24.2) cite incidences of ESRD that range from a low of 38 pmp in Northern Ireland to a high of 100 pmp in the United States. ESRD occurs in children at an annual rate of 0.5 to 5.5 pmp, with ESRD in infants less than one year of age contributing to only 0.2 pmp (9, 11). More than half of all children requiring dialysis or transplantation present between the ages of 11 and 16 years (12).

Etiology of ESRD

Although the list of renal-urologic diseases leading to ESRD is long (Table 24.1), glomerulonephritis is the single most common cause of renal failure in the adult population, accounting for 25% of patients who receive renal transplants in the United States and 31% of those performed in Europe (13). Chronic pyelonephritis and diabetic nephropathy (Kimmelstiel-Wilson syndrome) are the second and third leading causes of ESRD in adults, with the former contributing to 21% of all renal transplants (13) and the latter accounting for 15%-25% of all patients on dialysis (2). Diabetes mellitus is of particular concern because long-term follow-up studies have revealed that renal failure occurs in approximately 50% of patients with type I disease after a mean of 15 years following diagnosis (14) and in 10% of type II diabetes after a mean of only eight years postdiagnosis (15).

In contrast to the adult data, congenital anomalies, inherited disorders (congenital nephrotic syndrome-Finnish type, infantile polycystic kidney disease) and renal dysplasia are responsible for more than half of the cases of ESRD in children (16-18). Of the 3,342 children undergoing dialysis reported by the European Dialysis and Transplant Association's Pediatric Registry (19), 31.3% were diagnosed with glomerulonephritis, while 51% had renal hypoplasia, inherited disorders, or congenital malformations of the urinary tract.

Although the incidence of ESRD is reported as only 0.2 pmp in infants under one year of age, it is of interest to obstetricians that some of these cases are the result of perinatal asphyxia or neonatal renal hypoperfusion secondary to severe cardiopulmonary compromise, particularly in the premature newborn with hyaline membrane disease (20). Although the majority of these neonates who survive recover without sequelae, many are left with impaired renal function that may progress to ESRD, requiring treatment prior to adolescence.

Treatment of End-Stage Renal Disease

Treatment options for patients with ESRD today include hemodialysis, peritoneal dialysis, and renal transplantation. Hemodialysis and peritoneal dialysis replace the excretory function of the impaired kidneys by allowing the accumu-

Table 24.1 Indications for Renal Transplantation

Congenital Disorders	**Trauma Requiring Nephrectomy, Renal Vascular Diseases**
Aplasia	Renal artery occlusion
Hypoplasia	Renal vein thrombosis
Horseshoe kidney	
	Irreversible Acute Failure
Metabolic Disorders	Cortical necrosis
Hyperoxaluria	Hemolytic uremic syndrome
Nephrocalcinosis	Acute and subacute glomerulonephritis
Gout	Anaphylactoid purpura (Henoch-Schönlein syndrome)
Oxalosis	Acute tubular necrosis
Fabrey's disease	
Amyloidosis	**Irreversible Chronic Renal Failure**
Cystinosis	Chronic pyelonephritis
	Chronic glomerulonephritis
Hereditary Nephropathies	Diabetic nephropathy (Kimmelstiel-Wilson syndrome)
Alport's syndrome	Goodpasture's disease
Polycystic kidney disease	Hypocomplementemic nephrosclerosis
Medullary cystic disease	
	Other
Toxic Nephropathies	Multiple myeloma
Lead nephropathy	Macroglobulinemia
Analgesic nephropathy	Wegener's disease
	Scleroderma
Obstructive Uropathy	Systemic lupus erythematosus
Acquired	Polyarteritis nodosum (periarteritis nodosa)
Congenital	
Tumors Requiring Nephrectomy	
Renal carcinoma	
Wilms' tumor	
Tuberous sclerosis	

Reprinted with permission from Flye MW. Renal transplantation. In: Flye MW, ed. Principles of organ transplantation. Philadelphia: WB Saunders Company, 1989.

Table 24.2 Incidence of ESRD

Country	pmp	Patient Age Group
United States, 1983 (5)	100	All
Japan, 1979 (6)	70	All
Scotland, 1972 (7)	59	<65 years
N. Ireland, 1972 (8)	38	5–60 years

lated uremic wastes of the patient to diffuse across a semi-permeable membrane into the dialysate or dialysis fluid. This artificial membrane is made of cellulose acetate in the artificial kidney, whereas the peritoneum of the abdomen is the membrane in peritoneal dialysis. Hemodialysis is a safe, acceptable procedure that is generally performed three times per week for two to five hours either in a hospital, outpatient facility, or in the patient's home (21).

Peritoneal dialysis (PD) more commonly today implies continuous ambulatory peritoneal dialysis (CAPD), where, by means of an indwelling Tenckhoff catheter (22), patients perform peritoneal dialysis at home or at work without the assistance of medical personnel or specialized equipment.

Under aseptic conditions, the patient on a daily basis every six hours drains the abdominal cavity of the previously administered dialysate and infuses fresh, sterile dialysate from a two-liter reservoir hung overhead. During CAPD, the patient is generally able to perform normal daily activities with a minimum of disruption. CAPD is well tolerated clinically, but on rare occasions a patient may experience repetitive bouts of peritonitis, necessitating transfer to a hemodialysis program. A CAPD program is preferred by many nephrologists because it is more cost effective than hemodialysis, costing approximately $15,000 per year for each patient, compared to $35,000 per year for each patient placed on hemodialysis.

Renal transplantation is the surgical transfer of a living related donor (LRD) or cadaveric donor (CD) kidney to a patient with ESRD. The historical development of renal transplantation from its inception by Ullman in 1902 to the introduction of cyclosporin A (cyclosporine) in 1978 for host immunosuppression has been succinctly chronicled by Hamilton (23) (Table 24.3). During the first 50 years of renal transplantation experience, surgical skills were learned so that the donor kidney could be safely transplanted, but

Table 24.3 Landmarks in Kidney Transplantation

1902	First successful experimental kidney transplant (Ullman, 1902)
1906	First human kidney transplant—xenograft (Jaboulay, 1906)
1933	First human kidney transplant—allograft (Voronoy, 1936)
1950	Revival of experimental kidney transplantation (Simonsen, 1953; Dempster, 1953)
1950–53	Human kidney allografts without immunosuppression, Paris (Küss, et al., 1951; Servelle, et al., 1951; Dubost, et al., 1951) and Boston (Hume, et al., 1955)
1953	First use of live related donor, Paris (Michon, et al., 1953)
1954	First transplant between identical twins, Boston (Murray, et al., 1958)
1958	First description of leucocyte antigen "Mac" (Dausset, 1958)
1959–62	Radiation used for immunosuppression, Boston (Murray, et al., 1960) and Paris (Hamburger, et al., 1959; Küss, et al., 1960)
1960	Effectiveness of 6-MP in dog kidney transplants (Calne, 1960; Zukoski, et al., 1960)
1960	Prolonged graft survival in patient given 6-MP after irradiation (Küss, et al., 1962)
1962	First use of tissue matching to select a donor and recipients (Hamburger, et al., 1962; Terasaki, et al., 1965; Dausset, 1980)
1966	Recognition that positive crossmatching leads to hyperacute rejection (Kissmeyer-Nielsen, et al., 1966)
1967	Creation of Eurotransplant (van Rood, 1967)
1973	Description of the transfusion effect (Opelz, et al., 1973)
1978	First clinical use of cyclosporine (Calne, et al., 1978)
1978	Application of matching for HLA-DR and renal transplantation (Ting and Morris, 1978)

Reprinted with permission from Hamilton D. Kidney transplantation: a history. In: Morris PS, ed. Transplantation, principles and practice. London: Grune and Stratton, Inc., 1984.

Table 24.4 Treatment of ESRD; 70,960 Patients on Maintenance Therapy.

Treatment	Number of Patients	Percent
Hemodialysis	52,758	74.3
Peritoneal dialysis	3,953	5.6
CAPD (%)	76	
PD (%)	24	
Renal transplantation	14,249	20.1

Reprinted with permission from Broyer M, Brunner FP, et al. Combined report on regular dialysis and transplantation in Europe, XII, 1981. Proceedings of the European Dialysis Transplant Association 1982;19:2.

host rejection of the allograft made virtually all attempts at clinical success futile. Investigative interest was rekindled when Murray and co-workers (24) successfully performed the first renal transplant between identical twins whereby host rejection was adeptly avoided. Further research in allogenic graft rejection led to several breakthroughs in host immunosuppression, such as the introduction of azathioprine in 1962 (25), antilymphocyte globulin (ALG)—a polyclonal antibody—in the 1970s (26), and OKT3—a monoclonal antibody—in the 1980s (27). Over the past decade, azathioprine and cyclosporine, in conjunction with low-dose prednisone, have proved to be an effective triple-drug method of host immunosuppression in renal transplant patients (28), resulting in one-year patient survival rates in excess of 95%, exceeding the one-year survival rates of patients undergoing dialysis (3, 29).

Prior to the advent of this triple-drug therapy for host immunosuppression, the vast majority of ESRD patients were placed on dialysis. Broyer and co-workers (30) in 1982, reporting from the data of the European Dialysis and Transplant Registry (Table 24.4), demonstrated that 80% of 70,960 patients with ESRD were treated by hemodialysis, PD or CAPD, with only 20.1% referred for renal transplantation. In the United States in 1980, Davis (31), reporting from the Health Care Financing Administration, stated that there were 52,364 patients on dialysis and only 4,697 patients (8.2%) with renal transplants. The hesitation among care providers to refer patients for renal transplantation before 1980 was twofold. First, many ESRD patients, because of age or health status, were not considered candidates for a major operative procedure. Secondly, referring physicians were concerned about the limited success rates of renal allograft survival and function due to the relatively inadequate but morbid techniques available for host immunosuppression.

By the late 1970s, host immunosuppression consisted of azathioprine, high-dose steroids, and prophylactic antithymocyte globulin (ATG), often combined with splenectomy (32). This technique produced a two-year cadaveric graft survival rate of only 50% but was responsible for a morbidity-mortality rate of 15%-25%, largely from the complications of high-dose steroid administration, such as sepsis, gastrointestinal hemorrhage, hypertension, and hyperglycemia (32).

Utilization of the triple-drug regimen of azathioprine (1 mg/kg), low-dose prednisone (30 mg/day tapered to 10 mg/day after 45 days), and cyclosporine (3–5 mg/kg/day) in the early 1980s yielded one-year cadaveric graft survival rates of 81% with nephrotoxicity a rare complication (33). By 1983, the use of cyclosporine for host immunosuppression was widespread, and ever-increasing allograft and patient survival rates were being reported (34). As an example, Terasaki and co-workers (35) demonstrated that, since 1985, the half-life of cadaveric kidneys transplanted under cyclosporine protocols increased from 8 to 11 years, while the Task Force on Organ Transplantation (36) in 1986 reported one-year patient survival rates of 96% for LRD and 91% for cadaveric transplants.

In 1991, the United States Renal Data System, in its Annual Report (37), published the two-year patient and renal graft survival rates of 56,500 renal transplant recipients between 1983 and 1989. LRD and CD recipient survival rates are shown in Figure 24.1. The survival rates of LRD recipients, ages 20–44 years, increased from 91% in 1983 to 96% in 1988. For the age group 45–64 years, the survival rate increased from 81% in 1983 to 90% in 1988. For cadaveric recipients, age group 20–44 years, the survival rates increased from 85% to 90%, while for the age group 45–64 years, the rate improved from 75% to 84% over the same time period. The improved graft survival rates for LRD and CD transplants performed between the years 1983 and 1989 are reported in Figures 24.2 and 24.3. These data were in part responsible for the growing number of renal

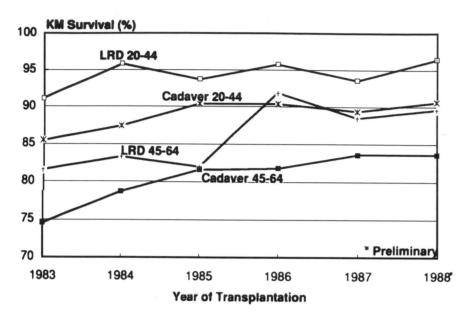

Figure 24.1 Two-year Kaplan and Meier statistical technique (KM) (38) patient survival (percent) for ESRD patients receiving a first transplant, by donor type (living related, cadaver) and age, adjusted for age, race, sex, and primary disease, 1983-1988. Data for 1988 are preliminary.

Reprinted with permission from 1991 Annual Data Report, United States Renal Data System. Am J Kidney Dis 1991; 18(Suppl 2) :61.

transplant procedures performed in the United States from 1983 through 1988 (Figure 24.4).

Further contributing to the interest in and the success of renal transplantation in the 1980s were the data of Vollmer et al. (39) and Evans et al. (40). Vollmer and associates, analyzing the case records of 1,038 patients with ESRD, compared the long-term survival rates of patients on dialysis with those receiving renal transplants (Figure 24.5). Patients receiving LRD kidneys survived significantly longer than comparable patients on maintenance dialysis. Cadaveric kidney recipient survival rates, although identical initially, began to exceed those of dialysis patients beyond

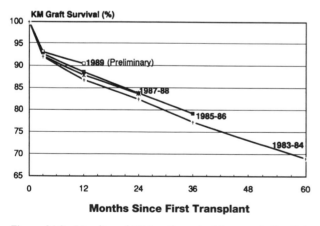

Figure 24.2 Unadjusted KM graft survival (percent), first living related transplant recipients, by time since first transplant, and year of transplantation, 1983-1989. Data for 1989 are preliminary.

Reprinted with permission from 1991Annual Data Report, United States Renal Data System. Am J Kidney Dis 1991;18(Suppl 2) :61.

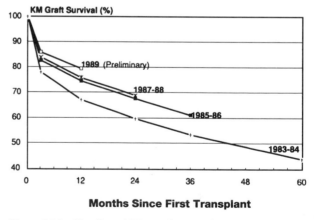

Figure 24.3 Unadjusted KM graft survival (percent), first cadaver transplant recipients, by time since first transplant, and year of transplantation, 1983-1989. Data for 1989 are preliminary.

Reprinted with permission from 1991 Annual Data Report, United States Renal Data System. Am J Kidney Dis 1991;18(Suppl 2) :61.

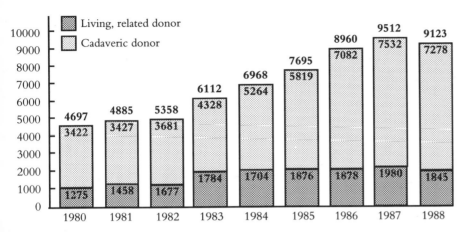

Figure 24.4 Kidney transplantation in the United States, 1980–1988.

Reprinted with permission from Health Care Financing Administration, Washington, DC, and United Network for Organ Sharing, Richmond, VA.

three years of treatment. Evans and co-workers published the results of a National Kidney Dialysis and Transplant Study that compared both objective and subjective quality-of-life issues in 859 patients with ESRD treated by hemodialysis, CAPD, and renal transplantation. In the areas of both physical and occupational rehabilitation, concerning employment and overall life satisfaction, patients with renal transplants fared better than comparable patients on any other form of treatment.

The success of renal transplant programs over the past decade culminated in the American Society of Transplant Physicians' statement (3, 41) that "all ESRD patients should be considered as candidates for transplantation unless there is a specific contraindication" (Table 24.5).

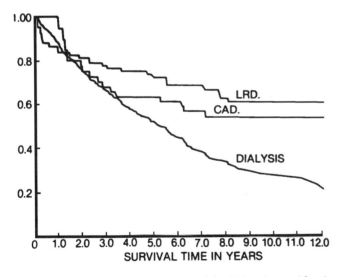

Figure 24.5 The probability of survival for 849 patients with primary renal disease, according to transplant classification. Estimates were obtained by using the method of Kaplan and Meier (38), taking into account the time-dependent nature of the treatment status.

Reprinted with permission from Vollmer WM, Wohl PW, Blagg CR. Survival with dialysis and transplantation in patients with end-stage renal disease. N Engl J Med 1983;308:1553.

Table 24.5 Contraindications to Renal Transplantation

Absolute

1. Active cancer (A patient fully treated for cancer with no recurrence for a minimum of one year may be considered as a transplant candidate.)
2. Active sepsis
3. Chronic, active hepatitis
4. Active gastrointestinal hemorrhage disorder: peptic ulcer disease, esophageal varices
5. Symptomatic AIDS

Relative

1. Substance abuse/noncompliance (Drug abuse/alcohol rehabilitation strongly suggested prior to transplantation.)
2. Asymptomatic HIV+ (Infectious disease evaluation indicated prior to consideration as transplant candidate.)
3. Severe cardiac dysfunction (If the cardiac problem can be corrected surgically [coronary artery bypass graft, percutaneous angioplasty, etc.], transplantation may be considered.)
4. Age over 65 years (Any patient older than 65 in generally good health may be considered as a transplant candidate.)

Organ Procurement

Patients with clinical and biopsy-proven ESRD who are candidates for renal transplantation are referred to an organ transplant center. In the United States, all centers, organizations, and institutions involved in organ procurement and transplantation belong to the United Network for Organ Sharing (UNOS), a tax-exempt medical, scientific, and educational organization.[1] UNOS, under a federal contract from the United States Department of Health and Human Services, operates the National Organ Procurement and Transplantation Network (OPTN), which, in turn, develops policies and oversees all procedures to ensure maximum utilization of organs donated for transplantation. Organ allocation is based on a point system established by UNOS for the purpose of assuring equal organ access for all patients throughout the United States. Patients with medical and/or surgical contraindications, who are not candidates for transplantation, are maintained on hemodialysis or CAPD for chronic treatment of their ESRD.

The majority of patients today in the United States are considered candidates for renal transplantations and fall into two major categories: those *with* and those *without* potential living related donors. Candidates with potential donors are scheduled for further evaluation and testing, whereas those without potential donors are placed on a national computerized waiting list maintained by UNOS in order to procure a cadaveric donor. Currently, patients on the UNOS list wait an average of 18–24 months before a suitable cadaveric donor is located. Such patients may require dialysis until renal transplantation is accomplished.

The workups of ESRD patients and potential living related donors are meticulous and may take up to two months to complete. The potential donor is physically and psychologically evaluated to determine suitability (42) (Table 24.6). Above all, the donor must be free of any renal

dysfunction or disease and obviously committed to the procedure. When an acceptable match results, the living donor transplantation may be electively scheduled with a minimum of surgical risk to either party (43).

It should be noted that in many transplant centers throughout the world today, cadaveric pancreatic-duodenal and renal transplantations are being performed simultaneously on patients with juvenile-onset, insulin-dependent (type I) diabetes mellitus and ESRD. This combined surgical procedure entails transplantation of a kidney on one side and a pancreas with its attached duodenal segment implanted into the dome of the bladder on the other side of the recipient's false pelvis (Figure 24.6). To date, fourteen such procedures have been performed by members of the Division of Transplantation, Department of Surgery, Georgetown University Medical Center, Washington, DC (Alijani MR, unpublished data, 1992).

The surgical goal of the renal transplant procedure is to place a donor kidney extraperitoneally in the recipient's iliac fossa. Through an oblique incision just above the

---

Table 24.6 Evaluation of Potential Living Donors

Family conference with transplant surgeon.
History and physical examination with multiple blood pressure readings.
Complete blood count with differential, platelets, prothrombin time, partial thromboplastin time.
Determinations of serum sodium, potassium, chlorine, carbon dioxide, serum glutamic oxaloacetic transaminase, bilirubin, uric acid, blood urea nitrogen (BUN), Cr, calcium, phosphorus, fasting blood sugar, HbsAg, cholesterol, triglycerides.
Urinalysis, 24-hour creatinine clearance, urine culture × 2.
ABO blood group, tissue typing, leukocyte crossmatch, mixed leukocyte culture.
Chest x-ray film.
Electrocardiogram.
Intravenous pyelogram.
Psychologic evaluation, when indicated.
Finally, if all other studies are normal, arteriogram (done on inpatient basis 48 hours prior to nephrectomy).

Reprinted with permission from Haag BW, Stuart FP. The organ donor: brain death, selection criteria, supply and demand. In: Flye MW, ed. Principles of organ transplantation. Philadelphia: WB Saunders Company, 1989.

---

[1] UNOS: National Organ Procurement and Transplantation Network, 1100 Boulders Parkway, Suite 500, PO Box 13770, Richmond, VA, 23225-8770.

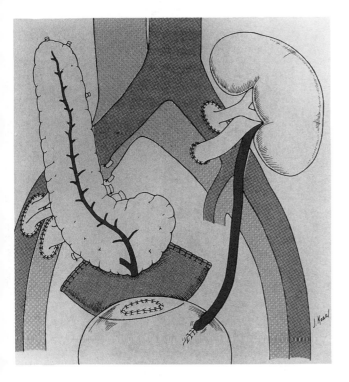

Figure 24.6   Combined pancreas-kidney transplantation with the duodenal segment technique.

Reprinted with permission from Sollinger HW, Knechtle SJ. The current status of combined kidney-pancreas transplantation. In: Sabiston DC, ed. Textbook of surgery, update 6. Philadelphia: WB Saunders Company, 1990.

inguinal ligament, the transplant surgeon identifies the peritoneal layer of the abdominal cavity and dissects it downward and medially until the dome of the bladder is visualized. Often, exposure of the bladder is enhanced by dividing and ligating the inferior epigastric vessels and the round ligament of the uterus. Transplantation is accomplished by anastomosing the donor renal artery to the proximal end of the divided hypogastric artery and the donor renal vein to the external iliac vein (Figure 24.7A) (44). The donor ureter is then attached to the recipient's bladder by ureteroneocystostomy. More recently, transplant surgeons have chosen to anastamose the donor renal artery directly to the external iliac artery, thus preserving the integrity of the hypogastric artery (Figure 24.7B).

Following successful transplantation, the recipient gener-

ally experiences an uncomplicated postoperative course and a return to normal renal function within five days with an LRD kidney or within 7–15 days after a cadaveric transplant (2).

Pregnancy after Renal Transplantation

Women in the childbearing age group on chronic dialysis for treatment of ESRD are relatively infertile. Because of their disease, patients experience amenorrhea, anovulatory cycles, and loss of libido. Often, the malaise of chronic anemia compounds their symptoms, necessitating multiple blood transfusions over a prolonged period of time and diminishing their quality of life. Recombinant human erythropoietin (45) only very recently available, has been utilized to successfully reverse the chronic anemia of ESRD and to eliminate the need for perpetual blood transfusions. Renal transplantation, available for well over three decades worldwide, reverses the loss of libido and renders the patient with ESRD fertile again, usually within six months after successful transplantation (46). Maintenance dialysis therapy, on the other hand, is associated with improved sexual function in only 6% of women (47). Whereas one in 200 women of childbearing age conceives while on dialysis (48), one in 50 becomes pregnant following transplantation (49, 50).

Klein (51), as well as Davison and Lindheimer (52), recommend that women contemplating pregnancy posttransplantation wait at least 18 months to two years to allow time for stabilization of graft function and for surveillance of graft rejection. During this time, as fertility is reestablished, women should use barrier contraceptive methods such as the diaphragm, cervical cap, or condoms in order to avoid hypertensive and thromboembolic risks of oral contraceptives and the possible infectious complications of the intrauterine device (IUD), particularly in immunosuppressed patients. Research indicates (49-53) further that women attempting to conceive should be free of proteinuria and hypertension and, of course, demonstrate no laboratory signs or clinical symptoms of allograft rejection (Table 24.7). Prior to conception, the recipient's serum creatinine level should be less than 2.0 mg/dL, and renal ultrasonography should demonstrate no abnormality in the

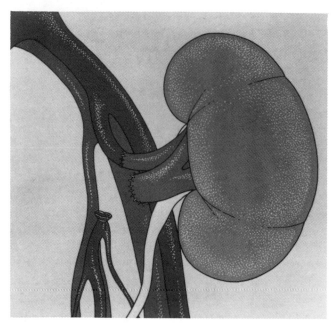

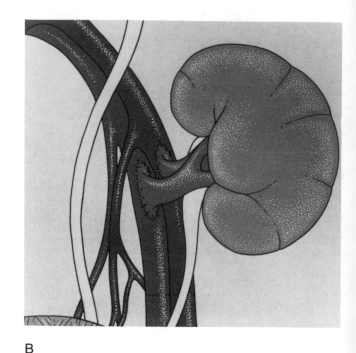

A

B

Figure 24.7   Technique of renal transplantation.

Reprinted with permission from Garovoy MR, Vincenti F, Amend WJC, et al. Renal transplantation, the modern era. New York: Gower Medical Publishing, 1987.

allograft; in particular, no dilatation should be apparent in the allograft's collecting system. Lastly, the recipient's doses of immunosuppressive medications should be at minimum daily levels.

Obstetricians, nephrologists, transplant surgeons, internists, and other physicians who attend renal transplant patients must thoroughly counsel fertile women regarding the risks of pregnancy. Theses risks are associated with morbidity and include deterioration or impairment of allograft function, pregnancy-induced hypertension (PIH), and premature labor and intrauterine growth retardation (IUGR). Penn and co-workers (49) addressed the risks of pregnancy in their 1980 publication of pertinent data on 56 pregnancies in 37 women with renal allografts treated at the University of Colorado and Denver VA Medical Centers from 1962 to 1979. Of interest, 25 of the women (67.5%) required renal transplantation because of ESRD secondary to chronic glomerulonephritis, while chronic pyelonephritis was the primary cause for renal failure in five (13.5%) of the

women. Twenty-nine women received LRD, and eight received cadaveric donor transplants. Five of the 37 women required two or more renal transplants before conception occurred. Forty-six of the 56 pregnancies (82%) occurred in the 29 women with LRD transplants, while only 10 (18%) occurred in the eight cadaveric recipients.

Table 24.7   Evidence of Allograft Rejection

Clinical Signs
Graft enlargement and tenderness
Low grade fever (37.8–38.0° C)
Decreasing urinary output
Hypertension
Retention of fluid
Increasing weight gain

Laboratory Signs
Rising BUN and serum creatinine
Increasing serum B_2 microglobulins

Of the 56 pregnancies reported, three were currently ongoing, nine resulted in early terminations (one reported ectopic gestation, one spontaneous and two elective abortions, five medically indicated abortions for impaired renal function and/or hypertension), and 43 resulted in livebirths ranging from 27 to 42 weeks' gestation. One pregnancy resulted in a 38-week antepartum stillbirth unrelated to medical or obstetrical causation. Thirty-four (79%) of the 43 livebirths were at 36 or more weeks' gestation, while nine (21%) were between 27 and 35 weeks. Thirty-five of the livebirths were appropriate for gestational age (AGA) in birthweight, two were large (LGA), and six (14%) were small for gestational age (SGA).

In 21 (37.5%) of the 56 pregnancies reported, hypertension and/or evidence of impaired renal allograft function predated conception, and five of these pregnancies were medically terminated in early gestation. In 10 pregnancies complicated by prior renal allograft impairment, superimposed preeclampsia was encountered in late gestation, while PIH occurred in five pregnancies with normal allograft function, raising the incidence of preeclampsia in this study to 27%. In four of the 56 pregnancies (7%), deterioration of renal allograft function was attributable to pregnancy, but in only one of the four pregnancies was renal allograft function normal prior to pregnancy.

Davison and Lindheimer (54), in a survey of 40 reports published over a 20-year period from 1963 to 1982, compiled the outcomes of 759 pregnancies in women with renal transplants. Over 80% of the reported cases occurred in women with cadaveric kidneys. Forty-two percent of the pregnancies reviewed were terminated by the end of the first trimester—14% spontaneously and 28% induced—for a variety of reasons, including unplanned pregnancy, concerns for maternal survival, unstable renal function, and hypertension. Of the remaining 58% of pregnancies, over 80% were completed successfully.

Their survey pointed out that proteinuria occurred near term in 30%–40% of patients but generally disappeared postpartum in those patients with normal allograft function. Normal graft functioning was most often determined by a serum creatinine level of less than 2 mg/dL and a rise in the glomerular filtration rate (GFR), as measured by the 24-hour creatinine clearance test (55). Transient reductions in the 24-hour creatinine clearance may occur during the third trimester (56-58) (Figure 24.8) but may also occur in normal pregnancy (59). Approximately 9% of renal transplant recipients experienced rejection episodes in the third trimester of pregnancy or postpartum (50), a rate comparable to that seen in nonpregnant recipients. The incidence of PIH was in the range of 30%, similar to that reported by Penn and co-workers (49), but only one reported case was found where a renal transplant recipient actually experienced eclampsia.

In addressing the neonatal outcomes of these 759 pregnancies, the authors reported a 20% incidence of SGA births, many of which were attributable to the maternal complications of severe renal impairment, vascular disease, and/or hypertension during pregnancy. Davison, however, referring to data from his own institution, Princess Mary

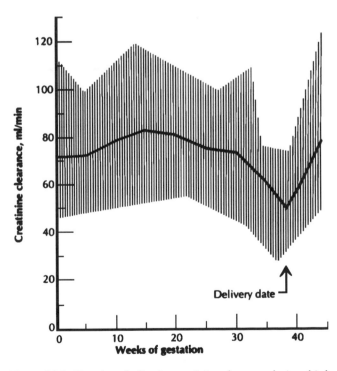

Figure 24.8 Transient decline in creatinine clearance during third trimester.

Reprinted with permission from Merkatz IR, Goldfarb JM. The renal transplant patient. In: Queenan JT, ed. Management of high-risk pregnancy. 1st ed. Oradell, NJ: Medical Economics Company, 1980.

Maternity Hospital, Newcastle upon Tyne, England, reported an SGA incidence in transplant patients of 40% without an apparent antecedent maternal or obstetrical cause. The authors also reported that a majority of AGA infants in their survey were of low birthweight secondary to preterm delivery.

Despite the significantly increased incidences of preterm and SGA births, over 60% of neonates delivered of transplant mothers experienced normal neonatal outcomes. Management of neonates who experienced problems relating to preterm or SGA births was identical to that of nontransplant offspring. Some special problems were occasionally encountered, however, including thymic atrophy, thrombocytopenia, transient leukopenia, and septicemia, often due to adrenocortical insufficiency secondary to maternal corticosteroid therapy. No predominant congenital or developmental abnormalities have been linked to children of renal transplant recipients.

In 1987, Davison (60) provided an updated survey of 1,569 pregnancies in 1,009 women with renal transplants (80% cadaveric, 20% LRD). His findings were very similar to the data reported in the 1982 survey (54) in that almost 40% of pregnancies were terminated in the first trimester (16% spontaneous, 22% elective or medically indicated, and 0.5% ectopic). The remaining 60% had successful pregnancy outcomes in 92% of the cases. Although neonatal outcome was complicated by a prematurity rate that approached 60%, and 20% of the offspring were SGA, over 50% of all neonates born to renal transplant recipients had no neonatal problems. Those with problems experienced respiratory distress syndrome, leukopenia, thrombocytopenia, adrenocortical insufficiency, and sepsis. The risk of CMV and viral hepatitis were of particular concern to neonatologists because of the longstanding maternal exposure to immunosuppressive medications and multiple blood transfusions.

Sturgiss and Davison (61), in a recent study of 22 pregnancies in 17 allograft recipients over 28 weeks' gestation, searched for preconception and early pregnancy clinical markers or clues that could prospectively predict pregnancy complications and adverse perinatal outcomes. The authors divided their 22 reported pregnancies into two groups: the first comprised of 10 pregnancies with adverse outcomes (five stillbirths, four SGA infants, and one neonatal death) and the second comprised of 12 pregnancies with satisfactory perinatal outcomes. Although the outcomes in each group were disparate, maternal allograft function, as determined by serial serum creatinine levels and 24-hour creatinine clearance studies, did not differ. The clinical marker that distinguished adverse from normal pregnancy outcome was hypertension, defined as a mean arterial pressure (MAP) above 107 mm Hg, equivalent to a blood pressure of over 140/90. MAP was statistically significantly higher at 16, 20, 24, and 28 weeks' gestation in pregnancies with an adverse outcome. When hypertension occurred before 28 weeks' gestation, it was always associated with a perinatal complication.

In a subsequent study, Sturgiss and Davison (62) matched 18 renal transplant recipients who conceived a total of 34 pregnancies with 18 nulliparous controls to determine the impact of pregnancy on long-term allograft survival and function. The patients were matched for age, date of transplantation, immunosuppressive medication, early rejection episodes, and LRD or cadaveric donor, and were followed over a mean period of 12 years (range 4–23 years). Periodic renal assessments, including plasma creatinine levels and determinations of the glomerular filtration rate (GFR) by infusion clearance of inulin and measurements of blood pressure, precluded a major deleterious effect of pregnancy on allograft survival and function. The authors further concluded that pregnancy in these patients did not result in nor aggravate a chronic hypertensive condition in transplant recipients. Although this study includes only 36 study patients, its data on long-term graft survival are unique and definitely supportive of childbearing in renal allograft recipients who wish to conceive.

Obstetrical Management of the Organ Recipient

Allograft recipients who report a resumption of their menstrual cycles following successful transplantation surgery must receive thorough contraceptive counselling from their nephrologists, transplant surgeons, and gynecologists in order to prevent an undesired pregnancy when there is high risk for poor pregnancy outcome. Only selected patients, carefully screened by their physicians regarding their medical conditions, should be counselled to conceive if they choose to do so. As reiterated by Lindheimer and Katz (63) in their recent editorial, certain preconditions must be met before a transplant recipient considers attempting pregnancy:

1. An LRD recipient should wait one year and a CD recipient two years before conception in order to verify normal allograft function.
2. Immunosuppressive therapy must be at low daily maintenance levels.
3. Plasma creatinine level must be less than 2.0 mg/dL and preferably less than 1.5 mg/dL.
4. Hypertension should be absent or easily controlled.
5. Proteinuria should be absent or minimal.
6. There should be no clinical or laboratory evidence of graft rejection.
7. No evidence of pelvicalyceal distention should be found on renal ultrasonography.

Patients who conceive must be referred as early in pregnancy as possible to an obstetrician-gynecologist, preferably a maternal-fetal medicine specialist, practicing in a tertiary level hospital. The obstetrician should closely coordinate all care and testing procedures in close consultation with the patient's nephrologist, transplant surgeon, and pediatrician so that all consulting physicians are apprised of the patient's progress throughout pregnancy. Antepartum visits should generally be scheduled at two-week intervals for the first half of pregnancy and weekly thereafter for the remainder of the gestational period. Appointments should be coordinated so that the patient is able to consult with her obstetrician and nephrologist or transplant surgeon during each visit to the hospital or outpatient facility.

In addition to the routine antepartum laboratory tests drawn on every patient, the pregnant transplant recipient should have the following tests performed every two weeks:

BUN
Creatinine
Hematocrit
White blood count
Follicle-stimulating hormone (FSH)

Luteinizing hormone (LH)
Estradiol
Beta 2 microglobulin
Urinalysis
Urine culture and sensitivity

A 24-hour urine collection should also be obtained every two weeks for determination of total protein excretion, creatinine clearance, and urinary levels of sodium, chloride, potassium, and creatinine.

An ultrasound of the allograft should be performed monthly to determine renal size, position, rotation, if any, during pregnancy, and to detect early evidence of calyceal-ureteral distention secondary to allograft rotation or obstruction. Technetium renal scanning (64) is also recommended once each trimester and postpartum to assess allograft perfusion and function.

Plasma protein, calcium and phosphate levels, and cytomegalovirus (CMV) titers should be checked at six-week intervals. Hepatitis screening is performed on the initial prenatal visit. Patients with positive CMV or hepatitis screen or persistent urinary tract infections should be referred to an infectious disease specialist to ensure proper treatment and disposition of the condition as early in pregnancy as possible.

All patients should be questioned thoroughly and examined carefully at each prenatal visit to detect the early warning signs and symptoms of preterm labor, PIH, and fetal growth retardation, the three most common obstetrical problems causing adverse pregnancy outcomes in allograft recipients.

A thorough level II ultrasonographic evaluation of the pregnancy should be performed every three weeks throughout pregnancy to determine fetal growth and development and to detect fetal growth retardation or other abnormalities such as the development of oligohydramnios, premature placental aging, or premature cervical effacement and dilatation.

Because every organ recipient is at high risk for an adverse pregnancy outcome, antepartum surveillance of fetal well-being should commence at 24–26 weeks' gestational age and continue serially throughout the remainder of pregnancy on at least a weekly basis. The physicians managing these patients should schedule the appropriate combination of antepartum testing techniques from the spectrum of tests available today—fetal kick counts, nonstress tests (NST) and contraction stress tests (CST) of the fetal heart rate, amniotic fluid index (AFI), fetal biophysical profile (BPP), and amniocentesis (for fetal lung maturity)—to ensure that continuation of the pregnancy is not detrimental to maternal or fetal health. As emphasized by Davison (60), "meticulous monitoring of fetal well-being is the key to a successful outcome."

Because approximately half of the renal transplant recipients reported to date have experienced preterm delivery, patients should be taught the signs and symptoms of premature labor. Daily home monitoring of uterine activity and/or daily telephone contact with designated obstetrical nurse specialists is advisable to detect the onset of preterm labor. When preterm labor is suspected, the patient should be admitted to the hospital for assessment and commencement of tocolysis, if necessary.

Careful monitoring of blood pressure, weight gain, and proteinuria is indicated throughout pregnancy because all allograft recipients are at risk for PIH, and many have underlying chronic hypertension. Hospitalization, bed rest, and close surveillance of both maternal and fetal well-being is mandatory to prevent an untoward pregnancy outcome.

Allograft recipients should await the spontaneous onset of labor and anticipate vaginal delivery as term approaches, unless a specific maternal or fetal indication for induction of labor or cesarean delivery pertains. Obstruction of the birth canal by the renal allograft is rare but has been reported (65). For the majority of allograft recipients who achieve viable pregnancies, vaginal delivery is safe (66).

Patients in labor or with premature rupture of membranes (PROM) should be admitted to the hospital and managed according to accepted obstetrical practice. However, specialized care as follows is warranted:

1. Maternal fluid and electrolyte balance must be maintained at all times. Adequate hydration is essential to maintain allograft perfusion and satisfactory urinary output.
2. Augmentation of corticosteroid therapy is indicated to cover the stress of labor, delivery, and the immediate postpartum period.
3. Careful monitoring of blood pressure recordings is necessary to detect PIH or superimposed preeclampsia.
4. Careful aseptic technique must be maintained whenever invasive procedures (venopuncture, urinary bladder catherization, intrauterine monitoring) are performed.
5. Meticulous observation of maternal temperature recordings is indicated to detect early onset of sepsis in an immunocompromised patient.
6. Prophylactic antibiotic coverage should be administered to the mother immediately following delivery of the baby.
7. Neonatal personnel must be at delivery to immediately care for the newborn at risk for complications such as respiratory distress syndrome (RDS), transient leukopenia, hypoglycemia, septicemia, and other problems common to premature or SGA neonates.

As indicated in all high-risk patients, continuous monitoring of the fetal heart rate and uterine contractions should be employed to evaluate fetal condition throughout labor.

Postpartum, the patient must be evaluated carefully to detect any signs, symptoms, or laboratory evidence of graft rejection. Following discharge from the hospital, the patient should be seen weekly by the transplant surgeon for the next two to three months to maintain surveillance of allograft function.

At the six weeks' postpartum examination, the obstetrician-gynecologist should thoroughly discuss contraception, and an appropriate method should be prescribed. Thereafter, renal transplant recipients should be examined every six months and carefully screened for human papillomavirus (HPV) infection and cervical neoplasia. As reported by Halpert (67) and others (68), immunocompromised patients have increased rates of HPV infection, cervical neoplasia, and cervical carcinoma that are respectively five-fold, eight-fold and thirteen-fold, over that seen in the general population. Gynecologic management of these or any other gynecologic disorder is identical to that of immunocompetent women.

References

1. Berlyne GM, Giovannetti S. When should entry into a regular hemodialysis programme occur? Nephron 1976; 16:81.

2. Flye MW. Renal transplantation In: Flye MW, ed. Principles of organ transplantation. Philadelphia: WB Saunders Company, 1989.

3. Perryman JP, Stillerman PU. Kidney transplantation. In: Smith SL, ed. Tissue and organ transplantation. St. Louis: Mosby Yearbook, 1990.

4. Canadian Renal Failure Registry. 1984 Report. Montreal: The Kidney Foundation of Canada, 1985.

5. Luke RG. Renal replacement therapy. N Engl J Med 1983; 308:1593.

6. Wing AJ, Selwood NH. Achievements and problems in the treatment of end stage renal failure. In: Jones NF, Peters DK, ed. Recent advances in renal medicine 2. London: Churchill Livingstone, 1982.

7. Pendreigh DM, Heasman MA, et al. Survey of chronic renal failure in Scotland. Lancet 1972;i:304.

8. McGeown M. Chronic renal failure in Northern Ireland, 1968–70. Lancet 1972;i:307.

9. Broyer M. Incidence and etiology of ESRD in children. In: Fine RN, Gruskin AB, eds. End stage renal disease in children. Philadelphia: WB Saunders Company, 1984.

10. Potter DE, Holliday MA, et al. Treatment of end-stage renal disease in children: a 15 year experience. Kidney Int. 1980; 18:103.

11. Alexander S. Treatment of infants with ESRD. In: Fine RN, Gruskin AB, eds. End stage renal disease in children. Philadelphia:WB Saunders Company, 1984.

12. Fine RN. Renal transplantation in children. In: Morris PF, ed. Kidney transplantation, principles and practice. 2nd ed. London: Grune and Stratten, Inc., 1984.

13. Brynger H, Brunner FP, et al. Combined report on regular dialysis and transplantation in Europe, X, 1979. Proceedings of the European Dialysis Transplants Association 1980; 17:2.

14. Goldstein DA, Massry SG. Diabetic nephropathy: clinical course and effect of hemodialysis. Nephron 1978;20:286.

15. Burton BT, Hirschman GH. Diabetic-renal-retinal syndrome. In: Diabetes in the USA: a demographic overview. Friedman EA, L'Esperance FA, eds. New York: Grune and Stratton, 1979.

16. Habib R, Broyer M, et al. Chronic renal failure in children. Causes, rate of deterioration and survival data. Nephron 1973;11:209.

17. Leumann EP. Die chronische Nieren in suffizienz in Kindesalter. Schweiz Med Wochensch 1976;106:244.

18. Helin I, Winberg J. Chronic renal failure in Swedish children. Acta Paediatr Scand 1980;69:607.

19. Donckerwolcke R, Broyer M, et al. Combined report on regular dialysis and transplantation of children in Europe, 1981. Proceedings of the European Dialysis Transplant Association 1982;19:61.

20. Arant BS. Renal disorders of newborn infant. In: Brenner BM, et al., eds. Contemporary issues in nephrology, volume 12, pediatric nephrology. New York: Churchill Livingstone, 1984.

21. Blagg CR. The role of dialysis in the management of end-stage renal disease. In: Cerilli GJ, ed. Organ transplantation and replacement. Philadelphia: J.B. Lippincott Company, 1988.

22. Tenckhoff H, Schechter H. A bacteriologically safe peritoneal access device. Trans Am Soc Artif Intern Organs 1968; 14:181.

23. Hamilton D. Kidney transplantation: a history. Morris PS, ed. Kidney transplantation, principles and practice, 2nd edition. London: Grune and Stratton, Inc., 1984.

24. Murray JE, Merrill JP, Harrison JH. Kidney transplantation between seven pairs of identical twins. Ann Surg 1958; 148:343.

25. Murray JE, Merrill JP, et al. Prolonged survival of human kidney homografts by immunosuppressive drug therapy. N Engl J Med 1963;268:1315.

26. Howard RJ, Condie RM, et al. The use of antilymphoblast globulin in the treatment of renal allograft rejection. Transplantation 1977;24:419.

27. Debure A, Chkoff N, et al. One-month prophylactic use of OKT3 in cadaveric kidney transplant recipients. Transplantation 1988;45:546.

28. Canafax DM, Sutherland DER, et al. Combination immunosuppression. Three drugs (azathioprine, cyclosporine, prednisone) for mismatched related and four drugs (+ ALG) for cadaver renal allograft recipients. Transplant Proc 1985; 17:2671.

29. Held PJ, Pauly MV, Diamond L. Survival analysis of patients undergoing dialysis. JAMA 1987;257:654.

30. Broyer M, Brunner FP, et al. Combined report on regular dialysis and transplantation in Europe, XII, 1981. Proceed-

ings of the European Dialysis Transplant Association 1982; 19:2.

31. Statement by Carolyne K. Davis, PhD, Administrator, Health Care Financing Administration, before the Subcommittee on Health, Committee on Finance, United States Senate, September 28, 1981.

32. Cerilli GJ. Management of the adult renal transplant patient. In: Cerilli GJ, ed. Organ transplantation and replacement. Philadelphia: J.B. Lippincott Co. 1988.

33. Cerilli GJ. Highlights of recent progress in transplantation. In: Cerilli GJ, ed. Organ transplantation and replacement. Philadelphia: J.B. Lippincott Co. 1988.

34. Kahn BD. Transplantation timeline. Transplantation 1991; 50:1.

35. Terasaki P, Mickey MR, et al. Long term survival of kidney grafts. Transplant Proc 1989;21:615.

36. Task Force on Organ Transplantation (April, 1986). Organ transplantation: issues and recommendations: report of the Task Force on Organ Transplantation. Rockville, MD: Health Resources and Services Administration (NTIS No HRP-0906976).

37. 1991 Annual Data Report, United States Renal Data System. Am J Kidney Dis 1991;18(Suppl 2):61.

38. Kaplan EI, Meier P. Nonparametric estimation from incomplete observations. J Am Stat Assoc 1958;53:457.

39. Vollmer WM, Wahl PW, Blagg CR. Survival with dialysis and transplantation in patients with end-stage renal disease. N Engl J Med 1983;308:1553.

40. Evans RW, Manninen DL, et al. The quality of life of patients with end-stage renal disease. N Engl J Med 1985;312:553.

41. American Society of Transplant Physicians (1988). Statement of criteria for selection of ESRD patients for renal transplantation. Alexandria, VA: American Council on Transplantation.

42. Haag BW, Stuart FP. The organ donor: brain death, selection criteria, supply and demand. In: Flye MW, ed. Principles of organ transplantation. Philadelphia: WB Saunders Company, 1989.

43. Leary FJ Deweerd JH. Living donor nephrectomy. J Urol 1973;109:947.

44. Garovoy MR, Vincenti F. Amend WJC, et al. Renal transplantation, the modern era. New York: Gower Medical Publishing Ltd, 1987.

45. Eschbach JW, Egrie JC, et al. Correction of the anemia of end-stage renal disease with recombinant human erythropoietin. N Engl J Med 1987;316:73.

46. Waltzer W. The urinary tract in pregnancy. J Urol 1981; 125:271.

47. Levy NB. Sexual adjustment to maintenance hemodialysis and renal transplantation: National Survey by questionnaire, preliminary report. Trans Am Soc Artif Intern Organs 1973;19:138.

48. Editorial. Pregnancy after renal transplantation. Br Med J 1976;1:733.

49. Penn I, Makowski E, Harris P. Parenthood following renal transplantation. Kidney Int 1980;18:22.

50. Rudolph J, Schweizer R, Bartos S. Pregnancy in renal transplant patients. Transplantation 1979;27:26.

51. Klein EA. Urologic problems in pregnancy. Obstet Gynecol Surv 1984;39:605.

52. Davison JM, Lindheimer MD. Renal disorders. In: Creasy RK, Resnick R, eds. Maternal-fetal medicine: principles and practice, 2nd ed. Philadelphia: W.B. Saunders Company, 1989.

53. Cunningham R, Buszta C, et al. Pregnancy in renal allograft recipients and long term follow-up of their offspring. Transplant Proc 1983;15:1067.

54. Davison JM, Lindheimer MD. Pregnancy in renal transplant patients. J Reprod Med 1982;27:613.

55. Merkatz IR, Goldfarb JM. The renal transplant patient. In: Queenan JT, ed., Management of high-risk pregnancy, 1st ed. Oradell: Medical Economics Company, 1980.

56. Merkatz IR, Schwartz GH, et al. Resumption of female reproductive function following renal transplantation. JAMA 1971;216:1749.

57. Rifle G, Traeger J. Pregnancy after renal transplantation: an international survey. Transplant Proc 1975;7:723.

58. Warren SE, Mitas JA, Evertson LR. Pregnancy after renal transplantation: reversible acidosis and renal dysfunction. South Med J 1981;74:1139.

59. Davison JM, Dunlop W, Ezimokhai M. 24-hour creatine clearance during the third trimester of normal pregnancy. Br J Obstet Gynaecol 1980;87:106.

60. Davison JM, Renal transplantation and pregnancy. Am J Kidney Dis 1987;1:374.

61. Sturgiss SN, Davison JM. Perinatal outcome in renal allograft recipients: prognostic significance of hypertension and renal function before and during pregnancy. Obstet Gynecol 1991;78:573.

62. Sturgiss SN, Davison JM. Effect of pregnancy on long-term function of renal allografts. Am J Kidney Dis 1992; XIX:167.

63. Lindheimer MD, Katz AI. Pregnancy in the renal transplant patient. Am J Kidney Dis 1992;XIX:173.

64. Goldstein HA, Ziessman HA, et al. Renal scans in pregnant transplant patients. J Nuc Med 1988;29:1364.

65. Nolan GH, Sweet RL, et al. Renal cadaver transplantation followed by successful pregnancies. Obstet Gynecol 1974; 43:732.

66. Davison JM. Dialysis, transplantation and pregnancy. Am J Kidney Dis 1991;XVII:127.

67. Halpert R, Fruchter RG, et al. Human papillomavirus and lower genital neoplasia in renal transplant patients. Obstet Gynecol 1986;68:251.

68. Schneider V, Kay S, Lee HM. Immunosuppression as a high-risk factor in the development of condyloma accumulation and squamous neoplasia of the cervix. Acta Cytol 1983; 27:220.

25

Gestational Diabetes

Donald R. Coustan, M.D.

GESTATIONAL diabetes, much more common than preexisting diabetes, complicates 2%–3% of pregnancies in the United States. Women with gestational diabetes are at increased risk of developing overt diabetes (usually type II) later in life. Their pregnancies also appear to be at risk for perinatal morbidity and perhaps even perinatal mortality.

The diagnosis of gestational diabetes has been defined as "carbohydrate intolerance with onset or first recognition during pregnancy" (1). Therefore, it is not necessary to defer diagnosis until it can be proven that the abnormality of carbohydrate metabolism has abated after delivery, as required by previous definitions. A woman with gestational diabetes who has persistent carbohydrate intolerance after delivery may then be reclassified as having impaired glucose tolerance, type I or type II diabetes.

Glucose tolerance testing protocols during pregnancy are not universally agreed upon. After an overnight fast and two days of adequate carbohydrate intake, a 100-g glucose challenge is administered in the United States, whereas 75 or 50-g challenges are used in many other countries. Diagnostic criteria used here are based upon the original work of O'Sullivan and Mahan in which fasting, one-, two-, and three-hour mean values were derived, and the threshold set at two standard deviations above each of the means (2). Any two thresholds met or exceeded denoted gestational diabetes, based upon the likelihood of the later development of overt diabetes. Their thresholds, based upon whole blood samples with glucose analysis by the Somogyi–Nelson methodology, are: fasting, 90 mg/dL; one hour, 165 mg/dL; two hours, 145 mg/dL; and three hours, 125 mg/dL.

In the years following the publication of these widely accepted criteria, most laboratories switched from whole blood to plasma or serum samples. Since such samples yield glucose values approximately 14% higher than whole blood, the National Diabetes Data Group (NDDG) in 1979 published an adaptation of these criteria for plasma or serum: fasting, 105 mg/dL; one hour, 190 mg/dL; two hours, 165 mg/dL; and three hours, 145 mg/dL (3).

These NDDG criteria have been endorsed by the American Diabetes Association (ADA) and the American College of Obstetricians and Gynecologists (ACOG) and are widely accepted. However, in our own center, we do ived a different set of criteria, based upon the fact that the Somogyi-Nelson technique detects about 5 mg/dL of reducing substances other than glucose. These substances are not detected by more specific current methods, such as glucose oxidase or hexokinase. Thus, the criteria we have proposed are: fasting, 95 mg/dL; one hour, 180 mg/dL; two hours, 155 mg/dL; and three hours, 140 mg/dL (4). Henceforth, NDDG refers to the criteria endorsed by the ACOG and other organizations, and C&C refers to our own criteria.

Screening Tests

Traditionally, the 100-g oral glucose tolerance test (OGTT) has been administered to pregnant women who meet certain criteria, or risk factors, based upon their past histories. Such risk factors include a previous large baby, a previous adverse obstetric outcome, a family history of diabetes, or glycosuria during the present pregnancy. A number of studies have shown that only approximately 50% of women with gestational diabetes have such risk factors (5). This finding is not surprising since many of the risk factors imply a previous pregnancy complicated by undiagnosed gestational diabetes. Therefore, a 50-g, one-hour glucose challenge was devised by O'Sullivan's group as a screening test (6). ACOG has recommended that this screening test be applied to all pregnant women aged 30 years or more, with younger women screened if historic risk factors are present (7). A plasma glucose level of 140 mg/dL or more one hour after the challenge would require that the woman undergo a three-hour, 100-g OGTT. The ADA has recommended that all pregnant women be screened (8). A recent study from our center demonstrated that following the ACOG protocol would lead to the diagnosis of only 35% of the cases of gestational diabetes (NDDG criteria) in a given population, while lowering the age for universal screening to 25 years would result in the diagnosis of 85% of cases, with little additional cost (5). Universal screening with a threshold of 140 mg/dL would lead to the diagnosis of 90% of cases in the population, while lowering the threshold from 140 mg/dL to 130 mg/dL would presumably diagnose all cases. It is possible, however, that some

women with gestational diabetes had screening test values below 130 mg/dL and thus went undetected.

There is no "perfect" number to use as a threshold, just as there is no "perfect" maternal age cutoff to use for screening. If the goal is to achieve maximal sensitivity, universal screening with a threshold of 130 mg/dL makes sense. If some sensitivity can be sacrificed, missing 35% of cases, in order to reduce the number of needed OGTTs from 23% of the population to approximately 10% of the population, the ACOG recommendations make sense.

Current recommendations are that screening be performed at 24–28 weeks' gestation in order to make the diagnosis in a timely fashion, yet late enough for the carbohydrate metabolic changes of pregnancy to be at or near their maximum. It is certainly permissible to screen earlier if there is a strong suspicion, provided a negative screening test is repeated at 24–28 weeks. If a particular patient manifests one abnormal value on the three-hour OGTT, this test should be repeated approximately one month later (9). Because of a lack of precision, screening with test strips and reflectance meters is not recommended (10).

Initial Management

Once the diagnosis of gestational diabetes has been made, it is imperative the patient be counselled without delay. Although there does not appear to be any long-lasting psychological effect, many patients with gestational diabetes become quite concerned and need explanations and reassurance (11). Although the original work of the O'Sullivan team disclosed a markedly increased perinatal mortality rate among untreated gestational diabetics, more recent studies have demonstrated that, with just about any intervention, the postnatal mortality rate is similar to that in the general obstetric population (12). It is useful to provide some written material for the patient to read and share with her family. One patient publication from the American Diabetes Association describes various aspects of the problem in detail (13). However, it is important that obstetricians familiarize themselves with the contents of such publications in order to be prepared to discuss any philosophical disagreements he or she has with the information presented.

Glucose Testing

The most important component of care for women with gestational diabetes is the periodic measurement of circulating glucose levels. A certain proportion of such patients, ranging from 10% to 80% depending upon the particular center, will manifest hyperglycemia severe enough to pose a risk to fetal survival. Although there is not total agreement as to what level of glucose is too high, we use the same thresholds for gestational diabetic patients as we would in an overt insulin-taking diabetic patient: a fasting glucose exceeding 100 mg/dL or a two-hour postmeal value exceeding 120 mg/dL. Some centers use 105 mg/dL as the fasting threshold, and some use 140 mg/dL as a one-hour postmeal threshold. The most important issue is that glucose must be measured periodically. Although in our center we obtain a "set" of glucose measurements (fasting, two hours after breakfast, two hours after lunch) once each week, many centers advise their patients with gestational diabetes to perform self-glucose monitoring at home four to six times daily, just as is standard in the overt diabetic. This approach, while not always practical, may represent the ideal.

Diet Counseling

Each patient should receive nutritional counseling from a trained dietician familiar with the needs of both pregnancy and gestational diabetes. We favor a diet that contains 30–35 kcal/kg of ideal body weight, divided into three meals and one or two snacks. The diet is high in protein (125 g/day). Other diets that are high in fiber or carbohydrate have also been suggested. Opinion is currently mixed as to whether hypocaloric diets are appropriate for obese women with gestational diabetes (14). There is no evidence for adverse effects of such diets if ketosis does not occur.

Therapeutic Insulin

When circulating glucose levels exceed the established thresholds, there is an increased likelihood of perinatal mortality, as evidenced by the data of Karlsson and Kjellmer (15). To reduce that risk, presumably associated with fetal hyperglycemia and resultant fetal hyperinsulinemia, it is necessary to add insulin to the dietary management already in place. Insulin therapy should produce lower maternal glucose levels, with lower fetal glucose and insulin levels. Therefore, fetal macrosomia, neonatal hypoglycemia, hyperbilirubinemia, and respiratory distress syndrome should also be less likely. When insulin is needed, if the patient is at 28 weeks' gestation or beyond, we generally start with a combination of 20 units of NPH insulin (human) and 10 units regular insulin (human), mixed in the same syringe and injected prior to breakfast each morning. This dose is certainly not excessive for a pregnant woman in the third trimester, particularly with gestational diabetes uncontrolled by diet. However, women who are in earlier stages of pregnancy are started on a regimen at half the above dose. Patients started on insulin are also generally asked to perform self-glucose monitoring four times daily in order to evaluate the appropriateness of the insulin dose. The regular insulin is reflected in the two hours postbreakfast glucose level, and the NPH in the afternoon level, with some carryover to the next morning.

If a particular patient has an acceptable glucose level in the afternoon, but an elevated level in the evening or prior to breakfast the next morning, a split regimen should be introduced (14). Although hypoglycemia is extremely unlikely in this group of patients, they should be informed about the possibility and instructed on measures to take to correct it (that is, a mixed carbohydrate and protein snack).

Macrosomia Prevention

When metabolic control is good, perinatal mortality should be no higher than in the general population. However, macrosomia continues to be a problem in a higher-than-average proportion of such cases (17). If it is true that fetal hyperinsulinemia is the cause of macrosomia, then the failure of good diabetic control to prevent this problem is perplexing. Perhaps our definition of "good control" is not good enough. It is based on the usual two standard deviations above the mean, but, in fact, most of us accept readings around the mean rather than two standard deviations above it. Even mild disturbances of maternal carbohydrate metabolism have been associated with macrosomia in the offspring (18). Another possibility is that we do not measure

ure glucose often enough to detect subtle disturbances in arbohydrate metabolism that can lead to fetal hyperinsulnemia.

A number of approaches have been used to try to prevent macrosomia. Prophylactic insulin, administered to gestational diabetic women even if they do not exceed the standard glycemic thresholds, has been shown to lower the likelihood of macrosomia and traumatic or operative delivery. Similarly, daily self-glucose monitoring with institution of insulin for even mild hyperglycemia (fasting >90 mg/dL or postprandial >100 mg/dL) has been successful (19).

Obstetric Management

here is controversy surrounding the use of antepartum sting in pregnancies complicated by gestational diabetes. here is evidence that such testing is not necessary prior to rm when diabetic control is optimal and no complications or example, hypertensive disorders or prior stillbirth) exist 0). Daily fetal activity determinations, however, are suggested even for these patients. In our own center, we begin ntepartum testing with weekly nonstress tests at approximately 36 weeks, or earlier if any complications exist. ther centers use biophysical profiles or contraction stress sts. Disagreement over routine testing of otherwise uncomplicated gestational diabetes does not extend to patients ith complications. If, for example, hypertension is also esent, most, if not all, authorities would agree that testing least twice weekly is indicated. The testing method pends upon the customary practice at a particular center.

Ultrasound examination is useful to evaluate fetal owth and look for hydramnios, in addition to the usual dications. We perform scans around the time of diagnosis d again near term to estimate the fetal weight and help ide the choice of mode of delivery.

ming and Mode of Delivery

ie presence of gestational diabetes is not an indication for ly delivery, but its complications may be. The presence pregnancy-induced hypertension, evolving macrosomia, other problems may dictate delivery before the onset of ontaneous labor. Because there may be a delay in pul-

monic maturation related to fetal hyperinsulinemia, we believe that elective induction or cesarean section (CS), even at term, should be deferred until amniocentesis can be done to demonstrate the presence of pulmonic maturity. However, if amniocentesis cannot be accomplished because of oligohydramnios, this can be taken as an indication to proceed with delivery in such a term patient with gestational diabetes.

Gestational diabetes is not an indication for CS. However, because fetal macrosomia may lead to cephalopelvic disproportion or, even worse, to shoulder dystocia, it is more common in such pregnancies. Unfortunately, there is no infallible method for predicting shoulder dystocia. Certain risk factors predispose to this complication, and the clinician should have a low threshold for CS in cases of gestational diabetes with a long second stage of labor requiring midpelvic instrumental delivery. The presence of a macrosomic fetus would also suggest a higher-than-usual risk. Unfortunately, no available method of estimating fetal weight has been shown to be highly reliable. Ultrasound is currently the usual method. Although not entirely satisfied with this system, we generally perform CS without a trial of labor in a woman with gestational diabetes if the estimated fetal weight is greater than 4,500 g. Between 4,000 and 4,500 g, we add clinical judgment as to the dimensions of the pelvis, the patient's previous obstetric history, and the normalcy of the labor progress.

When induction of labor is planned, insulin and breakfast should be omitted in the morning and IV fluids begun. We usually use 5% dextrose in half-normal saline at 125 mL/hour via infusion pump. The oxytocin is infused in normal saline via piggyback. Circulating glucose levels are measured every one to two hours, with a target of 70–120 mg/dL. If the level exceeds 120 mg/dL, regular insulin (10 units/L) is added to the infusate. The insulin concentration can be doubled or halved, as needed, to maintain euglycemia and thus reduce the risk of neonatal hypoglycemia. Although most women with gestational diabetes will not require insulin during labor, it is important to monitor glycemia in order to detect the few who do.

It is particularly important to avoid the rapid infusion of large volumes of glucose-containing solutions, since hyperglycemia in utero may be associated with fetal acidosis. Thus, if rapid IV hydration is necessary prior to institution of conduction anesthesia, nonglucose solutions should be used.

Follow-up Testing

Because of the increased likelihood of developing overt diabetes later in life, women with previous gestational diabetes should be tested with a 75-g, 2-hour oral glucose tolerance test at about the time of the six-week checkup. Criteria for the diagnosis of diabetes are: fasting plasma glucose 140 mg/dL on two occasions or two-hour value ≥200 mg/dL, and one other value (30, 60, or 90 minutes) ≥200 mg/dL. Criteria for the diagnosis of impaired glucose tolerance are: fasting plasma glucose <140 mg/dL, two-hour value between 140 and 200 mg/dL, and any other value (30, 60, or 90 minutes) ≥200 mg/dL. The ADA recommends annual testing thereafter, since approximately half of all individuals with diabetes are asymptomatic and undiagnosed.

References

1. Second International Workshop-Conference on Gestational Diabetes. Summary and recommendations. Diabetes 1985; 34(Suppl 2):123.

2. O'Sullivan JB, Mahan CM. Criteria for the oral glucose tolerance test in pregnancy. Diabetes 1964;13:278.

3. National Diabetes Data Group. Classification of diabetes and glucose intolerance. Diabetes 1979;28:1039.

4. Carpenter MW, Coustan DR. Criteria for screening tests for gestational diabetes. Am J Obstet Gynecol 1982; 144:768.

5. Coustan DR, Nelson C, Carpenter MW, et al. Maternal age and screening for gestational diabetes: a population-based study. Obstet Gynecol 1989;73:577.

6. O'Sullivan JB, Mahan CM, Charles D, et al. Screening criteria for high-risk gestational diabetic patients. Am J Obstet Gynecol 1973;116:895.

7. American College of Obstetricians and Gynecologists. Management of diabetes mellitus in pregnancy. ACOG Tech Bull 1986;92:1.

8. American Diabetes Association. Position statement on gestational diabetes. Diabetes Care 1986;9:430.

9. Neiger R, Coustan DR. The role of repeat glucose tolerance tests in the diagnosis of gestational diabetes. Am J Obstet Gynecol 1991;165:787.

10. Carr S, Coustan DR, Martelly P, et al. Precision of reflectance meters in screening for gestational diabetes. Obstet Gynecol 1989;73:727.

11. Spirito A, Williams C, Ruggiero L, et al. Psychological impact of the diagnosis of gestational diabetes. Obstet Gynecol 1989;73:562.

12. Coustan DR. Screening and diagnosis of gestational diabetes. In: Oates JN, ed. Diabetes in Pregnancy. Baillière's Clinical Obstetrics and Gynaecology 1991;5:293–314.

13. American Diabetes Association. Gestational diabetes: what to expect. Washington DC: ADA, 1989.

14. Knopp RH, Magee MS, Raisys V, et al. Metabolic effects of hypocaloric diets in management of gestational diabetes. Diabetes 1991;40(suppl 2):165.

15. Karlsson K, Kjellmer I. The outcome of diabetic pregnancy in relation to the mother's blood sugar level. Am J Obstet Gynecol 1972;112:213.

16. Coustan DR. Maternal insulin to lower the risk of fetal macrosomia in diabetic pregnancy. Clin Obstet Gynecol 1991; 34:288.

17. Widness JA, Cowett RM, Coustan DR, et al. Neonatal morbidities in infants of mothers with glucose intolerance in pregnancy. Diabetes 1985;34(Suppl 2):61.

18. Langer O, Mazze R. The relationship between large-for-gestational-age infants and glycemic control in women with gestational diabetes. Am J Obstet Gynecol 1988;159:1478.

19. Coustan DR. The use of prophylactic insulin in women with gestational diabetes. In: Weiss PAM, Coustan DR, eds. Gestational diabetes. Vienna: Springer-Verlag, 1988: 134–41.

20. Landon MB, Gabbe SG. Antepartum fetal surveillance in gestational diabetes mellitus. Diabetes 1985; 34(Suppl 2):50.

26

Diabetes Mellitus

Steven G. Gabbe, M.D.

THE time-honored method of managing the pregnant diabetic patient has been by means of elective premature delivery at some arbitrary date—usually between 36 and 38 weeks' gestation—in an attempt to prevent fetal demise. With advances in antepartum fetal monitoring and improved techniques for determining fetal maturity, however, management can now be varied to suit the individual patient, more diabetic patients can be brought to term, and perinatal mortality rates from stillbirth, prematurity, and birth injury can be markedly reduced. It is important that the obstetrician who occasionally manages diabetic patients become familiar with the uses and limitations of some of the newer methods now practiced in large obstetrics services that deliver many diabetic patients.

At present, the leading cause of perinatal mortality in pregnancies complicated by insulin-dependent diabetes mellitus is the fatal congenital malformation. The risk of major malformations in such pregnancies is increased three- to fourfold over the 2%–3% incidence noted in the general population. There is increasing evidence that these anomalies are due to marked alterations in maternal glycemic control during the critical period of fetal embryogenesis, five to eight weeks' gestation. Patients whose diabetes is poorly regulated are also at greater risk for a spontaneous abortion. For this reason, treatment of the woman with insulin-dependent diabetes who is considering a pregnancy should be initiated before conception (1). In this way, optimal glucose control can be achieved. In addition, thorough evaluation should be made to detect evidence of maternal retinopathy, nephropathy, or coronary artery disease.

Initial Evaluation

On the patient's first prenatal visit, it is important to take a careful history and physical examination paying special attention to the following:

1. Careful dating of the pregnancy by history and physical signs
2. Classification of the diabetic patient, using White's criteria (Table 26.1)
3. Progress and outcome of any previous pregnancies
4. Careful funduscopic examination for presence of retinopathy

5. Findings of urinalysis and culture
6. Baseline blood pressure measurement
7. Baseline glycosylated hemoglobin measurement
8. Thorough instruction about insulin dosage, importance of adhering to the prescribed diet, and home glucose monitoring

Regulating Maternal Glycemia

Careful control of maternal glucose levels significantly improves perinatal outcome. Except for brief periods after meals, these levels should normally remain below 100 mg/dL. Maternal hyperglycemia and rapid fluctuations in blood glucose produce similar changes in the fetal compartment. Fetal hyperglycemia leads to β-cell hyperplasia and hyperinsulinemia. Also, there is a significant correlation between maternal glucose levels and subsequent adiposity in the infant. Ketoacidosis at any time during pregnancy may lead to death in utero.

Maintenance of euglycemia depends, not only on diligent regulation of diet and insulin, but also on strict

attention to physical activity and stress. Capillary glucose levels of 60–140 mg/dL throughout the day should be the objective of therapy. Patients should eat three meals and three snacks each day, adding up to 30–35 cal/kg of ideal body weight. This regimen permits a total weight gain of about 25 lb.

The most successful regimen of insulin administration usually includes two injections daily of both NPH and regular insulin. Lewis and co-workers have found that the amount of NPH insulin given in the morning should exceed that of regular insulin by a 2:1 ratio (2). In the evening, equal amounts of NPH and regular insulin are given. If fasting or postprandial glucose levels are not acceptable, insulin doses are increased by 20%. Several days are then allowed to pass before further changes are made.

Gestational or class A diabetes (abnormal glucose tolerance test with normal fasting and postprandial plasma glucose levels) is usually managed by diet alone. Treatment with human insulin is initiated for elevations in fasting or postprandial glucose levels.

For insulin-dependent patients, a continuous insulin infusion during labor will stabilize maternal glucose levels. This simple approach may also reduce neonatal hypoglycemia (3).

Glycemic control cannot be accurately assessed by random blood glucose determinations or by testing urine specimens for glucose. Glycosuria may be misleading, as the increased glomerular filtration rate characteristic of pregnancy results in an eightfold rise in glucose excretion at term.

The patient should be taught to assess her capillary glucose levels by using glucose oxidase-impregnated reagent strips with a color-coded chart or a blood glucose reflectance meter. Determinations should be made in the fasting state before lunch, dinner, and bedtime. Measurements made two hours after meals may also be helpful. A blood glucose sample drawn 80 minutes after breakfast has been found to correlate well with the mean amplitude of glycemic excursions throughout the day.

A useful tool for assessing control over previous weeks and months is hemoglobin A_{1c}, a minor variant of hemoglobin A, produced by the addition of a single glucose moiety to the terminal valine of the β chain. This glycosylated

Table 26.1 White's Classification of Diabetes in Pregnancy

Class A_1	Class C
Abnormal glucose tolerance test with normal fasting plasma (<105 mg/dL) and postprandial (<120 mg/dL) glucose levels. Controlled with diet alone.	Insulin-treated diabetic. Onset between ages 10 and 20 years. Duration between 10 and 20 years. Background retinopathy.
Class A_2	**Class D**
Abnormal glucose tolerance test with abnormal fasting or postprandial glucose levels. Treated with diet and insulin.	Insulin-treated diabetic. Onset under age 10. Duration more than 20 years. Background retinopathy.
Class B	**Class F**
Insulin-treated diabetic. Onset over age 20. Duration less than 10 years. No vascular disease or retinopathy.	Diabetic nephropathy.
	Class H
	Cardiac disease.
	Class R
	Proliferative retinopathy.

hemoglobin is synthesized throughout the red blood cell's life cycle in amounts that reflect the degree of chronic hyperglycemia present. Levels correlate significantly with mean fasting glucose, mean daily glucose, and highest daily glucose values. In normal pregnancy, glycosylated hemoglobin declines during the first and second trimester, returning to baseline levels at term. Hemoglobin A_{1c} may be significantly higher in pregnant insulin-dependent and gestational diabetic patients.

Elevated maternal hemoglobin A_{1c} levels in the first trimester have been correlated with a significantly higher incidence of major malformations and spontaneous abortions (4, 5). Widness and co-workers have also shown a significant correlation between maternal third-trimester hemoglobin A_{1c} levels and increased birthweight (6).

The final assessment of maternal control is made after delivery. The neonate's activity and behavior in the nursery reflect the degree of hyperglycemia and hyperinsulinemia experienced in utero.

Detecting Maternal Diabetes

In the past, screening for gestational diabetes was limited to the patient with a family history of diabetes or an obstetric history marked by an unexplained stillbirth or a malformed or macrosomic neonate. Obesity, hypertension, or glycosuria also demanded additional investigation. However, this screening approach is too insensitive (7).

Many investigators now recommend that *all* obstetric patients be evaluated for diabetes at no later than 24 to 28 weeks' gestation (8, 9). Plasma glucose levels are measured one hour after a 50-g glucose load (upper limit of normal, 140 mg/dL). A patient who had an abnormal screening test result would then be given an oral glucose tolerance test (OGTT).

Classification A

Diabetic patients who show abnormal oral glucose tolerance but normal fasting blood sugars are classified A (10). These patients have no higher incidence of intrauterine fetal demise than "normal" obstetric patients (11). For this reason, class A diabetic patients are seen every week in the clinic and placed on an 1,800- to 2,200-calorie diet. They are not delivered earlier or managed any differently than nondiabetic patients, with the exception that fasting and postprandial glucose levels are repeated every week. If the fasting plasma glucose rises above 105 mg/dL or postprandial levels exceed 120 mg/dL, the patient is put on a program of human insulin, and fetal surveillance as described for insulin-dependent diabetics is instituted at 34 weeks. Most recently, some clinicians have also utilized self-blood-glucose monitoring in patients with gestational diabetes.

If a class A diabetic patient has required insulin in a previous pregnancy, has had a stillbirth, has hypertension, or develops preeclampsia during the course of her current pregnancy, she, too, is managed as an insulin-dependent diabetic with respect to fetal surveillance, although her classification is not changed.

Classifications B–R

As soon as an insulin-dependent patient is seen, these measures are implemented:

1. Instruction on diet and insulin
2. Education about the relationship between diabetes and pregnancy
3. Determination of baseline creatinine clearance, protein excretion and hemoglobin A_{1c}
4. Ophthalmologic consultation
5. Optimum control of diabetes
6. Sonography to date the pregnancy and search for congenital malformations

During the second trimester, a careful search for the presence of fetal malformations is performed by obtaining a maternal serum α-fetoprotein level at 16 weeks, a targeted ultrasound at 18 weeks, and fetal echocardiography at 20 weeks. In addition, the rate of uterine growth, development of early signs of preeclampsia, and incidence of infection of the urinary tract or other sites are closely monitored.

By accurately assessing fetal health and maturity, clinicians can prevent intrauterine deaths while safely prolonging pregnancy to avoid the hazards of iatrogenic prematurity. Antepartum heart rate testing using both the contraction stress test (CST) and the nonstress test (NST) has proved to be a reliable index of fetal well-being in a metabolically stable patient. Daily maternal assessment of fetal activity is a valuable screening test.

Class A diabetics who have had previous stillbirths or who have hypertension, as well as all insulin-requiring diabetics, need careful fetal surveillance with antepartum fetal heart rate (FHR) monitoring. At 28 weeks, we begin weekly NSTs and daily maternal assessment of fetal activity. Twice-weekly NSTs are ordered at 32 weeks. A nonreactive nonstress test must be followed by a contraction stress test. Our goal is to achieve at least 38 weeks' gestation as long as these tests of fetal well-being are reassuring. If, at 38 weeks, the cervix is favorable, there is no macrosomia, the lecithin/sphingomyelin (L/S) ratio is more than 2.0:1, phosphatidylglycerol (PG) is present, and the presenting part is cephalic, labor is induced. If the cervix is unfavorable and the fetus is not macrosomic, it appears reasonable to wait as long as fetal activity is normal and antepartum heart rate testing is reassuring.

Since there may be a spurious decrease in fetal activity not associated with fetal jeopardy, one should not intervene on the basis of reduced activity alone, but if a significant decrease in fetal activity occurs, one should repeat an NST. If the NST is reactive, avoiding intervention is reasonable, especially if the fetus doesn't have a mature L/S ratio. A fetal biophysical profile may also be helpful in such cases. However, in the face of a decrease in fetal movement associated with nonreactive NST and a positive oxytocin challenge test (OCT), intervention should be strongly considered, even if the L/S ratio is less than 2.0:1.

The accuracy of an L/S ratio of 2.0:1 as a predictor of fetal pulmonary maturity in pregnancies complicated by diabetes has been questioned. Lowensohn and Gabbe studied 93 patients with ratios of 2:1 or higher and observed a 5.4% incidence of respiratory distress syndrome (12). In addition, Simon reported only two cases (3.5%) of hyaline membrane disease in 63 infants of diabetic mothers with an L/S ratio ≥2.0 (13). The presence of phosphatidylglycerol is a further marker of fetal lung maturity.

Amniocentesis to determine the L/S ratio need not be done until the result will influence management. In uncomplicated diabetes, it is usually done at about 38 weeks or earlier only if abnormalities in antepartum fetal testing or deteriorating maternal condition would indicate delivery if the L/S were mature.

Finally, in order to avoid birth injury from fetal macrosomia, a liberal attitude toward cesarean section should be employed in such cases. Sonographic assessment of estimated fetal weight and growth of the abdominal circumference are of value in detecting fetal macrosomia (14, 15). If the estimated fetal weight exceeds 4,000 g, delivery by elective cesarean section should be considered at about 38 weeks after a mature L/S ratio has been determined (16).

Individualizing Ambulatory Care

Attention to maternal control, reliable indices of fetal status, and continuing patient education have permitted a program of ambulatory management for selected patients during the third trimester. These patients avoid the financial and emotional burdens of extended hospitalization just before delivery. The ambulatory patient must nevertheless remain in excellent control and be responsible and communicative. Adjuncts to this program are outpatient antepartum fetal testing and home assessment of blood glucose using a glucose reflectance meter.

Delivery may be timed according to degree of maternal control, previous obstetric history, and evaluation of the fetus, rather than by the White classification. Preterm delivery is indicated only if maternal hypertension or retinopathy worsens or there is clear evidence of fetal compromise.

CASE 26.1

A 28-year-old gravida 2, para 1, aborta 0 was first seen at weeks' gestation. The patient had had diabetes mellitus for 17 years, which was complicated by proliferative retinopathy and nephropathy. She had received laser therapy during the previous year, and no active neovascularization had recurred. Her serum creatinine level was 1.4 mg/dL, and her creatinine clearance 70 mL/minute. Her blood pressure was normal.

In a prior pregnancy, the patient had been delivered by cesarean section (CS) at 35 weeks' gestation for pre-eclampsia. Her infant weighed 1,600 g. Prior to delivery, an L/S ratio of 2.5 had been obtained. Nevertheless, the infant developed severe respiratory distress, which worsened progressively during the first seven days of life, leading to the death of the infant on day 8. Autopsy revealed truncus arteriosus.

When first seen during this pregnancy, the patient was found to have a glycosylated hemoglobin level of 10% (normal: 5%–8%). Her mean glucose level was 170 mg/dL, based on self-blood-glucose monitoring determinations. The patient had not had prepregnancy care and had been adjusting her insulin doses and diet independently. At her first prenatal visit, she was asked to test her glucose levels both before and after meals. Appropriate changes were then made in her insulin regimen to obtain excellent glucose control.

At 16 weeks' gestation, a maternal serum α-fetoprotein level was found to be 3.0 multiples of the median (MoM). A repeat value was 3.5 MoM. A targeted ultrasound study revealed a meningomyelocele in the thoracolumbar area of the fetal spine. No other anomalies were noted, and fetal echocardiography was normal.

The patient and her husband were counseled about the consequences of this neural tube defect. Because the patient had decided that this would be her final pregnancy, she elected to continue the pregnancy. Ultrasonographic monitoring of the fetus subsequently demonstrated mild dilation of the cerebral ventricles.

The patient's renal function and retinal status remained stable. At 38 weeks' gestation, amniocentesis revealed an L/S ratio of 3.0 with phosphatidylglycerol present. The patient underwent a repeat CS and was delivered of a 3,750-g baby girl with a meningomyelocele in the thoracolumbar area. A bilateral tubal ligation was performed at the time of CS. Surgery was performed upon the infant soon after birth to close the neural tube defect and insert a ventricular shunt. ∎

CASE 26.2

A 30-year-old gravida 4, para 3 was first seen at 18 weeks' gestation. Her past obstetric history included the vaginal delivery of a 4,100-g baby boy, who suffered a fractured humerus in the process. The patient's mother had diabetes mellitus. Plasma glucose was obtained one hour after a 50-g oral glucose load and was found to be 175 mg/dL. A three-hour oral glucose tolerance test was then ordered. The results were: fasting, 90 mg/dL; one hour, 243 mg/dL; two hours, 176 mg/dL; and three hours, 154 mg/dL. The diagnosis of gestational (class A1) diabetes mellitus was made.

The patient was started on a 2,200-calorie diet with strict avoidance of concentrated sweets. Fasting plasma and postprandial glucose determinations were obtained every week at the patient's visits to the diabetes clinic. The fasting values ranged from 80 to 96 mg/dL. Uterine growth was normal, and the patient remained normotensive. At 40 weeks' gestation, the patient's cervix was found to be long and closed. Estimated fetal weight was 3,500 g. Antepartum fetal evaluation was initiated with twice-weekly nonstress testing.

At 41 weeks, the patient went into spontaneous labor and was delivered vaginally of a 3,250-g baby boy. The Apgar scores were 7 at one minute and 9 at five minutes; the infant had no neonatal morbidity. ∎

References

1. Kitzmiller JL, Gavin LA, Gin GD, et al. Preconception care of diabetes: glycemic control prevents congenital anomalies. JAMA 1991;265:731–6.
2. Lewis SB, Murray WK, Wallin JD, et al. Improved glucose control in nonhospitalized pregnant diabetic patients. Obstet Gynecol 1976;48:260.
3. Linzey EM. Controlling diabetes with continuous insulin infusion. Contemp Ob/Gyn 1978;12:43.
4. Miller E, Hare JW, Cloherty JP, et al. Elevated maternal hemoglobin A_{1c} in early pregnancy and major congenital anomalies in infants of diabetic mothers. N Eng J Med 1981;

304:1331.

5. Mills JL, Simpson JL, Driscol SG, et al. Incidence of spontaneous abortion among normal women and insulin-dependent diabetic women whose pregnancies were identified within 21 days of conception. N Engl J Med 1988; 319:1617.

6. Widness JA, Schwartz HC, Thompson D, et al. Glycohemoglobin (HbA$_{1c}$): a predictor of birth weight in infants of diabetic mothers. J Pediatr 1978;92:8.

7. O'Sullivan JB, Mahan CM, Charles D, et al. Screening criteria for high-risk gestational diabetic patients. Am J Obstet Gynecol 1973;116:895.

8. Metzger B, et al. Summary and recommendations of the Third International Workshop-Conference on Gestational Diabetes Mellitus. Diabetes 1991;40:197–201.

9. Coustan DR, Nelson C, Carpenter MW, et al. Maternal age and screening for gestational diabetes: a population-based study. Obstet Gynecol 1989;73:557.

10. Gabbe S, Mestman J, Freeman RK, et al. Management and outcome of class A diabetes mellitus. Am J Obstet Gynecol 1977;127:465.

11. Goldberg JD, Franklin B, Lasser D, et al. Gestational diabetes: impact of home glucose monitoring on neonatal birth weight. Am J Obstet Gynecol 1986;154:546.

12. Lowensohn RI, Gabbe SG. The value of L/S ratios in diabetics: a critical review. Am J Obstet Gynecol 1979;134:703.

13. Simon NV, Levisky JS, Lenko PM. The prediction of fetal lung maturity by amniotic fluid fluorescence polarization in diabetic pregnancy. Am J Perinatol 1987;4:171.

14. Bochner CJ, Medearis AL, Williams J, et al. Early third-trimester ultrasound screening in gestational diabetes to determine the risk of macrosomia and labor dystocia at term. Am J Obstet Gynecol 1987;157:703.

15. Landon MB, Mintz MC, Gabbe SG. Sonographic evaluation of fetal abdominal growth: a predictor of the LGA infant in pregnancy complicated by diabetes mellitus. Am J Obstet Gynecol 1989;160:115.

16. Acker DB, Sachs BP, Friedman EA. Risk factors for shoulder dystocia. Obstet Gynecol 1985;66:762.

27

Hyperthyroidism and Hypothyroidism

Jorge H. Mestman, M.D.

Hyperthyroidism

The incidence of hyperthyroidism in pregnancy is around 0.2%. We have found the disease in about 1:2,250 patients. In the majority, it was first diagnosed during pregnancy, but symptoms had antedated the pregnancy by months and sometimes years.

Hyperthyroid pregnant patients seem to have no unusual problems, provided they are under treatment and in good metabolic control. In fact, there is clinical evidence that the severity of hyperthyroidism may be ameliorated during the second half of pregnancy. The perinatal mortality rate does not appear to be increased if the mother's thyroid state is well controlled, but patients with untreated thyrotoxicosis show a higher incidence of perinatal mortality and morbidity, and low-birthweight infants than do treated mothers. Congestive heart failure and even thyroid crisis have been reported in women with uncontrolled thyrotoxicosis in the last half of pregnancy (1).

Symptoms and Signs

Graves' disease is the most common cause of hyperthyroidism (Table 27.1). Hydatidiform mole may be suspected when symptoms of acute hyperthyroxinemia develop in the first trimester (2). Patients with severe hyperemesis gravidarum, with vomiting, dehydration, and weight loss, may have elevation of the free thyroxine index (FT_4I), and suppressed serum TSH values. Sometimes the free triiodothyroxine index (FT_3I) may also be elevated. However, they do not have other hypermetabolic symptoms, and the tests return to normal after treatment of hyperemesis gravidarum (3).

Table 27.1 Causes of Hyperthyroidism in Pregnancy

Graves' disease
Toxic adenoma
Toxic multinodular goiter
Hashimoto or chronic thyroiditis
Hydatidiform mole
Hyperemesis gravidarum
Subacute thyroiditis
Factitious (exogenous) hyperthyroidism

Hyperthyroidism is sometimes difficult to diagnose because many normal pregnant women show symptoms typical of hypermetabolism: excessive warmth, nervousness, and a slight tremor. Eye signs—such as lid lag or retraction, stare, and exophthalmos—and weight loss despite a good appetite are characteristic of thyrotoxicosis (Table 27.2). The triad of hyperthyroidism, exophthalmos, and diffuse goiter is characteristic of Graves' disease.

Patients with Graves' disease often have eye symptoms, including photophobia, frequent lacrimation, periorbital swelling, and occasional diplopia. Characteristic eye signs may be caused by sympathetic overactivity or infiltrative opthalmopathy. The former, which includes lid retraction with widening of the palpebral fissure, lid lag, staring, and infrequent blinking, usually regress when thyrotoxicosis is controlled.

Infiltrative ophthalmopathy, however, is unique to Graves' disease and sometimes progresses in spite of good control of thyrotoxicosis. Exophthalmos is the most common manifestation; injection of the bulbar conjunctiva and chemosis are not unusual. Careful examination reveals a weakness of the extraocular muscles. Convergence is also impaired.

Table 27.2 Common Clues to Thyrotoxicosis

Symptoms
Changes in personality
Dyspnea
Fatigue
Heat intolerance
Increased appetite
Increased sweating
Insomnia
Nervousness
Palpitations

Signs
Eye signs
Goiter
Hyperkinetic reflexes
Onycholysis
Proximal muscle weakness
Tachycardia
Tremor
Weight loss

In infiltrative dermopathy, an uncommon manifestation of Graves' disease, there is a fine, localized thickening of the skin, usually over the tibial aspect of the lower leg just above the ankle. The skin lesions are nonpitting and violaceous.

Occasionally, a patient will have unexplained tachycardia and weight loss without any other marked symptoms or physical findings. Goiter may be absent. This clinical picture, which is not uncommon in older patients, is seldom seen in the young, but does occur occasionally in pregnancy.

In untreated patients or those who are noncompliant, an intercurrent disease such as pyelonephritis, anemia, pregnancy-induced hypertension or amnionitis may trigger the development of congestive heart failure and even thyroid crisis (4). Blood tests every two to three weeks are essential, as is prompt hospitalization when patients do not respond to drug therapy. Most patients who fail to respond to antithyroid medication are noncompliant, since resistance to antithyroid therapy is usually rare (5). Patients seen for the first time in the third trimester who have marked metabolic symptoms should be hospitalized until the disease is under control.

Graves' disease may worsen in the first trimester and in the postpartum period. It may improve spontaneously in the second and third trimesters. These changes in the clinical course are the result of an alteration in the concentration of thyroid-stimulating hormone receptor antibodies (TSHRAb) that occurs during pregnancy (6).

Laboratory Tests

In pregnancy, elevation of total serum T_4 concentration is not diagnostic of hyperthyroidism, since high levels are normal as a consequence of elevations in thyroxine-binding globulin (TBG). An elevation in serum-free thyroxine concentrations confirms the diagnosis. Since determination of the actual amount of free hormone in blood is time-consuming, expensive, and not widely available, an alternate is calculation of FT_4I based on serum T_4 and resin triiodothyronine uptake (RT_3U). The FT_4I is calculated as follows:

$$FT_4 = \text{patient's } T_4 \times \frac{\text{Patient's } RT_3U}{\text{Mean normal } RT_3U}.$$

The FT$_4$I correlates very well with the actual amount of serum-free thyroxine, the biologically active hormone. It is elevated and is diagnostic of hyperthyroidism in more than 95% of hyperthyroid patients. Occasionally, the free thyroxine index may be normal or slightly elevated, in which case the serum determination of triiodothyronine by radioimmunoassay (T$_3$RIA) is helpful. Since the total amount of T$_3$ is elevated in pregnancy because of the elevation in TBG, a calculation of the FT$_3$I is required. The formula to use is as follows:

$$FT_3I = \text{patient's } T_3RIA \times \frac{\text{Patient's } RT_3U}{\text{Mean normal } RT_3U \text{ value}}$$

Ultrasensitive thyroid-stimulating hormone (TSH) (7) is an excellent test for diagnosing hyperthyroidism, since such patients have levels of less than 0.04 μU/mL. In normal euthyroid individuals, values for ultrasensitive TSH vary from 0.04 to 6 μU/mL. The test is not useful in sick patients, since the value may be suppressed in euthyroid subjects (8). It has been reported that the values may also be suppressed in normal pregnancy in the first trimester (9).

Antibodies to the TSH receptor are present in most patients with Graves' disease (TSHRAb) (10). High maternal levels of TSHRAb in the last trimester of pregnancy are helpful for predicting neonatal hyperthyroidism and for making the presumptive diagnosis of fetal hyperthyroidism (6, 11).

Treatment Strategies

To ensure delivery of a healthy infant who will develop normally, the following three management approaches have been suggested:

- Antithyroid medication alone
- Antithyroid medication plus thyroid supplementation
- Subtotal thyroidectomy after treatment with antithyroid medication or propranolol

There are arguments for and against each approach. The final decision will depend somewhat on the physician's experience. We prefer using antithyroid medication alone. Very few of our pregnant patients need surgery.

The agents most commonly used to treat thyrotoxicosis—methimazole (Tapazole) and propylthiouracil (PTU)

—are in the thioamide family. Their mode of action is complex. Primarily, they inhibit the coupling of tryosines, and, secondarily, they inhibit the formation of diiodotyrosine and monoiodotyrosine. Therefore, they are far more capable of inhibiting hormone synthesis than of inhibiting total iodine accumulation. In addition, propylthiouracil inhibits the peripheral conversion of T$_4$ to T$_3$. Our hospitalized patients receive the drug every six to eight hours. To avoid compliance problems, however, we prescribe twice-daily dosages to outpatients.

As soon as the diagnosis is confirmed, we start therapy with methimazole or PTU (100 mg of PTU are equivalent to 10 mg of methimazole). We have found no marked difference in response to either drug. The few reports of fetal scalp lesions, aplasia cutia, with maternal methimazole treatment have not been confirmed (12). We have seen no such lesions in our hospital.

The initial dose is either 300 to 400 mg of PTU or 30–40 mg of methimazole daily, according to the severity of symptoms (Figure 27.1). As soon as the patient's condition improves, the dosage is decreased by half. We follow up our patients every two weeks with T$_4$, T$_3$RIA, and RT$_3$U determinations to calculate the FT$_4$I and FT$_3$I.

Symptoms improve after two to three weeks of treatment. Two objective signs of improvement are a lowered pulse rate and gain in weight.

To control severe hypermetabolic symptoms, we use propranolol, 10–40 mg every six to eight hours until symptoms are controlled, along with antithyroid medications. It takes a few days to a week for propranolol to exert full metabolic control. Antithyroid drugs may be discontinued in the last few weeks of pregnancy with mild disease, in those maintained euthyroid on minimum doses of antithyroid medications, and in patients with small goiters.

Exceptions are patients with a long history of thyrotoxicosis, large goiter, extrathyroid manifestations such as exophthalmopathy, and patients with high titers of TSHRAb. In such cases, treatment should be continued throughout pregnancy and postpartum, with the minimal amount of antithyroid medication to keep thyroid tests within upper normal limits. In such patients, relapses are not uncommon when medication is stopped. If pregnancy occurs during treatment with antithyroid drugs, we lower the dosage as

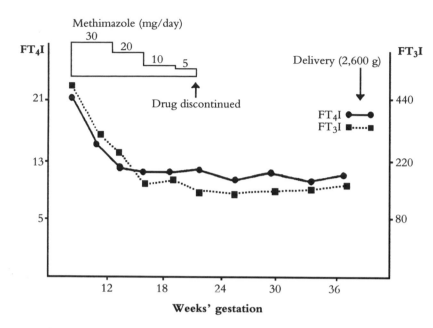

Figure 27.1 Effect of methimazole on thyroid tests. FT_3I = free triiodothyroxine index; FT_4I = free thyroxine index.

Reprinted with permission from Mestman JH. Management of thyroid diseases in pregnancy. In: Berkowitz RL, ed. Clinical perinatology. Philadelphia: WB Saunders, 1985:651–667.

soon as the patient becomes euthyroid, and management proceeds as described earlier.

Graves' disease may relapse within six weeks to twelve months after delivery. Thyroid tests should be done regularly during this time.

Several investigators advocate thyroid replacement therapy for patients on antithyroid drugs. They postulate that thyroid replacement may prevent hypothyroidism in the mother and fetus. Because thyroid hormones do not cross the placenta, and since their presence may mask the result of the mother's test, we feel that they are not indicated for treatment of hyperthyroidism in pregnancy. However, a recent paper suggests that adding thyroid hormone in patients with Graves' disease may prevent relapses of hyperthyroidism in the post partum period (13).

Breast-feeding is not generally recommended for mothers taking antithyroid medication. However, a few studies indicate that PTU may be used, since the concentration in mother's milk and infants' serum is low (14). If PTU is used, the dose should not exceed 200 mg/day, given in four doses after suckling. The infant should be followed up carefully with thyroid function tests (15).

Operative treatment of thyrotoxicosis in pregnancy is very seldom indicated, but, when necessary, it should be postponed until the second trimester and performed only after the patient has become euthyroid on antithyroid medication. Surgery is not recommended in the third trimester, when it may induce premature delivery. Propranolol may be used in preparation for surgery.

Complications of Drug Therapy: The incidence of adverse drug reactions to thioamides is low and uncommon in pregnancy (Table 27.3). The most common is skin rash, which occurs in about 5% of patients. If a drug reaction occurs with PTU, it may be possible to continue therapy with methimazole, because there is little cross-reactivity.

Fortunately, agranulocytosis, the most serious reaction, is uncommon. It appears within the first weeks or months

Table 27.3 Drug Reactions to Thioamides

Agranulocytosis*
Alopecia*
Arthralgia*
Fever†
Myalgia
Skin rash†
Thrombocytopenia

*Most serious, but very uncommon.
†More common (3%–5%).

of treatment, accompanied by fever and sore throat. When therapy is begun, the patient should be told to stop using the drug and notify the physician immediately if these symptoms should develop. Warning the patient is more important than taking routine leukocyte counts, because agranulocytosis may develop within a few days after normal leukocyte count. If it does occur, the drug should be discontinued immediately and the patient isolated and given glucocorticoids and antibiotics. Leukopenia may also be present in thyrotoxicosis, so it is advisable to get a complete blood count before starting therapy.

Pregnancy Outcome in Graves' Disease

Patients whose thyrotoxicosis is not controlled by medical or surgical therapy show a very high (up to 45%) incidence of fetal wastage, including spontaneous abortion, stillbirth, and neonatal death. In those whose disease is well controlled, the incidence is similar to that of normal pregnancy (16).

Antithyroid medication does cross the placenta, and fetal goiter has been reported when mothers received excessive amounts of it (2). Today, with better follow-up of patients, better availability of thyroid tests, and thyroid test values kept in the upper limits of normal, these complications are seldom reported.

Fetal hypothyroidism is rare in the offspring of mothers treated with antithyroid medication (17).

In patients who are kept euthyroid with antithyroid drug therapy, congenital malformations are uncommon (18). However, they are reported to be higher in mothers who were hyperthyroid at the time of conception (19). The growth of children exposed to PTU in utero is not adversely affected (20).

Fetal and Neonatal Effects

Fetal hyperthyroidism, a rare condition, should be suspected when fetal tachycardia and intrauterine growth retardation (IUGR) are noted in mothers with a history of Graves' disease and of previous delivery of an infant affected by neonatal hyperthyroidism (Table 27.4). The diagnosis could be confirmed by cordocentesis, although the technique may result in significant morbidity (21, 22). Treating the mother with PTU or methimazole benefits the infant, since the drug crosses the placenta, normalizing fetal tachycardia and IUGR (23).

Neonatal thyrotoxicosis is rare. It may occur in neonates of euthyroid mothers with a history of Graves' disease. It has been considered a self-limited disorder, lasting a few weeks, with a perinatal mortality rate of about 20%. A correlation has been found between maternal high titers of TSHRAb and neonatal hyperthyroidism (6).

At birth, the affected infant's weight is below 2,500 g; goiter and exophthalmos are often—but not always—present. The thymus, liver, spleen, and lymph nodes are frequently enlarged. Severe hypermetabolic symptoms and congestive heart failure are the most serious complications. These symptoms may appear several days after birth, particularly if the mother was receiving antithyroid drugs at the time of delivery. The child's symptoms may persist for six months or even longer (24).

Postpartum Thyroid Dysfunction

Women with chronic thyroiditis who remain euthyroid throughout pregnancy may develop postpartum thyroid dysfunction. A self-limited entity, it has been reported in 5%–10% of women. Clinically, it is characterized by mild symptoms of hyperthyroidism occurring four to eight weeks postpartum (Figure 27.2). In most of these cases, the free thyroxine index and the free T_3 index are elevated but return to normal spontaneously within a few weeks. In

---

Table 27.4 Clues to Diagnosis of Fetal Hyperthyroidism

Maternal
History of active or inactive Graves' disease
Persistent elevation of TSHRAb throughout pregnancy
Previous delivery of an infant with neonatal hyperthyroidism
Serum TSHRAb over 500% throughout pregnancy

Fetal
Advanced bone maturation
Craniosynostosis—coronal and/or sagittal sutures
Intrauterine growth retardation
Tachycardia

Neonatal
Hyperthyroidism
Intellectual and developmental impairment

TSHRAb: thyroid-stimulating hormone receptor antibody.

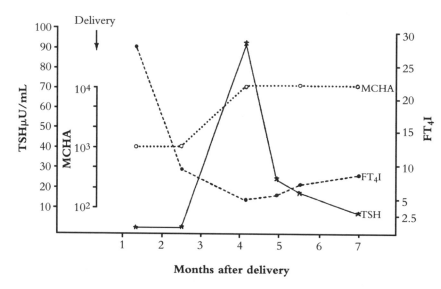

Figure 27.2 Postpartum hyperthyroidism and hypothyroidism. TSH = thyroid-stimulating hormone; MCHA = microsomal hemagglutination antibodies; FT₄I = free thyroxine index.

Reprinted with permission from Mestman JH. Management of thyroid diseases in pregnancy. In: Berkowitz RL, ed. Clinical perinatology. Philadelphia: WB Saunders, 1985:651–667.

more than 50% of patients, this period is followed by one of hypothyroidism with spontaneous recovery.

The disease may persist for two to six months and may recur in subsequent pregnancies (25). It is important to recognize postpartum thyroid dysfunction, since treatment is seldom indicated and spontaneous recovery is usual. The results of recent studies, however, suggest that permanent hypothyroidism may develop in a woman years after the original event (26, 27).

Hypothyroidism

Women who are hypothyroid frequently do not ovulate. Therefore, spontaneous pregnancies in untreated women are uncommon (28).

Hypothyroidism may be caused by a disease of the thyroid gland (primary hypothyroidism), by a hypothalamic or pituitary disease, with impairment in the secretion of TSH (secondary hypothyroidism), or by peripheral resistance in thyroid hormone action. In women of childbearing age, the most common causes are chronic or Hashimoto's thyroiditis, postsurgical ablation for Graves' disease or nodular goiter, postradioactive therapy for Graves' disease, or primary or idiopathic myxedema. Some authors consider the latter to be the end stage of Hashimoto's disease.

Clinical symptoms vary from patient to patient. Symptoms include fatigue, cold intolerance, mild weight gain, lethargy, lack of ambition, depression, arthralgia, muscle cramps, impaired hearing, hoarse voice, and constipation. Abnormal menses with excessive bleeding is common, and occasionally it may present as galactorrhea with amenorrhea. The presenting symptoms may be minimal or absent; rarely, they may be so severe that the patient presents with stupor or myxedema coma.

Clinical findings may be minimal. Periorbital edema is a frequent complaint, particularly on arising. The skin may be pale and yellowish. It generally is dry and rough and sometimes scaly. The scalp hair becomes thin and may fall out. Typically, the reaction phase of tendon reflexes is delayed. Examination of the neck may reveal the scar of a thyroidectomy or a diffuse or nodular goiter. Patients with primary myxedema or previous history of 131I therapy may have no palpable thyroid tissue.

A low FT₄I and a high serum TSH confirm the diagnosis of primary thyroid failure (1). Patients with Hashimoto's thyroiditis and primary myxedema have positive antiperoxidase (antimicrosomal) and antithyroglobulin antibody titers. In the first stage of thyroid failure, patients are asymptomatic; the FT₄I is normal, and TSH is elevated (subclinical hypothyroidism).

No major neonatal complications have been reported. A high incidence of preeclampsia, anemia, placental abruption, and postpartum hemorrhage was noted in one study (29). In our own experience, the incidence of PIH is increased, both in women with overt hypothyroidism and subclinical hypothyroidism. Correction of the hypothyroid decreases the incidence of PIH (30).

L-thyroxine is the treatment of choice, since it produces constant serum concentrations in both T_4 and T_3, has to be taken only once a day, and is well tolerated. The normal replacement dose varies between 0.1 and 0.2 mg/day. The goal of therapy is to normalize serum TSH and FT_4I. Some patients may need an increase in thyroid dosage in early pregnancy (31, 32).

C A S E   2 7 . 1

A 30-year-old gravida 3, para 2 was seen at 10 weeks' gestation with a four-month history of nervousness, heat intolerance, palpitations, and a four–pound weight loss. Her menstrual periods had been regular until two months previously.

Examination showed a somewhat anxious woman with blood pressure of 110/56 mm Hg and pulse 104 beats per minute and regular. The skin was warm; her palms were warm and moist. Eye examination showed no exophthalmos or bilateral lid lag and no involvement of the extraocular muscles. The thyroid gland was diffusely enlarged about two times normal, nontender, and slightly firm. Deep tendon reflexes were 3+. Pelvic examination was consistent with gestational age of 8 to 10 weeks.

Laboratory tests showed WBC 4,500/μL with normal differential. Total serum thyroxine was 17.6 μg/dL (normal = 5–13 μg/dL) and RT_3U was 35% (normal = 25%–35%), and the FT_4I was calculated accordingly:

$$FT_4I = 17.6 \times \frac{35}{30} = 20.5$$

$$\text{Total } T_3 \text{ RIA} = 394 \ \mu g$$

$$FT_3I = 394 \times \frac{35}{30} = 459$$

The normal values for the calculated FT_4I and FT_3I are the same as the normal values for total serum T_4 and total serum T_3, respectively.

Hydatidiform mole was ruled out. The most likely explanation for this patient's hyperthyroidism was thought to be Graves' disease. Treatment was started with methimazole 20 mg in the morning and 10 mg in the evening. Two weeks later, the patient felt no significant improvement, although the FT_4I had decreased to 15.4. By 14 weeks' gestation, clinical improvement had occurred, and the amount of methimazole was reduced to 10 mg bid.

By 18 weeks' gestation (8 weeks of therapy), the patient felt euthyroid. She had gained 4 lb, the pulse was 78 beats per minute, and the FT_4I was 10.2. A serum T_3RIA index was 180 (normal = 70–210). The amount of methimazole was reduced to 10 mg daily and was further reduced to 5 mg daily by 20 weeks' gestation because of absence of symptoms and normal FT_4I. At 22 weeks' gestation (12 weeks of therapy) the drug was discontinued altogether. The patient was seen at regular intervals. She gained 22 lb throughout pregnancy and remained euthyroid. The goiter size decreased slightly. She underwent spontaneous labor by 39 weeks and was delivered vaginally of a 2,600-g normal baby. No signs of hyperthyroidism were detected in the newborn, who was discharged home at 3 days of age.

The mother was followed in the postpartum period. She was allowed to breast-feed her child, but by four weeks postpartum symptoms of hyperthyroidism recurred, and she was advised not to breast-feed. Her FT_4I was elevated and she was started on methimazole 20 mg bid.

This case illustrates that patients with Graves' disease may ovulate normally (hence the need for contraception), that in some instances they may have rapid improvement after initiation of treatment, and that the disease may recur in the postpartum period. Patients should be followed at regular intervals with clinical assessment and laboratory evaluation of thyroid tests (the most practical of which is calculation of the FT_4I). ∎

CASE 27.2

A 22-year-old gravida 2, para 0, abortus 1, was seen in the emergency room at 12 weeks' gestation because of nausea and vomiting, weight loss, and ketonuria. On physical examination the patient was dehydrated, the pulse rate was 130 beats per minute, the blood pressure was 90/60 mm Hg, the skin was dry and cold, and the thyroid gland was not enlarged. There was no evidence of exophthalmopathy, and deep tendon reflexes were 2+. Past medical history and family history were negative for thyroid disease.

A free thyroxine index was 17.2 (normal = 5–13). The free T_3 index was 220 (normal = 70–200). An ultrasensitive TSH was less than 0.3 μU/mL (normal = 0.3–6 μU/mL). The patient was admitted to the hospital and treated with IV fluids, with improvement of her symptoms. Repeat thyroid tests a week later showed a free thyroxine index of 14, and a free T_3 index of 180. Three weeks later the patient was seen in the outpatient clinic. The vomiting had subsided, although she still had some nausea. She had gained five pounds. The free thyroxine index was 11. The free T_3 index was 162, and the ultrasensitive serum TSH was 1.2 μU/mL.

This patient is a typical example of a patient with hyperemesis gravidarum presenting with thyroid tests in the hyperthyroid range. She did not have physical signs of Graves' disease, and family history was negative. Furthermore, the thyroid gland was not enlarged, and she responded promptly to hydration therapy. Hyperemesis gravidarum may present with laboratory tests of hyperthyroidism, and sometimes the differentiation from true hyperthyroidism is difficult. If patients don't improve in a few weeks, antithyroid therapy should be considered. ∎

References

1. Mestman JH. Severe hyperthyroidism in pregnancy. In: Clark S, Phelan J, Cotton D, eds. Critical care in obstetrics. Oradell, NJ: Medical Economics, 1987:262–79.
2. Mestman JH. Diagnosis and mangement of hyperthyroidism in pregnancy. Curr Probl Obstet Gynecol 1981;4:1.
3. Goodwin TM, Montoro M, Mestman JH. Transient hyperthyroidism and hyperemesis gravidarum: clinical aspects. Am J Obstet Gynecol 1992;167:648–52.
4. Davis LE, Lucas MJ, Hankinds GD, et al. Thyrotoxicosis complicating pregnancy. Am J Obstet Gynecol 1989; 150:63.
5. Cooper DS. Propylthiouracil levels in hyperthyroid patients unresponsive to large doses. Evidence of poor patient compliance. Ann Intern Med 1985;102:328.
6. Zakarija M, McKenzie JM. Pregnancy-associated changes in the thyroid-stimulating antibody of Graves' disease and the relationship to neonatal hyperthyroidism. J Clin Endocrinol Metab 1983;57:1036.
7. Spencer CA, Lai-Rosenfeld AO, Guttler RB, et al. Thyrotropin secretion in thyrotoxic and thyroxine-treated patients: assessment by a sensitive immunoenzymometric assay. J Clin Endocrinol Metab 1986;63:349.
8. Ehrmann DA, Weinberg M, Sarne DH. Limitations to the use of a sensitive assay for serum thyrotropin in the assessment of thyroid status. Arch Intern Med 1989;149:369.
9. Guillaume J, Schussler GC, Goldman J. Components of the total serum thyroid hormone concentrations during pregnancy: high free thyroxine and blunted thyrotropin (TSH) response to TSH-releasing hormone in the first trimester. J Clin Endocrinol Metab 1985;60:678.
10. Morris JC III, Hay ID, Nelson RE, et al. Clinical utility of thyrotropin-receptor antibody asssays: comparison of radioreceptor and bioassay methods. Mayo Clin Proc 1988; 63:707.
11. McKenzie JM, Zakarija M. The clinical use of thyrotropin receptor antibody measurements. J Clin Endocrinol Metab 1989;69:1093.
12. Van Dijke CP, Heydendael RJ, De Kleine MJ. Methimazole, carbimazole, and congenital skin defects. Ann Intern Med 1987;106:60.
13. Hashizume K, Ichikawa K, Nishii Y, et al. Effect of administration of thyroxine on the risk of postpartum recurrence of hyperthyroid Graves' disease. J Clin Endocrinol Metab 1992;75:6–10.
14. Kampmann JP, Johansen K, Hansen JM, et al. Propylthiouracil in human milk. Revision of a dogma. Lancet 1980;1:736.
15. Cooper DS. Antithyroid drugs: to breast-feed or not to breast-feed. Am J Obstet Gynecol 1987;157:234.
16. Mestman JH, Manning PR, Hodgman J. Hyperthyroidism and pregnancy. Arch Intern Med 1974;134:434.
17. Cheron RG, Kaplan MM, Larsen PR, et al. Neonatal thyroid function after propylthiouracil therapy for maternal Graves'

disease. N Engl J Med 1981;304:525.

18. Millar LK, Wing DA, Leung AS, Kooning PP, Montoro MN, Mestman JH. Maternal and neonatal outcome in pregnancies complicated by hyperthyroidism. Am J Obstet Gynecol. In press.

19. Momotani N, Ito K, Hamada N, et al. Maternal hyperthyroidism and congenital malformation in the offspring. Clin Endocrinol 1984;20:695.

20. McCarroll AM, Hutchinson M, McAuley R, et al. Long-term assessment of children exposed in utero to carbimazole. Arch Dis Child 1976;51:532.

21. Wenstrom KD, Weiner CP, Williamson RA, Grant SS. Prenatal diagnosis of fetal hyperthyroidism using funipuncture. Obstet Gynecol 1990;76:513–17.

22. Porreco RP, Bloch CA. Fetal blood sampling in the management of intrauterine thyrotoxicosis. Obstet Gynecol 1990;76:509–12.

23. Cove DH, Johnston P. Fetal hyperthyroidism: experience of treatment in four siblings. Lancet 1985;1:430.

24. Fisher DA. Pathogenesis and therapy of neonatal Graves' disease. Am J Dis Child 1976;130:133.

25. Amino N, Mori H, Iwatani Y, et al. High prevalence of transient postpartum thyrotoxicosis and hypothyroidism. N Engl J Med 1982;306:849.

26. Roti E, Emerson CH. Clinical Review 29: postpartum thyroiditis. J Clin Endocrinol Metab 1992;74:3–5.

27. Jansson R, Dahlberg PA, Karlsson FA. Post-partum thyroiditis. Baillieres Clin Endocrinol Metab 1988;2:619.

28. Montoro M, Collea JV, Frasier SD, Mestman JH. Successful outcome of pregnancy in women with hypothyroidism. Ann Intern Med 1981;94:31.

29. Davis LE, Leveno KJ, Cunningham FG. Hypothyroidism complicating pregnancy. Obstet Gynecol 1988;72:108.

30. Leung AS, Millar LK, Koonings PP, Montoro M, Mestman JH. Perinatal outcome in hypothyroid pregnancies. Obstet Gynecol 1993;81:349–53.

31. Tamaki H, Amino N, Takeoka K, et al. Thyroxine requirement during pregnancy for replacement therapy of hypothyroidism. Obstet Gynecol 1990;76:230.

32. Mandel SJ, Larsen PR, Seely EW, et al. Increased need for thyroxine during pregnancy in women with primary hypothyroidism. N Engl J Med 1990;323:91.

28

Asthma in Pregnancy

J. Patrick Lavery, M.D.

ASTHMA is the most common obstructive airway disease associated with pregnancy, affecting approximately 1% to as high as 4% of all pregnant women (0.2%–1.3%) (1, 2). At the onset of pregnancy, it is impossible to predict the subsequent course of this disease in a particular patient. In a summary review on the course of asthma during pregnancy collected from nine series including 1,054 patients, Turner et al. (3) reported that 29% of cases improved, 49% remained the same, and 22% became worse as the pregnancy progressed. In a recent series from Long Beach Memorial Hospital 0.12% of all asthmatic gravidas required antenatal hospitalization for asthmatic symptoms (4). In general the more severe the asthma at the onset of pregnancy, the greater the likelihood of eventual and significant complications. Perinatal outcome is more likely to be compromised in the medication-dependent asthmatic (4).

The above retrospective and cumulative data are similar to the observations made in a large review of 366 pregnancies in 330 prospectively managed asthmatic patients. Schatz et al. (5) noted that there was improvement in 28%, no change in 33%, and worsening in 35% of the cases. Further, there was a consistent pattern of response to the disease in the 34 patients who experienced repeat pregnancies. DeSwiet (6) has suggested that only 1% of asthmatics will not be able to sustain the physiologic changes and stresses in pulmonary function that are related to the pregnancy.

When dealing with a pregnant asthmatic patient, the management goals are as follows:

1. Anticipate the development of respiratory difficulty by patient education, avoid exposure to known allergens, and treat early symptoms promptly.
2. Avoid acute emergency room visits for respiratory compromise or status asthmaticus by early and aggressive intervention.
3. Achieve the delivery of a term healthy newborn while preserving the mother's well-being.

Physiology

The physiologic changes in the respiratory system concurrent with pregnancy are mediated by hormonal and mechanical factors. During pregnancy, the vital capacity remains the same as in the nonpregnant state at 3,200 cc, but, because of a mean increase in the tidal volume from 450 cc to 600 cc, an increase in minute ventilation occurs during pregnancy ranging from 19% to 50% (7). This increase in tidal volume is thought to be mediated by a progesterone effect on airway resistance and increased sensitivity to CO_2. From a mechanical point of view, the functional residual capacity, which is the remaining unused air space in the lungs, is reduced by about 20%. This occurs primarily in the latter half of pregnancy, related to an elevation of the diaphragm (8). Overall airway resistance has been reported to decrease as much as 50% during normal pregnancy (9).

These pulmonary changes lead to altered blood gases and chemistries. There is a decrease in P_{CO_2} to 30 torr, while P_{O_2} ranges from 90 to 106 torr. Plasma bicarbonate will be reduced by secondary renal mechanisms to 18–22 mEq/L, with a relative alkalinization of the serum to a pH of 7.44 (10).

Anatomically, there is an increase in the subcostal angle from 68.5 degrees to 103.5 degrees during the course of pregnancy. This physical change is associated with an elevation of the diaphragm by approximately 4 cm and a 2-cm increase in maximal transverse chest diameter as measured by x-ray (11). These changes lead to a conversion from abdominal to thoracic breathing and in part contribute to the increased maternal oxygen consumption during pregnancy.

Pulmonary Function Testing

Pulmonary function testing (PFT) can be used to evaluate and detect pathologic changes associated with obstructive disease. Among the most common PFTs are the determination of the forced vital capacity (FVC) and the forced expiratory volume in the first second of exhalation (FEV-1). Bronchospasm associated with asthma decreases the FEV-1 although it may not affect the FVC. Because asthmatic patients have difficulty exhaling rapidly, the FEV-1/FVC ratio is an index of progressing severity of the condition. Normally, this ratio should exceed 75%. With restrictive disease, it will be less. Impaired forced expiratory volume can be demonstrated by serial spirometric measurements even before a patient recognizes an attack.

These function tests can be employed during pregnancy. It is desirable to obtain a baseline arterial blood gas as well. In patients who show an elevation in P_{CO_2} (35–38 torr), some degree of alveolar hypoventilation is usually present. Management will depend on the patient's clinical condition. Thus, function tests per se do not contribute much to clinical treatment. Indeed, when a patient is asymptomatic, some studies may be normal. Sims et al. (12) found no changes in respiratory function attributable to pregnancy when pregnant asthmatic patients were compared to normal controls and tested serially in pregnancy, the puerperium, and postpartum.

Endocrinology

The hormonal milieu of pregnancy is dramatically different from the nonpregnant state and undergoes change throughout the course of gestation. These changes will have an effect on pulmonary function. Progesterone appears to exert an early influence by increasing the parturient's sensitivity to CO_2, thus leading to mild hyperventilation or the so-called dyspnea of pregnancy. Later, smooth muscle relaxant effects may be appreciated. The full impact of progesterone despite its 50-100 fold increase above baseline values in pregnancy is still subject to debate with clinical findings open to various interpretations (13).

Estrogen levels rise throughout pregnancy, and there are some data to suggest that this may significantly decrease the diffusing capacity in the capillary bed due to an increased amount of pericapillary acid mucopolysaccharide secretions (14). Estrogens have an impact on gestational asthma by decreasing the metabolic clearance of glucocorticoids and hence increasing the level of cortisol. They also appear to potentiate isoproterenol-induced bronchial relaxation (15).

The level of plasma-free cortisol increases during gestation, as does the level of total plasma cortisol (16). While this should result in a general improvement in the patient's condition, this is not necessarily the case, as reflected in the response to pregnancy noted in the reviews cited earlier (3, 4, 5). It would appear that some individuals become refractory to cortisol despite the two- to threefold increase that takes place in serum levels. This may be attributable to a binding site competition for glucocorticoid receptors exerted by progesterone, deoxycorticosterone, and aldosterone, all of which are elevated during pregnancy (16).

Prostaglandins of all types are elevated in the maternal serum throughout pregnancy, but most particularly during labor at term. However, despite the finding of a 10%–30% increase in serum levels of the metabolites of prostaglandin F2a (PGF2A), a potent bronchoconstrictor, this does not result in a clinically consistent deleterious effect on asthmatic patients during labor (3).

Histamine is found in high concentration in fetal tissue. The response to this stimulus is the placental production of an histaminase (diamine oxidase) which reaches levels nearly 1,000-fold greater than those seen in nonpregnant women (18). Studies to date have not correlated these biochemical changes with clinical effects, but the potential stimulus to an asthmatic attack inherent with histamine may yet prove to be of some significance (3).

Fetal Oxygenation

Asthma may result in hypoxemia and/or hyperventilation, leading to hypocapnea and alkalosis. With extreme states of airway obstruction, hypercarbia may develop with acidosis. Any clinical disturbance can result in biochemical changes which can have significantly adverse effects on the fetus. Maternal hypoxia will lead to direct fetal hypoxia, and, when the maternal PO_2 goes below 70 torr, the degree of fetal oxygen deprivation becomes significant. Hyperventilation and decreasing PCO_2 will lead to maternal alkalosis and as much as a 24% decrease in fetal scalp PO_2 (19). The mechanisms suggested for such an effect include a decrease in uterine blood flow, placental shunting, and a shift in the maternal O_2 dissociation curve to the left provoked by the developing alkalosis. In the above studies, fetal oxygen delivery was thought to be compromised when the maternal pH exceeded 7.6 and the PCO_2 was 15 torr. It is uncommon to find such extreme values in clinical management (1).

Acute changes can occur with an asthmatic attack and be superimposed on the chronic state of mild alkalosis present throughout pregnancy. These changes are mediated by both mechanical and hormonal factors. Progesterone, by stimulating carbonic anhydrase B in the red blood cell, facilitates CO_2 transfer and leads to a reduction in PCO_2 independent of ventilation changes (6). Wulf et al. (19), by experimentally inducing a condition of maternal hyperventilation, showed that when maternal PCO_2 fell to 13.6 torr, there was a decrease in fetal scalp PO_2 from 24.8 to 19.3 torr despite a rise in maternal PO_2 from 90.8 to 99.7 torr. Moya et al. (20) had shown earlier that hyperventilation induced under anesthesia led to depressed infants. These observations on human subjects and others with sheep suggest that in acute airway obstruction in the asthmatic patient, the combination of hypoxemia and respiratory alkalosis may have adverse fetal effects and that, indeed, it may be the alkalosis that is the more detrimental (3).

Effect of Asthma on Pregnancy

The effect that asthma has on pregnancy has been reported to be of varying degrees of severity for mother and infant. The interpretation of this statement depends on the time the study was performed and the nature of the disease in the population studied. More recent series, where intensive and aggressive management have been exercised, appear to show more favorable outcome than suggested by earlier historical accounts. In two retrospective studies from the 1970s, both Bahna and Bjerkedal (21) (in a series of 381 asthmatic gravidas) and Gordon et al. (22) (in 277 cases) reported increased complications of both a maternal and fetal nature. These studies alluded to greater maternal complications, such as hyperemesis, hemorrhage, and preeclampsia. Gordon et al. (22) reported two maternal deaths. The fetal problems included increased birth hypoxia and perinatal mortality. Of further interest in the later study was the finding that 5.7% (22) of the infants of asthmatic mothers developed the disease within the first year of life.

More recent prospective series, such as that of Fitzsimmons et al. (23), showed a favorable outcome in 56 steroid dependent asthmatics. There were no maternal or neonatal deaths. However, there was a greater frequency of prematurity (19% versus 10%) and low-birthweight infants (29% versus 12%) when compared to a control population and particularly so when studied among women whose course was complicated by emergency room visits and episodes of status asthmaticus.

In another prospective series of 198 gestations among 181 asthmatic women, a greater incidence of mild pre-eclampsia was seen, as well as hypoglycemia among the infants of the severe asthmatics (24). No increase in mortality or prematurity was seen.

Despite these optimistic reports, caution must be exercised in the care of the severe asthmatic. Major life-threatening complications such as mediastinal emphysema and tension pneumothorax have been described (25). The use of bronchoalveolar lavage has been described under controlled ventilation to relieve life-threatening status asthmaticus, which can extend the length of gestation (26, 27).

Effect of Pregnancy on Asthma

The impact that pregnancy has on the asthmatic's clinical course is variable and unpredictable. Symptomatic dyspnea of pregnancy, which affects 60%–70% of pregnant women, can suggest aggravation of the asthmatic's condition (28). However, even with intense prospective management, there will be variable responses, as noted in the prospective study of 181 patients by Stennius et al. (24), where 18% improved, 42% worsened, and 40% remained the same.

Gluck and Gluck (29) have suggested that a rising IgE level may predict the likelihood of a worsening of the asthmatic state during the pregnancy. Conversely, those patients with decreasing IgE levels appeared to improve during the pregnancy. This concept was supported from data on 2,657 nonpregnant patients where there was a significant ($p < 0.0001$) correlation between serum IgE levels and the prevalence of asthmatic symptoms (30).

If patients are to experience an exacerbation in their symptoms, it appears that it will most likely occur in the third trimester or at the time of labor (5, 29). This raises the issue of whether changing hormonal factors, namely, declining progesterone and elevated prostaglandins, may possibly be influential in the exacerbation of the disease.

Recent work dealing with asthma and allergic rhinitis have linked enhanced IgE responsiveness and the apparent autosomal dominant inheritance of atopy with a gene locus on chromosome 11 (31).

Drugs in the Treatment of Asthma

Various pharmacologic agents, as well as immunotherapy, are employed in the treatment of asthma. Commonly employed agents are included in Table 28.1. With the exceptions noted in Table 28.2, the treatment of the pregnant asthmatic is similar to that of her nonpregnant counterpart. During pregnancy, the use of the lowest dose taken as infrequently as possible is desirable. However, because of the significant impact that exacerbations of asthma may have on the outcome of the pregnancy, excess caution may deprive the patient of needed pharmacologic benefits. Since avoidance of asthmatic attacks is a primary goal of therapy, early signs and symptoms should be vigorously treated.

Theophylline is one of the most common bronchodilators. The drug is metabolized primarily in the liver (90%) and, based on clinical reports and experience, is safe for use in pregnancy (10). In cases of acute therapy with parenterally administered theophylline, toxicity can be manifest by nausea, vomiting, abdominal pain, and tachycardia. Cardiac arrythmias and convulsions have been reported with rapid intravenous infusion (3). Of clinical importance are several papers that have shown decreasing clearance of theophylline in pharmacokinetic studies during the third trimester. Such changes warrant frequent (i.e., monthly) determination of theophylline levels to avoid potential toxicity, particularly toward the end of pregnancy (32, 33).

The use of immunotherapy was originally employed for asthma as early as 1911 (34). Immunotherapeutic techniques have been employed during pregnancy with no greater risk of prematurity, toxemia, abortion, perinatal death, or congenital malformations than for the general population (35, 36).

The use of beta-agonist inhalation bronchodilators is a common treatment for both chronic and mild acute asthmatic attacks. Among the more selective agents in this category that are commercially available is albuterol (Proventil-r). In a study of 259 prospectively studied patients using metaproterenol, also a beta agonist, as an inhalent, Schatz, et al. (37) found no significant increase in any of the several parameters that were investigated. These included perinatal mortality, congenital malformations, prematurity, low birthweight, and outcome when these patients were compared to patients not using such agents.

Table 28.1 Therapeutic Recommendations for Pregnant Asthmatics

Chronic Asthma: General Recommendations

Psychogenic support
Environmental control
Desensitization
Avoidance of sensitizing medications
Prophylactic antibiotics
Cromolyn sodium 20–40 mg q.i.d. aerosol
Influenza immunization in the second and third trimester

Acute Asthma: Specific Agents

Nebulized albuterol 0.5cc + 3 cc NS for 5–15 min
Parenteral epinephrine 0.2–0.5 cc, 1:1,000 solution SQ q 30 min
Aminophylline 500 mg/200 cc LR over 30 min
   (4–6 mg/kg/30 min); continue with 0.5 mg/kg/h
Anhydrous theophylline 100–250 mg P.O., q 6 h
   (therapeutic levels 10–20 μg/mL)
Phenobarbital 60 mg q 6 h (or other mild sedative)
Hydrocortisone 100–250 mg/200 cc LR; 4 mg/kg loading,
   0.5 mg/kg/h maintenance
Antibiotics when infectious component present
Hydration 125–150 cc/h
Oxygen p.r.n. based on blood gas determinations
Nebulized bronchodilators (see above)

General Medications

Antibiotics
Ampicillin 250 mg P.O. q.i.d.
Erythromycin 250 mg P.O. q.i.d.

Bronchodilators
Nebulized isoproterenol 1:200 q 3 h
Metaproterenol 10–20 mg P.O. q.i.d.
Terbutaline 2.5 mg P.O. b.i.d. to 5 mg P.O. t.i.d.
Aminophylline 250–500 mg P.O. b.i.d. to q.i.d.
Albuterol by inhalent q 3–4 h
Beclomethasone dipropionate inhaler 100 μg, two inhalations
   t.i.d.–q.i.d.

Systemic Steroids
Prednisone 60–80 mg q.d. in divided doses, tapered in 5–10 days;
   then 2.5–5 mg P.O. b.i.d. to q.d.

Expectorants
Elixer terpin hydrate 5 cc P.O. q 4–6 h
Guaifenesin 5 cc P.O. q 4–6 h

Table 28.2 Drugs to Avoid with Pregnant Asthmatics

Asthmatic Stimuli	Adverse Fetal Effects
Aspirin	Iodides, because of the effect on the fetal thyroid gland
Nonsteroidal antiinflammatory drugs (NSAIDs)	Tetracycline, because of the effect on fetal bones and dentition
Propranolol	
Prostaglandins, especially the abortifacient types (F2a)	
Known sensitizing drugs (PCN)	
Antihistamines	
Sulfa dioxide	
Tartrazine (FDA yellow #5)	
Azo and nonazo food dyes	

Acute therapy for asthmatic attacks has often incorporated the use of epinephrine. As this may affect a reduction in uterine blood flow by alpha stimulation, there is a theoretical reason to avoid its use. There was an increase in the frequency of malformations noted in 189 mother-child pairs seen in The Perinatal Collaborative Project with first-trimester use (38). However, the associated respiratory compromise may also have played a role in the developmental problems. Other reviews have not supported any teratogenic association with epinephrine (39).

As data have accumulated with the use of sodium cromoglycate, this drug appears to be particularly helpful in "allergic" asthma and has prophylactic benefit in exercise-induced asthma (40). It can be administered as a chronic medication by inhalation or for acute therapy in an aerosol form 20–30 minutes before exercise. No dysmorphogenic effects have been reported when used in pregnancy (41). With the use of the inhaled form, only 8% of the administered dose enters the maternal circulation (4). Early studies in animals had suggested that decreased fetal weights occurred when toxic levels were reached in the maternal serum from parenterally administered doses (42). No such findings have been reported in humans.

In a review of 11 series where corticosteroids were employed for the treatment of asthma during pregnancy, few if any untoward effects could be related to the steroid therapy (4). Of 532 pregnancies treated with steroids, the congenital malformation rate was 1.5%, a figure comparable to the rate of the general population. Thus, there is no reason to withhold steroid therapy in a pregnant asthmatic patient when it would otherwise be clinically warranted. Some reports have noted that, in patients on steroid therapy, a slightly greater frequency of prematurely born infants may occur (14.0%) than in the general population (43), as well as more low-birthweight infants (23). These findings, however, may be more related to the severity of the condition than to any pharmacologic effect. Steroid therapy has not been demonstrated to have an effect on fetal adrenal suppression when used throughout pregnancy at therapeutic levels (43). An additional benefit of steroid therapy is the potentiation of the effect of beta agonist bronchodilators (44). The use of inhaled corticosteroids (e.g., beclomethasone [Vanceril-r]) may allow for a reduction in the dose of orally administered corticosteroid (44, 45).

Treatment

The treatment of a pregnant asthmatic patient in the nonacute situation requires a cooperative effort on the part of the obstetrician and pulmonologist. Efforts through patient education and early pharmacologic intervention must be made to avoid the precipitation of an asthmatic attack. This includes the avoidance of drugs known to have adverse fetal effects, specific allergens, and drugs such as aspirin and nonsteroidal antiinflammatory agents, to which 5%–10% of asthmatic patients are sensitive (46) (see Table 28.2).

Foods containing sulfur dioxide and sulfites, tartrazine (FDA yellow #5), a coal tar food additive, and other azo and nonazo dyes have been implicated as stimuli to asthmatic and other allergic attacks.

Individualization is required in asthmatic management. There are, however, certain principles that should be considered when obstetrical care is initiated. These include:

1. Review and elimination of any asthmatic "triggers" known to the patient.
2. Discontinuation of smoking for both pulmonary and obstetrical reasons.
3. Encouragement of prompt communication when infectious problems are suspect in the respiratory tract, such as bronchitis, sinusitis, and rhinitis.
4. Discussion between obstetrician and pulmonologist to review potential individual problems and general management plans, including drug usage.
5. Consideration for the lowering medication doses within the frame of good medical response.
6. Baseline pulmonary function studies as well as blood gas determinations, particularly in the more severely affected patient.

Regularly administered agents such as theophylline should be monitored on a monthly basis to avoid potential toxicity, as well as to allow a reduction in dose when feasible. As noted earlier, if immunotherapy has been initiated or is in progress, this may be continued without anticipation of any adverse fetal effect (36).

In a well-controlled pregnancy, there is no need for early obstetrical intervention. Fetal growth should be monitored using ultrasound and clinical parameters (47), particularly in those patients severely affected by their disease or who are steroid dependent since they are at greater risk for fetal growth problems. Spontaneous onset of labor should be allowed. Preterm intervention would only be justified by an obstetrical indication. Preterm intervention would most likely be justified by obstetrical indications although the occasional life-threatening circumstance may warrant such intervention for maternal reasons.

Because of the increased ventilatory demands on the mother in labor (to 12 L/Min), delivery should take place in a facility prepared to deal with potentially significant pulmonary complications. Schatz et al. (5) reported that 10% of 350 asthmatic women experienced aggravation of their symptoms with the onset of labor.

Terbutaline, a beta-agonist, is often used for tocolytic therapy in preterm labor. It may be best to decrease dosage as term approaches. However, this literature review did not find any references to inordinate delays in the onset of normal labor when this agent was used as standard antiasthmatic therapy. Patients on chronic terbutaline therapy may, however, have increased blood glucose levels, and periodic determinations should be made, in addition to standard diabetic screening (48).

Wheeze, cough, and dyspnea characterize the onset of an acute attack. In the patient who experiences an acute asthmatic attack during pregnancy, the principal physiologic concerns for both mother and fetus are the need to maintain adequate oxygenation and to avoid alkalosis. Initially, the PO_2 is typically less than 80 torr, the PCO_2 less than 35 torr, and the pH above 7.4. As the attack continues, if a pregnant patient's PCO_2 exceeds 35 torr or the arterial pH drops below 7.35 (developing acidosis), hospitalization is warranted (see Table 28.3). A PCO_2 above 60 torr, particularly when associated with developing acidosis (falling pH), probably mandates intubation and assisted ventilation. An arterial PO_2 below 60 torr places the fetus in jeopardy and may necessitate delivery if the pregnancy is close to term, as the pregnancy itself may be compromising pulmonary function. A chest x-ray with abdominal shielding is in order if there is any suspicion of an infectious component and a possible pneumonia (39).

In acute asthmatic attacks with the potential of developing status asthmaticus, therapy should be initiated as follows:

1. Oxygen: humidified at 4–6 L/min.
2. Hydration: IV lactated Ringer's solution or normal saline (NS).
3. Alupent: (Proventil-r) 0.5 cc in 3.0 cc NS administered in a nebulizer over 5–15 minutes.
4. Aminophylline: a soluble salt containing 85% theophylline. The only parenteral form is given as 4–6 mg/kg loading dose and followed with 0.8–1.0 mg/kg/h to achieve a therapeutic level of 10–20 μg/mL. A continuous infusion rate of <0.5 mg/kg/h or 1 g/day will minimize the risk of toxicity. Theophylline levels should be drawn 24 hours after initiating the infusion to allow for a steady

state. Earlier determinations are warranted if the patient is already on theophylline therapy.

5. Steroids: Hydrocortisone 100–250 mg IV Q 8 hours. Change to oral prednisone 60–80 mg/day, tapering over 5–10 days after the attack.
6. Antibiotics: either ampicillin or erythromycin with any suspicion of an infectious component.
7. Intubation, assisted ventilation, and paralysis are rarely required except in life-threatening cases. Here, beta mimetic bronchial lavage has been utilized (26, 27).
8. Serial determinations of blood gases are necessary to monitor the state of oxygenation and to avoid hypercarbia and alkalosis.

If erythromycin as antibiotic therapy is continued for an extended period of time, it will decrease the clearance of theophylline, and the dose of theophylline may require reduction (40).

Delivery

There is no contraindication to the use of conduction anesthetics (e.g., spinal, epidural, caudal), and, indeed, if possible, such techniques would be preferable to general anesthesia for cesarean section. Tachycardia and other cardiac arrythmias are seen particularly in relation to the use of aminophylline, ephedrine, and epinephrine. Both hydroxyzine and droperidol appear to increase airway conductance and are probably safe premedications (49). With narcotic/nitrous oxide combinations, morphine, but not fentanyl, will release histamine, and hence the latter is preferable (50). With the need for general anesthesia, halogenated agents (e.g., halothane) are advantageous because of their broncholytic properties. Nitrous oxide has no specific bronchial effects (3).

Postoperative complications, particularly of a pulmonary nature, are seen with asthmatic patients more than with nonasthmatic patients (24% versus 14%) after operative delivery (51). Conduction anesthesia is not without its own hazards. When epinephrine is added as a vasoconstrictor, it may potentiate cardiac arrythmias in the parturient who is on beta agonist therapy. Bronchospasm was reported to occur in 1.9% of nonpregnant asthmatic patients utilizing regional anesthesia (52).

Table 28.3 Clinical and Laboratory Criteria for Hospitalization of a Pregnant Asthmatic

Test	Finding
PCO_2	>38 torr
PO_2	<70 torr
pH	<7.35
Pulse	>120 beats/minute
Respiratory rate	>30 breaths/minute

For vaginal births, shortening of the second stage by use of vacuum extraction or outlet forceps, though not required, may be beneficial if there is any respiratory compromise.

Patients beginning labor or facing a cesarean section who have had recent steroid therapy or who are currently receiving such medication should be supplemented by 100 mg of hydrocortisone IV and the dose repeated Q 8 hours for 24 hours through labor and delivery to avoid an Addisonian crisis. They may then return to their original regimen immediately after delivery (11).

Postpartum

Postpartum asthma management will proceed as clinically warranted. Dramatic changes in the asthmatic course are not expected. For patients who are interested in breast-feeding, there is no contraindication related to their disease. Theophylline will be present in maternal milk, but the quantity is ~10% of the maternally ingested dose (40). The maximum level in the milk occurs two hours after maternal ingestion (53). Likewise, prednisone is present in an insufficient concentration to have an effect on the newborn (3).

No data are available regarding cromolyn sodium, but because of the relatively low maternal serum level, the newborn exposure should be negligible. For the most part, the medical and psychological benefit of breast-feeding outweigh the theoretical risks (54).

Summary

The management of a patient with asthma during pregnancy requires attention to detail, frequent symptom review, and an alert anticipation of impending problems. Maternal and fetal complications are related to the severity of the asthmatic condition. Various reports show increased rates of preeclampsia, hyperemesis, abnormal labor, increased perinatal mortality, fetal growth retardation, prematurity and neonatal hypoxia (2). Outcome data and the influence of therapy are difficult to interpret because the severity of the disease and the specific therapy varies among the studies reviewed. Well-controlled asthma should not pose a threat to fetal or maternal well-being. Severe disease can have life-threatening implications for both. With a cautious, yet at times aggressive, approach to pulmonary management, a successful outcome can be achieved in an overwhelming majority of the cases treated.

References

1. Mabie WC, Barton JR, Wasserstrum N, et al. Clinical observations on asthma in pregnancy. J Matern Fetal Med 1992; 1:45–50.

2. Management of Asthma during Pregnancy. Report of the Working Group on Asthma and Pregnancy. NIH Publication, No. 93-3279A October 1992.

3. Turner ES, Greenberger PA, Patterson R. Management of the pregnant asthmatic patient. Ann Intern Med 1980;6: 905–18.

4. Perlow JH, Montgomery D, Morgan MA, et al. Severity of asthma and perinatal outcome. Am J Obstet Gynecol 1992; 167:963–67.

5. Schatz M, Harden K, Forsythe A, et al. The course of asthma during pregnancy, postpartum and with successive pregnancies: a prospective analysis. J Allergy Clin Immunol 1988; 81:509–17.

6. DeSwiet M. Pulmonary disorders. In: Creasy R, Resnick R, eds. Maternal-fetal medicine, principles and practice. 2nd ed. Philadelphia: WB Saunders, 1989:875–89.

7. Leontic EA. Respiratory disease in pregnancy. Med Clin North Am 1977;61:111.

8. Greenberger PA. Pregnancy and asthma. Chest 1985; 87 (Suppl):85s–87s.

9. Novy MJ, Edwards MH. Respiratory problems in pregnancy. Am J Obstet Gynecol 1967;99:1024.

10. Greenberger PA. Asthma in pregnancy. Clin Perinatol 1985; 12:571–84.

11. Greenberger PA, Patterson R. Management of asthma during pregnancy. N Engl J Med 1985;312:897–902.

12. Sims CD, Chamberlain GVP, DeSwiet M. Lung function tests in bronchial asthma during and after pregnancy. Br J Obstet Gynecol 1976;83:434–7.

13. Asthma, progesterone and pregnancy. Editorial. Lancet 1990; i:204.

14. Pecora LJ, Putnam LR, Baum GL. Effects of intravenous estrogens on pulmonary diffusion capacity. Am J Med Sci 1963; 246:48–52.

15. Schatz M, Hoffman C. Interrelationships between asthma and pregnancy. Clin Rev Allergy 1987;5:301–15.

16. Vagnucci A, Lee P. Diseases of the adrenal cortex. In: Brody SA, Ueland K, eds. Endocrine disorders in pregnancy. Norwalk: Appleton and Lange, 1989: Ch 12.

17. Holbrook RH, Ueland K. Endocrinology of parturition and preterm labor. In: Endocrine disorders in pregnancy. Norwalk: Appleton and Lange, 1989: Ch 6.

18. Gahl WA, Vale AM, Pitol HC. Spermidine oxidase in human pregnancy serum, probable identity with diamine oxidase. Biochem J 1982;201:161.

19. Wulf KH, Kunzel W, Lehman V. Clinical aspects of placental gas exchange. In: Longo LD, Bartels H, eds. Respiratory gas exchange and blood flow in the placenta. Bethesda, MD: Public Health Serv, 1972:505–21 (DHEW Pub No. NIH-73-361).

20. Moya F, Morishima HO, Shnider SM, James LS. Influence of maternal hyperventilation on the newborn infant. Am J Obstet Gynecol 1965;91:76–84.

21. Bahna SL, Bjerkedal T. The course and outcome of pregnancy in women with bronchial asthma. Acta Allergologica 1972; 27:397–406.

22. Gordon M, Niswander KR, Berendes H, Kantor AG. Fetal morbidity following potentially anoxigenic obstetric conditions. VII Bronchial asthma. Am J Obstet Gynecol 1970; 106:421.

23. Fitzsimons R, Greenberger PA, Patterson R. Outcome of pregnancy in women requiring corticosteroids for severe asthma. J Allergy Clin Immunol 1986;78:349–53.

24. Stenius-Aarniala B, Piirila P, Teramo K. Asthma and pregnancy: a prospective study of 198 pregnancies. Thorax 1988; 43:12–18.

25. Hague WM. Mediastinal and subcutaneous emphysema in a pregnant patient with asthma. Br J Obstet Gynaecol 1980; 87:440.

26. Munakata M, Abe S, Fujimoto S, Kawakami Y. Bronchoalveolar lavage during the third trimester pregnancy in patients with status asthmaticus: a case report. Respiration 1987;51:252–5.

27. Schreier L, Cutler RM, Saigal V. Respiratory failure in asthma during the third trimester: report of two cases. Am J Obstet Gynecol 1989;160:180–1.

28. Gilbert R, Epifano L, Auchincloss JH Jr. Dyspnea of pregnancy: a syndrome of altered respiratory control. JAMA 1962; 182:1073–7.

29. Gluck JC, Gluck PA. The effects of pregnancy on asthma: a prospective study. Ann Allergy 1976;37:164–8.

30. Burrows B, Martinez FD, Halonen M, et al. Association of asthma with serum IgE and skin test reactivity to allergens. N Engl J Med 1989;320:271–7.

31. Cookson WOCM, Faux JA, Sharp PA, et al. Linkage between immunoglobulin E responses underlying asthma and rhinitis and chromosome 11q. Lancet 1989;1:1292–5.

32. Carter BL, Driscoll CE, Smith GD. Theophylline clearance during pregnancy. Obstet Gynecol 1986;68:555–9.

33. Gardner MJ, Schatz M, Cousins L, et al. Longitudinal effects of pregnancy on the pharmacokinetics of theophylline. Eur J Clin Pharmacol 1987;31:289–95.

34. Freeman J. Futher observations on the treatment of hayfever by hypodermic innoculation of pollen vaccine. Lancet 1911; 2:814.

35. Fein BT, Kamin PB. Management of allergy in pregnancy. Ann Allergy 1964;22:341–8.

36. Metzger WJ, Turner E, Patterson R. The safety of immunotherapy during pregnancy. J Allergy Clin Immunol 1978; 61:268–72.

37. Schatz M, Zeiger RS, Harden KM, et al. The safety of inhaled beta agonist bronchodilators during pregnancy. J Allergy Clin Immunol 1988;82:686–95.

38. Heinonen OP, Slone D, Shapiro S. Birth defects and drugs in pregnancy. Littleton, Massachusetts: Publishing Sciences Group, Inc., 1977:287–389.

39. Greenberger PA, Patterson R. The management of asthma during pregnancy and lactation. Clin Rev Allergy 1987; 5:317–24.

40. Mawhinney H, Spector SL. Optimum management of asthma in pregnancy. Drugs 1986;32:178–87.

41. Wilson J. Utilsation du cromoglycate de sodium au cours de la grossesse. Resultats sur 296 femmes asthmatiques. Acta Therapeutica 1982;8(Suppl):45–51.

42. Dykes MHM. Evaluation of an antiasthmatic agent cromolyn sodium. JAMA 1974;227:1061–2.

43. Laurens RG, Honig EG. Corticosteroids in the treatment of asthma. South Med J 1986;79:1544–52.

44. Schatz M, Patterson R, Zeitz S, et al. Corticosteroid therapy for the pregnant asthmatic patient. JAMA 1975;233:804–7.

45. Greenberger PA, Patterson R. Beclomethasone dipropionate for severe asthma during pregnancy. Ann Intern Med 1983; 98:478–80.

46. Mathison DA, Stevenson DD, Simon RA. Precipitating factors in asthma. Chest 1985;87(Suppl):50s–54s.

47. Seeds JW. Impaired fetal growth: evaluation and clinical management. Obstet Gynecol 1984;64:577–84.

48. Main EK, Main DM, Gabbe SG. Chronic oral terbutaline

therapy is associated with maternal glucose intolerance. Am J Obstet Gynecol 1987;157:644.

49. Cottrell JE, Wolfson B, Siker ES. Changes in airway resistance following droperidol, hydroxyzine and diazepam in normal volunteers. Anesth Analg 1976;55:18–21.

50. Moss J, Rosow CE. Histamine release by narcotics and muscle relaxants in humans. Anesthesiology 1983;59:330–9.

51. Fung DL. Emergency anesthesia for asthma patients. Clin Rev Allergy 1985;3:127–41.

52. Shnider SM, Popper EM. Anesthesia for the asthmatic patient. Anesthesiology 1961;22:886–92.

53. Spector SL. The treatment of the asthmatic mother during pregnancy and lactation. Ann Allergy 1983;51:173–5.

54. Coutts, II, White RJ. Asthma in pregnancy. J Asthma 1991; 28:433–36.

29

Epilepsy

S. Roy Meadow, M.D.

RECURRENT seizures of unknown cause affect at least 1% of women of childbearing age. In the United States and Western Europe, the majority of these women regularly take anticonvulsant therapy that enables them to lead normal lives.

Response to Pregnancy

About 50% of epileptic women show no marked change in the frequency of convulsions when they become pregnant; another 30% have more seizures than usual. In this latter group are women who also tended to have seizures while menstruating (1–3). It seems that these patients are responding to some as-yet-undefined metabolic stimulus.

In addition, women who carry a male fetus are twice as likely to deteriorate as those carrying a female. Some women whose seizures increase during gestation suffer severe hyperemesis gravidarum early in pregnancy. Thus, they fail to retain the usual dose of oral anticonvulsant, and this may be the main reason for an increase in frequency of convulsions.

Another predisposing factor may be the induction, by pregnancy, of hydroxylating enzymes that lower the levels of anticonvulsant drugs. Fluid retention and the extra tissue of the fetus and placenta, which increase the volume of distribution of the anticonvulsant drug, may lower its level further.

The remaining patients actually have fewer seizures when pregnant. Finally, there are some curious case reports of women who have had seizures when carrying a male child and none when carrying a female (4).

Epilepsy occurring for the first time during pregnancy is uncommon. Gestational epilepsy tends to be focal more often than other forms. Pregnancy itself is not particularly epileptogenic.

Status epilepticus, although rare during pregnancy, requires prompt, aggressive treatment, just as at other times. It has been suggested that status epilepticus is more likely to be harmful to pregnant than nonpregnant women, but such reports are based on uncontrolled, inconclusive data.

Since the epileptic woman's clinical response to pregnancy varies considerably, she should be supervised closely and reevaluated for drug therapy. If she has troublesome morning sickness, delayed-release capsules may be helpful

Taken at bedtime, the anticonvulsant will be released slowly and—most important—will still be present in the blood the next morning, when she is vomiting and unable to take her usual morning dose.

Severe hyperemesis in a woman accustomed to substantial doses of anticonvulsants is likely to require hospitalization. Unless her vomiting can be controlled, she won't maintain adequate drug levels and can progress to status epilepticus.

Anemia

Epileptic women are often deficient in folic acid, so that, when they become pregnant, an overt anemia frequently develops. Moreover, most anitconvulsant drugs now in common use act as antagonists to folic acid.

A folate supplement, however, will correct the deficiency, which is most accurately determined by measuring the red blood cell level of folic acid rather than the serum folate level. A case can therefore be made for giving a small folate supplement to all women of childbearing age who take anticonvulsants regularly.

Some evidence suggests that additional folate interferes with anticonvulsant metabolism, for instance, by lowering the serum level of phenytoin sodium (5). Yet this does not happen in all patients. Moreover, most persons with epilepsy do not have more seizures when given a small folate supplement, and we cannot identify those few who should not receive folate therapy. Therefore, the risk of a folate supplement increasing the frequency of seizures is small and should not be exaggerated.

Since folate-deficiency anemia is common among pregnant epileptic women, regular blood counts should be done and the anemia should be treated with a folic acid supplement. It is particularly important to ensure that epileptic women are receiving, taking, and retaining the prophylactic iron and folic acid therapy that is usually given to all women during pregnancy. Probably, a low dose of 100 μg, with up to 1,000 μg allowed, is sufficient (6).

Vitamin D Deficiency

The anticonvulsant phenytoin induces the production of enzymes that hydrolyze vitamin D. Women who are prescribed long-term phenytoin and their fetuses have a greater risk of vitamin D deficiency than other pregnant women. They should receive supplementary vitamin D throughout pregnancy, in addition to iron and folic acid.

Pregnancy Complications

There is no major difference between epileptic and non-epileptic women in the incidence of complications of pregnancy. The spontaneous abortion rate is similar for both. The incidence of multiple births is similar as well. Finally, the fertility of both women and men with epilepsy is slightly reduced compared with those who do not have epilepsy.

Although the incidence of toxemia is also similar, there is no doubt that major seizures occurring in women with toxemia sometimes cause undue alarm. Confusion can arise over whether the seizures are a feature of idiopathic epilepsy or of eclampsia. Theoretically, there should be no confusion. Although the diastolic blood pressure may rise to 90 or 95 mm Hg during an epileptic seizure, it does not usually exceed 95, the level associated with an eclamptic convulsion.

Earlier reports of a higher incidence of premature babies born to epileptic mothers have not been confirmed. More recent surveys show a similar incidence of babies of low birthweight (less than 2,500 g) and preterm babies (less than 37 weeks' gestation) to both epileptic and nonepileptic women (7).

In the past 20 years, considerable interest has focused on the possibility of an increased incidence of congenital abnormalities among the offspring of epileptic mothers. There were early reports of babies with cleft lip and palate, unusual skull configurations, and congenital heart defects being born to women with epilepsy (7–11).

A study of 427 pregnancies in 186 epileptic women showed that epileptic mothers who take anticonvulsant drugs while pregnant are more than twice as likely as normal mothers to give birth to malformed babies (7). Of 365 pregnancies in 168 epileptic women taking anticonvulsants, 17 babies with major congenital malformations were born to 16 mothers. The most common defect was congenital heart disease, with an incidence of 18:1,000 births. Cleft lip and microcephaly were also common.

There were no malformations in the infants of 62 pregnancies in 27 epileptic mothers not taking anticonvulsants, and only seven such anomalies in controls. The primary anticonvulsive drugs implicated by the study are phenobarbital, phenytoin, and primidone, which were taken in 15 of the 17 cases in which congenital abnormaltities resulted.

Since those reports, a number of large surveys have been completed in several countries. The general pattern that emerges shows that an epileptic woman has two to three times the normal risk of having a baby with a major congenital anomaly. A healthy woman has a 3% chance of bearing an infant with a major congenital anomaly, whereas, for epileptic women, the risk is in the range of 6%–10%. This figure applies to defects generally, but defects of midline closure   clefts of the lip and palate (ten times more likely)—and septal defects of the heart (four times more likely) appear to be particularly common.

In addition, offspring of epileptic mothers have a relatively high incidence of such minor skeletal abnormalities as small reduction deformities of the phalanges and metacarpal and metatarsal bones. We also see unusually shaped skulls, such as are seen in trigonocephaly, in which the skull appears triangular when viewed from above.

Some investigators have attempted to link a particular anomaly with an individual drug, but it is doubtful that, apart from valproate sodium, one anticonvulsant produces significantly different abnormalities than another. In addition to being associated with the usual dysmorphic features, valproate is unusual in being linked with spina bifida (12). The International Clearinghouse for Birth Defects monitoring system suggests that the risk for a mother with epilepsy taking valproate during pregnancy of having a child with spina bifida is approximately 1.2%, compared with a risk of 0.06% for a woman who neither has epilepsy nor is receiving anticonvulsants (13). Carbamezapine has also been incriminated (14). More worrying have been reports that the offspring of mothers with epilepsy may make slower neurodevelopmental progress.

The direct cause of the increase in congenital anomalies is uncertain. However, among possible explanations are: (1) the teratogenic action of anticonvulsant drugs, (2) damage from seizures, and (3) genetic factors.

Anticonvulsant drugs cross the placenta freely (15, 16). Most have an antifolate action, and evidence suggests that folate depletion predisposes to congenital abnormalities (17).

There is no doubt that strong folate antagonists such as aminopterin cause human congenital abnormalities. Certainly, anticonvulsants have been shown to cause congenital abnormalities in mice and other animals, although this observation has not been directly linked with folate depletion. In addition, experimental anomalies have not been prevented by supplementary folate intake.

We know that the pregnant epileptic woman begins gestation with folate depletion and becomes further depleted as pregnancy proceeds. Vomiting, an inadequate or variable diet, or both, may exacerbate the problem.

Although much of the animal work and several of the reports of human congenital defects have implicated phenytoin sodium, there is no certainty that any one anticonvulsant is more likely to be teratogenic than another. In particular, the large retrospective surveys have not suggested that major anomalies are associated with any individual drug (11, 18).

The surveys do show that epileptic women not receiving anticonvulsants do not have an increased incidence of abnormal babies. However, untreated epileptic women as a group are likely to differ in several ways from treated women. They may have fewer, less severe seizures than those taking drugs regularly. That anticonvulsants in themselves predispose to congenital abnormalities is still unclear.

Prolonged seizures may damage the fetal brain at any age. In pregnancy, hypoxic damage to the fetus could occur as a result of severe maternal seizures. As yet, however, no careful prospective studies comparing the outcome of pregnancy with the frequency or severity of epileptic seizure have been done.

To obtain such information would require a detailed study of the many variables involved, including the type of seizure and the frequency, duration, and time of occurrence. It would also be helpful to learn whether the fetus is more vulnerable to maternal seizures at particular stages of development.

Finally, it is possible that the tendency to epilepsy and the tendency of the epileptic to have abnormal babies are linked. This is known to be the case for facial clefts and may be true for other abnormalities as well.

We know that epileptic mothers have an increased chance of bearing a baby with a major congenital abnormality, but fewer large surveys of children of epileptic fathers have been published. Those that are available suggest that such children have either a small or no increase in congenital abnormalities (18).

It is unfortunate but relevant that epilepsy still imposes social limitations on the choice of spouse, as well as opportunities for employment. Moreover, a considerable number of epileptic women marry epileptic men. Thus, we can at least suspect that the genetic heritage of the offspring is sometimes unfairly weighted toward abnormality.

Most congenital abnormalities result from several influences. A defect is expressed because of genetic, environmental, or intrauterine factors, either separately or in combination. This is likely to be so for the infants of epileptic mothers, too. Although anticonvulsants seem to be one of the factors predisposing to abnormalities, it would be wrong to discontinue or alter anticonvulsant therapy for pregnant mothers. It is important to remember, too, that many of the major congenital abnormalities, including clefts of the lip and palate and congenital heart lesions, can be corrected by surgery.

Hemorrhage Risk in Newborns

The perinatal mortality rate is twice as high among babies of epileptic mothers who are taking anticonvulsants regularly as in the offspring of nonepileptic mothers. This situation is due, not only to the higher incidence of severe congenital abnormalities but also to an increased incidence of spontaneous hemorrhage (7).

Coagulation deficiencies are more likely in newborns whose mothers are taking barbiturate or hydantoin anticonvulsants (19). Overt hemorrhages are uncommon but potentially very serious. A few fetuses die in late pregnancy from massive hemorrhage, but more often bleeding does not occur until after the baby is born.

The hemorrhages are unique in that they occur suddenly and massively in unusual sites, intrathoracically or retroperitoneally (20). The neonatal coagulation defect is similar to that found in vitamin K deficiency, and treatment is with vitamin K or fresh frozen plasma (21).

The mother should be given 10mg of vitamin K daily P.O. during the last two months of pregnancy. This regimen should prevent the occasional severe intrauterine fetal hemorrhage, as well as possible neonatal hemorrhage.

All epileptic mothers should be delivered in a unit with a full hematology service so that any coagulation problems or hemorrhage can be treated promptly. All babies born to epileptic mothers taking anticonvulsants should be given 1 mg of vitamin K IM immediately after birth.

Women with epilepsy require close supervision during pregnancy. A minority have more seizures when pregnant, and many develop folate deficiency anemia. The perinatal mortality rate is twice the normal rate, mainly because of an increased incidence of congenital malformations and spontaneous hemorrhage in the baby.

Although both malformations and hemorrhage may result from anticonvulsant therapy, the pregnant woman with epilepsy needs her usual anticonvulsant therapy. With careful medical supervision and management, she has a good chance of experiencing a normal outcome.

CASE 29.1   Epilepsy in a Primigravida

A 23-year-old primigravida had severe tonic-clonic epilepsy, for which she took 100 mg of phenytoin t.i.d. and 60 mg of phenobarbital t.i.d. Despite these anticonvulsants, she had a major seizure about every eight weeks. After becoming pregnant, she was first seen by her doctor with severe hyperemesis. Her seizures occurred daily and were not satisfactorily controlled until midpregnancy.

During this period, the patient was found to have a severe anemia (hemoglobin 8.1g/dL), which was judged to be the result of folate deficiency. Iron and folic acid were given orally for the rest of the pregnancy.

At 39 weeks' gestation, she was admitted to the hospital in status epilepticus. The seizures caused alarm until eclampsia was ruled out. Her urine contained only a trace of protein, and her blood pressure was only mildly raised. She was given paraldehyde IM, which stopped the seizures. Shortly afterward, she went into labor and gave birth to a 2,800-g boy. The baby was healthy, but he had a cleft lip and palate, an unusual facial appearance, a triangular skull (trigonocephaly), and divarication of the rectus abdominal muscles.

The patient had not been given oral vitamin K during the last two months of pregnancy. Her baby was given 1 mg of vitamin K IM immediately after birth to lessen the chance of hemorrhagic disease of the newborn.

The patient's epilepsy became worse during pregnancy, possibly because the severe hyperemesis prevented her taking her usual anticonvulsants. She had a severe folate-deficiency anemia, probably present before pregnancy and exacerbated by poor food intake because of hyperemesis and the demands of pregnancy. It is also relevant that the fetus was male.

The baby had multiple malformations. It is likely that the anticonvulsant medications were a contributory factor, but, as is so often the case, there were many adverse factors operating at each stage of the pregnancy. ■■

References

1. Rosciszewska D. Fertility and epilepsy. In: Hopkins A, ed. Epilepsy. London: Chapman & Hall, 1987:378.

2. Schmidt D. The effect of pregnancy on the natural history of epilepsy: review of the literature. In: Janz D, Dam M, Richens A, et al. eds. Epilepsy, pregnancy and the child. New York: Raven Press, 1982:3-14.

3. Schmidt D, Canger R, Avanzini G, et al. Change of seizure frequency in pregnant epileptic women. J Neurol Neuro-surg Psychiatry 1983;46:751.

4. Knight AK, Rhind EG. Epilepsy and pregnancy: a study of 153 pregnancies in 59 patients. Epilepsia 1975;16:99.

5. Hiilesmaa VE, Teramo K, Granstrom ML, et al. Serum folate concentrations in women with epilepsy. Br Med J 1983; 187:577.

6. Strauss RG, Bernstein R. Folic acid and Dilantin antagonism in pregnancy. Obstet Gynecol 1974;44:345.

7. Speidel BD, Meadow SR. Maternal epilepsy and abnormalities of the fetus and newborn. Lancet 1972;2:839.

8. Meadow SR. Anticonvulsant drugs and congenital abnormalities. Lancet 1968;2:1296.

9. Meadow SR. Congenital abnormalities and anticonvulsant drugs. Proc Roy Soc Med 1970;63:48.

10. Elshove J, Van Eck JMH. Congenital malformations, particularly cleft lip with or without cleft palate, in children with epileptic mothers. Ned Tijdschr Geneeskd 1971;115:33.

11. Delgado-Escueta AV, Janz D, Beck-Mannagetta G. Pregnancy and teratogenesis in epilepsy. Neurology 1992;42(Suppl 5): 7–160.

12. Tein I, MacGregor DL. Possible valproate teratogenicity. Arch Neurol 1985;42:291.

13. Bjerkedal T, Czeizel A, Goujard J, et al. Valproic acid and spina bifida. Lancet 1982;2:1096.

14. Rosa FW. Spina bifida in infants of women treated with carbamazepine during pregnancy. N Engl J Med 1991;324: 674–7.

15. Melchior JC, Svensmark O, Trolle D. Plancental transfer of phenobarbitone in epileptic women, and elimination in newborns. Lancet 1967;2:860.

16. Mirkin BL. Diphenylhydantoins: placental transport, fetal localization, neonatal metabolism, and possible teratogenic effects. J Pediatr 1971;78:329.

17. Hibbard ED, Smithells RW. Folic acid metabolism in human embryopathy. Lancet 1965;1:1254.

18. Janz D, Dam M, Richens A, et al., eds. Epilepsy, pregnancy and the child. New York: Raven Press, 1982.

19. Mountain KR, Hirsch J, Gallus AS. Neonatal coagulation defect due to anticonvulsant drug treatment in pregnancy. Lancet 1970;1:265.

20. Kohler HG. Haemorrhage in the newborn of epileptic mothers. Lancet 1966;1:267.

21. Davis VA, Argent AC, Staub H, et al. Precursor prothrombin status in patients receiving anticonvulsant drugs. Lancet 1985;1:126.

30

Chronic Hypertension

Frederick P. Zuspan, M.D.

WITHIN the chronic hypertensive diseases, the most common diagnosis is essential vascular hypertension, for which there is no known cause. There are other causes for chronic hypertension, however, but these are less prevalent in younger women.

Chronic hypertension in pregnancy is diagnosed if there is a sustained elevation of arterial blood pressure greater than 140/90 mm Hg prior to the 20th week of gestation. The diagnosis of chronic hypertension is often made retrospectively and can be suspected if the diastolic blood pressure during pregnancy or prior to the twentieth week of gestation is greater than 80 mm Hg.

Classification of chronic hypertension in pregnancy can be mild, moderate, or severe and depends upon the absolute level of blood pressure with or without evidence of end organ damage. If the patient has superimposed preeclampsia, this is one of the most severe problems that mother and fetus will encounter.

There are many classifications of chronic hypertension, one of which is shown in Table 30.1.

Blood Pressure Regulation

The brachial artery blood pressure is highest in the sitting position and lowest when on the side. Uterine size and compression of the inferior vena cava and aorta are factors

Table 30.1 Chronic Hypertensive Disease

Primary: essential or idiopathic, most common type observed.

Secondary (to a specific or known cause)
  Renal: parenchymal (glomerulonephritis, chronic pyelonephritis, interstitial nephritis, polycystic kidney); renal vascular

  Adrenal: cortical—Cushing's syndrome, hyperaldosteronism medullary—pheochromocytoma; other—coarctation of aorta, thyrotoxicosis

Chronic hypertensive disease with superimposed preeclampsia (after the 20th week of pregnancy)

Reprinted with permission from Zuspan FP, O'Shaughnessy RW. Chronic hypertension in pregnancy. In: Pitkin RM, ed. Yearbook of obstetrics and gynecology. Chicago: Year Book Medical Publishers; 1989.

that alter blood pressure readings as the uterus enlarges. It is imperative to take the blood pressure reading during pregnancy with the patient lying on her side. Consistency in taking measurements will assure that a first- and second-trimester reading can be compared with a third-trimester reading (Table 30.2).

Women who have chronic hypertensive disease in pregnancy are instructed in self-blood-pressure determination using a two-headed stethoscope. The blood pressure is taken in the upper arm while the patient is in the lateral recumbent position with a 15- to 30-degree tilt. The upper arm should be brought across the chest to near the level of

the heart. An aneroid gauge manometer is preferred.

It is important to record the systolic, the fourth, and the fifth Korotkoff sounds. The fourth Korotkoff sound is preferable since pregnancy is a high cardiac output condition, but, if all three values are recorded, there is no confusion in understanding each value.

If the mean arterial blood pressure (MAP) is persistently greater than 100 mm Hg, the prognosis for the fetus begins to worsen. MAP can be calculated by the formula

$$\text{MAP} = (\text{Systolic} + 2\ \text{Diastolic})\ /3$$
or
$$\text{Diastolic} + [(\text{Systolic} - \text{Diastolic})\ /3]$$

Studies have shown that fetal loss is directly proportional to the elevation of the mean arterial blood pressure (Figure 30.1).

The circadian rhythm of all humans for blood pressure recordings indicates that the blood pressure is lowest during sleep, and next lowest upon awakening. It is highest in the afternoon and then gradually decreases as activity decreases. We ask the patient to take her blood pressure at least two times during the work week and once on the weekend. We would prefer to have the blood pressure taken prior to the noon rest of 45 minutes.

Suspicion and Diagnosis of Disease

It is often difficult, if a patient does not have overt hypertension (that is, a blood pressure of greater than 140/90 mm Hg prior to the twentieth week of gestation), to be certain that chronic hypertension is an underlying factor. If one or more of the following factors are present, chronic hypertension may be suspected:

- Diastolic blood pressure in a nonpregnant state or prior to the twentieth week of gestation that consistently exceeds 80 mm Hg. It is important to remember that "white coat" hypertension (that is, an increase in office blood pressure) does not make this reading accurate.
- Antecedent history of hypertension during pregnancy or to a stress event.
- History of secondary causes of hypertension (for

Table 30.2 Recommendations on Care

Patient should be seen at least every two weeks during prenatal visits.

Encourage her to take blood pressure (BP) readings before and after 45 minutes of bed rest at noon.

Encourage additional bed rest of at least one hour before the evening meal.

Emphasize that lying on her side is the only acceptable method to increase uterine blood flow to the baby.

If the home BP recording is consistently greater than 84 mm Hg in the first half of pregnancy, consider pharmacotherapy to control BP. (There is no proof that pharmacotherapy will alter fetal salvage, but it should control major alterations in maternal BP and be protective for the mother.)

Reemphasize that in a well-balanced diet, it is essential to have at least 70 g of protein per day to maintain a zero-nitrogen balance and to restrict salt intake by using fresh or frozen food.

Reestablish and reaffirm the specific estimated date of delivery by ultrasound.

Ultrasound will probably need to be done on at least three occasions, perhaps in the first trimester for pregnancy dating, then at 28 weeks, and again at 32 to 34 weeks to rule out IUGR.

Careful dating of gestational age is important since one of the precepts in caring for the chronic hypertensive patient is not to permit her to go beyond term.

A second precept is to prevent the patient from developing preeclampsia; if it does develop, this should be diagnosed by an increase in BP and the development of proteinuria.

example, chronic renal disease).

- A positive family history of hypertension.
- Hypertension in previous pregnancies.

Home blood pressure monitoring permits the patient to be her own advocate and further reinforces the role of bed rest as well as the control of her situation. It diminishes the use of antihypertensive drugs during pregnancy as well as decreasing the need for hospitalizations.

Management Protocol

Ideally, preconceptional counseling would be important for the woman who has chronic hypertension. She may well have had a tragic experience with a previous pregnancy and may have developed preeclampsia. It is important to establish baseline data on this patient, including prepregnancy laboratory work, and to teach her self-blood pressure monitoring prior to conception. If the patient is taking a specific type of medication and she contemplates pregnancy, her medication should be changed to one acceptable during the pregnancy. If she is taking diuretics, their dosage should

gradually be diminished and eventually eliminated prior to conception.

An appropriate diet that curtails heavy salt (NaCl) use is also recommended. The easiest way this can be achieved is to encourage the patient to utilize fresh or frozen food and avoid liquids or foods in cans or bottles. This basically amounts to a 4-g NaCl diet, which is sufficient restriction for the pregnant chronic hypertensive patient. Table 30.2 gives additional instructions.

Therapy during Pregnancy

The major therapy for women who have chronic hypertensive diseases of pregnancy is bed rest (Figure 30.1). This should be encouraged for 45 minutes at noontime and for one hour prior to the evening meal. The physician, nurse, and patient must understand that this is the only way to increase uterine blood flow. There are no drugs that will increase the flow.

Studies have shown that uterine blood flow is increased in the left lateral recumbent position. The mechanism for this increased flow is most likely the decreased

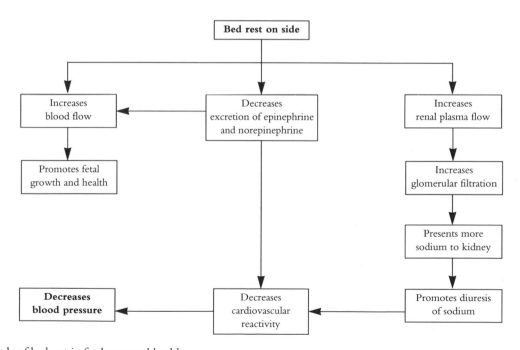

Figure 30.1 Role of bed rest in fetal–maternal health.

Table 30.3 Commonly Used Drugs

Name	Type	Usual dose
Propranolol	β blocker	20–40 mg b.i.d. to q.i.d.
Atenolol	β blocker	25–50 mg b.i.d. to t.i.d.
Labetalol	β blocker with α component	100 mg b.i.d. to t.i.d.
Hydralazine*	Direct action	20–30 mg b.i.d. to q.i.d.

*More useful in parenteral doses because tachyphylaxis will often occur.

excretion of stress hormones (epinephrine and norepinephrine), increased renal plasma flow, and increased glomerular filtration rate to the kidneys. This sequence presents more sodium to the kidney and promotes the "physiologic diuresis" of sodium that, in turn, decreases cardiovascular reactivity and maintains a stable or decreased blood pressure. All of this ultimately ends up promoting fetal growth and health. Therapeutic doses of magnesium sulfate are prescribed only if the patient develops superimposed preeclampsia.

When the diastolic blood pressure exceeds 90 mm Hg, therapy is administered specifically for the mother (Table 30.3). It has never been shown to improve fetal condition. The drug of choice for the past 20 years has been methyldopa in divided doses of 750 to 2,000 mg per day. More recently, clinicians have chosen such beta blockers as aten-

olol and propranolol or the alpha and beta blocker labetalol. Beta blockers should be used cautiously because they are associated with IUGR. ACE inhibitors are associated with congenital renal anomalies and are contraindicated.

All drugs cross the placenta and enter the fetal circulation. Newborns usually make good adjustments to these drugs unless prematurity is a factor. These drugs have not been known to cause birth defects.

Bromocriptine mesylate should not be used for lactation suppression if the patient has hypertension. It has been recommended that breast-feeding should be avoided if beta blockers are used postpartum in marked amounts.

Antepartum Fetal Evaluation

Antepartum fetal evaluation begins at the start of the pregnancy (Table 30.4). A tape should be used to measure from the symphysis to the uterus to assess fetal growth. Periodic ultrasound scans should be scheduled. Biochemical testing has been of no value, and only biophysical testing is currently used.

Careful dating of gestation is important. Intrauterine growth retardation is usually not seen until after the 30th or 32d week of gestation. The patient should not be permitted to go beyond term, and often delivery prior to the 38th week of gestation is necessary (Table 30.5). If the patient develops preeclampsia, hospitalization and early delivery are in order.

Table 30.4 Ruling Out Hypertension

Serial ultrasound to date gestation should initially be done around 10–12 weeks, again at 20–24 weeks, and next at 30–32 weeks to observe for IUGR.

Nonstress tests (NST) should be done on each visit from 30 weeks on, and nipple stimulation or oxytocin contraction test (OCT) may be needed if the NST is unsatisfactory. The vibroacoustic stimulation test will facilitate the NST.

Fetal movement activity count is used after 34th week of gestation. The patient is instructed to lie on her side for two 1-hour periods and do fetal kick counts. If the counts are greater than six per hour, this indicates fetal health.

If preterm delivery and lack of pulmonary maturity are present, glucocorticoids utilizing betamethazone or dexamethazone may be given to decrease respiratory distress syndrome.

Table 30.5 Labor and Delivery Considerations

It would be advisable to deliver the patient no later than term and before superimposed preeclampsia or IUGR.

Continuous electronic fetal monitoring during labor is advised.

Early rupture of membranes for scalp electrode application and judicious use of scalp pH as needed.

Regional anesthesia with epidural is satisfactory and ideal, but guard against hypotension if the patient has had antihypertensive medication during pregnancy. An adequate fluid load prior to anesthesia is essential.

A pediatrician should be available to evaluate the baby. Assume that all antihypertensive agents cross the placenta. The newborn usually does quite well if it is not premature.

Chronic hypertension is associated with a four- to eightfold increase in abruptio placentae. Care should be taken when the patient complains of abdominal discomfort to rule this out.

Long-term Considerations

Women who have chronic hypertension should not be prescribed oral contraceptives once they leave the hospital or at their six-week examination. Some form of barrier contraception is preferable. Many of these women have completed their childbearing and can be offered a permanent form of contraception.

The majority of women who have mild or moderate hypertension should do well during pregnancy and can expect to have a liveborn baby. If complications occur, then it is necessary to handle each individual problem appropriately.

Suggested Reading

Rayburn WF, Zuspan FP, Biehl EJ. Self blood pressure monitoring during pregnancy. Am J Obstet Gynecol 1984;148:159.

Redman CWG, Bellin LJ, Bonnar J, et al. Fetal outcome in trial of antihypertensive treatment in pregnancy. Lancet 1976; 2:753.

Reiss RE, O'Shaughnessy RW, Quilligan EJ, et al. Retrospective analysis of blood pressure course during preeclamptic and matched controls. Am J Obstet Gynecol 1987;156:894.

Rubin PC, Butters L, Clark D, et al. Obstetric aspects of the use of pregnancy-associated hypertension of the β-adrenoceptor antagonist atenolol. Am J Obstet Gynecol 1984; 150:389.

Sibai BM, Abdella TN, Anderson GD. Pregnancy outcome in 211 patients with mild chronic hypertension. Obstet Gynecol 1983;61:571.

Zuspan FP. Chronic hypertension in pregnancy. Clin Obstet Gynecol 1984;27:854.

Zuspan FP, O'Shaughnessy RW. Maternal physiology and diseases; chronic hypertension in pregnancy. In: Pitkin RM, Zlatnik FJ, eds. Yearbook of obstetrics and gynecology. Chicago: Year Book Medical Publishers, 1989:11.

31

Systemic Lupus Erythematosus

Robert Resnik, M.D.

LESS than 50 years ago, systemic lupus erythematosus (SLE) was considered an extremely rare and dramatic clinical entity. The classic findings consist of a facial butterfly rash, fever, malaise, and involvement of such organs as the pleura, pericardium, joints, hematologic system, and kidneys. Those afflicted with the disease usually died within a few months.

Today, we know that SLE is much more common than previously believed and that the vast majority of patients have mild and unobtrusive symptoms. Lupus is ten times more common in women than in men and most often occurs in the first few decades of life. Consequently, it may occasionally coincide with pregnancy, causing complications.

The clinical manifestations of SLE tend to be rather vague and insidious. For example, the well-known malar rash in a butterfly pattern is seen in only 50% of patients and may be quite faint. However, approximately 95% of all lupus patients will, at some point, develop systemic symptoms, including fatigue, malaise, low-grade fever, anorexia, and weight loss. Joint and muscle pain are also quite common, as are cardiopulmonary symptoms, predominantly pleurisy and pericarditis. But perhaps most consistently associated with SLE are hematologic abnormalities, such as hypochromic microcytic anemia, leukopenia, and, less frequently, thrombocytopenia.

Laboratory Tests

Because SLE is a diffuse multisystem autoimmune disease, sufferers often have a wide array of autoantibodies and circulating immune complexes. The hallmark and primary indicator is the antinuclear antibody (ANA), but some patients will also have leukopenia and hypergammaglobulinemia. Antiplatelet antibodies and anticardiolipin antibodies (ACL) occur less often, although patients may have false-positive serology if antiphospholipid antibodies are present.

Anti-DNA antibodies are frequently correlated with SLE activity, such as lupus nephritis flare-ups. In addition, serum complement levels of C3 or C4 may decrease, possibly because these components are consumed by immune complexes during the antigen-antibody reaction of disease activity. Thus, because anti-DNA and complement are associated with SLE, it is advisable to obtain baseline studies in all patients early in pregnancy, even if their disease is in remission.

Clinical Effects

Generally, active-phase SLE is exacerbated by pregnancy. Roughly 50% of such patients will become worse, while very few will improve. However, about two-thirds of patients in remission before conception show no worsening of disease during pregnancy (1–4).

Some investigators have observed that flare-ups of severe nephritis are common in patients insufficiently treated with steroids (2). Others believe that pregnancy has no substantial effect on the disease state, although they note that thrombocytopenia and preeclampsia are more common (5). Indirectly, these syndromes are probably linked with SLE via their association with anticardiolipin antibodies, lupus anticoagulant, or both.

The effects of SLE on the fetus are more variable. They largely correspond to the degree of severity of the disease and the presence of specific antibodies directed at either maternal or fetal tissues.

Overall, patients with SLE have a higher incidence of spontaneous abortion, intrauterine growth retardation, and stillbirth. Preterm birth is also more common, though it is generally a consequence of medically indicated preterm deliveries resulting from specific maternal or fetal complications.

Conversely, outcomes among women whose disease is in remission are generally quite favorable. These women often fare better because they usually do not suffer complications from specific antibodies.

Lupus Anticoagulant and Anticardiolipin Antibodies

The lupus anticoagulant was first described as a circulating coagulation inhibitor occurring in association with SLE (6). Patients with this inhibitor have abnormal coagulation pro-files (specifically, a prolonged activated partial thromboplastin time) that do not improve when normal plasma is added. Lupus anticoagulant is an acquired antibody (IgM or IgG) directed toward the phospholipid component of the cell wall. The ACL is another antiphospholipid protein that may coexist with lupus anticoagulant and may be found in the blood of women with SLE.

Both antibodies are strongly associated with a history of venous or arterial thrombosis. It is important to note that, while either or both antibodies may be present in known SLE cases, they may also occur in women lacking specific criteria to confirm an SLE diagnosis.

The association between these antibodies and fetal loss is a recently recognized phenomenon. The presence of lupus anticoagulant is associated with a higher risk of embryonic and fetal death than any other condition known. Recent data demonstrate that, among 264 pregnancies in 68 women with lupus anticoagulant, the combined abortion and perinatal mortality rate was 94%. Two-thirds of the losses were from recurrent spontaneous abortions. Of the 17 liveborn infants in the accumulated series, 41% were delivered preterm and 18% were severely growth retarded (7).

Because many women with these antibodies have never had symptoms to suggest SLE, the clinician should test for the antibodies in any woman with a history of the following:

- Recurrent fetal losses
- Connective tissue disorder
- Venous or arterial thrombosis
- False-positive serology
- Thrombocytopenia

The presence of anticardiolipin antibody may be confirmed by direct laboratory evaluation. Lupus anticoagulant is usually screened by measuring the activated partial thromboplastin time (APTT). Although the partial thromboplastin time may be prolonged by an intrinsic clotting factor deficiency, testing with a 1:1 addition of normal plasma will help to differentiate between the two disorders. If the coagulation abnormality is caused by an intrinsic factor deficiency, the activated partial thromboplastin time will return to the normal range. If a circulating anticoagulant is the source of the problem, the APTT will remain abnormal.

A number of small, uncontrolled clinical trials seems to suggest that, for women with lupus anticoagulant, the combination of high-dose corticosteroid therapy and low-dose aspirin improves fetal outcome. The usual daily regimen is 40–60 mg of prednisone combined with 80 mg of aspirin every other day. The rationale for the use of corticosteroid is to suppress antibody production; the low-dose aspirin is used to inhibit the production of thromboxane A2, a vasoconstrictive prostaglandin associated with platelet aggregation and thrombocytopenia. Although not successful in all cases, this treatment often appears to improve fetal outcome markedly (8–10). More recently, it has been shown that anticoagulation with heparin may be as, if not more, effective than corticosteroid therapy (11).

More controversial is management of the patient with only anticardiolipin antibodies. Currently, it is not known how corticosteroids react during treatment of this condition or whether they are beneficial or deleterious. However, most investigators agree with the use of low-dose aspirin.

Anti-Ro Antibodies

In the early 1980s, the association between congenital heart block and SLE was well recognized, and we now know that almost all infants with congenital block are born to mothers who have anti-Ro (SSA) antibodies. It is important to remember that half of these women will be clinically normal, without any evidence of SLE. Furthermore, the vast majority of women with anti-Ro antibodies will not have children with heart block. Therefore, the presence of the anti-Ro antibody does not appear to represent a major risk to the neonate, although mothers of neonates with the disorder usually have the antibody (12).

It is very important, however, to detect the cardiac lesion in the fetus so that a pediatric cardiologist can be available to provide immediate care and artificial pacing shortly after birth, if necessary. The mortality rate for neonates with congenital heart block may be as high as 25%. Fortunately, the condition is easily detectable prenatally by auscultation and M-mode echocardiography.

It is notable that some neonates will have transient serologic abnormalities or skin lesions, others will have congenital heart block, and a few will suffer all three abnormalities. Fortunately, the serologic abnormalities and skin lesions usually resolve during the first year of life.

Pregnancy Management

At the first prenatal visit, patients with SLE should undergo routine prenatal laboratory work. They should also have a platelet count and be tested for blood urea nitrogen (BUN) creatinine, anti-DNA antibody, anticardiolipin, and anti-Ro levels. In addition, partial thromboplastin time should be measured to check for lupus anticoagulant. C3 and C4 levels may be useful during flare-ups.

Serial ultrasounds should be performed to determine if fetal growth is adequate. Also, fetal function should be assessed by biophysical profiling or contraction stress testing as soon as appropriate.

Corticosteroids remain the mainstay of treatment for patients with SLE. Generally, mild flares such as rashes and arthritis can be managed with relatively low doses of prednisone. However, higher doses are indicated if major organ system involvement—such as nephritis, central nervous system disorders, or vasculitis—should occur. Low-dose aspirin may also be of value. Potent immunosuppressive agents are another option, but they should be used only when severe flares are unresponsive to other types of therapy.

Preeclampsia and Lupus Nephritis

It is often difficult to differentiate between preeclampsia and lupus nephritis when patients develop hypertension and proteinuria. If there are no other symptoms of SLE, preeclampsia is the likely diagnosis. However, decreases in serum complement and increases in anti-DNA antibodies suggest lupus nephritis. If the patient suffers from nephritis corticosteroids should be used liberally.

If the syndrome appears to represent preeclampsia, traditional obstetric management is appropriate, including maternal and fetal indications for delivery. Patients developing thrombocytopenia independent of hypertension or proteinuria usually will have lupus anticoagulant or anticardiolipin antibodies. The platelet count generally returns to normal following delivery.

References

1. Hayslett JP. Effective pregnancy in patients with SLE. Am J Kidney Dis 1982;2:223.

2. Tozman ECS, Urowitz MB, Gladman DD. Systemic lupus erythematosus and pregnancy. J Rheumatol 1980;7:624.

3. Zulman MI, Telal N, Hoffman GS, et al. Problems associated with the management of pregnancy in patients with systemic lupus erythematosus. J Rheumatol 1980;7:37.

4. Lockshin MD, Reinitz E, Druzin ML, et al. Lupus pregnancy. Case-control prospective study demonstrating absence of lupus exacerbation during or after pregnancy. Am J Med 1984;77:893.

5. Lockshin MD, Harpel PC, Druzin ML, et al. Lupus pregnancy. II. Unusual pattern of hypocomplementemia and thrombocytopenia in the pregnant patient. Arthritis Rheum 1985; 28:58.

6. Conley CL, Hartmann RC. A hemorrhagic disorder caused by circulating anticoagulant in patients with disseminated lupus erythematosus. J Clin Invest 1952;31:621.

7. Gant NF. Lupus erythematosus, the lupus anticoagulant and the anticardiolipin antibody. Wyeth Laboratories Supplement No. 6, Appleton-Century-Crofts. 1986;(May/June):7.

8. Lubbe WF, Butler WS, Palmer SJ, et al. Fetal survival after prednisone suppression of maternal lupus anticoagulant. Lancet 1983;1:1361.

9. Lubbe WF, Butler WS, Palmer SJ, et al. Lupus anticoagulant in pregnancy. Br J Obstet Gynaecol 1984;91:357.

10 Lubbe WF, Liggins GC. Lupus anticoagulant and pregnancy. Am J Obstet Gynecol 1985;153:322.

11. Branch DW, Silver RM, Blackwell JL, et al. Outcome of treated pregnancies in women with antiphospholipid syndrome: an update of the Utah experience. Obstet Gynecol 1992;80:614.

12. Watson RM, Braunstein BL, Watson AJ, et al. Fetal wastage in women with anti-Ro (SSA) antibody. J Rheumatol 1986;13:90.

32

Toxoplasmosis in Pregnancy

John L. Sever, M.D., Ph.D.
Antonio V. Sison, M.D.

Introduction

The first case of congenital toxoplasmosis in humans was reported by Janku, an ophthalmologist in Prague, in 1933 (1). He recognized parasitic cysts in the retina of a child with congenital hydrocephalus and microphthalmia with coloboma in the macular region. The organism is a coccidian, *Toxoplasma gondii*, named after the North African rodent (the gondii) from which the organism was first isolated. It is ubiquitous in nature and is an important cause of abortion in sheep and swine.

Primary maternal toxoplasmosis during pregnancy occurs in approximately 1:900 pregnancies in the United States. This estimate is based on a prospective study of sera from 23,000 pregnant women done in early and late gestation (2). The study, which was conducted by the National Institutes of Health (NIH), showed that 38% of the women tested had antibody to *Toxoplasma gondii*, indicating previous infection with the organism. The presence of antibody correlated with increasing patient age and was twice as frequent among blacks as among whites. Women who had lived in Puerto Rico were twice as likely as black women to have the *Toxoplasma gondii* antibody. None of these mothers tested had evidence of significant clinical disease.

Follow-up of the children delivered by the women from this study showed that acute infection with *Toxoplasma gondii* during pregnancy resulted in cases of microcephaly and low IQ. One child had obvious findings of congenital toxoplasmosis and was positive to toxoplasma-specific IgM at birth. Several others showed no more than one of the clinical features associated with fetal damage. The main clinical findings in the affected child were typical of congenital toxoplasmosis and included hypotonia, hepatosplenomegaly, lethargy, nystagmus, chorioretinitis, and microcephaly. Only primary infection in the pregnant woman results in congenital infection in the infant. Approximately one-third of mothers who acquire primary toxoplasmosis while pregnant transmit the infection to their infant.

In some studies done in the United States, the incidence of congenital toxoplasmosis has been estimated to be as high as 1:750 births. However, the higher estimates probably relate to 1) the high rate of infection in the indigent populations which were studied and 2) the inclusion of both asymptomatic and subclinically infected children.

Clinical Findings

Maternal infection with *Toxoplasma gondii* is usually asymptomatic, although 10%–20% of infected mothers present with lymphadenopathy. Posterior cervical lymphadenopathy is the most frequent finding associated with acute maternal toxoplasmosis. The infection can also result in a mononucleosislike syndrome with fatigue and lassitude and, rarely, in encephalitis. Patients who are immunosuppressed, such as those infected with the human immunodeficiency virus type 1 (HIV-1), are particularly at risk for acute toxoplasmosis and for developing severe sequelae (3–5).

Newborns with congenital toxoplasmosis become infected in utero by the transplacental route. The clinical findings are shown in Table 32.1. Chorioretinitis is the single most common clinical manifestation of symptomatic toxoplasmosis in the newborn. The frequency of congenital toxoplasmosis following acute maternal infection is directly related to which trimester of pregnancy the woman developed the infection. In general, the risk of fetal infection

Table 32.1 Clinical Findings with Congenital Toxoplasmosis

Chorioretinitis
Hydrocephaly
Jaundice
Hepatosplenomegaly
Microcephaly
Glaucoma
Convulsions
Fever
Hypothermia
Lymphadenopathy
Vomiting
Diarrhea
Cataracts
Microphthalmia
Optic atrophy
Pneumonia

increases with each trimester of pregnancy. Similarly, the severity of damage associated with congenital toxoplasmosis is related to the timing of maternal infection (6). Severe fetal disease or fetal death occurs in about 10% of cases when infection occurs in the first trimester, drops to about 5% when infection occurs in the second trimester, and is extremely rare with infection in the third trimester. Mild damage is more frequent in the second and third trimesters (about 5%). Subclinically evident infections increase from about 2% with first-trimester infections to 50% with third-trimester infections.

Transmission

Cats

The definitive host for *Toxoplasma gondii* is the cat. About half of the cats tested in this country have antibodies to *Toxoplasma*. It is thought that cats become infected by eating infected wild rodents and birds. A week after infection, the cat begins to shed oocysts in its feces. Shedding of oocysts persists for about two weeks before the cat spontaneously recovers. These animals are susceptible to reinfection and may also shed *Toxoplasma* oocysts when infected with other organisms.

Cat feces are extremely infectious. The fecal oocysts are spread through the air and, when inhaled, are likely to cause infection. Sporulation of the organism occurs after 1–5 days in the litter and may be prevented by changing the litter daily. If the oocysts are deposited on soil, the particles remain on top and tend to float on rainwater. The oocysts remain viable for more than a year but are inactivated by freezing, drying, heating above 50°C, or exposure to ammonia, iodine, or formalin. Care must be taken in disposing of cat litter.

Meat

The "Christiaan Barnard" epidemic is an example of transmission through ingestion of infected meat. Several years ago, Dr. Barnard visited Cornell University Medical College to talk about heart transplant surgery. A large number of students tried to get lunch in the cafeteria before the lecture began. When the cafeteria became swamped with customers, the cook hurriedly served rare or raw hamburgers. A few of the students contracted clinical or subclinical toxoplasmosis.

The ingestion of infected meat is an important cause of toxoplasmosis in Europe, where the use of refrigeration is more limited and meat is usually not frozen. In this country, much of the meat is frozen at some point during storage or transport. Freezing is probably one of the factors responsible for the difference in incidence of toxoplasmosis here and in Europe. Worldwide, about 1% of cattle, 20% of hogs, and 30% of sheep have toxoplasmosis, according to estimates based on isolation of the organism from animal muscle tissue. Meat should therefore be cooked thoroughly at adequate temperatures to avoid the transmission of toxoplasma.

Diagnosis

Mother

Clinical diagnosis of acute toxoplasmosis is not reliable due to the nonspecific findings associated with the infection. Nevertheless, acute toxoplasmosis should be considered in any pregnant woman who presents with lymphadenopathy, particularly involving the posterior cervical chain, and/or mononucleosislike symptoms. The vast majority, however, of those acutely infected with *Toxoplasma gondii* are asymptomatic.

The diagnosis of primary infection with *Toxoplasma gondii* during pregnancy requires either 1) the demonstration of a seroconversion to this organism, 2) a significant rise in antibody titer obtained from maternal sera taken at two different times, or 3) the detection of toxoplasma-specific IgM antibody. Adults with primary infection develop IgG and IgM antibody to toxoplasma rapidly. Toxoplasma-specific IgG antibody develops within two weeks after infection and persists for life. Toxoplasma-specific IgM develops within 10 days after infection and remains elevated for six months to more than six years (7).

Since IgM antibody remains elevated for many months, this test may not provide useful information to document recent primary infection in pregnant women. The enzyme-linked immunosorbent assay (ELISA) test for IgM frequent-

ly shows the development of high titers of antibody which persist for many years. Indirect immunofluorescence antibody (IFA) tests for toxoplasma-specific IgM usually show high titers for only about six months after infection, following which, the titer rapidly drops. The IFA test then is frequently more useful than ELISA in differentiating remote from recent primary infection in a pregnant woman.

Approximately 50% of placentas of congenitally infected infants will show *Toxoplasma gondii* cysts on histological slides, and their presence supports the diagnosis of acute infection in the mother during pregnancy. The organism has also been isolated from placental tissue of acutely infected mothers in 2%–25% of cases (8). Recovery was more frequent when infection occurred later in pregnancy.

Child

Clinically symptomatic newborns will present with findings, as shown in Table 32.1. The most frequent clinical findings are chorioretinitis, jaundice, fever, and hepatosplenomegaly. Demonstration of toxoplasma-specific IgM in the affected infant confirms the diagnosis of congenital infection, although approximately 20% of infected newborns are not detectable by toxoplasma-specific IgM at birth. Presence of the cysts of *Toxoplasma gondii* in histological sections of the placenta also strongly supports the diagnosis of fetal infection.

Prenatal Diagnosis

Antenatal diagnosis of fetal toxoplasmosis has relied on culture of amniotic fluid or fetal blood obtained at the time of diagnostic amniocentesis or cordocentesis, respectively. The specimen is commonly cultured in mice or fibroblast cells (9, 10). The main difficulties with culture techniques have been that some assays may take up to several weeks to get complete results, and very few laboratories are able to perform the assay. Nevertheless, detection of the organism in fetal blood by culture appears to be the most useful prenatal method of diagnosis.

Toxoplasma-specific IgM, when present in fetal blood from cordocentesis, has also been used to diagnose fetal infection prenatally. Unfortunately, fetal-specific IgM antibody frequently does not develop until after 21–24 weeks' gestation and is only positive in about 50% of infected cases. Thus, this test has less value than culture for the in utero diagnosis of toxoplasmosis.

Preliminary reports suggest that gene amplification techniques such as the polymerase chain reaction (PCR), used to detect *Toxoplasma gondii* DNA, has been shown to be useful in the detection of fetal infections in utero (11, 12). Grover et al. compared PCR to detection of fetal toxoplasma-specific IgM in fetal blood and inoculation of amniotic fluid into mice and tissue culture (12). The study showed that PCR identified five of five samples from amniotic fluid from four proven cases of congenital infection. In comparison, detection of IgM in fetal blood and inoculation of amniotic fluid into tissue culture identified only three and four of 10 samples from confirmed infected infants, respectively. Therefore, PCR may prove to be a reliable method of prenatal diagnosis for congenital toxoplasmosis.

More recent literature has shown that detection of toxoplasma-specific IgA may be a reliable method for the diagnosis of toxoplasmosis in the newborn (13). Stepick-Biek et al. detected toxoplasma-specific IgA antibodies in 12 pregnant women who seroconverted during pregnancy and in eight of nine infants with evidence of congenital toxoplasmosis (13).

The laboratory methods presently available for the detection of *Toxoplasma gondii* are summarized in Table 32.2.

Treatment and Prevention

Mother

Treatment of the clinical findings associated with acute toxoplasmosis is primarily supportive. The prognosis in general following acute infection is good, except in the setting of profound immunosuppression (such as in acquired immunodeficiency syndrome) where patients can develop severe neurological sequela.

In addition, pregnant women with acute infection should be treated with a combination of pyrimethamine, folinic acid, and a sulfonamide. Although not definitive, treatment with this regimen may prevent maternal-to-fetal transmission of the infection. The standard dose is 25 mg of pyrimethamine by mouth given daily and 1 g of sulfadi-

Table 32.2 Laboratory Methods of Detection of Acute Toxoplasmosis

Pregnant Women (adults)

Acute infection
Demonstration of:
1. Recent seroconversion
2. Toxoplasma-specific IgM **or**
3. Rise in titer of toxoplasma-specific antibody
4. *Toxoplasma* cysts in placental histological sections supports the diagnosis

Chronic (or remote infection)
Demonstration of:
1. Serology positive to *Toxoplasma gondii* antibody
and
2. Toxoplasma-specific IgM negative status

Infant/Fetus

Fetus (prenatal diagnosis)
1. Amniotic fluid (culture, PCR)
2. Fetal blood by cordocentesis (culture, PCR)

Newborn
Demonstration of:
1. Toxoplasma-specific IgM in newborn sera **or**
2. Toxoplasma-specific IgA

azine by mouth four times daily for one year. Pyrimethamine is a folic acid antagonist and therefore may have teratogenic effects when given in the first trimester. Whenever possible, treatment with pyrimethamine in the first trimester should be weighed against potential risk of drug teratogenicity to the infant. Folinic acid, given as a dose of 6 mg intramuscularly or by mouth every other day should be used to correct the depletion of folic acid induced by pyrimethamine.

Sulfonamides are known to displace bilirubin from its binding sites and therefore put the infant of a mother who had been on the medication within the last month of her pregnancy at risk for hyperbilirubinemia. However, there has never been a reported case of kernicterus in an infant following administration of sulfonamide to its mother in the last month of pregnancy. Nevertheless, its benefit should be weighed against its possible side effects in the neonate.

Spiramycin is another agent used in the treatment of

acute toxoplasmosis and can be obtained in the United States through the Centers for Disease Control (CDC). It is more commonly used in Europe, and, hence, there are no good controlled studies of its efficacy in this country.

Serosusceptible pregnant women should be counselled to avoid eating raw or undercooked meats which may contain the Toxoplasma gondii cysts and to avoid close contact with cat feces, such as changing cat litter. Other important preventive measures for the pregnant woman at risk include: routinely boiling water for consumption, vigorously washing fruits and vegetables, and consuming meat that has been either cooked to at least 150°F, smoked, or cured. Although serological testing to Toxoplasma gondii is currently not a routine test done in pregnancy, it may be important in the following settings: pregnant women who 1) have symptoms suggestive of acute infection, 2) are infected with HIV-1, and 3) who may have been recently exposed to the organism while pregnant.

Infant

Symptomatic infection in the newborn should be treated with pyrimethamine at a dose of 1 mg/kg/day by mouth for 34 days, followed by 0.5 mg/kg/day for 21–30 days, and sulfadiazine at a dose of 25 mg/kg by mouth for one year. As with adults, folinic acid at 2–6 mg intramuscularly or by mouth should be given three times a week whenever the infant is taking pyrimethamine. The congenitally infected infant is not infectious and therefore need not be isolated.

Newborns who do not have clinical evidence of infection and are toxoplasma-specific IgG antibody positive may have passively acquired this antibody transplacentally from their mothers. In the absence of any other findings suspicious for congenital infection (positive toxoplasma-specific IgM, placental Toxoplasma cysts on histology, any prenatal testing that was positive), the infant may be observed and, if uninfected, should demonstrate decreasing titers of IgG antibody to Toxoplasma.

Conclusion

Approximately one third of pregnant women have antibody to Toxoplasma gondii, indicating previous infection. Primary maternal toxoplasmosis occurs in about 1:900 pregnancies.

The risk of fetal infection following primary infection in a pregnant woman and the severity of fetal damage is related to the timing of infection. The earlier in the gestation the infection, the lower the risk of infection but the more severe the damage to the fetus.

The main sources of infection are infected cat feces and uncooked meats. Pregnant women should be advised to avoid exposure to these major sources of infection.

Laboratory diagnosis of acute toxoplasmosis in an adult requires demonstration of either 1) seroconversion to an antibody positive status, 2) greater than fourfold rise in antibody titer to Toxoplasma, or 3) presence of toxoplasma-specific IgM. However, the IgM may persist for six months to several years and therefore cannot differentiate between very recent to remote primary infection. Isolation of the organism in fetal blood is presently the most accurate method of diagnosing toxoplasmosis in the fetus in utero. Twenty percent of infected newborns will not demonstrate toxoplasma-specific IgM and, hence, it is essential to carefully observe infants who are IgM negative for infection.

Treatment of acute toxoplasmosis in pregnant women involves supportive therapy, as well as administration of a combination of pyrimethamine, a sulfonamide, and folinic acid.

References

1. Janku J. Pathogenesa a pathologicka anatomie tak nazraneho vrozeneho Kolobomu zlute skrrny v oku normalne velikem a mikro phthalmickem s nalezem parazitu v sitnikci. Cas Lek Ces 1923;62:1021–1138.
2. Sever JL. Perinatal infections affecting the developing fetus and newborn. In: The prevention of mental retardation through the control of infectious diseases. Washington D.C.: U.S. Public Health Service, 1968. Publication No. 1692.
3. Navia BA, Petito CK, Gold WM, et al. Cerebral toxoplasmosis complicating the acquired immune deficiency syndrome: clinical and neuropathological findings in 27 patients. Ann Neurol 1986;19:224.
4. Luft BJ, Brooks RG, Conley FK, et al. Toxoplasma encephalitis in patients with acquired immune deficiency syndrome. JAMA 1984;252:913.
5. Mills J. Pneumocystis carinii and Toxoplasma gondii infections in patients with AIDS. Rev Infect Dis 1986;8:1001.

6. Sever JL, Larsen JW, Grossman JH. Toxoplasmosis. In: Handbook of perinatal infections, 2nd ed. Boston: Little, Brown, and Company, 1989:160.

7. Fung JC, Tilton RC. TORCH serologies and specific IgM antibody determination in acquired and congenital infections. Ann Clin Lab Science 1985;15:204.

8. Desmonts G, Couvreur J. Toxoplasmosis in pregnancy and its transmission to the fetus. Bull NY Acad Med 1974;50:146.

9. Desmonts G, Daffos F, Forestier F, et al. Prenatal diagnosis of congenital toxoplasmosis. Lancet 1985;1:500.

10. Derouin F, Thulliez P, Candolfi E, et al. Early prenatal diagnosis of congenital toxoplasmosis using amniotic fluid samples and tissue culture. Eur J Clin Microbiol 1988;7:423.

11. Burg JL, Grover CM, Pouletty P, et al. Direct and sensitive detection of a pathogenic protozoan, *Toxoplasma gondii*, by polymerase chain reaction. J Clin Microbiol 1989; 27:1787.

12. Grover CM, Thulliez P, Remington JS, et al. Rapid prenatal diagnosis of congenital *toxoplasma* infection by using polymerase chain reaction and amniotic fluid. J Clin Microbiol 1990;28:2297.

13. Stepick-Biek P, Thulliez P, Araujo FG, et al. IgA antibodies for diagnosis of acute congenital and acquired toxoplasmosis. J Infect Dis 1990;162:270.

33

Rubella

Dorothy M. Horstmann, M.D.

RUBELLA is primarily a mild disease of childhood; in prevaccine times, the peak incidence was in the five- to nine-year-old age group. In temperate climates, it is a disease of late winter and spring, with highest attack rates between March and May. For every clinical case, there are one or more subclinical infections that induce lasting protection. Before the introduction of vaccines, serologic surveys in the United States and countries with similar climates indicated that approximately 85% of young women had experienced natural infection and were immune by age 15 to 19.

Figure 33.1 summarizes the clinical and laboratory responses to infection with rubella virus. After exposure, the virus enters and multiplies first in the upper respiratory tract, in mucosal cells, or in local lymph nodes. After 7–10 days—and as long as a week before the appearance of rash—the virus appears in the bloodstream and throat. When antibodies appear, viremia ceases, but shedding from the throat continues for 5–7 days or longer.

The incubation period of rubella is 14–21 days, most commonly 16–18 days. In children, rash is usually the first evidence of the disease; accompanying signs and symptoms—low grade fever, malaise, and lymphadenopathy—are mild. Adolescents and adults often experience a more severe illness, with a prodrome lasting several days. Tender swollen postauricular and posterior cervical lymph nodes, which may also be present as long as a week before onset of the rash, are the most typical features. Fever, malaise, sore throat, coryza, cough, and conjunctivitis may accompany the rash. The pink, macular eruption starts on the face and spreads rapidly to the chest, abdomen, and extremities.

Differentiation from other exanthems is often difficult. In distinguishing rubella from enterovirus infections and infectious mononucleosis, the invariable rash on the face and the characteristic lymphadenopathy are the most helpful signs. The disease is milder and of much shorter duration than measles, and complications are infrequent. Transient arthralgia or arthritis occur chiefly in women and increase in frequency with advancing age. The fingers and wrists are most often involved, but elbows, knees, and ankles may also be stiff and swollen. Joint problems last 1–2 weeks but may persist for several years. Reoccurrences occasionally occur. Rare complications include encephalitis and thrombocytopenic purpura.

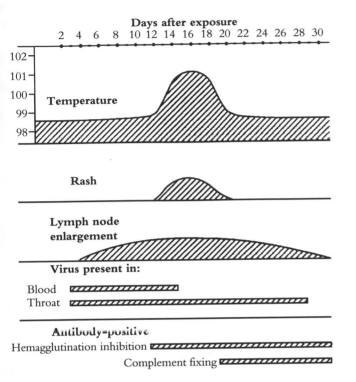

Days after exposure

Figure 33.1   Time relationship between clinical signs of rubella, virus shedding, and antibody development.

Rubella elicits antibody responses that are detectable by a variety of serologic tests, including hemagglutination inhibition (HI), neutralization (NT), complement fixation (CF), fluorescent, precipitating, and hemolysin in gel tests, as well as enzyme-linked immunosorbent assay (ELISA) and radioimmunoassay (RIA) (1). Over the years, the HI test has been the one most widely used, but it has been largely superseded by ELISA and latex agglutination (LA) tests (2, 3). The LA test has certain advantages: It is rapid (results are read after eight minutes), it requires no special technical training or equipment, and all reagents are available in a commercial kit. An extensive evaluation in which several hundred sera were tested by LA, HI, ELISA, and NT tests indicated that LA compared favorably with the others in sensitivity and accuracy (2).

As with other viral infections, the first antibodies to appear after primary infection with rubella virus are of the immunoglobulin M (IgM) class. Immunoglobulin G (IgG)

follows and rises rapidly. IgM declines and disappears after 4–8 weeks or so, but IgG remains elevated for life.

Congenital Infection

Rubella was considered an inconsequential disease until 1941, when an Australian ophthalmologist discovered the association between maternal rubella and fetal defects (3). His paper, while focusing primarily on congenital cataracts in affected offspring, included precise descriptions of cardiac and other anomalies, which together were subsequently labeled the rubella syndrome.

Early estimates of the incidence of congenital defects associated with maternal infection were extremely high. It required some years and at least three large prospective epidemiologic studies in Sweden, England, and the United States before it was possible to determine the actual risk to the fetus when infection occurs during pregnancy. Based on these and other studies, and on virologic and serologic data obtained during and after the great 1964 epidemic in the United States, the following points can be made (4–8):

- Both clinically apparent and totally silent maternal infection can result in fetal infection.
- The consequences for the fetus when rubella occurs in the first trimester may be either no infection, inapparent infection with no clinical consequences, or damage to many organs and tissues, with mild to severe involvement.
- There appears to be little or no risk of congenital defect when maternal infection occurs preconceptually (9); if it occurs shortly after conception the embryo is at high risk due to infection of the placenta resulting from maternal viremia. When exposed during the first month of gestation the fetus rarely escapes infection (10).
- Approximately 20% of infants born to mothers infected during the first three months of pregnancy will have signs of congenital rubella at birth, most commonly cataracts and congenital heart disease (Table 33:1). An additional 30%–54% will develop clinical evidence of infection, mainly hearing defects, during the first few years of life.

Table 33.1 Abnormalities Associated with Congenital Rubella

Common	Less Frequent	Rare
Cardiovascular lesions	Central nervous system defects	Brain calcification
Patent ductus arteriosus	Coarctation of the aorta	Cardiac septal defects
Pulmonary artery hypoplasia	Diabetes	Chronic arthritis
Deafness or impaired hearing*	Interstitial pneumonitis	Chronic progressive rubella panencephalitis
Eye lesions	Jaundice	Endocrine problems
Cataracts	Meningoencephalitis	Hyper- or hypothyroidism
Retinopathy	Micrognathia	Genitourinary anomalies
Growth retardation	Microphthalmia	Glaucoma
Hepatosplenomegaly	Myocardial necrosis	Hepatitis
	Psychomotor retardation*	Humoral immune defects
	Radiolucencies of the long bones	Microcephaly
	Thrombocytopenic purpura	

*Not detected until one year of age.

- Fetal infection rates determined by serologic tests reveal far higher levels of intrauterine infection (8, 11). When infants born to mothers with confirmed rubella were followed clinically and serologically, 80% were found to be infected when maternal infection occurred during the first 12 weeks of pregnancy, 54% during 13–16 weeks, and 25% at the end of the second trimester. Thirty-five percent of infants infected during the 13–16th week of gestation developed deafness. No rubella defects were found in those infected after the 16th week. Although there is approximately 20% viral transmission to the fetus in the third trimester, congenital defects are extremely rare in this group (11).

- Infections in early weeks of pregnancy are associated with an increased abortion rate: approximately twice that of controls.

Rubella virus reaches the placenta and the fetus primarily through the bloodstream, but infected chorionic cells that break off and settle in various fetal organs are also a likely source. Placental infection may occur without transmission to the fetus. Once the virus has established itself in fetal tissue, however, the infection remains chronic and continues throughout gestation and into the first months of life. Decreasing amounts of virus are excreted from the throat up to approximately one year of age; the agent has been recovered from a lens removed from a child almost three years of age (12).

The mechanisms by which the virus induces pathologic changes in fetal organs and tissues are not clearly understood. The small size that is frequently a striking feature of term infants infected in utero results from an actual diminution in the total number of cells in the various organs (13). One hypothesis is that the reduced size of infants with congenital disease is caused by the dropping out of infected clones of cells, which are known to have a shortened life span (14).

Cataracts, patent ductus arteriosus, and impaired hearing are the most frequent abnormalities and are often found together (11). But many other anomalies may also be associated with congenital rubella (5–7). Often multiple systems are involved, especially when infection occurs in the second month of gestation. Severely involved infants have a poor prognosis, with a high mortality rate in the first year of life. At autopsy, inflammatory lesions have been found on occasion in virtually every organ and tissue in the body.

Beginning at about 16 weeks' gestation, maternal IgG is transmitted to the fetus, and by 20 weeks, the infected fetus begins to make its own IgM antibody; neither can eliminate the virus in utero, even though maternal IgG and fetal IgM can neutralize the virus in vitro. The presence of rubella-specific IgM at birth indicates intrauterine infection, but its absence does not rule out such infection. Congenital rubella has occasionally been associated with immune system defects that result in failure of antibody production.

Establishing the Diagnosis

Sometimes women are seen early in their pregnancies with illnesses suggestive of rubella or with histories of possible exposure. The first priority is to obtain a blood sample to determine serologically whether the patient is susceptible. A past history of the disease is unreliable because many other viral infections induce rubella-like rashes. Nor is absence of such history conclusive evidence of susceptibility, since over half of all rubella infections are subclinical, yet result in long-lasting immunity.

If immune status is determined by the HI test on a blood specimen drawn within a few days of exposure, the presence of antibody indicates that the patient is immune as a result of infection some time in the past; she can therefore be reassured that she is not at risk. A titer of 1:16 or higher is conclusive evidence of immunity. When a value of 1:8 is obtained, the test should be repeated to be certain that the titer represents specific antibody and not inadequate removal of the nonspecific inhibitors that are present in all human sera and interfere with HI but not other serologic tests. Another possibility is that a 1:8 value represents an early rise in antibody resulting from exposure several weeks previously followed by inapparent infection. A repeat specimen should be examined after 5–7 days, by which time the titer will have risen sharply if the patient is currently infected. A second blood sample should be collected approximately three weeks later and tested *along with the first specimen*. (The usual practice is to freeze the serum, but it may be kept in a refrigerator for several weeks.) If infection has occurred, antibodies will be present in the second serum.

If, instead of the standard HI test, the more sensitive ELISA or other newer tests are used, the results may be reported in several ways. However, if titrations are carried out, the findings are generally comparable with HI results (1, 2).

The laboratory can also help the clinician when a patient reports exposure (or an atypical illness) several weeks earlier. When a single serum specimen reveals a titer of 1:64 or higher, the question arises: Were the antibodies acquired recently or several years ago? This point can often be re-solved by determining whether IgM is present in the serum. In the convalescent phase of infection, IgM accounts for up to 40% of the rubella-specific antibody; it declines steadily and is rarely detectable after 5–10 weeks. The presence of rubella IgM indicates a recent or current infection. When all the rubella antibody is of the IgG class, the patient can be considered immune.

The serologic diagnosis of rubella is also complicated by the variability of results from one laboratory to another. This is true of several of the tests, particularly HI. It has certain pitfalls, and not all laboratories seem able to get reproducible results. To compound the problem, the commercial kits used by many smaller laboratories are of different types and give different results. A test done in one laboratory on serum collected soon after exposure may give a titer of 1:8 or 1:16, while results on a second specimen obtained two weeks later and tested in another laboratory may be 1:128. In such a situation, a mistaken diagnosis of rubella infection could be made on the basis of an apparently rising titer. The correct answer can only be obtained by testing both specimens at the same time. If the difference between the two sera is not more than twofold (within the range of error of the test), recent or current infection can be ruled out.

It is also possible to confirm the diagnosis by isolating the virus from the throat, but virus isolation is complicated and slow; a serologic test is the method of choice. If acute and convalescent blood specimens collected approximately 10 days apart and *tested together at the same time* reveal a fourfold or greater rise in titer, the diagnosis of rubella is confirmed. If the first specimen was obtained several days or more after onset, a maximum titer may have been reached already, so that a rising level cannot be demonstrated. In such a situation, the detection of rubella-specific IgM can establish the diagnosis. When the sera have been collected too late to show increasing antibody levels, detection of a rising titer of CF antibodies (which appear 7–10 days after onset) may also confirm the diagnosis (1).

Use of Gamma Globulin

In the past, immune serum globulin (ISG) was often given to pregnant women exposed to rubella in the hope of preventing infection should the patient be susceptible. The results were unsatisfactory. Both inapparent infection and clinical rubella have been documented in women given optimum doses of ISG soon after exposure. Part of the reason for this failure lies in the fact that the time of exposure is dated in terms of the onset of rash in the case. Since shedding of the virus from the throat (and viremia) occur as long as a week *before* the rash appears, infection may have occurred much earlier. Thus, ISG is often given too late to prevent infection in exposed pregnant women. Some experimental evidence suggests that, if given in adequate dosage immediately before or after exposure, gamma globulin may have a modifying effect, preventing the disease but not the infection (15, 16).

The prophylactic effectiveness of ISG is thus unpredictable and unreliable; furthermore, by masking the infection, its administration may result in a false sense of security. ISG should not be used routinely, but there is perhaps a place for it in the case of the patient who will not consent to termination of the pregnancy even if infection occurs. The recommended dose is 20 mL IM, to be given as soon as possible after exposure.

Immunization

The main objective of vaccination against rubella is to prevent miscarriages, stillbirths, and the seriously damaging fetal malformations that result from maternal infection during pregnancy. The last major rubella epidemic in the United States occurred in 1964; it was followed by the birth of approximately 20,000 infants with the congenital rubella syndrome. In addition some 6,250 cases of spontaneous abortion and 5,000 therapeutic abortions occurred. By 1969, seven years after the first isolation of the virus, two vaccines were available: one prepared in duck cells (HP77-DE5), the other in rabbit kidney cells (Cendehill). They were used until 1979, when RA27/3, grown in human diploid cells, was introduced. RA27/3 has the advantage of avoiding the possible side effects of vaccine viruses grown in animal cells. Since 1980 it has been marketed as Meruvax-2 (Merck, Sharp & Dohme) and is the only rubella vaccine available in the United States. It can be given alone or in combination with measles and mumps vaccines. All three rubella vaccines have been shown to induce long lasting immunity (18, 19).

Rubella vaccines induce seroconversion in approximately 95% of susceptible individuals. The attenuated virus is shed from the throat briefly but transmission to susceptible close contacts does not occur (20). The virus is also detectable in the blood of up to 80% of antibody negative vaccines (21).

Vaccination in childhood is rarely followed by symptoms or signs of rubella: fever, rash, lymphadenopathy; only 0.5% to 3% have been noted to experience transient arthralgia. As in the natural disease, young adult women are prone to have joint involvement: 10%–15% or more have been reported to develop arthralgia and arthritis, generally beginning 3 to 25 days after immunization and lasting up to 11 days (17). In some, joint involvement recurs or is persistent for years; such vaccinees have lymphocytes that are chronically infected. The virus has also been recovered from breast milk of women immunized postpartum; transmission to the infant has occurred but the infection is asymptomatic, transient, and usually does not evoke a lasting serologic response.

Vaccination during Pregnancy

While emphasizing the importance of immunizing susceptible young women, it has been stressed since the beginning that pregnancy is a contraindication to giving rubella vaccine, for the virus is capable of infecting the placenta and the fetus. Recovery of the virus from the products of conception obtained at abortion revealed a 3% (1/32) isolation rate when the current RA27/3 vaccine had been given, and 20% (17/85) following administration of Cendehill or HPV77 (22). From the beginning, however, it was inevitable that pregnant women would be vaccinated inadvertently, as happened soon after vaccines were licensed. In 1971, the Centers for Disease Control set up the Vaccine in Pregnancy Registry and began following up pregnant women who had received vaccine either within three months before or three months after conception. By 1979, 538 women had been entered in the registry, and 220 of them had carried the pregnancy to term. All of the infants born to these women, 94 of whom were known seronegatives at the time of vaccination, were normal, none showing any abnormalities indicating intrauterine infection with rubella virus. Data collected after 1979 show similar results when RA$_{27/3}$ vaccine had been given during pregnancy: All of the 212 infants born to 210 women who were known seronegatives were normal at birth (23). The evidence indicates that the risk of damage to the fetus when a woman is vaccinated shortly before or after conception is slight: based on a 95% confidence limit, the theoretical maximum risk for RA$_{27/3}$ vaccine is 1.7%; for all known susceptible women given any of the three types of vaccine since 1971, it is 1.2%. The risk is therefore much lower than the overall 2%–3% rate of major birth defects. Termination of pregnancy because of inadvertent vaccination is not considered necessary (23). The Vaccine in Pregnancy Registry was discontinued by the Centers for Disease Control in April, 1989.

Risks in the Vaccine Era

When rubella vaccines became available in the United States in 1969, the decision was made to focus primarily on prepubertal children. The objective was to prevent congenital rubella indirectly by inducing a high degree of herd immunity, thus blocking circulation of the virus in the segment of the population in which most infections occurred: young children, who commonly served as sources of infection for pregnant women. At the same time, it was also considered desirable to vaccinate women of childbearing age who lacked serologic evidence of immunity. Good obstetric practice currently includes testing for immunity to rubella on the first prenatal visit, followed by vaccination of susceptibles shortly after delivery, before leaving the hospital. Even though pregnancy is uncommon during the first postpartum months, contraception may be advisable during this period.

As a result of widespread immunization of children, circulation of the virus declined dramatically, resulting in reduction of the number of cases by up to 99%. Before 1969 approximately 50,000 were reported each year. By 1983 the figure had fallen to 1,000 and by 1987 to 300. The total for 1988 was 225. Congenital rubella syndrome declined similarly from 20–70 cases annually in the 1970s to 2 cases in 1989 (24). Accompanying this success was a shift

in age incidence of the disease. Instead of the highest rate occurring in school children as in pre-vaccine times, approximately half the cases were in children 1–5 years old and 50% or more were in those 15 years or older. Numerous small outbreaks occurred in universities, colleges, and places of employment, particularly hospitals.

Since the all time low of 225 cases of rubella in 1988, a resurgence of the disease has occurred: there has been a rise in incidence of rubella and the congenital rubella syndrome (25). The number of cases nearly doubled in 1989, rose to 1093 in 1990 and 1401 in 1991 (26). A parallel rise in CRS occurred with an increase to 11 cases in 1990. The figures reflect the continuing 10%–20% susceptibility rate of adolescents and young adults that has not changed significantly over the years. They also emphasize the necessity to improve rubella prevention among children and adults, particularly women of childbearing age, for it is clear that rubella virus still lurks around. When it finds its way into pockets of seronegative individuals, outbreaks ensue and the risk of rubella and congenital rubella syndrome become a hazard. It is thus imperative that immunization of all women of childbearing age be made a high-priority goal, one that is well recognized as being difficult to achieve. Currently, a mainstay of the effort is serologic testing of pregnant women early in prenatal care and postpartum immunization of those lacking antibody. Similarly, young adults who are students in schools and colleges or who work in hospitals are also important targets. Monitoring progress through serologic surveillance will continue to be vital to increasing the success of the universal immunization strategy.

References

1. Herrmann KL. Available rubella serologic tests. Rev Infect Dis 1985;7:S108.
2. Meegan JM, Evans BK, Horstmann DM. Comparison of the latex agglutination test with the hemagglutination test, enzyme-linked immunosorbent assay, and neutralization test for detection of antibodies to rubella virus. J Clin Microbiol 1982;16:644.
3. Wittenburg RA, Roberts L, Elliot B, Little ML. Comparative evaluation of commercial rubella virus antibody kits. J Clin Microbiol 1985;21:161.
4. Gregg NM. Congenital cataract following German measles in the mother. Trans Ophthalmol Soc Aust 1941;3:35.

5. Cooper LZ. The history and medical consequences of rubella. Rev Infect Dis 1985;7:S2.

6. Peckham C. Congenital rubella in the United Kingdom before 1970: the prevaccine era. Rev Infect Dis 1985;7:S11.

7. Sever JL, South MA, Shaver KA. Delayed manifestations of congenital rubella. Rev Infect Dis 1985;7:S164.

8. Miller E, Cradock-Watson JE, Pollack TM. Consequences of confirmed rubella at successive stages of pregnancy. Lancet 1982;1:871.

9. Enders G, Miller E, Nickerl-Packer U, Cradock-Watson JE. Outcome of confirmed periconceptual maternal rubella. Lancet 1988;1:1445.

10. South MA, Sever JL. Teratogen update: The congenital rubella syndrome. Teratology 1985;31:297.

11. Munro ND, Smithells RW, Sheppard S, Jones G. Temporal relationship between maternal rubella and congenital defects. Lancet 1987;2:201.

12. Menser MA, Harley JD, Herzberg R, et al. Persistence of virus in lens for three years after prenatal rubella. Lancet 1967; 2:387.

13. Naeye RL, Blanc W. Pathogenesis of congenital rubella. JAMA 1965;194:1277.

14. Simons MJ. Congenital rubella: an immunological paradox? Lancet 1968;2:1275.

15. Green RH, Balsamo MR, Giles JP, et al. Studies on the natural history and prevention of rubella. Am J Dis Child 1965; 110:348.

16. Schiff GM, Young BC, Stefanovic GM, Stamler EF, Knowlton DR, Brundy BJ, Dorsett PH. Challenge with rubella virus after loss of detectable vaccine-induced antibody. Rev Infect Dis 1985;7:S157.

17. Preblud SR. Some current issues relating to rubella vaccine. JAMA 1985;254:253.

18. Larson HE, Parkman PD, Davis WJ, et al. Inadvertent rubella virus vaccination during pregnancy. N Engl J Med 1971; 284:870.

19. Horstmann DM, Schluederberg A, Emmons JE, et al. Persistence of vaccine-induced immune responses to rubella: comparison with natural infection. Rev Infect Dis 1985; 7:S80.

20. Halstead SB, Diwan AJ. Failure to transmit rubella virus vaccine. A close contact study in adults. JAMA 1971;215:634.

21. O'Shea S, Best JM, Banatuala J. Viremia, virus excretion, and antibody responses after challenge in volunteers with low levels of antibody to rubella virus. J Inf Dis 1983; 148:639.

22. Bart SE, Stetler HC, Preblud SR, et al. Fetal risk associated with rubella vaccine: an update. Rev Infect Dis 1985; 7:S95.

23. Centers for Disease Control. Rubella vaccination during pregnancy—United States 1971–1988. MMWR 1989;38:290.

24. Centers for Disease Control. Rubella Prevention. Recommendations of the Immunization Practices Advisory Committee (ACIP). MMWR 1990;39:1.

25. Lindegren ML, Fehrs LJ, Hadler SC, Hinman AR. Update: Rubella and congenital rubella syndrome, 1980–1990. Epidem Rev 1991;13:341.

26. Centers for Disease Control. Summary of Notifiable Disease in the United States, 1991. MMWR 1992;40:10.

34

Cytomegalovirus Infections in Pregnancy and the Neonate

Antonio V. Sison, M.D.
John L. Sever, M.D., Ph.D.

CYTOMEGALOVIRUS (CMV) is the most common congenital viral infection, affecting approximately 1% of all live births. About 35,000 infants are born infected with CMV annually in this country (1). *Congenital* CMV infections are acquired by the fetus in utero when the mother develops primary CMV infection while pregnant, or with reactivation of a prior maternal infection. Although reactivated disease in the pregnant woman accounts for more than half of the congenital infections, primary maternal CMV infection is much more likely to result in a severely affected and symptomatic infant (2). Passive in utero transfer of maternally derived CMV-specific IgG antibody appears to provide some protection to the fetus when CMV is reactivated during pregnancy (3).

The great majority of infants with congenital CMV are asymptomatic (90%), but some have some evidence of disease in the newborn period (10%). About 10% of the symptomatic group present with full-blown cytomegalic inclusion disease. An additional 10% of infected infants who are asymptomatic at birth later present with symptoms related to CMV infection. The most common late-onset symptoms in these cases are mental retardation and deafness (4). These infants usually shed high titers of virus in the urine and saliva for a number of months.

CMV infections can be acquired by the child during the postpartum period through 1) exposure of the infant to infectious maternal body fluids such as cervical secretions, urine, saliva, and breast milk (5, 6), 2) following blood transfusion or tissue transplantation from an infected donor (7, 8), or 3) most frequently, through contact with infected individuals, such as in the newborn nursery, day-care centers, or from other family members in the household (9). These cases are called *acquired* CMV infections, in contrast to congenital infections.

Acquired infections usually result in less virus excretion and less antibody response than congenital CMV. However, viral shedding in the urine and saliva of the infant can last for several months. The great majority of acquired infections are asymptomatic, but infection can result in pulmonary disease (e.g., pneumonitis) in a few cases in infants.

Epidemiology of Maternal, Congenital, and Perinatal CMV Infections

Maternal Infection

Seroprevalence to CMV among adult populations shows significant geographic variability. Rates range from 40% to 100% depending on the region surveyed (10). Countries or regions with low socioeconomic status usually demonstrate very high seroprevalence rates (10). The incidence of congenital CMV is directly associated with maternal seroprevalence rates (1, 11). This is due to the fact that previously infected pregnant women may develop reactivation of the infection which may then result in fetal transmission. The risk of seroconversion for a pregnant seronegative woman is approximately 2% during pregnancy (12).

Table 34.1 summarizes the different routes of transmission of CMV for both infant and adult populations. Pregnant women acquire CMV infection primarily through exposure to infected children (13). The infected children shed virus in urine, saliva, and nasopharyngeal secretions and are infectious for a prolonged period of time (14). In a study of day-care centers in Iowa, the average duration of viral shedding among 12 infected infants was 13 months (14). Pregnant women who work in conditions that require intimate contact with infants, such as newborn nurseries and day-care centers, are therefore at high risk for acquiring primary infection.

Among adolescents and adults, heterosexual contact provides an additional source of infection. For example, Chandler, et al. reported a direct correlation between primary CMV infection in women and indicators of sexual activity, such as a high number of sexual partners and early age of intercourse (15). Both cervical secretions and semen have been shown to act as sources for viral transmission (16).

Infant Infection

In the United States, of the 35,000 infants that are congenitally infected each year, about 3,500 to 5,000 have some damage due to CMV. An additional 1%–15% of seronegative infants become infected by six months of age from exposure to infected parents, relatives, other children, and health-care givers. These acquired infections may produce pneumonia in very young or immunocompromised infants, but otherwise they are asymptomatic and cause no late-onset effects.

Biology, Humoral Responses and Mechanisms of Fetal Infection

Cytomegaloviruses are members of the herpesvirus group. The virus was first described by two investigators: Weller et al. in 1953 and Rowe et al. in 1956 (17, 18). The virus has a diameter of about 180 nm and is encapsulated by an icosahedral capsid containing 162 capsomeres. Within the capsid is double stranded DNA of about 240 kilobases which is enclosed by a lipid bilayer envelope. Gene expression and subsequently translation is controlled by early regulatory genes called α, which in turn regulate expression of later genes called β and γ (19). The name "cytomegalic inclusion disease" comes from the ability of the virus to induce cellular cytomegalia or "swelling" and intracellular inclusions in infected host cells.

The inbred guinea pig has served as a useful animal model for the study of congenital CMV infections (20). Griffith et al. inoculated seronegative pregnant guinea pigs with varying doses of virus during the different trimesters of the animal's pregnancy. They found that infectious virus was detectable in both fetal and placental tissues, not only at the

Table 34.1 Routes of Transmission of CMV

Neonate and Infant
Congenital (in utero)
Acquired
   Contact with infectious source
      Mother (urine, saliva, cervical secretions, breast milk)
      Other infected contacts (nursery, day-care center, household)
   Blood transfusion
   Tissue transplant

Adult
Contact with infectious source
   Infants and children (nasopharyngeal secretions, urine, saliva)
   Sexual contact (semen, cervical secretions)
Blood transfusion
Tissue transplant

time of maternal viremia, but also as late as 3–4 weeks after inoculation, suggesting that initial infection may be followed by development of a reservoir in the infected host (e.g., in the placenta) from which virus may later be recovered (20). A study by Goff et al. has shown similar findings (21).

In humans, Britt and Vugler reported higher levels of CMV-specific IgG antibodies in cord sera of infants who were clinically symptomatic of CMV infection than those with subclinical or asymptomatic infections (22). Alford et al. studied serial IgG precipitin antibody responses in pregnant women who either had CMV mononucleosis or subclinical infection with CMV and, similar to the previous report, found a more intense and prolonged antibody response in mothers (regardless of symptoms) who delivered infected infants (23). This difference suggests that antibody response (whether maternal or fetal) may play less of an important role in transmission and subsequently in the development of symptomatic disease than other viral factors, such as the amount of maternal viremia or the timing in pregnancy during which infection and subsequent maternal-to-fetal transmission occurs.

Amishessami-Aghili et al. successfully infected human placental cells in explant culture with CMV in vitro and therefore suggested that the placenta may be an important host to CMV and may serve as a chronic source of viral infection of the fetus in vivo (24).

Clinical Manifestations

Mother

The vast majority of pregnant women with primary CMV infection are asymptomatic. Symptomatic disease, if present, usually appears as a mononucleosislike syndrome, including some lymphadenopathy, lassitude, malaise, pharyngitis, and fever. Viremia is very transient, and virus is very commonly shed from the nasopharynx, urine, and breast milk (when postpartum). CMV-specific antibody (IgM) develops within a few days following infection and remains detectable for a few months. CMV-specific IgG develops rapidly and persists for life. There is no evidence that pregnancy affects the course or extent of symptoms with CMV.

Following primary infection, the virus goes into a latent phase. Intermittent periods of reactivation frequently occur, and virus is again excreted in the nasopharynx, cervix, urine, saliva, and breast milk. Most recurrent infections, as with primary infections, are asymptomatic. Immunocompromised individuals, such as those infected with HIV-1 or those with malignancies, may have high titers of CMV in blood, and disease due to CMV may appear in the eyes, lungs, and brain.

Infant

Table 34.2 summarizes the important clinical findings in infants and children with symptomatic CMV disease. While the great majority of infants with congenital CMV are asymptomatic, infants with symptomatic infection at birth usually have findings associated primarily with the reticuloendothelial and central nervous system (CNS) systems. The severe cases of congenitally acquired symptomatic infection result from primary rather than recurrent infection in the pregnant woman and from infections occurring early in pregnancy. The most common findings in these cases include hepatosplenomegaly, jaundice, a generalized petechial rash, and microcephaly. Less common findings include chorioretinitis with or without optic atrophy, pneumonitis, cerebral calcifications, microphthalmia, microcephaly, seizures, and cerebral and cerebellar atrophy. The mortality of newborns with symptomatic disease is approximately 30%.

Approximately 10% of infants that are asymptomatic at birth will later develop symptoms related to their CMV infection. The most common findings include mental retardation and hearing loss. Other defects include motor defects, leading to spastic diplegia, and dental abnormalities (such as a yellow and hypocalcified enamel). Some clinical findings may be subtle, such as learning disabilities, behavioral problems, expressive language difficulties, and hearing loss. The hearing loss is usually bilateral and may be progressive, which makes follow-up audiometric testing of these infants (whether symptomatic or not) very important (1).

Congenital infection is usually followed by a prolonged period of shedding of large quantities of virus from the nasopharynx and urine. These children have significantly higher levels of virus excretion than is seen with acquired

Table 34.2 Clinical Manifestations of Congenital CMV Infections in Infants and Children

I. Early Findings

Common
Hepatosplenomegaly
Purpura/petechiae
Microcephaly
Jaundice
Hemolytic anemia
Hepatitis
Thrombocytopenia

Less Common
Chorioretinitis (with or without optic atrophy)
Microphthalmia
Cerebral calcifications
Seizures
Cerebral/cerebellar atrophy
Interstitial pneumonitis
Dental abnormalities
Hernias
Prenatal findings
    Intrauterine growth retardation (IUGR)
    Small for gestational age (SGA)
    Fetal death in utero (FDU)

II. Late-Onset Findings

Common
Mental retardation
Hearing loss

Less Common
Optic atrophy
Spasticity
Dental defects
Neuromuscular defects
Learning disability
Psychomotor retardation

infections. Viral shedding in congenitally infected infants is most pronounced in the first six months of life.

Infants and children infected after birth are almost all asymptomatic. However, those with immunosuppressive infections such as HIV-1 may be at risk for CMV-related chorioretinitis, CNS, and pulmonary infections.

Diagnosis

Mother

The great majority of primary maternal infections with CMV are asymptomatic and unrecognized. When symptoms do occur, they may also go unrecognized because they appear as a mild, infectious, mononucleosislike illness, with lymphadenopathy, fatigue, and slight fever. Even though CMV is hepatotropic, elevations in liver enzymes are rarely seen in primary or recurrent infections. About one-third to two-thirds of all pregnant women have IgG antibody to CMV, indicating previous infection. Detection of CMV-specific IgM in the acute phase of infection is useful for making the diagnosis of CMV infection, but only 80% of women with primary infection demonstrate this antibody (25). In addition, more than a third of mothers with recurrent CMV from latent infection will be positive for CMV-specific IgM. CMV-specific IgM antibody may persist from 4–9 months, and some test methods may give false-positive results because of cross-reactions with other herpes viruses, antinuclear antibody, or rheumatoid factor (26).

Virus culture is the gold standard for the diagnosis of CMV infection. Virus is usually detected in the cervix, nasopharynx, and urine of infected individuals. However, cultures are positive with both primary and recurrent infections. The laboratory methods for diagnosing CMV in adults are summarized in Table 34.3.

Prenatal Diagnosis

Sonography may be useful for identifying some abnormalities in the fetus that may be related to CMV infection. Nonspecific sonographic findings of fetal hydrops, intrauterine growth retardation, polyhydramnios, fetal ascites, and specific central nervous system anomalies (e.g., ventriculomegaly) suggest an intrauterine infection, possibly CMV, and should be evaluated further with amniocentesis or cord blood sampling.

The first successful recovery of CMV by culture in amniotic fluid was reported in 1971 by Davis et al. from a symptomatic gravida at 21 weeks' gestation (27). Lynch et al. reported the successful prenatal diagnosis of fetal infec-

Table 34.3 Laboratory Methods for the Detection of
CMV in Mothers and Infants

Mother
Maternal blood
 CMV-specific IgG (acute and convalescent sera)
 CMV-specific IgM
 Culture
 Nonspecific laboratory findings
  Atypical lymphocytes
  Elevated liver enzymes
  Heterophile negative status
  Thrombocytopenia
  False-positive rheumatoid factor (30%)
  False-positive antinuclear antibody (20%)
Nasopharynx, cervix, urine, and breast milk culture

Prenatal
Amniotic fluid
 Culture
 Total and CMV-specific IgM
Chorionic villus sampling
 Culture
 PCR
Fetal blood sampling
 Culture
 CMV-specific IgM
 Gamma-glutamyl transpeptidase level

Postnatal
Cord or infant blood
 CMV-specific IgG (serial titers)
 CMV-specific IgM
 Culture
 Nonspecific laboratory findings
  Thrombocytopenia
Infant urine
 Culture
Nasopharyngeal secretions
 Culture

tion by a combination of amniotic fluid culture, measurement of total and CMV-specific IgM and gamma-glutamyl transpeptidase in fetal blood samples (28). Hogge et al. reported a CMV-specific IgM antibody titer of 1:256 from a fetal blood sample done at 36 weeks in a severely hydropic infant (29). Unpublished data from Hogge et al. have also

shown the successful detection of CMV DNA by the polymerase chain reaction (PCR) in chorionic villi and fetal tissues from pregnancies that were terminated due to other evidence of fetal infection (30). Further studies are needed on the sensitivity and specificity of these methods in identifying infected infants antenatally.

Postnatal Diagnosis in Infants

Most congenital infections in infants are asymptomatic. Symptomatic infants will commonly present with hepatosplenomegaly, jaundice, and petechiae. Table 34.3 summarizes laboratory methods for detecting CMV infections prenatally and postnatally. Serological testing of infants includes detection of CMV-specific IgG and IgM antibody in cord and infant blood. The presence of CMV-specific IgG antibody in the infant may be due to maternal antibody which crosses the placenta and hence is not diagnostic of fetal infection. However, persistently elevated CMV-specific IgG antibody in the infant over time strongly suggests endogenous production of this antibody and hence establishes the diagnosis of congenital infection (26). On the other hand, CMV IgM antibody is present in cord blood in about 80% of cases. Since maternal IgM does not cross the placenta, presence of this antibody either in cord or infant blood establishes the diagnosis of CMV infection. Other nonspecific laboratory abnormalities include atypical lymphocytosis, elevation in serum aspartate transaminase, thrombocytopenia, and hyperbilirubinemia (1). As with adult infections, viral culture of the infant's nasopharynx and urine is the most accurate method of diagnosing infection in the newborn.

Treatment and Prevention

Mother

Pregnant women with clinical symptoms from CMV infection are treated symptomatically. Susceptible pregnant women have a 2% risk of seroconverting while pregnant. Because this is a relatively low risk of infection and there is a somewhat low rate of possible damage to the fetus and because no effective therapy is available to infected infants, routine serological testing of pregnant women is generally not recommended.

Probably the single most important method of preventing primary infection during pregnancy is minimizing exposure in high-risk areas, such as nurseries, day-care centers, and other places that have a high concentration of young children. Susceptible pregnant women who work in these areas should be advised of their increased risk for infection. Careful handwashing techniques, as well as proper handling of potentially infectious body fluids, should be instituted to minimize spread of the infection. Clinicians should also be aware that primary infection can be acquired by other routes, such as through sexual contact, blood transfusion, and tissue transplants.

There are no current protocols for the use of antiviral agents (acyclovir and ganciclovir) during pregnancy to decrease the risk of mother-to-child transmission of CMV.

A live attenuated CMV vaccine (Towne strain) is available and has been used in renal transplant patients (31). Possible benefits and risks of this vaccine for children or susceptible pregnant women have not been established. Very recent advances have enabled the synthesis of CMV envelope proteins which may be used for immunization using recombinant DNA techniques (32). The use of this recombinant protein as a vaccine is investigational.

Infant

Clinically evident infection in newborns and infants is treated symptomatically. In the most severe cases of neonatal infection, antiviral agents such as acyclovir and ganciclovir have been used to suppress the infection, but discontinuation of the medication results in reappearance of the infection. Foscarnet (phophonoformic acid) has also been used in primary symptomatic neonatal disease and has been effective in reducing viral shedding.

Infants with primary infection (whether congenital or acquired) have a pronounced and protracted period of viral shedding and are infectious during this period. Once diagnosed as infected, these infants should therefore be isolated while in the nursery and careful handling of body fluids from these infants should always be instituted.

Conclusions

Cytomegalovirus is the most common congenitally acquired viral infection. About 2% of all pregnant women experience a primary infection and 1% of all live births are affected.

The great majority of primary and recurrent CMV infections in the pregnant woman and the newborn are asymptomatic and therefore remain undetected. Almost all cases of symptomatic disease in the infant result from primary infection in the woman while pregnant, with the most severe neonatal cases being associated with primary infection in the woman during the first half of pregnancy.

Asymptomatic but infected newborns carry a 10% risk of developing long-term sequelae from the infection. The most common late-onset findings in these cases are mental retardation and hearing loss. Infants diagnosed as having CMV should therefore be followed closely for development of such symptoms.

Diagnosis of maternal and neonatal CMV is established by the detection of CMV-specific IgM, although this assay is only 80% sensitive and the antibody may persist for up to nine months. Viral culture is still the gold standard for diagnosis of CMV in mother or infant. The most common sites of recovery include the cervix, nasopharynx, and urine in women and the latter two sites in children. Prenatal diagnosis of CMV is possible by culture of amniotic fluid. Detection of CMV-specific IgM by enzyme-linked immunosorbent assay (ELISA) and viral DNA by PCR techniques in fetal blood samples show promise but are presently only investigational. The prognostic value of these in-utero tests remains to be determined.

Treatment of clinically evident disease in mothers and children is symptomatic. Antiviral drugs only reduce viral shedding during the period that they are given and are generally not recommended.

References

1. Alford CA, Stagno S, Pass RF, et al. Congenital and perinatal cytomegalovirus infections. Rev Infect Dis 1990;12:S745.

2. Stagno S, Cloud G, Pass RF, et al. Primary cytomegalovirus infections in pregnancy: incidence, transmission to fetus, and clinical outcome. JAMA 1986;256:1904.

3. Stagno S, Pass RF, Dworsky ME, et al. Congenital cytomegalovirus infection. The relative importance of primary and recurrent maternal infection. N Engl J Med 1982; 306:945.

4. Stagno S, Pass RF, Dworsky ME, et al. Congenital and perinatal cytomegalovirus infections. Semin Perinatol 1983;7:31.

5. Reynolds DW, Stagno S, Hosty TS, et al. Maternal cytomegalovirus excretion and perinatal infection. N Engl J Med 1973;289:1.

6. Stagno S, Reynolds DW, Pass RF, et al. Breast milk and the risk of cytomegalovirus infection. N Engl J Med 1980;302: 1073.

7. Yeager AS, Grumet FC, Hafleigh EB, et al. Prevention of transfusion acquired cytomegalovirus infections in newborn infants. J Pediatr 1981;98:281.

9. Pass RF, Hutto C. Group day care and cytomegalovirus infections of mothers and children. Rev Infect Ris 1986;8:599.

10. Kicch U, Jung M, Jung F, eds. Cytomegalovirus infections of man. New York: Karger, 1971.

11. Medearis TN. Observations concerning human cytomegalovirus infection and disease. Bull Johns Hopkins Hosp 1964;266:1233.

12. Griffiths PD, Campbell-Benzie A, Heath RB. A prospective study of primary cytomegalovirus infection in pregnant women. Br J Obstet Gynecol 1980;87:308.

13. Pass RF, Little EA, Stagno S, et al. Young children as a probable source of maternal and congenital cytomegalovirus infection. N Engl J Med 1987;316:1366.

14. Murph JR, Bale JF. The natural history of acquired cytomegalovirus infection among children in group day-care. Am J Dis Child 1988;142:843.

15. Chandler SH, Holmes KK, Wentworth BB, et al. The epidemiology of cytomegaloviral infection in women attending a sexually transmitted disease clinic. J Infect Dis 1985; 152:597.

16. Ho M. Epidemiology of cytomegalovirus infections. Rev Infect Dis 1990;12:S701.

17. Weller TH. Serial propagation of agents producing inclusion bodies derived from varicella and herpes zoster. Proc Soc Exp Biol Med 1953;83:340.

18. Rowe WP, Hartley JW, Waterman S, et al. Cytopathogenic agent resembling human salivary gland virus recovered from tissue cultures of human adenoids. Proc Soc Exp Biol Med 1956;92:418.

19. Merigan TC, Resta S. Cytomegalovirus: where have we been and where are we going? Rev Infect Dis 1990;12:S693.

20. Griffith BP, McCormick SR, Booss J, et al. Inbred guinea pig model of intrauterine infection with cytomegalovirus. Am J Pathol 1986;122:112.

21. Goff E, Griffith BP, Booss J. Delayed amplification of cytomegalovirus infection in the placenta and maternal tissues during late gestation. Am J Obstet Gynecol 1987;156: 1265.

22. Britt WJ, Vugler LG. Antiviral antibody responses in mothers and their newborn infants with clinical and subclinical congenital cytomegalovirus infections. J Infect Dis 1990; 161:214.

23. Alford CA, Hayes K, Britt W. Primary cytomegalovirus infection in pregnancy: comparison of antibody responses to virus-encoded proteins between women with and without infection. J Infect Dis 1988;158:917.

24. Amirhessami-Aghili N, Manalo P, Hall MR, et al. Human cytomegalovirus infection of human placental explants in culture: histologic and immunohistochemical studies. Am J Obstet Gynecol 1987;156:1365.

25. Stagno S, Tinker MK, Irod C, et al. Immunoglobulin M antibodies detected by enzyme-linked immunosorbent assay and radioimmunoassay in the diagnosis of cytomegalovirus infections in pregnant women and newborn infants. J Clin Microbiol 1985;21:930.

26. Fung JC, Tilton RC. TORCH serologies and specific IgM antibody determination in acquired and congenital infections. Ann Clin Lab Science 1985;15:204.

27. Davis LE, Tweed GV, Chin TDY, et al. Intrauterine diagnosis of cytomegalovirus infection: viral recovery from amniocentesis fluid. Am J Obstet Gynecol 1971;109:1217.

28. Lynch L, Daffos F, Emanuel D, et al. Prenatal diagnosis of fetal cytomegalovirus infection. Am J Obstet Gynecol 1991; 165:714.

29. Hogge WA, Thiagarajah S, Benbridge AN, et al. Fetal evaluation by percutaneous blood sampling. Am J Obstet Gynecol 1988;158:132.

30. Hogge WA, Buffone GJ, Hogge JS, Prenatal diagnosis of cytomegalovirus (CMV) infection: a preliminary report. (Unpublished personal communication from authors.)

31. Plotkin SA, Friedman HM, Fleisher GR, et al. Towne-vaccine-induced prevention of cytomegalovirus disease after renal transplants. Lancet 1984;1:528.

32. Hudecz F, Gonczol E, Plotkin SA. Preparation of highly purified human cytomegalovirus envelope antigen. Vaccine 1985;3:300.

35

Varicella–Zoster Infection

David A. Baker, M.D.

CHICKENPOX can usually be diagnosed by the characteristic rash, a cluster of tiny blisters on reddened skin that dry and scab over in about five days. A stained smear that shows multinucleated giant cells containing eosinophilic nuclear inclusion bodies confirms the clinical diagnosis. However, varicella-zoster virus cannot be distinguished from herpes simplex virus merely by observing stained material from lesions.

Though isolating the virus may be difficult, fluorescent antibody staining offers a rapid diagnosis. There are also several serologic tests for varicella, not all of equal value. One drawback to the complement-fixation (CF) test is its insensitivity; many adults who are immune to varicella may be CF negative. Newer, more specific tests include immune adherence hemagglutination and a radioimmunoassay (1–5).

Complications of Chickenpox

Varicella Pneumonia

Fever, cough, chest pain, and respiratory distress within a week of developing an itchy rash strongly suggest a pneumonic process (6). At this point, a chest x-ray should be taken. The majority of adults who are not immunosuppressed recover from varicella pneumonia without severe pulmonary damage. The mortality for those with normal resistance is about 10% (7). But prompt attention is necessary, with oxygen-supportive therapy and testing for superimposed bacterial pneumonia.

Some investigators consider varicella more fulminant in pregnancy, but others have not substantiated this claim. The latter suggest that the pregnant woman's clinical course is similar to that of the nonpregnant adult (8, 9).

Skin Infection

Another complication of varicella may be superimposed infection of skin lesions by streptococci and staphylococci (10). Systemic or local antibiotics may be required.

Fetal Damage

In most cases, varicella is a self-limiting infection in the mother. The fetus, however, may be severely affected, depending on when the mother became infected. Approximately 15% of women of childbearing age are susceptible. Of those seronegative mothers infected in the first 14 weeks of gestation, approximately 2%–10% produce children with congenital defects: low birthweight, neurologic and ocular anomalies, limb defects, skin scars, and Horner's syndrome (11–14).

The viremia in primary varicella infection is the proposed mechanism by which the virus reaches the placental-fetal compartment. If maternal infection occurs late in pregnancy, neonatal varicella may result (15). It appears that transplacental passage of maternal antibodies decreases the severity of neonatal varicella.

Babies born within five days after the mother acquires acute varicella, or those who are exposed in the first 3–4 weeks of life, are at highest risk of being infected. Whenever possible, delivery should be delayed in a mother who has acute varicella until she can produce antibodies and transmit them to the fetus through the placenta.

Herpes Zoster

Shingles may occur at any age but usually affects an older population. The infection is limited to a specific body distribution (dermatome) and results when the varicella-zoster virus is reactivated. Attacks can be triggered by an injury, emotional stress, exposure to cold, sunburn, treatment with certain drugs, or development of another disease such as tuberculosis or cancer. Pain and paresthesia usually precede the cutaneous eruptions by several days. The distribution of the rash is distinctive (unilateral, not crossing the midline) and in two-thirds of cases involves the chest and waist area (3).

The lesions go through the same stages as do those of varicella and usually form crusts by 10 days. Unless defense mechanisms are compromised, the disease is self-limiting, clearing in 2–4 weeks. Complications include postherpetic neuralgia and secondary bacterial infection. Patients with malignant disease and those who are immunosuppressed have an increased incidence and severity of herpes zoster (16). Second attacks, however, are uncommon.

Prevention and Therapy

As with many other viral infections, prevention has high priority. This disease is extremely contagious, and pregnant women and newborns should not be exposed to it. Varicella-zoster immunoglobulin (VZIG) is available to those patients who have been exposed to the virus and are prone to developing serious complications (17). Because information concerning varicella in pregnancy is limited, it is recommended that VZIG be administered to all exposed pregnant patients who haven't had the infection.

Infants born to mothers who develop varicella late in pregnancy and infants exposed soon after birth are candidates for VZIG. The IM dose—1.25 mL/10 kg of body weight, which must be given within 96 hours after exposure to chickenpox—protects for 3–4 weeks.

In addition to preventive therapy with VZIG, there is a safe and effective antiviral therapy for established varicella zoster virus infections. Because of the severe morbidity and mortality of disseminated varicella infections and varicella pneumonia, these infections should be treated with IV acyclovir at a dose of 7.5 to 10 mg/kg every 8 hours for 5–7 days (18).

In specific cases of severe zoster, therapy with acyclovir has been effective in preventing certain serious complications. Larger oral doses of acyclovir, 800 mg five times a day, have to be administered (19).

CASE 35.1 Acute Varicella

For the past three days, a 24-year-old black woman, 38 weeks into her second pregnancy, has had a rash that started on her face and trunk. She has had a low-grade fever and has felt tired for the past five days. Three weeks ago, her son was diagnosed as having chickenpox and stayed home from school for a week. Over the past two months, several of his classmates have also had chickenpox.

The mother was fortunate that her baby was normal. Ideally, she should have contacted her doctor at the time of exposure in order to receive HZIG.

The woman's symptoms are typical of acute varicella, a highly contagious disease transmitted by close contact, with an incubation period of approximately three weeks. The period of communicability persists for about seven days, beginning one day before the onset of the rash and lasting six days thereafter. The attack rate among susceptible household contacts is 96%. Usually, varicella is more severe in adults than in children. The severity of the skin rash and systemic manifestations are directly related (1, 2). ▪

References

1. Haynes RE. Varicella zoster infections. In: Galasso CG, et al., eds. Normal and compromised hosts in antiviral agents and viral diseases of man. New York: Raven Press, 1979.

2. Asano Y, Nakayama H, Yazaki T, et al. Protection against varicella in family contacts by immediate inoculation with live varicella vaccine. Pediatrics 1977;59:3.

3. Oxman MN. Varicella. In: Braude AL, ed. Medical microbiology and infectious diseases. Philadelphia: WB Saunders Co, 1981.

4. Kalter ZG, Steinberg S, Gershon AA. Immune adherence hemagglutination: further observations on demonstration of antibody to varicella-zoster virus. J Infect Dis 1977;135: 1010.

5. Richman DD, Cleveland PH, Oxman MN, et al. A rapid ^{125}I-staphylococcal protein A radioimmunoassay for antibody to varicella-zoster virus. J Infect Dis 1981;143:693.

6. Krugman S, Goodrish CH, Ward R. Primary varicella pneumonia. N Engl J Med 1957;257:843.

7. Triebwasser JH, Harris RE, Bryant RE, et al. Varicella pneumonia in adults. Medicine 1967;46:409.

8. Harris RE, Rhoades ER. Varicella pneumonia complicating pregnancy. Report of a case and review of the literature. Obstet Gynecol 1965;25:734.

9. Amstey MS. Varicella in pregnancy. J Reprod Med 1978;21:89.

10. Wald ER, Levine MM, Togo Y. Concomitant varicella and staphylococcal scaled skin syndrome. J Pediatr 1973;83: 1017.

11. Paryani SG, Arvin AM. Intrauterine infection with varicella-zoster virus after maternal varicella. N Engl J Med 1986; 314:1542.

12. Fuccillo DA. Congenital varicella. Teratology 1978;15:329.

13. Brice JE. Congenital varicella resulting from infection during the second trimester of pregnancy. Arch Dis Child 1976; 51:474.

14. Klauber GT, Flynn FJ, Altman BD. Congenital varicella syndrome with genitourinary anomalies. Urology 1976;8:153.

15. Hyatt HW. Neonatal varicella. J Natl Med Assoc 1967;59:32.

16. Reboul F, Donaldson SS, Kaplan HS. Herpes zoster and varicella infections in children with Hodgkins disease: an analysis of contributing factors. Cancer 1978;41:95.

17. Medical World News. 1982;Feb 1:8.

18. Brown ZA, Baker DA. Acyclovir therapy during pregnancy. Obstet Gynecol 1989;73:526.

19. McKendrick MW, McGill JI, White JE, et al. Oral acyclovir in acute herpes zoster. Br Med J 1986;293:1529.

36

Herpes Simplex Infection

Marvin S. Amstey, M.D.

GENITAL herpesvirus infection during pregnancy is usually confined to a localized area. Mild-to-moderate systemic symptoms may arise and clear within several weeks. At least 30%–50% of infections affect only the relatively insensitive cervix and upper vagina and are therefore entirely asymptomatic (Figure 36.1).

Although the risk to the mother is small, the risk to the neonate is great. From 25%–40% of infants born to mothers with primary genital herpesvirus infection will develop disseminated herpesvirus infection, from which mortality in neonates is 30%–40%. For this reason, active management is important early in pregnancy, during labor and delivery, and postpartum. However, only 2%–3% of infants born to mothers with recurrent genital herpesvirus infections are at risk for disseminated disease.

The anatomic site of infection was once thought to constitute a major difference between herpes simplex virus types 1 and 2. It is now believed, however, that many types of herpesvirus infect the genital tract and that all of them carry degrees of risk for the newborn. Recent data show that at least one-third of genital herpetic infection results from type 1 and 10%–20% of oral-labial infection from type 2.

Herpes simplex virus, like other viruses within the herpes group (including cytomegalovirus and varicella zos-

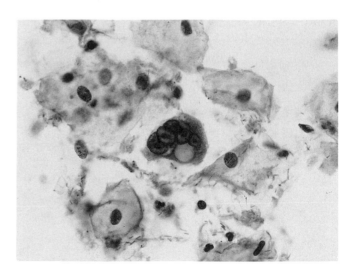

Figure 36.1   Pap smear of squamous cells infected with herpesvirus.

ter), has a latent phase. It reactivates even when the humoral and cell-mediated immune systems are intact.

At the first prenatal visit, a history of any genital herpesvirus infection in either the patient or her sex partner should be obtained. If the history is positive, the couple should be informed that their baby will be exposed to risk by coming into contact with the virus at birth. They should be told that most women who have a history of herpetic recurrences can nevertheless deliver vaginally. Only if a lesion is apparent, or suggested by symptoms, is it likely that sufficient virus is present to harm the newborn. For a woman carrying the virus but symptom free, the risk for disseminated infection in the newborn is reduced to a range of 1/1,000–1/2,500.

Weekly antenatal cultures do not predict whether the infant will be positive for herpesvirus on the day of birth (Figure 36.2) (1). This finding led the Infectious Disease Society for Obstetrics and Gynecology to recommend abandoning weekly cultures of asymptomatic women (2).

Some data are now accumulating that would indicate acyclovir treatment for pregnant women with primary infections and any women with disseminated infections. Such treatment was given to 274 pregnant women reported in a 1987 study (3) and in several instances noted anecdotally since then. In no instance was fetal toxicity reported. In addition, a number of animal studies have shown no harm from acyclovir. At present, however, therapy with this drug

during pregnancy has not been approved by the Food and Drug Administration. Therefore, it should be limited to pregnant women who have severe systemic disease, such as meningitis or encephalitis. Use for a localized primary genital infection is not recommended during pregnancy.

Managing Delivery

If a lesion is present at the onset of labor or ruptured membranes, or if prodromal symptoms of a herpetic lesion are present, every attempt must be made to keep the baby away from the infected area. Cesarean delivery can reduce but not eliminate the risk of transmittal from the mother. Ideally, cesarean section should be performed before membrane rupture or within 4–6 hours afterward. Cesarean delivery may still be beneficial in preventing neonatal herpesvirus infection regardless of the duration of membrane rupture. The rationale is that the amount of virus and the time of exposure to it are probably in direct proportion to the risk of neonatal infection (4).

If a woman has a viral lesion at or near term but before labor begins, it is useful to obtain repeat cultures every 3–7 days to ensure that virus is absent when labor begins.

Protecting the Neonate

Once the infant has been delivered, attention should focus on preventing neonatal infection. In the past, it was felt that the baby should be isolated from the mother until maternal lesions had cleared completely, but most practitioners now believe that this policy induces needless anxiety for the mother and her family. Instead, she should be instructed about the danger of infection, making sure she understands the need to protect the newborn from any contact with her lesions. She should be encouraged to wash her hands frequently, keep her perineum clean and dry it thoroughly with a hair dryer after washing or bathing. This policy allows the new mother to handle and breast-feed her baby and to take it home when she leaves the hospital.

In the hospital, the newborn should be kept in an isolated section of the nursery to protect other neonates from potential exposure. Isolation also alerts the nursery staff to

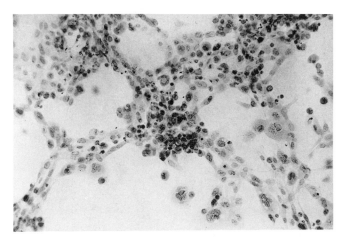

Figure 36.2 Herpesvirus-infected tissue culture.

the need for frequent hand washing and other precautions in handling this infant. The mother needn't be isolated from other patients.

If research should develop a rapid, cost-effective, sensitive test for herpesvirus infection, the management plan described above will be modified accordingly. As data accumulate about the efficacy and safety of acyclovir or some drug yet to be made available, we may find ourselves using such therapy to prevent the recurrence of viral eruption during pregnancy, thus assuring protection of the neonate.

References

1. Arvin A, Hensleigh P, Prober C, et al. Failure of antepartum maternal cultures to predict the infant's risk of exposure to herpes simplex virus at delivery. N Engl J Med 1986; 315:796.

2. Gibbs R, Amstey M, Sweet R, et al. Management of genital herpes infection in pregnancy. Obstet Gynecol 1988; 71:779.

3. Andrews E. Acyclovir in pregnancy registry: an observational epidemiological approach. Presented at the Wellcome International Antiviral Symposium, Monte Carlo, December 1987.

4. Prober C, Corey L, Brown Z. The management of pregnancies complicated by genital infections with herpes simplex virus. Clin Infect Dis 1992;15:1031–8.

37

Group B Streptococcus Infection

Mara J. Dinsmoor, M.D.

THE Group B *Streptococcus* (GBS), also known as *Streptococcus agalactiae*, has only recently been appreciated as an important perinatal pathogen. Reports of neonatal sepsis, septic abortion, and chorioamnionitis associated with GBS first appeared in the early 1960s. Since that time, its role in puerperal and neonatal infections has been increasingly recognized. In fact, the infection appeared to be increasing in incidence in the 1970s. Overall, costs for maternal and neonatal GBS disease have been estimated to be over $700 million annually.

Although there has been an apparent decrease in the case-fatality rate for neonatal GBS infections, they continue to affect approximately 7600 neonates and 7600 adults annually (1). The incidence of neonatal GBS infection remains higher than that of neonatal herpes, congenital syphilis, or congenital rubella, diseases for which prenatal surveillance is routinely performed (2). Unfortunately, routine surveillance for GBS is of dubious value. We continue to look toward a means of effective prevention of GBS disease, especially in the neonate.

Maternal Disease

Maternal GBS carriage is generally asymptomatic and is no more frequent in pregnancy than in the nonpregnant state. Carriage rates are fairly constant during the three trimesters, although GBS carriage may be intermittent, transient, or chronic. The carriage rate varies between 10% and 30%, depending on the population studied and culture technique used to confirm it.

Although GBS is transmitted sexually, carriage does not appear to be related to number of partners or to promiscuity. Higher carriage rates are found when cultures are taken serially, are taken from the lower vagina or rectum or from multiple sites rather than the cervix alone, or are grown in selective media such as Todd-Hewitt broth. Approximately one-third of the maternal isolates are serotype Ia, Ib, or Ic, one-third are type II, and one-third are type III (3).

In addition to asymptomatic carriage, GBS has been associated with several maternal disease states. GBS is isolated in 1%–5% of pregnant patients who have urinary tract infections. Ten percent to 15% of women with intraamniotic infection at term have GBS in the amniotic fluid. GBS is also associated with 10%–20% of cases of postpartum endometritis. The latter is characterized by an early onset (usually 12–24 hours postpartum), high fever, tachycardia, abdominal distension, and a high incidence of associated bacteremia (35%) (4). Lastly, approximately 10%–20% of maternal bacteremias in an obstetric population are due to GBS.

Although GBS is associated with maternal disease, it causes the most morbidity and mortality in the nursery. Generally, after delivery, 40%–70% of neonates of colonized mothers will also be colonized. In the first 48 hours after delivery, maternal and neonatal colonization rates are approximately equal. However, neonatal colonization persists for weeks to months. Several studies have documented the high concordance of serotypes between mother and colonized neonate (3). Both neonatal colonization and symptomatic infection are increased with heavy maternal colonization. The frequency of neonatal colonization is not affected by other maternal factors, although preterm and low-birthweight infants are at increased risk.

Neonatal Sepsis

Early-onset GBS disease is acquired via vertical transmission from a colonized mother. It occurs in three of 1,000 births, in 1%–2% of deliveries to colonized mothers, and in up to 10% of deliveries to heavily colonized mothers. The incidence of early-onset GBS sepsis is increased in association with prolonged rupture of membranes (18–24 hours), prolonged labor, maternal intrapartum fever or postpartum endometritis, preterm delivery, and low levels of maternal type-specific antibody (5) (Table 37.1).

The onset of symptoms is usually within 12 hours of delivery, but may become manifest several days later, resulting in septicemia in 30%–40%, meningitis in 30%, and pneumonia in 30%–40%. The five serotypes of GBS (Ia, Ib, Ic, II, and III) are equally represented, except in cases of meningitis, where more than 80% of the isolates belong to serotype III (3, 6). Although the mortality from GBS sepsis exceeded 50% in the 1970's, it had decreased to approximately 30% in preterm infants and 15% in term infants in the 1980's (6). A recent series estimated an overall case-fatality rate of 4.1% in the U.S. (1). Generally, the mortality rate in preterm infants is several fold higher than that in term infants, with delay in diagnosis contributing significantly to the latter (6).

The mode of acquisition of late-onset disease, that occurring more than 5–7 days after delivery, is uncertain. Vertical transmission, nosocomial acquisition in the nursery, or community acquisition may all play a role. The incidence of late-onset GBS disease is approximately one to two per 1,000 births. Manifestations include meningitis (85%), bacteremia, and bone and joint infections. Serotype III is responsible for a majority (more than 90%) of these infections. Mortality is lower than with early-onset disease (15%–30%), but 30%–50% of infants with meningitis will have long-term neurologic sequelae.

Chemoprophylaxis

Currently, all proposals to prevent neonatal GBS involve either chemoprophylaxis or immunoprophylaxis. Chemoprophylaxis encompasses antibiotic treatment of mother or neonate. Immunoprophylaxis includes treatment of the neonate with immunoglobulin or maternal vaccination.

After a report of a decrease in the incidence of early-onset neonatal GBS sepsis when a hospital began to use IM penicillin for prevention of gonococcal ophthalmia, there was brief enthusiasm for treating newborns with a single dose of parenteral penicillin. Such treatment at birth did decrease the incidence of colonization with GBS and of disease caused by all penicillin-susceptible organisms in one study (7). However, this finding was associated with an increase in the incidence of disease caused by penicillin-

Table 37.1 Risk Factors for Neonatal Group B Streptococcus Sepsis.

Maternal Factors	Neonatal Factors
Heavy colonization	Prematurity (<37 weeks)
Intrapartum fever	Multiple gestation
Prolonged membrane rupture (>18–24 hours)	
Low levels of type-specific antibody	
Prior child with GBS disease	

resistant pathogens. In a prospective, randomized study, investigators found that treatment of neonates weighing less than 2,000 g with IM penicillin within 60 minutes of birth did not significantly reduce the incidence or fatality rate of neonatal GBS sepsis (8). These findings may be at least partially explained by the observation that the majority of cases of early-onset GBS are established in utero, with 67%–88% of affected infants already bacteremic at birth (5, 8). As a result, most approaches to preventing neonatal GBS sepsis currently revolve around preventing vertical transmission by treating the colonized mother prior to delivery.

Antepartum Screening and Treatment

There are several problems with performing prenatal cultures on all pregnant women and treating those who are colonized. First, 10%–30% of pregnant women would require treatment with antibiotics, leading to potential problems with resistance or adverse reactions. Furthermore, eradicating GBS is difficult, if not impossible.

In a prospective study, there were no significant differences noted in maternal colonization at delivery or in neonatal colonization when women who had antepartum GBS colonization were treated with ampicillin in the third trimester. In fact, 30% of the treated women were recolonized at delivery (9). In addition, there is no evidence that prenatal treatment of GBS colonization improves pregnancy or neonatal outcome.

Screening for GBS at 38 weeks of gestation and treating colonized women and their husbands with penicillin or erythromycin until delivery significantly decreased the incidence of neonatal colonization in one study. This protocol, however, would be ineffective in preventing colonization of preterm infants, the group at highest risk for invasive disease (9).

Antepartum Screening and Intrapartum Treatment

Another approach might be to treat at the time of delivery those women with positive prenatal cultures for GBS. Unfortunately, prenatal GBS cultures are not predictive of colonization status at any other time in pregnancy. Only 57%–67% of women with positive prenatal cultures for GBS still carry GBS at delivery, whereas 4%–9% with negative prenatal cultures are positive at delivery (10, 11).

In a number of studies, intrapartum antibiotic treatment of colonized mothers has been shown to decrease the incidence of neonatal colonization in both term and preterm populations (11–13). In one study, intrapartum treatment with IV ampicillin (2 g initially, followed by 1 g every six hours) of women colonized prenatally reduced neonatal colonization from 35% in untreated patients to 2% in treated patients ($P < 0.001$) (12). Heavy neonatal colonization was reduced from 22% to zero ($P < 0.0001$). Another report showed that intrapartum treatment (1 g of ampicillin every six hours) of women with antepartum GBS colonization reduced neonatal colonization from 46% to zero ($P < 0.001$) (14). However, testing for GBS weekly from 36 weeks' gestation to delivery, as done in this study, is potentially costly, while ineffective in preventing colonization of the preterm infant.

Neonatal GBS colonization and bacteremia were significantly reduced in a randomized trial in which women with positive prenatal cultures for GBS and premature labor or ruptured membranes for more than 12 hours were treated intrapartum with IV ampicillin, and the corresponding neonates were given four doses of IM ampicillin over 48 hours (2). Neonatal colonization was reduced from 51% to 9% (40/79 versus 8/85, $P < 0.001$) and bacteremia from 6% to zero ($P = 0.024$). The investigators estimated that this management plan would prevent 50% of cases and 75% of deaths from early-onset disease, while treating only 13.6% of their patients (2, 5).

Intrapartum Screening and Treatment

Clearly, the problem lies in correctly identifying women who are colonized and who are carrying fetuses at risk for neonatal sepsis. Although antepartum cultures are not predictive of maternal colonization at the time of delivery, the results of cultures performed at the time of admission are usually not available quickly enough to allow intervention.

Selecting those patients at high risk for neonatal GBS sepsis (those with preterm labor or preterm premature rupture of the membranes) has been proposed (15). At the time of admission, GBS cultures would be performed, and the patient would be treated with ampicillin if in active labor. Only those patients whose GBS culture was known to be negative at the time of labor would not be given antibiotics. Using this protocol, culturing and therapy would be used in only the 9% of patients who deliver prematurely, the population in whom 90% of the GBS-associated deaths occur. This proposal has not been studied in a prospective fashion. A reliable rapid diagnostic test for the presence of GBS would greatly simplify this scheme and reduce the number of culture-negative patients treated unnecessarily.

Several methods for the rapid detection of GBS colonization have been evaluated. Depending on the methodology used, results can be available in 30 minutes to 19 hours. Although promising in early studies, none of the commercially available assays has proven to be adequately sensitive for clinical use thus far, with sensitivities ranging from 11–88%, with most in the 30–40% range (16).

There has been only one prospective randomized study using a rapid test for intrapartum detection of GBS colonization; 8,977 consecutive women in labor were tested. Those who were heavily colonized were randomized to treatment with IV penicillin G or to an untreated control group (17). Neonates born to the treated women had a significantly lower incidence of early onset disease (1.5% versus 9.0%, $P < 0.01$). The incidence of GBS disease in women with a negative test was only 0.07%. Unfortunately, 38% (157/412) of the women with positive tests delivered before completing the test. Two (1.3%) of these neonates had early-onset disease.

In a nonrandomized study, 260 women with preterm premature rupture of the membranes and no labor were tested with a rapid agglutination test for GBS (18). Of 84 colonized women, 36 received ampicillin until delivery. There were no cases of chorioamnionitis or neonatal sepsis in the treated group, compared with 11 (23%) cases of chorioamnionitis and 13 (27%) cases of neonatal GBS disease in the untreated group.

Neonatal Immunoglobulin

In studies using an animal model of GBS sepsis, treatment with intravenous immunoglobulin (IVIG) increased sur-vival, although high-dose IVIG combined with penicillin led to decreased survival (19). A preparation with enhanced activity against GBS also increased survival, even with established infections. In small studies, treatment with IVIG in human neonates has been shown to reduce mortality from bacterial sepsis, and its prophylactic use has reduced the incidence of bacterial sepsis (19). Although preliminary studies are promising, IVIG cannot be considered standard therapy at present.

Maternal Vaccines

In recent years, much work has gone into developing a maternal vaccine to prevent maternal and neonatal GBS disease. The rationale for this method of immunoprophylaxis is based on the fact that maternal antibody to the GBS type III capsular polysaccharide is found in most colonized women delivered of healthy infants and not in those delivered of infants who subsequently develop invasive GBS disease. It is thought that passive transfer of maternal IgG antibody across the placenta to the neonate confers protection.

To be effective, a vaccine must be safe and must induce the formation of antibody. Then it must be demonstrated that the increased antibody levels are actually protective against clinical disease.

In one report, 40 pregnant women, 35 with low preimmunization antibody levels to the type III capsular polysaccharide and five with antibody levels that were already considered protective, at a mean gestational age of 31 weeks, were given a single dose of GBS type III capsular polysaccharide (20). Of the 35 with low preimmunization antibody levels, 20 responded with increased antibody levels, and all five with protective antibody levels had significant increases in specific antibody levels, for an overall response rate of 63%. These antibody levels persisted at delivery and at three months postpartum. Approximately 60% of the antibody was of the IgG subclass, and the antibody levels in the umbilical cords at birth correlated directly with those of the mother. The elevated antibody levels persisted for at least three months in a majority of the neonates. In vitro testing of infant serum demonstrated efficient opsonization, phagocytosis, and bacterial killing. Whether a modified vaccine will lead to an increased response rate and whether the vaccine will protect either the mother or neonate against clinical disease remains to be seen.

Recommendations

Although the development of an effective vaccine and neonatal immunoglobulin therapy both appear promising, the clinician is currently limited to maternal chemoprophylaxis to prevent the colonization and infection of susceptible neonates. Antepartum treatment of GBS colonization does not appear to be effective, nor does neonatal chemoprophylaxis. Routine antepartum screening for GBS cannot be recommended, and, as refinement of rapid diagnostic tests continues, this practice may become totally obsolete. It would appear that intrapartum chemoprophylaxis of selected patients holds the most promise.

The American College of Obstetricians and Gynecologists currently recommends treating patients who are GBS colonized and who have one of the following risk factors: preterm (<37 weeks) labor or rupture of the membranes, prolonged rupture of the membranes (>18 hours), prior child with symptomatic GBS infection or maternal fever during labor (21). If a risk factor is present and the culture result is not available, consideration should be given to using antibiotic prophylaxis empirically. Most centers currently treat preterm pregnancies with unknown culture results, although the treatment of term patients with prolonged rupture of the membranes and unknown GBS status is more controversial. Regardless of GBS culture results, all women with clinical intraamniotic infection should be treated with antibiotics in the intrapartum period, preferably with ampicillin and an aminoglycoside. This will not only provide prophylaxis against GBS disease, but also reduce neonatal sepsis in general (22). Colonized women who develop an intrapartum fever (with or without additional signs of intraamniotic infection) should be given antibiotic prophylaxis, as should those with multiple gestations. Most experts also recommend intrapartum antibiotic prophylaxis for all subsequent pregnancies following the birth of a GBS-infected neonate.

The usual treatment of GBS colonization during labor consists of 2 g of ampicillin IV followed by 1 g every four hours. Ampicillin is rapidly transported across the placenta and quickly establishes therapeutic levels in the fetus. If preterm labor is successfully stopped, there is no evidence that continued treatment of GBS colonization is necessary, in that it does not appear to affect pregnancy outcome. In colonized patients with preterm premature rupture of the membranes, continuing oral treatment for 7–10 days, or until labor occurs, should be considered, at which time IV therapy would be initiated. In the presence of ruptured membranes, there is increased risk of maternal GBS infection and the possibility of early intrauterine infection of the fetus. However, prolonged treatment after ruptured membranes may simply lead to infections with penicillin-resistant organisms.

In any case, it is not necessary to repeat the culture to "test for cure," as recolonization is common. Rather, after antibiotic treatment, if preterm labor recurs or the patient has prolonged rupture of the membranes, she would be retreated with IV ampicillin during labor. If accurate rapid diagnostic methods become widely available, these management protocols may be modified so that only those women with positive intrapartum tests are treated.

References

1. Zangwill KM, Schuchat A, Wenger JD. Group B streptococcal disease in the United States, 1990: Report from a multistate active surveillance system. Morb Mort Wkly Rpt 1992;41 (SS-6):25.
2. Boyer KM, Gotoff SP. Prevention of early onset neonatal group B streptococcal disease with selective intrapartum chemoprophylaxis. N Engl J Med 1986;314:1665.
3. Baker CJ. Summary of the workshop on perinatal infection due to group B streptococcus. J Infect Dis 1977;136:137.
4. Faro S. Group B beta-hemolytic streptococci and puerperal infections. Am J Obstet Gynecol 1981;139:686.
5. Boyer KM, Gadzala CA, Burd LI, et al. Selective intrapartum chemoprophylaxis of neonatal group B streptococcal early onset disease. I. Epidemiologic rationale. J Infect Dis 1983 148:795.
6. Baker CJ, Edwards MS. Group B streptococcal infections. In Remington JS, Klein JO, eds. Infectious diseases of the fetus and newborn infant. 3rd ed. Philadelphia: W.B Saunders, 1990:742.
7. Seigel JD, McCracken GH, Threlkeld N, et al. Single-dose

penicillin prophylaxis against neonatal group B streptococcal infections. N Engl J Med 1980;303:769.

8. Pyata SP, Pildes RS, Jacobs NM, et al. Penicillin in infants weighing two kilograms or less with early-onset group B streptococcal disease. N Engl J Med 1983;308:1383.

9. Hall RT, Barnes W, Krishnan L, et al. Antibiotic treatment of parturient women colonized with group B streptococci. Am J Obstet Gynecol 1976;124:630.

10. Boyer KM, Gadzala CA, Kelly PD, et al. Selective intrapartum chemoprophylaxis of neonatal group B streptococcal early-onset disease. II. Predictive value of prenatal cultures. J Infect Dis 1983;148:802.

11. Allardice JG, Baskett TF, Seshia MMK, et al. Perinatal group B streptococcal colonization and infection. Am J Obstet Gynecol 1982;142:617.

12. Boyer KM, Gadzala CA, Kelly PD, et al. Selective intrapartum chemoprophylaxis of neonatal group B streptococcal early-onset disease. III. Interruption of mother-to-infant transmission. J Infect Dis 1983;148:810.

13. Yow MD, Mason EO, Leeds LJ, et al. Ampicillin prevents intrapartum transmission of group B streptococcus. JAMA 1979;241:1245.

14. Morales WJ, Lim DV, Walsh AF. Prevention of neonatal group B streptococcal sepsis by the use of a rapid screening test and selective intrapartum prophylaxis. Am J Obstet Gynecol 1986;155:979.

15. Minkoff H, Mead P. An obstetric approach to the prevention of early-onset group B β-hemolytic streptococcal sepsis. Am J Obstet Gynecol 1986;154:973.

16. Yancey MK, Armer T, Clark P, Duff P. Assessment of rapid identification tests for genital carriage of group B streptococci. Obstet Gynecol 1992; 80:1038.

17. Tuppurainen N, Hallman M. Prevention of neonatal group B streptococcal disease: intrapartum detection and chemoprophylaxis of heavily colonized parturients. Obstet Gynecol 1989;73:583.

18. Morales WJ, Lim D. Reduction of group B streptococcal maternal and neonatal infections in preterm pregnancies with premature rupture of membranes through a rapid identification test. Am J Obstet Gynecol 1987;157:13.

19. Fischer GW. Therapeutic uses of intravenous gammaglobulin for pediatric infections. Ped Clin North Am 1988;35:517.

20. Baker CJ, Rench MA, Edwards MS, et al. Immunization of pregnant women with a polysaccharide vaccine of group B streptococcus. N Engl J Med 1988;319:1180.

21. American College of Obstetricians and Gynecologists. Group B steptococcal infections in pregnancy. Technical Bulletin #170, July 1992.

22. Gibbs RS, Dinsmoor MJ, Newton ER, et al. A randomized trial of intrapartum versus immediate postpartum treatment of women with intra-amniotic infection. Obstet Gynecol 1988;72:823.

38

Viral Hepatitis

Manley Cohen, M.D.
Hartley Cohen, M.D.

VIRAL hepatitis can occur at any time during pregnancy, whereas some liver diseases are more likely to manifest themselves during different trimesters. Liver diseases during pregnancy, occurring with or without jaundice, may be peculiar to pregnancy, incidental to or intercurrent in it, or complicated by it (1).

Jaundice occurs in one in 1,500 pregnancies and is most frequently the result of viral hepatitis, a major cause of death and morbidity in Third World countries (2, 3). It is a major problem throughout the world, and, since most cases can be prevented by vaccination, we need to ensure that those at risk get the vaccine.

Variety of Viruses

Many hepatotropic viruses can cause acute liver disease: hepatitis A virus (HAV), hepatitis B virus (HBV), hepatitis C virus (HCV), hepatitis E virus (HEV), herpes simplex virus (HSV), cytomegalovirus (CMV), and Epstein-Barr virus (EBV). Acute hepatitis, displaying histologic and clinical hallmarks of viral disease but no demonstrable virus, is called non-A, non-B, non-C hepatitis.

Viral hepatitis may be complicated by chronic, progressive disease. The viruses responsible are HBV, HCV, and agents that cause non-A, non-B hepatitis. Chronic HBV infection may be exacerbated by the delta agent, a separate virus requiring HBV to facilitate its penetration (4).

Why the incidence and severity of viral hepatitis in pregnant women vary in different parts of the world is unknown. Investigators in India during an epidemic of non-A, non-B hepatitis found an incidence of 2.8% in men, 2.1% in nonpregnant women, and 17.3% in pregnant women. Moreover, the incidence during the second (19.4%) and third (18.6%) trimesters was significantly higher than during the first trimester (8.8%) (5). In Europe and the United States, however, acute viral hepatitis is probably equally frequent throughout the three trimesters, with an incidence similar to that of the general population (2, 6).

Clinical Features

Most patients with hepatitis have no symptoms. Their infection is usually detected only because of the chance finding of high transaminase levels or through markers of earlier disease. About a third of all patients who have symptoms will have jaundice.

Many patients do complain of lassitude, fatigue, nausea, vomiting, loss of appetite, or abdominal discomfort. Often, they have fever. Initially, a flulike illness may be diagnosed mistakenly, especially if there is no evidence of jaundice. Less frequently, there may be arthralgias and a rash that suggest HBV infection.

Time of onset helps differentiate vomiting of early pregnancy from that of viral hepatitis. In hepatitis, vomiting worsens as the day progresses, whereas in normal early pregnancy it is usually most troublesome in the morning. During the third trimester, it is difficult to distinguish clinically viral hepatitis from acute fatty liver of pregnancy, although the latter disease usually has a more abrupt, severe onset. Typical laboratory findings for alanine aminotransferase (ALT, formerly SGPT) and aspartate aminotransferase (AST, formerly SGOT) in viral hepatitis are above 1,000

U/L. Such high values are unusual in acute fatty liver of pregnancy, where values rarely exceed 500 U/L. Moreover, a marked leukocytosis, common in acute fatty liver of pregnancy, is not typical of acute viral hepatitis.

Serologic Diagnosis

A number of radioimmunoassays and other tests are now available to assist in diagnosing viral hepatitis. In 1977, HAV accounted for about 25% of all hospitalized cases, HBV for about 50% (Figure 38.1) (7). In one study of pregnant women hospitalized because of acute icteric hepatitis, the frequency of HAV was 7%, that of HBV 79%, and that of non-A, non-B 14% (Figure 38.2) (8).

Knowing the hepatitis serology of a pregnant patient, or of her obstetrician for that matter, may help answer some practical questions about infectivity (9). How likely is a carrier mother to transmit the disease to her infant or to

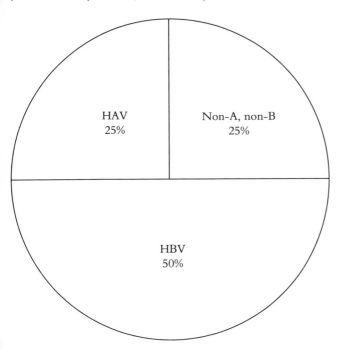

Figure 38.1 Etiology of hepatitis in hospitalized patients.

Reprinted with permission from Dienstag JL, Alaama A, Mosley JW, et al. Etiology of sporadic hepatitis B surface antigen-negative hepatitis. Ann Intern Med 1977;87:1.

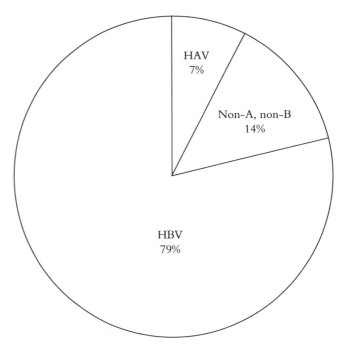

Figure 38.2 Acute icteric hepatitis in hospitalized pregnant women.

Reprinted with permission from Tong MJ, Thursby M, Rakela J, et al. Studies on the maternal-infant transmission of the viruses which cause acute hepatitis. Gastroenterology 1981;80:999.

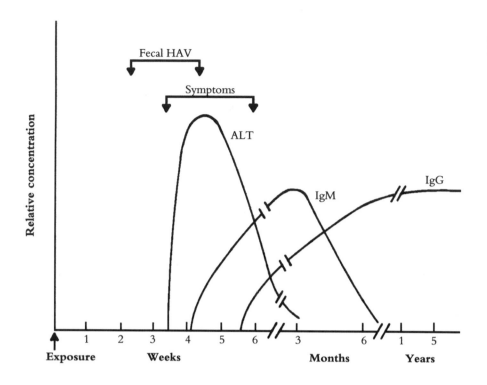

Figure 38.3   Course of hepatitis A disease. ALT = alanine aminotransferase; HAV = hepatitis A virus; IgG = immunoglobulin G; IgM = immunoglobulin M.

HAV: hepatitis A virus
ALT: alanine aminotransferase
IgM: immunoglobulin M
IgG: immunoglobulin G

the obstetrician who delivers her, especially if a finger is pricked during surgery or while sewing up an episiotomy? What is a patient's risk of getting hepatitis from an obstetrician who is a symptom-free carrier?

Hepatitis A

Hepatitis A is an acute disease, usually self-limited, with a 1% mortality from fulminant hepatic failure (Figure 38.3). Except for the rare patient whose disease lasts over a year and is associated with persistent IgM antibody to HAV (anti-HAV IgM), there is no chronic form. Although hepatitis A virus can be detected in feces before the onset of symptoms, this test is available only in research laboratories. Diagnosis depends on the detection of anti-HAV IgM, which occurs at the onset of clinical disease and usually persists for not more than six months. Detection of anti-HAV

IgG merely indicates earlier HAV infection and only serves to exclude acute hepatitis A.

Hepatitis B

The course of hepatitis B is complicated (Figure 38.4). HBV is a DNA virus, about 42 nm in diameter, whose outer protein coat is the antigen HBsAg, which is replicated in liver cell cytoplasm. HBV's central core contains DNA that is double-stranded for two-thirds and single-stranded for one-third of its length; it also contains a DNA polymerase and hepatitis B core antigen (HBcAg). The DNA is replicated in the hepatocyte nucleus.

Since more HBsAg is produced than is needed to cover the formed core, the excess can be seen as spheres and cylinders on electron micrographs of serum. Another antigen, the HBeAg, is soluble and appears to be related to

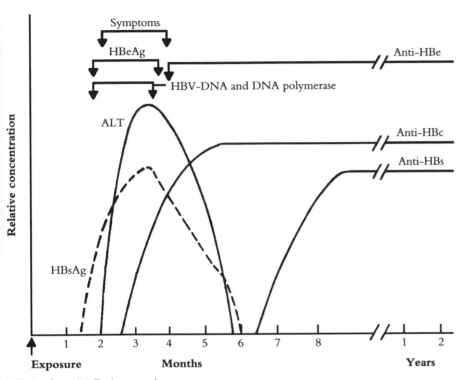

Figure 38.4   Course of hepatitis B disease. ALT = alanine aminotransferase; Anti-HBc = antibody to hepatitis B virus core antigen; Anti-HBe = antibody to hepatitis B virus e antigen; Anti-HBs = antibody to hepatitis B virus surface antigen; HBeAg = hepatitis B virus e antigen; HBsAg = hepatitis B surface antigen; HBV-DNA = deoxyribonucleic acid specific for hepatitis B virus.

HBeAg: hepatitis B virus e antigen
Anti–HBe: antibody to hepatitis B virus e antigen
HBV-DNA: deoxyribonucleic acid specific for hepatitis B virus
ALT: alanine aminotransferase
Anti–HBc: antibody to hepatitis B virus core antigen
Anti–HBs: antibody to hepatitis B virus surface antigen
HBsAg: hepatitis B surface antigen

the virus core. All three antigens—HBsAg, HBcAg, and HBeAg—are capable of stimulating production of antibodies by the infected host.

Although tests for the numerous HBsAg subtypes are available only in research laboratories, they are useful for epidemiologic studies. For example, an infant who contracts HBsAg from its carrier mother will have the same subtype. Such transmission is common, particularly if the HBsAg-carrier mother also harbors HBeAg.

Detection of HBeAg and the HBV-specific DNA polymerase suggests both high viral replication rates and the presence in the circulation of many complete HBV particles (Dane particles) demonstrable on electron microscopy. It has been assumed that such chronic carriers are more likely to transmit the disease than HBsAg carriers (mothers or obstetricians) who have anti-HBe. The presence of anti-HBe in the chronic HBsAg carrier originally was thought to indicate a healthy noninfective state. However, this is not always the case, because 31%–44% of carriers with anti-HBe may have liver disease, and transmission of HBV to chimpanzees by sera containing HBsAg and anti-HBe has been documented. Furthermore, HBV-associated HBeAg, although not free HBeAg, has been found in sera of patients who have the homologous anti-HBe (10).

Even the presence of anti–HBs, usually an indication of earlier infection, immunity, and noninfectivity and a good prognostic sign, may rarely be associated with the continuing presence of HBV-DNA. In these instances, part or all of the HBV-DNA has been incorporated into the host DNA. Patients who have HBV-DNA are at risk of developing hepatoma (11).

Nevertheless, in practical terms, most HBsAg-carrier health-care workers are not a great threat to patients (12). If they have circulating HBeAg, they probably are potential sources of infection. If they have circulating anti-HBe, they are even less likely to transmit the virus (13). But some such subjects are indeed infectious and harbor Dane particle-associated HBeAg, despite their having anti-HBe in their sera (10).

Non-A, Non-B Viral Hepatitis

In about 25% of patients hospitalized with "viral hepatitis," no serologic test confirms acute HAV or HBV infection, and the infections have been designated non-A, non-B hepatitis. Depending on the presenting features, CMV and EBV infections also should be excluded by spot tests for mononucleosis, EBV titers, and acute and convalescent CMV titers. A few may have "cryptic hepatitis B" in which HBsAg, anti-HBs, and anti-HB core are not expressed, but HBV-DNA can be detected in serum or liver tissue. Others may have nonviral toxic liver injury that cannot be distinguished from a viral hepatitis.

There are at least two major forms of non-A, non-B viral hepatitis. One, hepatitis C, is transfusion related. About 50% of infected patients will develop chronic disease. A serologic test for circulating antibodies to hepatitis C was released in 1989 and even more sensitive tests are now routine in 1993 (14). Therefore, posttransfusion viral hepatitis should drop to below its pre-1989 incidence of 3%–12%.

Hepatitis E, enteric non-A, non-B hepatitis, which appears to be waterborne, is widespread in India and Southeast Asia, as well as in Africa and South America (15, 16). It is usually a mild illness, except in young pregnant women who have a high case-fatality rate from fulminant hepatic failure. About 10% get chronic liver disease if the hepatitis was sporadically acquired (17, 18). As it is probably spread by contaminated water supplies, control measures include good sanitation and personal hygiene. No commercial assay for hepatitis E is available in early 1993.

Though the risk of death from fulminant hepatic failure is greater after labor, we urge pregnant patients, even in very early pregnancy, to avoid travel to Third World countries (19).

At present, non-A, non-B, non-C viral hepatitis is diagnosed by exclusion and has no specific treatment or vaccine. A rare cause of viral hepatitis is herpes simplex virus. Pregnant women seem to be at an increased risk for infection, which usually has a fulminant and fatal course (20, 21).

Managing the Pregnant Patient

Every pregnant woman should be tested routinely for HBsAg, and the infant immunized, depending on the results (22). We recommended such screening and immunization for mother and child at a time when the Centers for Disease Control (CDC) was recommending that only high-risk women (Table 38.1) be tested, for reasons of cost effectiveness. If only those who are at high risk are tested, 50% of carrier pregnant women are missed because patients may not admit to drug abuse or even be aware that their partners are bisexual or have chronic liver disease (22). Testing mothers and vaccinating infants at risk has recently

Table 38.1 Pregnant Women at High Risk for HBsAg Positivity

Those with acute or chronic liver disease

Those who have had accidental needle sticks with HBV-contaminated blood

Those whose sexual partners are bisexual, though mainly homosexual, men

Those who are or who have been IV drug abusers

Those who live in households of IV drug abusers, carriers, or hemodialysis patients

Spouses of patients with chronic or acute hepatitis B

Those who have had repeated blood transfusions, or who have been rejected as blood donors

Those from areas of high-HBV endemicity: Asia, Pacific islands, Alaska, Haiti, sub-Saharan Africa, whether immigrant or US-born

Those who are daughters of mothers who had acute or chronic perinatal liver disease or jaundice

Health-care workers with occupational exposure to blood or its products in medical, dental, and laboratory settings (dialysis nurses and laboratory technicians)

been shown to be both medically and economically effective in the United Kingdom (23). Despite this, in many Third World countries, even high-risk pregnant women are not tested because of the "prohibitively high cost of the vaccine" for the neonate (24).

This shortsighted view ignores the even higher costs of morbidity, economic loss to the community, and death from preventable chronic hepatitis and hepatoma. Thus, a disease that can be prevented by vaccination 90% of the time continues to spread. These untreated neonates have a 20%–50% chance of dying of cirrhosis or hepatocellular carcinoma (23). In November 1991, the CDC recommended routine vaccination of all infants, with the addition of HBIG for those born of mothers who are HBsAg positive (25).

There are no special ways to care for pregnant patients with viral hepatitis. Their activity need not be restricted, except as their own exercise tolerance dictates. Most can be spared hospitalization, unless their disease is severe enough to prolong prothrombin time or they cannot take food orally and vomit excessively. Those with fulminant disease require intensive care. Termination of pregnancy is not warranted, although there is no study to evaluate whether this ameliorates the illness. Liver transplantation may need consideration in severe fulminant progressive liver failure. Precautionary hospital measures are discussed in a recent report (26).

Effect on the Fetus

Most infants of mothers with hepatitic viral disease are delivered at term. Prematurity and neonatal death occur in cases of severe or fulminant maternal hepatitis (5, 27, 28), but nonfulminant disease generally does not increase the probability of fetal wastage. Risk of prematurity, however, may be increased (29). Theoretically, fetal exposure to high levels of maternal unconjugated bilirubin may result in kernicterus. This was not observed, however, in two cases (30, 31). Moreover, in icteric viral hepatitis, very high unconjugated bilirubinemia is rare.

Effects on the fetus depend on trimester and whether or not the virus crosses the placenta. There appears to be no increased risk of congenital abnormalities (29, 32), although reports of chromosomal aberrations in newborns of chronic HBsAg-positive mothers leave lingering doubts (33).

Vertical Transmission of Hepatitis

Congenital abnormalities occur rarely, if at all, as a result of maternal viral hepatitis, possibly because the hepatitis viruses rarely cross the placenta. There are few reports of HBsAg-positive newborns. Indeed, even HBsAg positivity may indicate only transfer of the 22-nm HBsAg particle and may not necessarily imply transfer of the 42-nm HBV (34).

A study of 51 neonates also argued against transplacental transmission of HBV from HBsAg-positive carrier mothers, some of whom were HBeAg positive, since none of the neonates had anti-HBc IgM, a marker of recent or active HBV infection (35). However, in an earlier study of 25 neonates, although 24 only became HBsAg positive four weeks after delivery, one was HBsAg positive at birth, and this case may have represented intrauterine transplacental transmission of HBV (8).

When the mother has HBsAg-positive hepatitis during pregnancy and seems to recover before delivery, it is rare to find HBsAg in the infant's cord blood (36, 37). These exceptions, however, tend to confirm occasional antepartum intrauterine transmission.

Vertical transmission of HBV occurs 80%–100% of the time if the mother is HBeAg positive as well as HBsAg positive, but only 25% of the time in the absence of HBeAg (38); the percentage is even less in the United States (39). It is rare when the mother had hepatitis B during pregnancy and completely recovered before delivery. It is more frequent with maternal acute hepatitis in the last trimester than with chronic maternal HBsAg infection that is HBeAg-negative (40). The neonatal infection is usually manifested postpartum rather than at birth, and cord blood HBsAg is not a good predictor of disease (37, 41). Immunoprophylaxis with hepatitis B immune globulin (HBIG) and vaccination of the infant prevents vertical transmission, even from HBeAg-positive mothers, in 90% of cases.

Vertical transmission of HBV perpetuates the chronic-carrier state and results in chronic liver disease that may progress to childhood cirrhosis. Neonates usually become HBsAg positive between one and four months and frequently become chronic carriers who transmit the disease to the next generation. The majority do not develop overt signs of liver disease, but have transient and fluctuating increases in their transaminase levels and usually chronic persistent hepatitis, histologically (27). They may develop hepatomas in later life. About 10% of infected neonates will become overtly jaundiced and have acute self-limiting hepatitis; they then often become HBsAg negative and develop HBs antibodies.

The role of cesarean section in preventing mother-to-infant transmission of hepatitis B virus is controversial (42, 43). Intrauterine infection of the fetus is rare. The major way infants become infected is by swallowing HBV during delivery. Supporting this conclusion is the finding of HBsAg in 95% of gastric contents sampled from neonates of infected mothers. By contrast, HBsAg has been found in only 33% of amniotic fluid samples, 50% of cord blood samples, and 70% of breast milk samples of carrier mothers (41).

Infants who received vaccine became infected at a rate of 39% if delivered vaginally, and 33% if delivered by cesarean section (CS)—an insignificant difference (42). Infants who also received HBIG at a dose of 50 IU had a 20% infection rate after vaginal delivery, reduced to only a 6% infection rate if they were delivered by cesarean. There was a similar 6% infection rate after vaginal delivery when three times the dose of HBIG (150 IU) was given (44). Also, only a 5% frequency of infections was observed after vaginal delivery using 200 IU anti-HBs (HBIG) (45).

Cesarean section should be reserved for cases where it is unequivocally better for mother or infant or both. It is felt that the data at this time do not support CS to prevent vertical transmission of hepatitis B. Equally good results are obtained by early high-dose HBIG (150 to 200 IU within two hours of birth), combined with active immunization in vaginally delivered infants.

Whether delivered by CS or vaginally, about 6% of treated infants will probably still become infected, which is much better than the 100% if left untreated, or the 20%–40% if inadequately treated. The neonatal infection is usually manifested postpartum rather than at birth, and cord blood HBsAg, positive in about 50% of samples, is not a good predictor of disease in the infant (37, 45).

Vertical transmission of the delta agent with HBV has been reported (46). Such transmission might increase the likelihood of developing chronic active hepatitis, which is more likely to progress to cirrhosis.

The trimester during which the mother has hepatitis is important in non-A, non-B hepatitis. Infants of three mothers who had non-A, non-B in the second trimester did not develop hepatitis, whereas six of nine mothers who had it in the third trimester or perinatal period gave birth to babies who had elevated transaminase levels at 4–8 weeks of age (8). None of the infants was jaundiced or had clinical evidence of liver disease. Of particular concern is that two of these six infants have had persistent transaminase abnormalities, suggesting the possibility of chronic liver disease; however, the follow-up period is too short for it to be determined.

HAV does not cause chronic disease, but its vertical transmission is of importance in causing acute hepatitis in neonates. This may be amenable to prophylaxis. In one study, only one of six infants delivered to mothers with acute HAV during pregnancy or at delivery had a transient (less than one month) minimal transaminase elevation (8). Whether this represents transplacental transmission of HAV is unclear. A recombinant vaccine has been released in Europe (47).

Active and Passive Immunization

The first vaccine against HBV licensed by the Food and Drug Administration (FDA) in 1982 gave hope that hepatitis B would go the way of smallpox and diphtheria. Made by purifying HBsAg from HBsAg-positive serum, it is neither a live nor a killed virus and contains no DNA. The vaccine is effective even in high-risk homosexuals (48). Early concerns that it might transmit the acquired immunodeficiency syndrome (AIDS) are unfounded (49). Second-generation vaccines made by recombinant DNA technology are available. Special formulations are required for hemodialysis or immunocompromised patients because of the large volume and aluminum content of the regular recombinant vaccines (22, 49).

The Immunization Practices Advisory Committee (ACIP) of the CDC constantly revises its recommendations for protection (vaccination) against viral hepatitis as new information becomes available and publishes these in *Mor-*

bidity and Mortality Weekly Report (MMWR). ACIP currently recommends preexposure prophylaxis for all health-care workers exposed to blood or to mentally disabled people (who have poor hygiene), homosexually active men, drug abusers, hemodialysis patients, recipients (hemophiliacs) of certain blood products, and special high-risk populations including heterosexually active persons with multiple partners, as well as international travellers to HBV endemic areas (Asia, Africa). One cannot always identify high-risk individuals for preexposure prophylaxis, however. The CDC now recommends universal vaccination for all infants born to some other unvaccinated groups of people (22, 49).

Franks and co-workers of the CDC recommended in 1989 that all neonates of Southeast Asian immigrants routinely be vaccinated against HBV, because only 54% of the cases of HBV infection among US-born children of such refugees were attributable to perinatal infection. The other 46% were considered to be due to child-to-child transmission within and between households (50). We agree with the 1991 recommendations which now extend this policy and recommend universal vaccination of all newborns, regardless of their mother's serology (25).

HBIG at birth confers passive immunity (antibodies to HBsAg, that is, anti-HBs), lasting about four weeks. Anti-HBs does not impede the immune response to the vaccine, nor does preexisting HBsAg positivity incur an adverse effect from the vaccine (51–53). Thus, prescreening of neonates of HBsAg positive mothers is unwarranted. It may delay vaccination, and, more importantly, there is poor correlation between cord blood positivity and subsequent confirmed HBV infection.

The optimal dose and timing of vaccinations is still under study. Although one study (45) suggests that the timing (one week, one month, or three months of age) of the first dose of HBV vaccine is not critical, we feel that the vaccine should be administered in addition to any HBIG required, but at different sites, intramuscularly, shortly after birth in the delivery room, if possible, with booster vaccinations at one or three months and six months. We feel that HBIG should be given in a high dose (200 IU anti-HBs) of 0.5 mL/kg body weight, preferably in the delivery room and as soon as possible after delivery, with subsequent doses of 0.16 mL/kg every four weeks for six months (23,

54). This regimen is probably more effective than other HBIG schedules. Current CDC guidelines recommend only 0.5 mL IM of HBIG within 12 hours of birth, but state that "other schedules have also been effective."

We recommend a vaccine dose of 20 μg in a small volume (23). The Centers for Disease Control recommends 2.5 to 10 μg in 0.25 to 0.5 mL of vaccine at birth and at one and six months (47).

Economic Factors for Preventing HBV

The cost of preventing perinatal transmission in the US has been discussed (25, 55). A British study estimates £36,000 as the cost for nonselective testing of 6,000 pregnant women at the Royal Free Hospital during three years. This, together with vaccination, prevented chronic hepatitis B in up to eight children who would have had a 20%–50% lifetime risk of cirrhosis or hepatoma. Inpatient treatment for ten patients with uncompensated cirrhosis averaged £12,000 per patient at 1988 prices. The indirect costs may be ten to 20 times higher. Thus, unselective screening and vaccination as indicated are economically cost effective in the United Kingdom and, we would hope, is now routine in most US hospitals.

We believe universal screening in the United States is cost effective. Economic studies are urgently needed in countries where testing and vaccination are not offered (24). Programs for universal screening of pregnant women were in progress in Hawaii, certain Canadian provinces, Italy, West Germany, New Zealand, Australia, and Japan in June of 1988 (22).

The CDC now recommends universal screening for HBsAg of all pregnant women, universal vaccination of all neonates and also HBIG if the mother is HBsAg positive, both given within 12 hours of birth (47).

The obstetrician's job is not done when he or she identifies an HBV-carrier pregnant patient. Depending on state law, they may be required to report the case to health authorities, though this is usually done by the laboratory. The obstetrician needs to counsel the patient and ensure that household members and sexual partners of HBV carriers be tested to determine susceptibility. If these contacts are susceptible, they should be vaccinated—as well, of course, as the neonate (22).

Although there are minor differences in opinion about dosages and schedules, screening is endorsed by the CDC, the American College of Obstetricians and Gynecologists, and the American Academy of Pediatrics (22).

Inadvertent Needle Stick

HBIG is produced from donors with very high titers of anti-HBs. It effectively protects against hepatitis in those exposed to HBV by needle, sexual contact, or vertical transmission from HBsAg-positive mothers. Health-care workers who get inoculated (by needle stick) with HBsAg blood need it if they are not already immune. In such cases, since most physicians and nurses do not know if they are immune, we immediately draw their blood for hepatitis testing and then inject the first of two doses of HBIG, which is in short supply and expensive. The second dose is given one month later, but only if the subject had no anti-HBs or other hepatitis markers (HBsAg, anti-HBc) when originally tested. To be effective, the first dose must be given as soon as possible after exposure and probably no later than 72 hours. In addition, 1.0 mL (20 μg) of vaccine is given (within seven days and one and six months later) if indicated by lack of hepatitis serologic markers, as recommended by the CDC (22, 56).

Studies evaluating immune serum globulin (ISG) for the treatment of pre- and postexposure to non-A, non-B hepatitis have been disappointing. At best, it ameliorates the severity and reduces the incidence of jaundice and progression to chronic liver disease (57, 58). Since ISG appears safe, it seems reasonable to administer it to the neonate of a mother who has had non-A, non-B hepatitis during the third trimester or perinatal period. The injection should probably be repeated after a month.

Although HAV does not cause chronic disease, ISG administration to the infant born to a mother with perinatal HAV hepatitis may be justified in order to diminish the small possibility of acute HAV hepatitis in the newborn.

Breast-feeding

Some, but not all, studies have detected HBsAg in breast milk (50%–70%) of mothers who are chronic HBsAg carriers (41, 59–60). Some consider it contraindicated for HBsAg-positive mothers, but others disagree (60–63). Provided that infants of HBsAg positive mothers receive both passive and active immunization, we believe that breast-feeding is permissible. No data, however, confirm this view.

Precautionary Hospital Measures

The CDC has issued guidelines for the care of hospitalized patients with viral hepatitis (26, 64). It suggests that, because HAV is excreted primarily in feces during the incubation period before the disease is recognized, no special precautions are needed. For all hospitalized patients, whether or not they have hepatitis, the CDC recommends that feces, secretions, bedpans, and instruments in contact with the intestinal tract be handled only with gloved hands. Additional precautions, including private rooms, separate toilet facilities, and gowning and gloving of staff when entering these patients' rooms, are considered unnecessary by the CDC. Most hospitals, however, have their own precautionary policies, which may differ from these recommendations. There is no particular reason why the pregnant mother or her newborn need be cared for differently. Table 38.2 gives guidelines for the care of HBsAg positive mothers and their newborn infants. We feel that universal precautions for all patients to prevent the spread of both HIV and HBV should be followed.

Since the fecal-oral route of hepatitis B transmission is rare, if it occurs at all, enteric precautions are of dubious value. Blood precautions are important, however, for patients with either acute or chronic HBV infection. It might be wise for the obstetrician and nursing staff to double glove when delivering a pregnant patient with HBV to minimize the possibility of accidental needle punctures. Particular care is necessary in cleaning all instruments that have been in contact with blood. Similar precautions for non-A, non-B are appropriate. When a patient with suspected viral hepatitis is admitted, both enteric and blood precautions are appropriate until the cause of the hepatitis has been established.

Table 38.2 Care of HBsAg-Positive Mothers and their Newborns

Observe blood precautions for pre- and postdelivery care.

Cesarean section is probably not indicated to prevent hepatitis transmission.

Use care during labor and delivery to avoid staff exposure to mother's blood.

Handle blood- or lochia-soaked dressings with gloved hands and disinfect sitz baths.

Give newborns of HBsAg-positive mothers at least 0.5 mL of IM HBIG in the delivery room and again at three and six months, following CDC recommendations. Inject the first dose of at least 0.5 mL (10μg) HBV vaccine in the delivery room and repeat at one and six months.

Isolation of newborns is not necessary after thorough bathing and rinsing.

Separation of newborn and mother is not indicated.

Breast-feeding should not be routinely discouraged, unless mother's nipples are cracked.

Strict isolation of the carrier with gowning, masking, and gloving not indicated, but staff must observe precautions related to blood, lochia, and dressings.

Routine infant immunization schedules need not be modified.

The CDC recommends obtaining HBsAg test at six months (optional) and, if positive, omitting the six-month dose of vaccine as the infant is infected. Obtain HBsAg and anti–HBs test at 12–15 months: a positive HBsAg indicates therapeutic failure; a positive anti–HBs indicates therapeutic success. The expense may not be justified.

References

1. Sherlock S. Jaundice in pregnancy. Br Med Bull 1968;24:39.

2. Haemmerli UP. Jaundice during pregnancy, with special emphasis on recurrent jaundice during pregnancy and its differential diagnosis. Acta Med Scand 1966;179 (Suppl 444):1.

3. Kwast BE, Steven JA. Viral hepatitis as a major cause of maternal morbidity in Addis Ababa, Ethiopia. Int J Gynaecol Obstet 1987;25:99.

4. Rizzetto M. The delta agent. Hepatology 1983;3:729.

5. Khuroo MS, Teli MR, Skidmore S, et al. Incidence and severity of viral hepatitis in pregnancy. Am J Med 1981;70:252.

6. Krejs GJ, Haemmerli UP. Jaundice during pregnancy. In: Schiff L, Schiff ER, eds. Diseases of the liver. 5th ed. New York, NY: Harper & Row, 1982:1561.

7. Dienstag JL, Alaama A, Mosley JW, et al. Etiology of sporadic hepatitis B surface antigen-negative hepatitis. Ann Intern Med 1977;87:1.

8. Tong MJ, Thursby M, Rakela J, et al. Studies on the maternal-infant transmission of the viruses which cause acute hepatitis. Gastroenterology 1981;80:999.

9. Lettau LA, Smith JD, Williams D, et al. Transmission of hepatitis B with resultant restriction of surgical practice. JAMA 1986;255:934.

10. Raimondo G, Recchia S, Lavarini C, et al. Dane particle-associated hepatitis B e antigen in patients with chronic hepatitis B virus infection and hepatitis B e antibody. Hepatology 1982;2:449.

11. Shafritz DA, Shouval D, Sherman HI, et al. Integration of hepatitis B virus DNA into the genome of liver cells in chronic liver disease and hepatocellular carcinoma. Studies in percutaneous liver biopsies and post-mortem tissue specimens. N Engl J Med 1981;305:1067.

12. Alter HJ, Chalmers TC. The HBsAg positive health worker revisited. Hepatology 1981;1:467.

13. Rosendahl C, Kochen MM, Kretschmer R, et al. Avoidance of perinatal transmission of hepatitis B virus: is passive immunization always necessary? Lancet 1983;1:1127.

14. Kuo G, Choo Q-L, Alter JH, et al. An assay for circulating antibodies to a major etiologic virus of human non-A, non-B hepatitis. Science 1989;244:362.

15. Nouasria B, Aouati A, Bernaj J, et al. Fulminant viral hepatitis and pregnancy in Algeria and France. Ann Trop Med Parasitol 1986;623:263.

16. Ramalingaswami V, Purcell RH. Waterborne non-A, non-B hepatitis. Lancet 1988;1:571.

17. Dienstag JL, Alter HJ. Non-A, non-B hepatitis: evolving epidemiologic and clinical perspective. Semin Liver Dis 1986;6:67.

18. Gayert GL, Bottoms SF, Sokol RJ. Anicteric presentation of fatal herpetic hepatitis in pregnancy. Obstet Gynecol 1985;65:585.

19. Bal V, Amin SN, Rath S, et al. Virological markers and antibody responses in fulminant viral hepatitis. J Med Virol 1987;23:75.

20. Flewett TH, Parker PG, Philip WM. Acute hepatitis due to herpes simplex virus in an adult. J Clin Pathol 1969;22:60.

21. Goyette RE, Donowho EM Jr, Hieger LR, et al. Fulminant herpes virus hominis hepatitis during pregnancy. Obstet Gynecol 1974;43:191.

22. Advisory Committee on Immunization Practices. Protection against viral hepatitis. MMWR 1990;39(RR-2).

23. Brook MG, Lever AML, Kelly D, et al. Antenatal screening for hepatitis B is medically and economically effective in the prevention of vertical transmission: three years experience in a London hospital. Q J Med 1989;71:313.

24. Siegel-Itzkovich J. National tragedy incubating. Jerusalem Post. 1989 May 25:7.

25. Advisory Committee on Immunization Practices. Hepatitis B virus: A comprehensive strategy for eliminating transmission in the United States through universal childhood vaccination. MMWR 1991;40:RR-13.

26. Centers for Disease Control. Guidelines for prevention of transmission of human immunodeficiency virus and hepatitis and hepatitis B virus to health-care and public-safety workers. MMWR 1989;38(S-6).

27. Schweitzer IL, Dunn AE, Peters RL, et al. Viral hepatitis B in neonates and infants. Am J Med 1973;55:762.

28. Borhanmanesh F, Haghighi P, Hekmat K, et al. Viral hepatitis during pregnancy. Severity and effect on gestation. Gastroenterology 1973;64:304.

29. Hieber JP, Dalton D, Shorey J, et al. Hepatitis and pregnancy. J Pediatr 1977;91:545.

30. Lipsitz PJ, Flaxman LM, Tartow LR, et al. Maternal hyperbilirubinemia and the newborn. Am J Dis Child 1973; 126:525.

31. Waffarn F, Carlisle S, Pena I, et al. Fetal exposure to maternal hyperbilirubinemia. Neonatal course and outcome. Am J Dis Child 1982;136:416.

32. Siegel M. Congenital malformations following chickenpox, measles, mumps, and hepatitis. Results of a cohort study. JAMA 1973;226:1521.

33. Jhaveri RC, Verma RS, Rosenfeld W, et al. Chromosomal abnormality in the newborns of hepatitis B surface antigen (HBsAg) carrier mothers. Clin Pediatr 1980;19:66.

34. Boxall EH, Flewett TH, Dane DS, et al. Hepatitis B surface antigen in breast milk [Letter]. Lancet 1974;2:1007.

35. Goudeau A, Yvonnet B, Lesage G, et al. Lack of anti-HBc IgM in neonates with HBsAg carrier mothers argues against transplacental transmission of hepatitis B virus infection. Lancet 1983;2:1103.

36. Schweitzer IL, Wing A, McPeak C, et al. Hepatitis and hepatitis-associated antigen in 56 mother-infant pairs. JAMA 1972;220:1092.

37. Schweitzer IL, Mosley JW, Ashcaval M, et al. Factors influencing neonatal infection by hepatitis B virus. Gastroenterology 1973;65:277.

38. Wong VC, Lee AK, Ip HM. Transmission of hepatitis B antigens from symptom free carrier mothers to the fetus and the infant. Br J Obstet Gynaecol 1980;87:958.

39. Gerety RJ, Schweitzer IL. Viral hepatitis type B during pregnancy, the neonatal period, and infancy. J Pediatr 1977; 90:368.

40. Skinhoj P, Cohn J, Bradburne AF. Transmission of hepatitis type B from healthy HBsAg-positive mothers. Br Med J 1976;1:10.

41. Lee AK, Ip HM, Wong VC. Mechanisms of maternal-fetal transmission of hepatitis B virus. J Infect Dis 1978;138:668.

42. Lee SD, Lo KJ, Tsai YT, et al. Role of cesarean section in prevention of mother-infant transmission of hepatitis B virus. Lancet 1988;2:833.

43. Beasley RP, Stevens CE. Vertical transmission of HBV and interruption with globulin. In: Vyas GN, Cohen SN, Schmid R, eds. Viral hepatitis. Philadelphia: Franklin Institute Press, 1978:333.

44. Beasley RP, Hwang LY, Lee GC, et al. Prevention of perinatally transmitted hepatitis B virus infections with hepatitis B immune globulin and hepatitis B vaccine. Lancet 1983; 2:1099.

45. Schalm SW, Pit-Grosheide P. Prevention of hepatitis B transmission at birth. Lancet 1989;1:44.

46. Smedile A, Dentico P, Zanetti A, et al. Infection with the delta agent in chronic HBsAg carriers. Gastroenterology 1981;81:992.

47. Mishra L, Seeff LB. Viral hepatitis, A through E, complicating pregnancy. Gastroenterology 1992;21(4):873–88.

48. Francis DP, Hadler SC, Thompson SE, et al. The prevention of hepatitis B with vaccine. Report of the Centers for Disease Control multi-center efficacy trial among homosexual men. Ann Intern Med 1982;97:362.

49. Advisory Committee on Immunization Practices. Update on hepatitis B prevention. MMWR 1987;36(23):353.

50. Franks AL, Berg CJ, Kane MA, et al. Hepatitis B virus infection among children born in the United States to Southeast Asian refugees. N Engl J Med 1989;321:1301.

51. Maupas P, Chiron JP, Barin F, et al. Efficacy of hepatitis B vaccine in prevention of early HBsAg carrier state in children. Controlled trial in an endemic area (Senegal). Lancet 1981;1:289.

52. Szmuness W, Oleszko WR, Stevens CE, et al. Passive-active immunization against hepatitis B: immunogenicity studies in adult Americans. Lancet 1981;1:575.

53. Dienstag JL, Stevens CE, Bhan AK, et al. Hepatitis B vaccine administered to chronic carriers of hepatitis B surface antigen. Ann Intern Med 1982;96:575.

54. Beasley RP, Hwang LY, Stevens CE, et al. Efficacy of hepatitis B immune globulin for prevention of perinatal transmission of the hepatitis B virus carrier state: final report of a randomized double-blind, placebo-controlled trial. Hepatology 1983;3:135.

55. Koretz RL. Universal prenatal hepatitis B testing: is it cost-effective? Obstet Gynecol 1989;74:808.

56. Centers for Disease Control. Recommendation of the Immunization Practices Advisory Committee (ACIP): postexposure prophylaxis of hepatitis B. MMWR 1984;33:285.

57. Knodell RG, Conrad ME, Ginsberg AL, et al. Efficacy of prophylactic gamma-globulin in preventing non-A, non-B post-transfusion hepatitis. Lancet 1976;1:557.

58. Knodell RG, Conrad ME, Ishak KG. Development of chronic liver disease after acute non-A, non-B post-transfusion hepatitis. Role of gamma-globulin prophylaxis in its prevention. Gastroenterology 1977;72:902.

59. Linneman CC Jr, Goldberg S. HBsAg in breast milk. Lancet 1974;2:155.

60. Derso A, Boxall EH, Tarlow MJ, et al. Transmission of HBsAg from mother to infant in four ethnic groups. Br Med J 1978;1:949.

61. Beasley RP, Stevens CE, Shiao IS, et al. Evidence against breast-feeding as a mechanism for vertical transmission of hepatitis B. Lancet 1975;2:740.

62. Krugman S. Viral hepatitis: recent developments and prospects for prevention. J Pediatr 1975;87:1067.

63. Beasley RP, Stevens CE, Shiao IS, et al. Breast-feeding and hepatitis B [Letter]. Lancet 1975;2:1089.

64. Favero MS, Maynard JE, Leger RT, et al. Guidelines for the care of patients hospitalized with viral hepatitis. Ann Intern Med 1979;91:872.

39

Parvovirus B19 Infection

Philip B. Mead, M.D.

Background and Incidence

Parvovirus B19, a single-stranded DNA virus, was discovered in 1975 and first linked to human disease in 1981 when it was found in the blood of a child with sickle cell anemia in hypoplastic crisis. B19 can cause asymptomatic infection and has been associated with five distinct clinical syndromes: erythema infectiosum (EI) or fifth disease, acute arthritis in adults, transient aplastic crisis (TAC) in patients with sickle cell disease or other chronic hemolytic states, chronic anemia in immunodeficient patients, and fetal hydrops.

Pathophysiology

The rash of EI and clinical manifestations of B19 arthritis are thought to be immune phenomena. The more serious hematologic manifestations of B19 infection result from selective infection and lysis of erythroid precursor cells with interruption of normal red cell production. In people with normal hematopoiesis, B19 infection produces a self-limited red cell aplasia that is clinically inapparent. In patients who have increased rates of red cell destruction or loss, and who depend on compensatory increases in red cell production to maintain stable red cell indices, B19 infection may lead to aplastic crisis.

The pathogenesis of B19 fetal hydrops appears to involve hematologic, hepatic, and cardiac factors. B19 infection of erythroid precursor cells causes arrest of red cell production. The fetus is particularly vulnerable because its red cell survival is short and its red cell volume is rapidly expanding. The resulting severe anemia causes high-output cardiac failure followed by generalized edema. Extramedullary erythropoiesis leads to hypoproteinemia and portal hypertension. B19 infection of myocardial cells has been observed, suggesting that direct damage to myocardial tissue may also contribute to heart failure in the fetus.

Adapted from Mead PB, Hager WD, editors. Infection Protocols for Obstetrics and Gynecology. Montvale, New Jersey: Contemporary Ob/Gyn, 1992.

Epidemiology

B19 is transmitted effectively after close contact exposures, presumably by respiratory secretions. The virus can also be transmitted parenterally by transfusion of blood or blood products.

Patients with EI are likely to be most contagious prior to the onset of rash, and unlikely to remain contagious for more than a few days after the appearance of the rash. Patients with TAC appear to be infectious prior to the onset of clinical symptoms through the subsequent week.

Cases of EI occur sporadically and, as part of community outbreaks, are often associated with elementary or junior high schools. Community outbreaks are common from midwinter to early summer and often last for several months or until school recesses. The incubation period of EI is usually between 4 and 14 days but can be as long as 20 days.

The secondary attack rate for infection among susceptible household contacts of patients with EI is 50% to 90%. In school outbreaks, 10% to 60% of students may develop EI; 16% to 54% of susceptible teachers and other staff may develop serologic evidence of B19 infection. In one large school outbreak, the minimal rate of B19 infection in susceptible personnel during the outbreak was 19%. In two studies, approximately 37% of susceptible health-care workers became infected with B19 after being exposed to children with TAC.

Diagnosis

Seroprevalence

The reported seroprevalence ranges from 2% to 15% in children 1 to 5 years old, 15% to 60% in children 5 to 19 years old, and 30% to 60% in adults. In one study of school personnel, previous B19 infection rates ranged from a low of 45% in nonteaching high school staff to a high of 68% in day-care providers. Overall, 58% of school personnel had evidence of previous B19 infection.

The most sensitive test for detecting recent infection is the IgM antibody assay. B19 IgM antibody can be detected by ELISA or radioimmunoassay in approximately 90% of cases by the third day after symptoms begin. The IgM anti-

body titer begins to fall 30 to 60 days after the onset of illness, but antibody can persist at a low level for four months or longer. B19 IgG antibody appears around the seventh day of illness and persists for years.

To summarize diagnostic serology: The absence of B19 IgM and IgG indicates no previous infection and a susceptible individual. The presence of only B19 IgG indicates previous infection and an immune individual, although the infection may have occurred as recently as four months earlier. The presence of only B19 IgM indicates a very recent infection, probably within the preceding seven days, whereas the presence of both B19 IgM and IgG suggests recent exposure, from seven days to six months previously. Physicians should be aware that the laboratory will report results of both B19 IgM and IgG antibody determinations. Therefore, only a single specimen taken between four days and four weeks after onset of symptoms is necessary for the serologic diagnosis of acute infection.

Fifth Disease

Erythema infectiosum is often called fifth disease after an otherwise short-lived numerical classification system of childhood rashes devised around 1900. In children, EI is a mild exanthematous disease with few constitutional symptoms. After a brief prodrome of low-grade fever, facial erythema ("slapped cheek") develops, followed by a lacy reticular rash on the trunk and extremities.

Adults may have a rash on their extremities, but facial erythema is uncommon. Acute arthralgias and arthritis of the hands, knees, and wrists may occur as the sole manifestation of infection in adults. A flulike illness is also common, as is numbness and tingling of the peripheral extremities. Approximately 25% of adults infected with B19 will have a nonrash illness, and 25% will be asymptomatic.

Sequelae of Fifth Disease and Pregnancy

Hydrops fetalis and stillbirth were first reported in 1984 as having an association with B19 infection. Since then, more than 400 cases of B19 infection during pregnancy have been described. The results were as follows: normal seronegative newborns (most cases), normal seropositive newborns, and spontaneous abortion or stillbirth due to fetal hydrops. Cases of maternal infection and subsequent fetal death have occurred during each trimester. Stillbirth occurred one to 16 weeks after maternal infection.

There is no evidence that the rate of congenital anomalies following B19 infection exceeds background rates. B19-associated congenital anomalies have not been reported among several hundred liveborn infants of B19-infected mothers. One aborted fetus born to a B19-infected woman had eye anomalies and histologic evidence of damage to multiple tissues. An anencephalic fetus has also been reported in a B19-infected woman, but the timing of the infection made it unlikely that B19 contributed to the defect.

Preliminary results from a study of 174 pregnant women in the United Kingdom suggest that the risk of fetal death attributable to B19 infection after documented maternal infection is less than 10%. Using this figure and the information on susceptibility and attack rates previously presented, one can estimate the risk of fetal death after maternal exposure to B19 as follows:

Mother exposed to a household member:
50% susceptible × 70% attack rate × 10% = 3.5%;

Teacher/staff exposed at school:
42% susceptible × 19% attack rate × 10% = 0.8%.

These assumptions are based on preliminary or imprecise data and await further refinement.

Management

For pregnant women with exposure to confirmed or probable cases of B19 infection, or with symptoms compatible with fifth disease, B19 IgM and IgG antibody determinations should be obtained on a single specimen taken between four days and four weeks after onset of symptoms or, if there are no symptoms, approximately two weeks after exposure.

If maternal infection is documented by the presence of B19 IgM, maternal serum α-fetoprotein (MSAFP) levels should be monitored and serial ultrasound scans performed. At Medical Center Hospital of Vermont, these tests are done every two weeks until 20 weeks' gestation. A preliminary study and two additional case reports suggest that MSAFP levels become elevated when the fetus is affected and that this change occurs before fetal hydrops is detectable by ultrasound. Elevations in MSAFP have been discovered up to six weeks before fetal death and four weeks before abnormalities were apparent by ultrasound. In these preliminary reports, fetal loss did not occur when the MSAFP level remained within normal limits for gestational age. After the twentieth gestational week, lack of normative data for MSAFP levels limits the continued use of this monitoring tool. Normal values for maternal serum AFP through 36 weeks gestation have been published (Lau and Linkins; Simpson et al.; Bremme et al.) but these data have not been used to monitor women exposed to B19 for the development of fetal hydrops.

Early ultrasound features of fetal hydrops include a dilated heart and ascites; generalized edema and pleural effusions are late signs. If MSAFP levels are normal after the twentieth week of gestation, ultrasonography should be continued every one to two weeks until 16 weeks after the maternal illness occurred. If MSAFP levels are elevated, weekly ultrasonography to diagnose fetal hydrops or ascites should be implemented. If fetal hydrops or ascites is suggested by ultrasonography, cordocentesis should be considered to obtain the following studies: hematologic indices, fetal B19 IgM (which may be negative despite fetal infection), and B19 virus studies (by DNA hybridization and electron microscopy).

The prenatal diagnosis of intrauterine infection with B19 by the polymerase chain reaction (PCR) technique has recently been documented. The PCR assay was a sensitive indicator of fetal infection with parvovirus B19 when applied to specimens of amniotic fluid and fetal blood. Amniotic fluid may prove to be the optimal sample for PCR since it is technically easier to obtain than fetal blood. Amniocentesis can be performed earlier in pregnancy, allows collection of a larger sample, and poses less risk of fetal injury or death.

Optimal management of nonimmune fetal hydrops due to B19 infection documented by cordocentesis or amniocentesis and PCR assay has not been determined. Past treatments have included in utero fetal transfusion and direct fetal digitalization. Recent reports of spontaneous resolution of B19 fetal hydrops (Morey et al.; Humphrey et al.; Kovacs et al.; Sheikh et al.; Torok et al.; Pryde et al.) have demonstrated that fetal hydrops in association with parvovirus B19 infection does not always lead to poor long-term outcomes, an observation in sharp contrast with earlier reports. A conservative approach, combining twice weekly fetal nonstress tests, serial sonograms, and fetal movement recording, has recently been proposed by Sheikh et al. These authors consider delivery when the fetus is at or beyond 32 weeks of gestation in cases where hydrops is increasing, arrhythmias are present, or fetal heart rate patterns show no variability or late decelerations. If severe prematurity precludes delivery, cordocentesis for reevaluation of hemoglobin is performed, and if the fetus is severely anemic (hemoglobin equal to or less than 5 gm/dl), transfusion is considered.

Other Considerations

Pathologists should study any hydropic fetus with nonimmune hemolytic anemia for possible B19 parvovirus infection, especially if hepatitis or nucleopathic changes in the erythroblasts are identified.

Pregnant health-care workers should avoid patients with EI until at least 24 hours after onset of rash, as well as patients likely to be viremic for their entire hospitalization. The latter are patients with hereditary or acquired chronic hemolytic anemias who develop aplastic crisis or who are admitted with a fever of unknown origin.

No B19 vaccine for active immunization is available at this time. No studies of prophylaxis with commercially available immune globulin preparations have been conducted, and this use is not currently recommended by the Centers for Disease Control. The role of hyperimmune serum globulin in the prevention or modification of fetal B19 infection is presently undefined but seems worthy of investigation, based on limited adult experience.

Finally, there are at present no Public Health Service guidelines for counseling pregnant women about the occupational risks of B19 infection. Serologic testing can document the natural immunity of the majority of school and day-care staff. The remaining susceptible women are left with the difficult choice between a less than 1% risk of fetal hydrops versus prolonged, recurrent, and unplanned absences from work during community outbreaks of fifth disease.

Suggested Reading

Bell LM, Naides SJ, Stoffman P, et al. Human parvovirus B19 infection among hospital staff members after contact with infected patients. N Engl J Med 1989;321:485.

Centers for Disease Control. Risks associated with human parvovirus B19 infection. MMWR 1989;38(6):81.

Gillespie SM, Cartter ML, Asch S, et al. Occupational risk of human parvovirus B19 infection for school and day-care personnel during an outbreak of erythema infectiosum. JAMA 1990;263:2061.

Humphrey W, Magoon M, O'Shaughnessy R. Severe nonimmune hydrops secondary to parvovirus B19 infection: spontaneous reversal in utero and survival of a term infant. Obstet Gynecol 1991;78:900.

Kovacs BW, Carlson DE, Shahbahrami B, et al. Prenatal diagnosis of human parvovirus B19 in nonimmune hydrops fetalis by polymerase chain reaction. Am J Obstet Gynecol 1992; 167:461.

Kurtzman G, Frickhofen N, Kimball J, et al. Pure red-cell aplasia of 10 years' duration due to persistent parvovirus B19 infection and its cure with immunoglobulin therapy. N Engl J Med 1989;321:519.

Lau HL, Linkins SE. Alpha-fetoprotein. Am J Obstet Gynecol 1976;124:533.

Morey AL, Nicolini V, Welch CR, et al. Parvovirus B19 infection and transient fetal hydrops. Lancet 1991;337:496.

Peters MT, Nicolaides KH. Cordocentesis for the diagnosis and treatment of human fetal parvovirus infection. Obstet Gynecol 1990;75:501.

Pickering LK, Reves RR. Occupational risks for child-care providers and teachers. JAMA 1990;263:2096.

Pryde PG, Nugent CE, Pridjian G, et al. spontaneous resolution of nonimmune hydrops fetalis secondary to human parvovirus B19 infection. Obstet Gynecol 1992;79:859.

Rogers BB, Singer DB, Mak SK, et al. Detection of human parvovirus B19 in early spontaneous abortuses using serology, histology, electron microscopy, in situ hybridization, and the polymerase chain reaction. Obstet Gynecol 1993; 81:402.

Sheikh AU, Ernest JM, O'Shea M. Long-term outcome in fetal hydrops from parvovirus B19 infection. Am J Obstet Gynecol 1992;167:337.

Torok TJ, Wang Q-Y, Gary GW, et al. Prenatal diagnosis of intrauterine infection with parvovirus B19 by the polymerase chain reaction technique. Clin Infect Dis 1992;13:149.

40

HIV Infection

Howard L. Minkoff, M.D.
Deepak Nanda, M.D.

THE acquired immunodeficiency syndrome (AIDS) era has entered its second decade, claiming more than 100,000 American victims. An increasing number of infected individuals are reproductive-age women, many of whom have been recently or soon will be pregnant. The children born to that cohort, unfortunately, frequently acquire their mothers' infections and eventually succumb to their consequences.

Increasingly, obstetricians are becoming involved in prenatal programs designed to identify infected women. To date, the majority of women so identified have chosen to maintain their pregnancies. Therefore, we must be prepared to provide appropriate prenatal care for HIV-infected women.

Identifying Infected Patients

Appropriate care of HIV-infected women depends on knowing their serostatus. That identification is particularly important in empowering women's reproductive decisions: for example, in enabling a woman infected with HIV to make an informed choice regarding abortion.

Ideally, counseling and testing a high-risk woman should precede pregnancy so that appropriate contraceptive advice can be given. Unfortunately, many infected women do not receive prenatal care until the third trimester. Even for those women, however, and for those tested early in pregnancy who choose to continue their pregnancy, prenatal care will be somewhat altered by serostatus. So, too, will the clinician's sensitivity to a variety of the early symptoms of HIV disease be altered.

To identify infected women, a program of prenatal counseling and testing should be available to all women. In high-prevalence cities such as New York and Newark (New Jersey), counseling and testing should be recommended to all women. Studies in these communities have demonstrated that programs based on physician–elicited risks fail to identify a substantial percentage of seropositive women. In lower-prevalence communities, a discussion of risks should be part of routine care. Testing should be offered to all women, who can then self-select and have access to the test even if they do not wish to acknowledge socially unacceptable behaviors.

Any institution planning to implement an HIV testing program should be prepared to care for persons identified through the program. Psychosocial support services should be developed and staff education instituted to assure that infected persons receive appropriate treatment and that the staff's fears are allayed. Finally, before testing begins, clinicians should become familiar with relevant statutes regarding confidentiality, consent, and partner notification.

Care of Seropositive Women

The initial step is to provide adequate post-test counseling. This counseling must address psychosocial, as well as medical, aspects of the diagnosis. The patient should be helped to understand, for example, that her serostatus may lead to discrimination against her and that casual contacts, such as landlords, need not be notified. Sexual partners, however, should be informed.

From a medical standpoint, it is important to draw a clear distinction between HIV infection and AIDS. The patient should be instructed in ways to avoid transmitting the virus to others: safe sex practices, no sharing of razors, and the like. The natural history of HIV disease and long-term follow-up plans should be incorporated into the counselling as well.

Perinatal counseling focuses on the potential consequences of pregnancy on HIV disease (relative rate of disease progression) and the impact of HIV disease status on pregnancy outcome, particularly current estimates of HIV transmission rates. Pregnancy may accelerate the progression of HIV disease because gestation can affect immune function and because other viral diseases are often more fulminant in the setting of pregnancy. Empiric data, however, do not demonstrate a marked clinical effect of pregnancy on the natural history of HIV disease.

Preliminary reports of pregnant and nonpregnant HIV-infected women have shown at most a slightly increased rate of CD4 depletion in the pregnant cohort. Those women whose CD4 counts drop to extremely low levels (for example, <200 mm^3) are at risk for opportunistic infections and should be advised accordingly.

Although a definitive comment about disease progression during pregnancy cannot yet be made, pregnancy can affect the diagnosis and management of HIV disease. Early signs of disease, such as fatigue and anemia, may be masked by pregnancy. The choice of therapeutic agents may need to be modified in the early stages of pregnancy. These factors should be discussed with the patient as a routine part of counselling.

Projecting Outcome

The effect of HIV infection on pregnancy outcome remains unclear. Preliminary data have failed to demonstrate marked differences between infected and uninfected women in short-term results, such as birthweights and preterm birth rates.

The focus of most current perinatal HIV research is the transmission rate of the virus from the mother to the fetus. That rate probably depends on such considerations as maternal immune status, genetic factors, and strain virulence.

The picture is further clouded by the lack of a definitive test to determine the status of the child at birth. Passively acquired maternal antibody is detectable in cord blood for up to 18 months. Tests that would be more specific for neonatal infection—IgM or antigen studies, for example—are still under development. Finally, some infants who lose antibody and are clinically well may still have culturable virus.

Despite these disclaimers, accumulated statistics enable health-care professionals to give the mother some broad-based estimates of transmission rates. A large number of studies have demonstrated a 14%–50% risk of perinatal transmission. More recent studies with longer follow-up put the rate in the lower part of that range (25%–35%). The prognosis for the child diagnosed with HIV disease is extremely poor. Most children infected with HIV die within the first few years after birth.

Prospective parents must consider all this information when deciding whether the woman should undergo an abortion. At present, a large majority of HIV-infected women have chosen to continue their pregnancies, despite the risks involved. It is important that clinicians be adequately prepared to provide ongoing prenatal care for these patients.

Antepartum Considerations

HIV infection is a sexually acquired and perinatally transmitted disease. Therefore, HIV-infected women should be screened for other organisms that they may have acquired by similar means and that can also be transmitted to the fetus. Screening is particularly important to protect the many children who will not acquire HIV infection from other infections to which they may be exposed by their mother. Thus, all HIV-infected women should be tested for hepatitis and chlamydial infection and should have syphilis serologies and gonorrhea cultures taken.

In addition, mycobacterium tuberculosis should be ruled out. Cytomegalovirus infection and toxoplasmosis, both relatively common among people infected with HIV, are sometimes difficult to diagnose and can have serious perinatal consequences. Baseline antibody titers should be obtained early in gestation and repeated if nonspecific symptoms develop.

Particular attention should be paid to symptoms that may not be especially ominous under other circumstances, such as fatigue and anemia. The patient should be carefully instructed not to ignore any symptoms and to come in for an evaluation immediately if she develops fever, sweats, cough, or diarrhea. Measuring CD4 levels each trimester can be helpful in assessing patient risks. Women with markedly depressed levels should receive *Pneumocystis carinii* pneumonia prophylaxis.

Opportunistic infections rarely develop during pregnancy. If they do, however, patient management should be coordinated with an infectious-disease consultant. The serious nature of such infections militates against any modification of therapy because of pregnancy. The unknown risk of the newer agents must be balanced against the life-threatening nature of the infections.

Intrapartum Therapy

A central goal of management of the infected parturient in labor and delivery is to prevent nosocomial acquisition of HIV by obstetric and neonatal personnel. In this setting, it is particularly appropriate to implement universal precautions for infection control.

Current information does not support any modification of mode of delivery in order to reduce the perinatal transmission of HIV. Many children with AIDS have been delivered by cesarean section (CS). In at least one study center, all HIV-infected women were delivered by CS. The incidence of infection among the children was about the same as, or slightly higher than, in settings where CS was performed wholly for obstetric indications.

In the hours prior to birth, the fetus is bathed in infected vaginal secretions. The last barrier to HIV infection among fetuses not infected transplacentally is intact skin. Therefore, it seems prudent to avoid such procedures as placing internal scalp electrodes if satisfactory alternative techniques for fetal monitoring can be found.

Universal blood and needle precautions should be maintained for mother and child, who may remain together. Although bonding should be promoted, the mother should be discouraged from breast-feeding. A few cases reported from Australia and Rwanda, in East Africa, suggest that mothers who contracted HIV infection from postpartum blood transfusions transmitted the virus to their neonates in breast milk. These women, who were recently infected, may have been antigenic and particularly infectious. While the risk of this occurrence is small, it seems appropriate not to encourage patients to assume any risk in parts of the world where acceptable alternatives to breast milk exist.

Although the relative immunocompromise of HIV-infected individuals could potentially increase postpartum or postoperative morbidity, particularly infections, no empiric data support this supposition. The few reports available on the postpartum course of infected parturients have not noted anything remarkable about the postpartum period.

Any physician who identifies HIV infection in a woman undergoing prenatal HIV testing has a responsibility to make sure that appropriate follow-up is arranged after she has been discharged from the hospital. We have entered the era when many prophylactic protocols are available for HIV-infected persons with evidence of immunocompromise and for their children. Patients should be discharged into the care of individuals who are familiar with these protocols as well as the many other unique aspects of caring for the HIV-infected woman.

Ethical and Legal Considerations

Obstetricians are especially aware that the exigencies of law and the less clearly defined issues of ethics impinge on their careers. Besides malpractice issues, many of the most controversial areas of law and medicine have involved obstetrics and neonatology. Despite this experience, however, the ethical and legal controversies that swirl around the issue of AIDS may still be the most challenging we will face. Among the areas yet to be addressed in a satisfactory way are confidentiality, including charting, and the duty to warn patients' sexual partners of seropositivity.

Clinicians should be aware of the relevant statutes within their own jurisdiction. Whatever the law, however, it is important that clinicians attempt to limit knowledge of a patient's serostatus to those with a medical need to know. Discrimination in housing, jobs, and the like is a growing problem for persons whose serostatus is known beyond the medical environment.

The clinician has an obligation to try to persuade the seropositive patient to notify her sex partner(s). It is important to explain that, even if sexual contact has preceded HIV testing, infection may not yet have occurred, but may occur later—possibly much later. It is far from clear whether the physician should contact exposed partners or utilize the local health department. A consultation with local health authorities may shed light on this.

Suggested Reading

Blanche S, Rouzious C, Guthard-Moscat ML, et al. A prospective study of infants born to women seropositive for human immunodeficiency virus type 1. N Engl J Med 1989;320:1643.

European Collaborative Study. Risk factors for mother-to-child transmission of HIV 1. Lancet 1992;339:1007–12.

Gerberding JL. Recommended infection-control policies for patients with human immunodeficiency virus infection. N Engl J Med 1986;315:1562.

Glatt AE, Chirgwin K, Landesman SH. Treatment of infection associated with human immunodeficiency virus. N Engl J Med 1988;318:1439.

Johnson J, Nair P. Early diagnosis of HIV infection in the neonate. N Engl J Med 1987;316:273.

Johnstone FD, MacCullum L, Brettle R, et al. Does infection with HIV affect the outcome of pregnancy? Br Med J 1988;296:467.

Landesman S, Holman S, McCalla S, et al. HIV serosurvey of postpartum women at a municipal hospital in New York City. In: Proceedings of the 3rd International AIDS Conference, Washington, D.C., June 2, 1987.

Miles SA, Balden E, Magpantay L, et al. Rapid serologic testing with immune-complex-dissociated HIV p24 antigen for early detection of HIV infection in neonates. N Engl J Med 1993;328:297–302.

Minkoff HL. Care of pregnant women infected with human immunodeficiency virus. JAMA 1987;258:2714.

Minkoff HL, Nanda D, Menez R, et al. Pregnancies resulting in infants with acquired immunodeficiency syndrome: description of the antepartum, intrapartum and postpartum course. Obstet Gynecol 1987;69:285.

Mok JQ, Rossi A, De Ades A, et al. Infants born to mothers seropositive for human immunodeficiency virus: preliminary findings from a multi-center European study. Lancet 1987; 1:1164.

Ryder RW, Nsa W, Hassig SE, et al. Perinatal transmission of the human immunodeficiency virus type 1 to infants of seropositive women in Zaire. N Engl J Med 1989;320:1637.

Rogers MF, Ou CY, Rayfield M, et al. Use of the polymerase chain reaction for early detection of the proviral sequences of human immunodeficiency virus in infants born to seropositive mothers. N Engl J Med 1989;320:1649.

Scott GB, Fischl MA, Klimas N, et al. Mothers of infants with the acquired immunodeficiency syndrome: evidence for both symptomatic and asymptomatic carriers. JAMA 1985;253:363.

PART SIX Pregnancy Complications

41

Genetic Causes of Spontaneous Abortion

Joe Leigh Simpson, M.D.

GENETIC factors are responsible for most losses in clinically recognized pregnancies and probably most losses before preclinical recognition. Although pregnancy is not generally apparent clinically until at least 5–6 weeks after the last menstrual period, sensitive β-hCG assays can confirm pregnancies earlier. During this early interval, fetal losses occur frequently.

Miller and co-workers performed the first study of preclinical losses by following 197 ovulating women (aged 25–35 years) (1). Beginning 21 days after the previous menses and continuing until menstruation or pregnancy, they performed urinary β-hCG assays on alternate days in 623 cycles. Pregnancy was defined by a single value of 5 μg/L or two values of 2 μg/L. In 152 of the 623 cycles, the diagnosis of pregnancy was made. However, in only 102 (67%) of the 152 was pregnancy appreciated clinically. Of the 102 conceptions showing clinical evidence of pregnancy, 14 (14%) were later lost. Overall frequency of losses (clinical and subclinical) was 43%.

Several later studies showed somewhat different results. Differences among these studies were generally attributable to vicissitudes in β-hCG assay sensitivities; thus, the more recent studies are of greater interest because assay technology has progressed. In 1988, Wilcox and co-workers performed daily urinary hCG assays, beginning around expected time of implantation. Of all pregnancies, 31% (62 of 198) were lost (2). The preclinical loss rate was 22% (43/198), whereas the clinically recognized loss rate was 12% (19/155). These total loss rates are consistent with data derived by Mills and others (3). In this trial, a National Institutes of Child Health collaborative study, women were identified before pregnancy. Serum β-hCG assays were performed 28–35 days after the previous menses. The fetal loss rate (preclinical and clinical) in normal women proved to be only 16.1%. Some of these losses would probably be classified as preclinical, but most were overtly clinical. That the loss rate here was slightly lower than in Wilcox's study would be expected because surveillance began several days later. It follows that the fourth week of gestation (second week of embryonic development) is a time of high mortality for embryos.

That the prevalence of preclinical losses is high, albeit of uncertain magnitude, can be deduced from other observations as well. Pregnancy rates are no more than 20%–25% after transfer of morphologically normal embryos fertilized in vitro, even ignoring the common practice of transferring multiple embryos to most recipients. Mechanical problems in transfer procedures doubtless contribute to the relatively poor outcome, but surely this is not the sole explanation.

Clinically Recognized Losses

Fetal loss rates of 12%–15% are well documented in both retrospective and prospective cohort studies. Traditionally, most losses have been said to occur after eight weeks' gestation. However, this assumption was based on such criteria as passage of tissue (products of conception), opening of the cervical os, uterine contractions, or bleeding. Fetal demise was thought to coincide with these physical signs. Stevenson and co-workers thus reported that 45% of losses occurred between gestational weeks 7 and 11 and that 30% occurred between gestational weeks 12 and 15. Only a few clinical losses were recognized before 7 weeks (4).

More recently, ultrasonographic studies have made it clear that fetal demise occurs weeks in advance of overt clinical signs. Most fetuses aborting at 10 to 12 weeks actually died weeks earlier. Among data that led to these conclusions were studies of patients who routinely undergo ultrasonography (5–7).

Although informative, studies involving obstetric patients may suffer from methodologic shortcomings because precise information concerning timing of conception is unavailable and because the potential for selection bias exists. For example, women registering at 7–10 weeks' gestation could be unusually health conscious and thus at low risk for abortion.

To address the issue of selection bias, my co-workers and I analyzed the prospective cohort identified for the collaborative National Institutes of Child Health and Human Development Diabetes in Early Pregnancy (DIEP) Project (8). Because these women were recruited before conception, biases of selection should be minimized. Among control subjects, there were 220 ultrasonographically proved normal pregnancies of eight weeks' gestation. The loss rate was 3.2%, similar to that reported from studies of obstetric registrants.

When does fetal demise occur in the 3% of pregnancies lost after eight weeks? Tabor and co-workers observed background losses of only 0.7% in 30- to 34-year-old women confirmed by ultrasound to have viable pregnancies at 16 weeks (9). Thus, most of the 3% lost after eight weeks appear to be lost in the third and fourth month of gestation.

Preclinical Losses

The one unequivocal explanation is morphologic abnormalities in early embryos. In turn, the most likely explanation for morphologic abnormalities is genetic factors. The first indication that this was the case came from the studies of Hertig and colleagues, who over many years recovered eight preimplantation embryos (less than six days from conception) (10). Four of these embryos were morphologically abnormal and presumably would not have implanted. If implanted, they would not have survived long thereafter. Similarly, nine of 26 implanted embryos (6–14 embryonic days) were morphologically abnormal, presumably also unlikely to develop further.

Most recently, cytogenetic studies in ostensibly normal human embryos fertilized in vitro (IVF) indicate chromosomal abnormalities in approximately 25% of IVF embryos (11, 12). This finding is consistent with estimates of chromosomal abnormalities in ostensibly normal sperm (approximately 10%) (13, 14) and ostensibly normal oocytes (13%–15%) (15, 16). If one observes chromosomal abnormalities of this magnitude in morphologically normal embryos, one would expect even higher rates in morphologically abnormal embryos. Thus, chromosomal abnormalities are probably responsible for most of the early morphologic abnormalities documented by Hertig's group.

First-trimester Losses

By far the most frequent explanation for the 12%–15% of clinically recognized first-trimester pregnancy losses is cytogenetic abnormalities. Approximately 50% of such losses show chromosomal abnormalities.

Autosomal trisomy comprises the largest single class of abnormal chromosomal complements in spontaneous abortions. Of all abnormal complements, 53% are trisomic; thus

Table 41.1 Chromosomal Complements in Spontaneous Abortions

Complement	Frequency	%
Normal		
46, XX or 46, XY		54.1
Triploidy		7.7
69,XXX	2.7	
69,XYY	0.2	
69,XXY	4.0	
Other	0.8	
Tetraploidy		2.6
92,XXXX	1.5	
92,XXYY	0.55	
Not stated	0.55	
Monosomy X		8.6
Structural abnormalities		1.5
Sex chromosomal polysomy		0.2
47,XXX	0.05	
47,XXY	0.15	
Autosomal monosomy (G)		0.1
Autosomal trisomy		
Chromosome number		22.3
1	0	
2	1.11	
3	0.25	
4	0.64	
5	0.04	
6	0.14	
7	0.89	
8	0.79	
9	0.72	
10	0.36	
11	0.04	
12	0.18	
13	1.07	
14	0.82	
15	1.68	
16	7.27	
17	0.18	
18	1.15	
19	0.01	
20	0.61	
21	2.11	
22	2.26	

Continued

Table 41.1 *Continued*

Complement	Frequency	%
Double trisomy		0.7
Mosaic trisomy		1.3
Other abnormalities or not specified		0.9

These complements are in clinically recognized first-trimester abortions.

Pooled data from several series: Simpson JL, Bombard AT. Chromosomal abnormalities in spontaneous abortions: frequency, pathology and genetic counselling. In: Edmonds K, Bennet MJ, eds. Spontaneous abortion. London: Blackwell, 1987.

approximately 25% of all abortuses are trisomic (Table 41.1). Trisomy for every chromosome except chromosome 1 has been reported, and trisomy for that chromosome has been observed in an eight-cell embryo (17).

Autosomal trisomy has a cytologic counterpart: autosomal monosomy. The latter is rarely, if ever, observed in humans. Natural history of autosomal monosomy in humans may thus be comparable with that in the mouse, a species in which Gropp observed that monosomies fail to survive implantation (18).

Polyploidy is the presence of more than two haploid chromosomal complements. Triploidy ($3n = 69$) and tetraploidy ($4n = 92$) occur frequently in abortuses. Pathologic features include cystic generation of placental villi, intrachorial hemorrhage, and hydrophobic trophoblasts (pseudomolar degeneration). Triploid abortuses are usually 69, XXY or 69,XXX, generally resulting from dispermy.

Tetraploidy is uncommon, rarely progressing beyond 2–3 weeks' embryonic life (4–5 weeks' gestation).

Monosomy X is the single most common chromosomal abnormality in spontaneous abortions. Monosomy X occurs in 8.6% of all conceptions (approximately 20% of chromosomally abnormal abortions). In fetuses surviving until later in gestation, anomalies characteristic of the Turner stigmata may be observed: horseshoe kidney, cystic hygromas, and generalized edema.

Of interest is the study of Guerneri and co-workers, who identified a sample of abortuses immediately after

Table 41.2 Relationship between Karyotypes of Successive Abortuses

Complement of First Abortion	Complement of Second Abortion					
	Normal	Trisomy	Monosomy X	Triploidy	Tetraploidy	De novo Rearrangement
Normal	142	18	5	7	3	2
Trisomy	31	30	1	4	3	1
Monosomy X	7	5	3	3	0	0
Triploidy	7	4	1	4	0	0
Tetraploidy	3	1	0	2	0	0
De novo rearrangement	1	3	0	0	0	0

From Warburton D, Kline J, Stein Z, et al. Does the karyotype of a spontaneous abortion predict the karyotype of a subsequent abortion? Evidence from 273 women with two karyotyped spontaneous abortus. Am J Hum Genet 1987;41:465.

ultrasound diagnosis of demise (19). Tissue for cytogenetic analysis was obtained by chorionic villus sampling (CVS), rather than relying later in gestation upon recovery of spontaneously expelled products. With CVS, not only could a far higher proportion of specimens be successfully cultured than in earlier studies, but more (77%) chromosomal abnormalities were found than in studies based upon analysis of spontaneously expelled fetuses (19). This suggests that abortuses failing to grow in culture are disproportionately represented by chromosomal abnormalities. The true prevalence of chromosomal abnormalities in first-trimester abortuses may thus be closer to 80% than 50%.

Second- and Third-trimester Losses

Recent appreciation of the high frequency of unrecognized missed abortion in the first trimester invalidates earlier efforts to correlate precisely the frequency of chromosomal abnormalities with gestational age. But the frequency of chromosomal errors in losses recognized between 16 and 28 weeks is surely less than that observed in losses recognized earlier (20, 21). One also observes chromosomal abnormalities more similar to those observed in liveborn infants.

Stillborn Infants

The frequency of chromosomal abnormalities in stillborn infants is about 5%, far less than that observed in earlier abortuses, but higher than that in liveborns (0.6%) (22, 23).

Chromosomal abnormalities have been detected in infants considered normal by gross examination (autopsy). Presumably, maceration of tissues after fetal demise greatly diminishes the ability of physicians to appreciate dysmorphia. For this reason, cytogenetic evaluation could be recommended routinely for all unexplained stillborns, especially intrapartum demises. Approximately half of all trisomy 18 fetuses manifest intrapartum fetal distress, necessitating cesarean section.

Numerical Abnormalities in Successive Pregnancies

Aneuploidy may be responsible, not only for sporadic losses, but also for recurrent losses. Such reasoning is based on observations that the complements of successive abortuses in a given family are more likely to be either consistently normal or consistently abnormal (Table 41.2). That is, abortuses in a given family show nonrandom distribution with respect to chromosomal complements. If the complement of the first abortus is abnormal, the likelihood is high (80%) that the complement of the second abortus will also be abnormal (24, 25). These data suggest that certain couples are predisposed towards chromosomally abnormal conceptions, most of which result in spontaneous abortion. Presumably, the mechanism involves mutant genes. Indeed, in humans, consanguinity increases the risk of aneuploidy (26).

If a couple were predisposed to recurrent aneuploidy they might logically be at increased risk for aneuploid liveborns. The trisomic autosome in a subsequent pregnancy might be characterized, not by lethality (for example, trisomy 16), but rather by compatibility with life (for example, trisomy 21). Available data do not allow one to state whether liveborn aneuploid is increased following liveborn aneuploid abortions. However, several studies suggest that the risk of liveborn trisomy 21 following a trisomic abortus is about 1% (27).

Structural Rearrangements

Structural chromosomal abnormalities are a well-accepted explanation for repetitive abortions and a less common explanation for losses in general. The most common rearrangement responsible for pregnancy loss is a translocation (Figure 41.1). Individuals with balanced translocations are phenotypically normal, but their offspring (abortuses or liveborns) may show duplications or deficiencies as a result of normal meiotic segregation. About 60% of the translocations are reciprocal, and 40% are Robertsonian (centric fusion translocations, like translocations between chromo-

somes 14 and 21).

Cytogenetic studies of couples experiencing recurrent fetal losses but no other adverse perinatal outcomes reveal the frequency of translocations to be about 2% of couples (28). Investigations restricted to couples experiencing, not only abortions, but also stillborn infants or anomalous liveborn infants will yield relatively more translocations (Table 41.3). Females are about twice as likely as males to show a balanced translocation (29). Whether prevalence rates are influenced by numbers of previous losses remains uncertain.

If a balanced translocation is detected, antenatal cytogenetic studies should be offered in subsequent pregnancies. Actually, the frequency of unbalanced (abnormal) fetuses detected at amniocentesis or chorionic villus sampling would be less if the balanced translocation were ascertained through repetitive abortions (perhaps 3%) than if ascertained through an anomalous liveborn (approximately 12%) (30).

A second parental chromosomal rearrangement that causes fetal loss is inversion. In this rearrangement, the order of genes is reversed. Although the cytologic origin of an inversion is different from that of a translocation, the

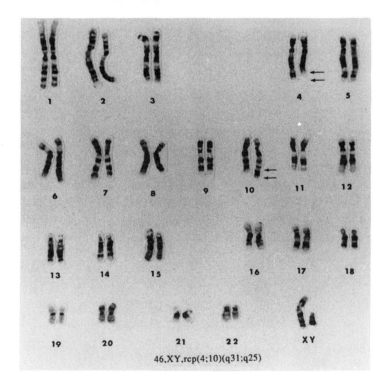

46,XY,rcp(4;10)(q31;q25)

Figure 41.1 This balanced translocation was detected in a woman who had experienced multiple spontaneous abortions.

(From: Simpson JL, Tharapel AT. Scientific Foundations of Obstetrics and Gynecology, ed 4. London: Heinemann, 1992).

Table 41.3 Frequency of Translocations

	Female	Male
Repeated spontaneous abortions	89/3,723	57/3,651
with or without normal liveborn	2.4%	1.6%
Repeated spontaneous abortions	20/432	7/409
with stillborn or abnormal liveborn	4.6%	1.7%
Repeated spontaneous abortions	100/3,074	65/3,069
without subcategorization	3.3%	2.1%

From Simpson JL, Meyers CM, Martin AO, et al. Translocations are infrequent among couples having repeated spontaneous abortions but no other abnormal pregnancies. Fertil Steril 1989;51:811.

clinical importance remains similar. Heterozygotes for inversions may be normal if genes are neither lost, gained, nor altered as a result of the breaks leading to the inversion. However, individuals with inversions suffer abnormal reproductive consequences if crossing over occurs during meiosis I. Crossing over may or may not occur within an inversion loop, but it is likely to do so if the loop encompasses a large portion of the chromosome. If crossing over occurs, certain gametes are unbalanced.

Inversion is an infrequent cause of fetal loss, even among repeated aborters. Nonetheless, inversions are highly deleterious and warrant prenatal studies. The actual risk varies according to the type of inversion. Inversions in which break points exist on opposite sides of the centromere are termed pericentric; those in which break points are on the same side of the centromere are termed paracentric (Figure 41.2).

A single crossover within a paracentric inversion results in both dicentric and acentric products, both of which eventually lead to loss of such large portions of the chromosome that survival is not possible. Both acentric and dicentric gametes contribute to fetal wastage. However, both outcomes are usually lethal; thus, paracentric inversions are rarely associated with anomalous livebirths.

By contrast, pericentric inversions are likely to cause not only abortions, but also anomalous liveborns. The unbalanced products that follow crossing over within a pericentric inversion are similar to the products that are associated with parental translocation. Thus, anomalous liveborns can occur. Empiric risk varies according to many factors, but usually approximates 10%–15% (31).

Approximately 0.6% liveborns have a chromosomal abnormality, but approximately 1.0% have a congenital anomaly as a result of a single mutant gene (Mendelian). An equal number are abnormal as a result of a disorder inherited in polygenic/multifactorial fashion. Yet few early spontaneous abortions can be shown to be caused by Mendelian or polygenic multifactorial mechanisms. This probably reflects the paucity of these two factors as etiologic agents

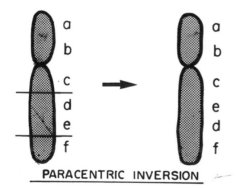

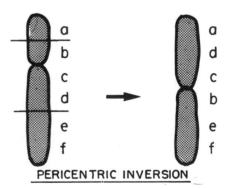

Figure 41.2   Differences are apparent between a paracentric (left) and pericentric (right) inversion.
(From: Simpson JL. Disorders of Sexual Differentiation. New York: Academic Press, 1976.)

less than experimental difficulty in verifying existence of such factors in pregnancy wastage. Many genes are essential for differentiation, and it can be assumed that their perturbations could confer lethality, leading to preclinical and early clinical losses.

Not all anomalies in liveborns are inherited because of monogenic factors. Polygenic/multifactorial factors also exist. Such factors are presumably also responsible for midtrimester losses of fetuses. This cause is most likely to apply to anatomic malformations limited to a single organ system (for example, anencephaly). Such a mechanism could be responsible as well for losses earlier in pregnancy. As an example, neural tube defects are estimated to be present in 1% of fetal losses (32).

REFERENCES

1. Miller JF, Williamson E, Glue J, et al. Fetal loss after implantation: a prospective study. Lancet 1980;2:554.

2. Wilcox AJ, Weinberg CR, O'Connor JF, et al. Incidence of early loss of pregnancy. N Engl J Med 1988;319:189.

3. Mills JL, Simpson JL, Driscoll SG, et al. Incidence of spontaneous abortion among normal women and insulin-dependent women whose pregnancies were identified within 21 days of conception. N Engl J Med 1988;319:1617.

4. Stevenson AC, Dudgeon MY, McClure HI. Observations on the results of pregnancies in women resident in Belfast. II. Abortions, hydatidiform moles and ectopic pregnancies. Ann Hum Genet 1959;23:395.

5. Wilson RD, Kendrick V, Wittman BK, et al. Risk of spontaneous abortion in ultrasonographically normal pregnancies. Lancet 1984;2:920.

6. Gilmore DH, McNay MB. Spontaneous fetal loss rate in early pregnancy. Lancet 1985;1:107.

7. Cashner KA, Christopher CR, Dysert GA. Spontaneous fetal loss after demonstration of a live fetus in the first trimester. Obstet Gynecol 1987;70:827.

8. Simpson JL, Holmes LB, Ober CL, et al. Low fetal loss rates after ultrasound-proved viability in early pregnancy. JAMA 1987;258:2555.

9. Tabor A, Philip J, Masden J, et al. Randomized controlled trial of genetic amniocentesis in 4606 low-risk women. Lancet 1986;1:1287.

10. Hertig AT, Rock J, Adams EC, et al. Thirty-four fertilized human ova, good, bad and indifferent, recovered from 210 women of known fertility. A study of biologic wastage in early human pregnancy. Pediatrics 1959;25:202.

11. Plachot M, Junca AM, Mandelbaum J. Chromosome investigations in early life. II. Human preimplantation embryos. Hum Reprod 1987;2:29.

12. Papadopoulos G, Templeton AA, Fisk N, et al. The frequency of chromosome anomalies in human preimplantation embryos after in vitro fertilization. Hum Reprod 1989;4:91.

13. Martin RH, Balkan W, Burns K, et al. The chromosome constitution of 1,000 human spermatozoa. Hum Genet 1984;63:605.

14. Brandiff B, Gordon L, Ashworth L, et al. Chromosomal abnormalities in human sperm: comparisons among four healthy men. Hum Genet 1984;66:193.

15. Martin RH, Mahadevan MM, Taylor PJ, et al. Chromosomal analysis of unfertilized human oocytes. J Reprod Fertil 1986;78:673.

16. Wramsby H, Fredga K, Liedholm P. Chromosome analysis of human oocytes recovered from preovulatory follicles in stimulated cycles. N Engl J Med 1987;316:121.

17. Watt JL, Templeton AA, Messinis I, et al. Trisomy 1 in an eight cell human pre-embryo. J Med Genet 1987;24:60.

18. Gropp A. Chromosomal animal model of human disease. Fetal trisomy and development failure. In: Berry L, Poswillo DE, eds. Teratology. Berlin: Springer-Verlag, 1975:17–35.

19. Guerneri S, Bettio D, Simoni G, et al. Prevalence and distribution of chromosome abnormalities in a sample of first trimester internal abortions. Hum Reprod 1987;2:735.

20. Ruzicska P, Cziezel A. Cytogenetic studies on midtrimester abortuses. Hum Genet 1971;10:273.

21. Warburton D, Kline J, Stein Z, et al. Cytogenetic abnormalities in spontaneous abortion of recognized conceptions. In: Porter IH, Hatcher NH, Willey AM, eds. Perinatal genetics: diagnosis and treatment. Orlando: Academic Press, 1980:23–40.

22. Bauld R, Sutherland CR, Bain AD. Chromosome studies in investigation of stillbirths and neonatal deaths. Arch Dis Child 1974;49:782.

23. Kuleshov NP. Chromosome anomalies of infants dying during the perinatal period and premature newborn. Hum Genet 1976;34:151.

24. Hassold T. A cytogenetic study of repeated spontaneous abortions. Am J Hum Genet 1980;32:723.

25. Warburton D, Kline J, Stein Z, et al. Does the karyotype of a spontaneous abortion predict the karyotype of a subsequent

abortion? Evidence from 273 women with two karyotyped spontaneous abortus. Am J Hum Genet 1987;41:465.

26. Alfi OS, Chang R, Azen SP. Evidence for genetic control of non-disjunction in man. Am J Hum Genet 1981;32:477.

27. Alberman ED. The abortus as a predictor of future trisomy 21. In: De la Cruz FF, Gerald PS, eds. Trisomy 21 (Down syndrome). Baltimore: University Park Press, 1981:69.

28. Simpson JL, Meyers CM, Martin AO, et al. Translocations are infrequent among couples having repeated spontaneous abortions but no other abnormal pregnancies. Fertil Steril 1989;51:811.

29. Simpson JL, Elias S, Martin AO. Parental chromosomal rear-rangements associated with repetitive spontaneous abortions. Fertil Steril 1981;36:584.

30. Daniels A, Hook EB, Wulf G. Risks of unbalanced progeny at amniocentesis to carriers of chromosome rearrangements: data from United States and Canadian Laboratories. Am J Med Genet 1989;31:13.

31. Sutherland GR, Gardiner AJ, Carter RF. Familial pericentric inversion of chromosome 19 inv (19) (p13q13) with a note on genetic counseling of pericentric inversion carriers. Clin Genet 1976;10:53.

32. Byrne J, Warburton D. Neural tube defects in spontaneous abortion. Am J Med Genet 1986;25:327.

42

Nongenetic Causes of Recurrent Fetal Loss

Sandra Ann Carson, M.D.

ALTHOUGH 60% of miscarriages are chromosomally abnormal, the remaining 40% have led to a variety of theoretic etiologies, most leading to therapeutic misconceptions (1). Treatment should begin with clearing away these misconceptions by educating the patient about the many factors involved in recurrent pregnancy loss.

In the United States, 4% of reproductive-age women experience two spontaneous abortions, and 3% experience three (2). The likelihood of having one spontaneous abortion is 15%, and, if a woman has had no previous liveborn children, the likelihood that she will have another spontaneous abortion is 35%. The risk never increases after that. Similarly, 25% of women who have had at least one liveborn child will experience two, three, or more spontaneous abortions (3).

Therefore, the likelihood of finding an abnormality in a patient who has had one spontaneous abortion should be the same as in someone who has had six. However, testing after only one spontaneous abortion is impractical and certainly unwise because 65% of women will go on to have a term pregnancy.

The evaluation of couples experiencing recurrent pregnancy losses should probably begin after three spontaneous abortions (Table 42.1). Couples over age 35 may wish to begin an evaluation after two spontaneous abortions. Once begun, it is preferable to complete the entire evaluation rather than choose one test or another. For example, there is no reason to perform hysterosalpingography and not a karyotype or an endometrial biopsy.

Anatomic Abnormalities

Müllerian abnormalities are often cited as the cause of spontaneous abortion. The prevalence of abortions in patients with such defects may be as high as 20%–25% (4). However, most studies have a large ascertainment bias. Diagnosis by hysterosalpingogram (HSG) or hysteroscopy is usually performed after patients have already experienced spontaneous abortions or infertility. Few HSGs are performed in women who have had children and have no further problems. One small study suggests metroplasty may benefit patients with recurrent losses (4).

Hysteroscopic lysis of uterine septa has virtually re-

Table 42.1 Medical Evaluation of Patients

Karyotype on both partners
Hysterosalpingogram
Thyroid hormone profile
Serum prolactin
Endometrial biopsy for histologic dating and *Ureaplasma urealyticum* culture
Systemic lupus erythematosus screen
Lupus anticoagulant
Anticardiolipin antibodies

placed metroplasty as treatment for uterine septa. One team reported only one spontaneous abortion in 11 pregnancies after hysteroscopic metroplasty in 16 women with histories of recurrent pregnancy loss (4).

The incompetent cervical os has also been associated with recurrent second-trimester spontaneous abortion. The diagnosis is made after a history of pregnancy loss preceded by painless cervical dilation in the late first or second trimester. Alternatively, in the nonpregnant state, an incompetent cervix is one that will allow passage of a No. 8 Hegar dilator without resistance. HSG is no longer used to make the diagnosis.

Weekly cervical exams in early pregnancy may detect the onset of dilation and allow placement of a cerclage, which is the standard treatment. Reported success rates have been as high as 80% (5). However, two randomized trials failed to demonstrate any therapeutic benefit of the procedure (6, 7). These studies did include patients with both first- and second-trimester losses, and the evaluation of many women was incomplete. These variations suggest the conclusions may not be valid.

After a complete evaluation of recurrent spontaneous abortion, if the only cause uncovered is incompetent cervix, a cerclage may be placed when the cervix first begins to dilate. Onset is determined with weekly cervical exams in the first trimester. With improved ultrasonic diagnosis, cervical cerclage may be attempted in the first trimester after fetal viability has been documented.

Women with normal scans at eight or more gestational weeks may benefit from a cerclage when dilation begins. No data exist on the actual therapeutic value of the procedure in this group. It makes intuitive sense that, if the cerclage is beneficial, it should be placed early. The patient must understand, however, that a genetic abnormality in the fetus will not be thwarted by the surgical procedure, and, if such an abnormality exists, the cerclage will have been unnecessary.

Leiomyomas have also been implicated through a variety of mechanisms: thin endometrial surface predisposing to implantation in a poorly decidualized site; rapid growth related to increasing pregnancy hormones leading to degeneration, necrosis, and consequent uterine contractions with fetal expulsion; or encroachment on the space required by a developing fetus causing fetal deformations or even premature delivery. If all other factors are ruled out, myomectomy may be warranted, but, as in pregnancies with Müllerian fusion abnormalities, careful patient selection is important.

DES Exposure

In utero diethylstilbestrol (DES) exposure has caused a variety of abnormalities in the reproductive tract that may impair reproductive performance. The classic T-shaped uterus may impair conception and, in association with uterine hypoplasia, lead to spontaneous pregnancy loss. Women exposed to DES in utero have a higher rate of spontaneous pregnancy loss (8). Even those women whose mothers took DES but had no prior spontaneous abortions have a higher risk of loss.

Unfortunately, there is no therapy for this group of women. They should undergo a complete evaluation to rule out other possibly treatable causes of losses.

Endocrinologic Defects

Well- or moderately well-controlled diabetes mellitus is no longer thought to be a cause of recurrent spontaneous abortion. However, diabetics do have an increased risk of pregnancy loss if their glycemic control is poor (9).

Although decreased conception rates occur in women with overt thyroid disease, subclinical thyroid disease has not been shown to result in fetal loss (10). Thyroid testing is now very sensitive and specific and subclinical thyroid disease is easily detectable by serum measurements.

A corpus luteum insufficiency supposedly results from a progesterone deficiency or an inability of the uterus to develop an endometrium mature enough to support placentation. Unfortunately, no randomized, prospective study comparing progesterone therapy with placebo has been performed. Thus, it is assumed that the corpus luteum defect is a true entity and may cause pregnancy loss. The diagnosis is made by two out-of-phase biopsies performed in the late luteal phase.

When using the criteria defined by Noyes and co-workers, histologic dating should lag at least two days behind the actual postovulation date, as defined by counting backward from the first day of the next menstrual period (11). Numerous studies have used alternative dating procedures, but none of the results have correlated the defect with pregnancy outcome. Similarly, alternative procedures to endometrial biopsy have been suggested (12, 13). However, these tests have been shown effective only in predicting an in-phase endometrial biopsy, rather than predicting pregnancy outcome.

Clinicians are left to assume that luteal phase deficiency is a cause of pregnancy loss and that it may be treated with either progesterone or clomiphene citrate. Progesterone will restore an "in-phase" endometrium in 50% of patients, and clomiphene will correct another 12% (14). However, it is unclear whether this actually prevents pregnancy loss.

Treatment of luteal phase defect is either with progesterone or with clomiphene citrate. Only natural progesterone should be administered, either by 25-mg vaginal suppositories twice each day or by daily 12.5-mg IM injections. Progesterone therapy should begin three days after the LH peak and continue for eight weeks.

Patients should be informed that reports in the literature ascribe teratogenicity to synthetic progestins but that natural progesterone is unlikely to produce birth defects; however, guarantees should be avoided. The medicolegal hazards of teratogenicity may be avoided by using follicular phase stimulation with clomiphene citrate, which does not require subsequent progesterone augmentation. Both therapeutic regimens require a repeat endometrial biopsy in a treatment cycle to assure that the defect is corrected.

Endometriosis

Women with endometriosis appear to have a higher chance of spontaneous abortion if conception occurs prior to treatment rather than after conservative surgery (15, 16). The mechanism by which endometriosis increases the spontaneous abortion rate is unknown. The disease has been associated with luteal phase defect, autoimmune disorders, and increased peritoneal prostaglandin concentrations, all of which may also be associated with spontaneous abortion. However, one study shows the incidence of spontaneous abortion to be inversely related to severity of endometriosis: a 49% loss in mild disease to 24% loss in severe disease (17). This relationship suggests that endometriosis is not a primary cause of spontaneous abortion but that, more likely, the initiation of endometriosis is itself related to a factor that causes spontaneous abortion. Further growth of endometriosis would then be unlikely to be associated with recurrent abortion, but rather with infertility.

Unless a patient with recurrent spontaneous abortion has had an entire evaluation that discloses no abnormality, it is not necessary to routinely perform evaluative laparoscopy. But if a patient has a problem, such as severe dysmenorrhea, that suggests endometriosis, then laparoscopic therapy is in order.

Infection

A variety of organisms have been implicated as causes of recurrent spontaneous abortion. The pathogenesis of a single abortion may involve interference with fetal differentiation, fetal demise during the active stages of infection with fever, or even treatment of the mother for infection. However, it is difficult to postulate a mechanism for recurrent fetal demise unless the microorganism continues to live within the maternal system, reinfecting each subsequent fetus and causing its demise.

The only controlled studies in this area are for *Ureaplasma urealyticum*. Clinical investigators found significantly more subsequent abortions in the untreated couples (18).

Arguably, no other organism was screened for in these studies, so results may reflect a therapeutic effect on another coexistent organism. Indeed, empiric antibiotics have been shown to decrease the recurrent spontaneous abortion rate (10%) in treated couples over that of untreated couples (38%) (19).

Immunologic Abnormalities

Immunologic processes are clearly altered during pregnancy or the mother would not be able to harbor a fetus half of whose proteins would be antigenic to her in her nonpregnant state. However, the exact mechanism of this tolerance is unknown. Thus, it is not surprising that women with autoimmune disease are more prone to pregnancy loss.

Systemic lupus erythematosus (SLE) is the most common autoimmune disease of young women and is associated with a pregnancy loss rate up to 46% (20). One retrospective study of 20 women with SLE showed the pregnancy loss rate of 40% to be significantly higher than the 12.5% in 80 matched controls (21).

Lupus anticoagulant is an antibody causing in vitro anticoagulation, but in vivo thrombosis (22). Along with related anticardiolipin antibodies, it may react against trophoblast, result in subplacental clots, and interfere with further placentation. Anticardiolipin antibodies may be associated, not only with first-trimester loss, but also with complications and thrombosis in all trimesters. A literature survey of 242 untreated pregnancies in 65 women with lupus or anticardiolipin antibodies revealed 220 losses (23). This suggests that screening is advisable for patients with recurrent losses. Patients testing positive may be treated with low-dose aspirin and prednisone during pregnancy (24, 25).

The immunologic tolerance of the mother to the fetus may result from a protective blocking antibody or suppressive factor stimulated by the foreign antigens of the fetus. After their first pregnancy, 20% of women develop antipaternal antileukocytotoxic antibodies, as do 65% of multiparous women (26–28). These may actually serve to protect the fetus and, therefore, maternal-paternal histoincompatibility would stimulate such factors and contribute to term pregnancy. Which histocompatibility antigen is important in this recognition and situation is unclear.

The major histocompatibility antigens were initially suggested to be those antigens that, if shared, could lead to recurrent losses (29). However, in some studies, couples sharing HLA antigens have shown no spontaneous abortion despite ten or more pregnancies (30). There has been no HLA typing on abortuses to determine if they inherited the shared antigen.

Rather than the HLA antigens, it may be that normal pregnancy requires maternal-fetal histocompatibility for trophoblast-linked antigens (31). Couples that experience repetitive spontaneous abortions share TLX antigens more frequently than couples without pregnancy wastage (32). Circumstantial evidence suggests that immunotherapy to enhance diminished maternal immunologic tolerance may be successful in preventing recurrent loss. For example, blood transfusion before kidney transplantation aids in preventing subsequent rejection (33). Although women who share HLA antigens and have a history of recurrent abortions have been immunized by paternal leukocytes, third-party leukocytes, and even trophoblast membranes, only one large prospective randomized trial for the efficacy of immunotherapy has been published (34–37). In this trial, 77% of immunized women went on to deliver liveborn children, compared with 37% of untreated women. Although these results are certainly impressive, pregnancy complications, such as intrauterine growth retardation, may be increased in immunized pregnancies. Thus, at this time, immunotherapy should be restricted to research trials.

Toxins

Environmental exposure to high doses of irradiation and chemotherapeutic agents results in spontaneous abortion. A host of environmental toxins has been implicated in losses, but few studies have taken account of confounding variables. In general, it is good advice to tell pregnant women to limit the amount of their exposure to any noxious agent.

Spontaneous abortion rates in women who smoke increase in proportion to the number of cigarettes smoked (38). When counselling women about the risk of smoking, clinicians should be careful not to invoke guilt by suggesting that previous habits caused pregnancy losses.

Similarly, alcohol intake increases the chance of spontaneous abortion in proportion to the amount consumed. This increase is still significant after correcting for such confounding variables as smoking, age, and parity (38).

Intercourse, falls, or blows to the abdomen do not cause loss in an otherwise healthy pregnancy, which can sustain such direct injury as chorionic villus sampling or amniocentesis. However, a threatened pregnancy may be hastened to detach and abort if a stimulant to uterine contractions is given, be it oxytocin, prostaglandin from semen, or abdominal injury. Thus, the patient is likely to equate the pregnancy loss with such an event rather than associate an occult spontaneous demise weeks earlier with the true cause.

Maternal Illness

Any life-threatening disease may be associated with increased abortion rates. It is rare that a woman with a serious chronic illness becomes pregnant, but in some cases the disease process worsens after pregnancy occurs. Wilson's disease, phenylketonuria, cyanotic heart disease, and hemoglobinopathies are all associated with increased fetal loss. These diseases need not be screened for in a patient presenting with recurrent abortion, as they are not likely to be subclinical or first appear with recurrent losses.

Maternal Age Effect

Spontaneous abortion increases with maternal age. Clearly, the incidence of trisomic conception increases with maternal age and so too do the number of trisomic abortions. However, karyotypic abnormalities do not explain the total increase in spontaneous abortions related to age. Women aged 40–44 have approximately twice the likelihood of a euploid loss as do women of age 20 (39). Decreased uterine vascularization and luteal phase inadequacy may be the mechanisms of age-related effects.

Clinical Recommendations: Summary

After three spontaneous abortions, couples should be offered formal evaluation; older couples may begin after two. It is important to stress that the entire evaluation should be completed and all factors considered. Even in the midst of an evaluation, if some factor tests positive, the evaluation should be continued to the end. Furthermore, once therapy is initiated, testing should be repeated to check therapeutic efficacy.

Both partners are karyotyped to detect the 2% of chromosomal rearrangements that occur in these patients. If another abortion occurs while treatment or investigation is in progress, then the abortus should be karyotyped.

Ultrasound, hysterosalpingography, or hysteroscopy will exclude Müllerian abnormalities, submucous leiomyoma, and intrauterine adhesions. If a defect is found that can be corrected hysteroscopically and no other anomaly is detected, it is prudent to perform the procedure. If the correction requires transabdominal surgery, the couple may want to attempt another pregnancy before undertaking the risk of major surgery.

An incompetent cervix should be followed during pregnancy and a cerclage performed when diagnosis is made if the ultrasound scan is normal at eight gestational weeks. The loss rate for viable pregnancies is only 3% after eight weeks if cardiac activity is demonstrated on ultrasound. Genetically abnormal fetuses are usually lost prior to that time.

Thyroid testing and prolactin measurements should be performed, even though abnormalities are rare, because these disorders are easily diagnosed and treated. Although there is no need to screen patients for diabetes mellitus, known diabetics should have their glycemic control monitored with glycosylated hemoglobin measurements.

An endometrial biopsy should be performed for both histologic dating and *U urealyticum* cultures. Two endometrial biopsies that are out of phase signal a need for treatment; after therapy is initiated, the biopsy should be repeated to assure that normality has been restored.

Patients should be screened for SLE and circulating lupus anticoagulant, and anticardiolipin antibodies should be assayed. Parental histocompatibility antigens are expensive and most likely not a sole cause of recurrent abortion. HLA types should not be done routinely. Immunologic therapy should remain for those centers investigating efficacy and side effects of such.

Finally, women should be advised to stop or decrease

their consumption of alcohol and smoking. This advice should be given in an informative rather than an accusatory manner to assuage guilt over past losses.

Any succeeding pregnancy is likely to be stressful to the couple. Weekly visits for cervical examination also allow patient-physician contact for emotional support. Our data indicate that frequent ultrasonic surveillance in these patients is beneficial in detecting anomalies that may be treatable or have important implications in further prenatal diagnosis and obstetric management (40).

References

1. Carson SA, Simpson JL. Spontaneous abortion. In: Eden RD, Boehm F, eds. Fetal assessment: physiological, clinical and medicolegal principles. East Norwalk, CT: Appleton-Century-Crofts, 1989.

2. US Department of Health and Human Services. Reproductive impairment among married couples. US vital and health statistics. Hyattsville, MD: National Center for Health Statistics, 1982: Series 23, No. 11:5–31.

3. Warburton D, Fraser FC. Spontaneous abortion risks in man: data from reproductive histories collected in a medical genetics unit. Am J Human Genet 1964;16:1.

4. Heinonen P, Saarikoski S, Pystynen P. Reproductive performance of women with uterine anomalies: an evaluation of 182 cases. Acta Obstet Gynecol Scand 1982;61:157.

5. Rock J, Jones HW Jr. The clinical management of the double uterus. Fertil Steril 1977;28:798.

6. Lazar P, Gueguen S. Multicentered controlled trial of cervical cerclage in women at moderate risk of preterm delivery. Br J Obstet Gynaecol 1984;91:731.

7. Rush RW, McPherson K, Jones L, et al. A randomized controlled trial of cervical cerclage in women at high risk of spontaneous preterm delivery. Br J Obstet Gynaecol 1984; 91:724.

8. Herbst AL, Senekjian EK, Frey KW. Abortion and pregnancy loss among diethylstilbestrol-exposed women. Sem Reprod Endocrinol 1989;7:124.

9. Mills JL, Simpson JL, Driscoll SG, et al. NICHD-DIEP Study: incidence of spontaneous abortion among normal women with insulin-dependent diabetic women whose pregnancies were identified within 21 days of conception. N Engl J Med 1988;319:1617.

10. Montoro M, Collea JV, Frasier D, et al. Successful outcome of pregnancy in women with hypothyroidism. Ann Intern Med 1981;94:31.

11. Noyes RW, Hertig ATR, Rock J. Dating the endometrial biopsy. Fertil Steril 1950;1:3.

12. Horta JL, Fernandez JG, de Leon BS, et al. Direct evidence of luteal insufficiency in women with habitual abortion. Obstet Gynecol 1977;49:705.

13. Smith SK, Lenton EA, Landgren BM, et al. The short luteal phase and infertility. Br J Obstet Gynaecol 1984;91:1120.

14. Daly DC, Walters CA, Soto-Albors CE, et al. Endometrial biopsy during treatment of luteal phase defects is predictive of therapeutic outcome. Fertil Steril 1983;40:305.

15. Petersohn L. Fertility in patients with ovarian endometriosis before and after treatment. Acta Obstet Scand 1970;49:331.

16. Rock JA, Guzick DS, Sengos C, et al. The conservative surgical treatment of endometriosis: evaluation of pregnancy success with respect to the extent of disease as categorized using contemporary classification systems. Fertil Steril 1981; 35:131.

17. Wheeler JM, Johnston BM, Malnak LR. The relationship of endometriosis to spontaneous abortion. Fertil Steril 1983; 39:656.

18. Stray-Pedersen B, Eng J, Reikvan TM. Uterine T-mycoplasma colonization in reproductive failure. Am J Obstet Gynecol 1978;130:307.

19. Toth A, Lesser ML, Brooks-Toth CW, et al. Outcome of subsequent pregnancies following antibiotic therapy after primary or multiple spontaneous abortions. Surg Gyneco Obstet 1986;163:243.

20. Gimovsky ML, Montoro M, Paul RH. Pregnancy outcome in women with systemic lupus erythematosus. Obstet Gyneco 1984;63:686.

21. Fraga A, Mintz G, Orozco J, et al. Sterility and fertility rates fetal waste, and maternal morbidity in systemic lupus erythematosus. J Rheumatol 1974;1:293.

22. Gastineau DA, Kazimier FJ, Nichols WL, et al. Lupus anticoagulant: an analysis of the clinical and laboratory features of 219 cases. Am J Hematol 1985;19:265.

23. Scott JR, Roe NS, Branch DW. Immunologic aspects of recurrent abortions and fetal death. Obstet Gynecol 1987 70:645.

24. Branch DW, Scott JR, Kochenour NK, et al. Obstetric complications associated with the lupus anticoagulant. N Engl Med 1985;313:1322.

25. Harris EN. Clinical and immunological significance of anti phospholipid antibodies. In: Beard RW, Sharp F, eds. Earl

pregnancy loss: mechanism and treatment. Proceedings of the 18th Study Group of the Royal College of Obstetricians and Gynaecologists. London: Royal College of Obstetricians and Gynaecologists, 1988:43–60.

26. Weksler BB, Pett SB, Alsono D, et al. Differential inhibition by aspirin of vascular and platelet prostaglandin synthesis in atherosclerotic patients. N Engl J Med 1983;308:800.

27. Beard RW, Baude P, Mowbray JF, et al. Protective antibodies and spontaneous abortion. Lancet 1983;1:1090.

28. Gill TH III. Immunogenetics of spontaneous abortion in humans. Transplantation 1983;35:1.

29. Power DA, Mason RJ, Stewart GM, et al. The fetus as an allograft: evidence for protective antibodies to HLA-linked paternal antigens. Lancet 1983;2:701.

30. Ober CL, Martin AO, Simpson JL, et al. Shared HLA antigens and reproductive performance among Hutterites. Am J Hum Genet 1983;35:994.

31. Faulk WP, Coulam CB, McIntyre JA. The role of trophoblast antigens in repetitive spontaneous abortions. Semin Reprod Endocrinol 1989;7:182.

32. Faulk WP, McIntyre JA. Trophoblast survival. Transplantation 1981;32:1.

33. Norman DJ, Barry JM, Fischer S. The beneficial effect of pretransplant third–party blood transfusions on allograft rejection in HLA identical sibling kidney transplants. Transplantation 1986;41:125.

34. Beer AE, Quebbeman JF, Ayers JW, et al. Major histocompatibility complex antigens, maternal and paternal immune responses, and chronic habitual abortions in humans. Am J Obstet Gynecol 1981;141:987.

35. Takakuwa K, Kanazawa K, Takeuchi S. Production of blocking antibodies by vaccination with husband's lymphocytes in unexplained recurrent aborters: the role in successful pregnancy. Am J Reprod Immunol Microbiol 1986;10:1.

36. Mowbray JF, Gibbing C, Liddell H, et al. Controlled trial of treatment of recurrent spontaneous abortion by immunization with paternal cells. Lancet 1985;1:941.

37. McIntyre JA, Faulk WP, Nichols-Johnson VR, et al. Immunological testing and immunotherapy in recurrent spontaneous abortion. Obstet Gynecol 1986;67:169.

38. Kline J, Shrout P, Stein ZA, et al. Drinking during pregnancy and spontaneous abortion. Lancet 1980;2:176.

39. Boué J, Boué A, Lazar P. Retrospective and prospective epidemiological studies of 1500 karyotyped spontaneous human abortions. Teratology 1975;12:11.

40. Carson SA, Schriock ED, Emerson DS, et al. Detection of anomalies in pregnancies following evaluation for recurrent spontaneous abortions: justification for routine ultrasonographic surveillance? Presented at Annual Meeting of the American Fertility Society, San Francisco, CA, November 13–16, 1989. Abstract P-58, p. S85.

43

The Incompetent Cervix

Jennifer R. Niebyl, M.D.

INCOMPETENT cervix, which occurs in 0.1% to 1% of all pregnancies, may be responsible for approximately 20%–25% of midtrimester abortions. The classic history is one of gradual, painless dilation and effacement. The patient is usually unaware of any contractions when she appears with bulging membranes and a dilated cervix.

Later, membranes may rupture, and the patient may have a short labor and be delivered of an immature fetus. Although incompetent cervix may cause premature delivery in the patient's first pregnancy, in subsequent pregnancies, loss characteristically occurs in the second trimester.

There is a possibility of subtle warning signs and symptoms, including vaginal or lower abdominal pressure, frequent urination, and discharge (occasionally bloody). The patient who appears with a dilated cervix may have noticed some of these manifestations for several days.

Possible Causes

Congenital incompetent cervix is associated with such uterine anomalies as bicornuate uterus and may be increased in patients who have been exposed to diethylstilbestrol in utero. In these women, there is presumably a higher proportion of muscular tissue in the cervix.

Causes of acquired incompetent cervix may be traumatic dilatation and curettage (D&C), large cone biopsy, or obstetric lacerations from precipitous labor or operative delivery. Multiple pregnancy may also be a cause of this problem, but incompetence will not usually recur in subsequent singleton pregnancies.

Epidemiologic studies suggest that midtrimester spontaneous abortions are more frequent in women who have had previous induced abortion by D&C under general anesthesia. These were more commonly performed in the early 1970s, when suction abortion first became legal.

The relative risk of midtrimester abortion for women who had a D&C done before 1973 is higher than for women whose abortions were performed after 1973 (1). This point is true because Laminaria tents came to be used more frequently in the nulliparous cervix after 1973. Use of these tents causes less cervical trauma than use of Hegar's dilators (2). After 1973, too, the more graduated Kay-Pratt dilators replaced Hegar's dilators, and local anesthesia was used much more often.

Approaches to Diagnosis

Patients who have had a small cone biopsy of the cervix are more at risk for cervical stenosis than for second-trimester abortion or prematurity. For those who have had a large cone removed, the opposite is true (3).

In one Swedish study, cervical conization was followed by a sevenfold increase in late spontaneous abortions: from 0.6% to 4.1% (4). In this population, 15% of all pregnancies after biopsy were complicated by cervical dilation requiring cerclage and 5% with cervical stenosis leading to cesarean section (CS). In another study from Sweden, premature deliveries increased from 4% to 31% after conization, the highest risk group being young nulliparous women (5).

The diagnosis is based on clinical history. Other methods of testing the nonpregnant cervix are unreliable. Directly measuring the cervical canal on X-ray film or passing a No. 8 Hegar's dilator during the luteal phase is not always predictive: An apparently normal cervix may become incompetent, or a defective-appearing one may retain a pregnancy. Although more patients with preterm deliveries have wide cervical canals, this condition can also be seen in patients with histories of normal pregnancy or preterm labor without clinically apparent incompetent cervix (6). Hysterography before a subsequent planned pregnancy is appropriate to rule out other uterine anomalies, myomata, or synechiae.

If the patient is already pregnant, her records should be reviewed carefully. Weekly vaginal examinations may detect dilation and effacement. Teaching the patient to report early symptoms is essential. Ultrasound may help visualization of a dilated internal os before clinical examination reveals a dilated external os. In one series, when the internal os width was measured sonographically during pregnancy, it was found to be significantly larger in patients with cerclage planned than in controls (2.57 cm versus 1.67 cm) (7). All patients with measurements below 1.9 cm went to term. The vaginal probe may give more predictive measurements than abdominal ultrasound, as it eliminates the artifact caused by bladder filling (8).

Women who had normal obstetric histories were found to have smaller measurements than those with a history of abortion or trauma (9). Five women with this history who presented with premature rupture of the membrane (PROM) had a mean cervical os width of 2.9 cm, compared with 1.8 cm for the whole group.

For women exposed to diethylstilbestrol (DES), Michaels and co-workers advocated weekly ultrasound surveillance and used cerclage only selectively (10). Routine cervical cerclage has been recommended by Ludmir and co-workers for all DES-exposed patients because of poor outcome with expectant management in their series (11).

Therapy Methods

For a patient with a classic history, uncontrolled trials suggest that cerclage is effective. Two procedures, the McDonald and Shirodkar, are best performed at 12–14 weeks' gestation, after fetal heartbeat is confirmed with ultrasound. For McDonald cerclage, a purse-string suture—silk or nonabsorbable surgical suture—that will allow easy removal when necessary should be used (Figure 43.1). For Shirodkar cerclage, a submucosal band should be placed with anchoring sutures of 4-0 silk (Figure 43.2). Shirodkar sutures may be left in place if the patient plans another pregnancy (which, of course, would require a cesarean delivery).

In rare cases, when the cervix is scarred, amputated, or deeply lacerated, transabdominal cerclage should be performed (Figure 43.3) (12). This approach is necessary only when vaginal procedures have failed or cannot be done because the cervix is extremely short or absent.

Transabdominal cerclage can be highly successful in patients with failed vaginal cerclage, history of deep cone biopsy, cervical laceration, and short cervix (such as with DES exposure) (11, 13).

Success has been reported with Smith-Hodge pessaries and a silicone plastic cuff (Baylor balloon) (14–16). Although historic controls were used, as in many cerclage studies, results were also very good with these techniques. The pessary may need to be increased in size as the pregnancy progresses (15).

Medical preventive therapies, such as 17α-hydroxy-progesterone caproate or β-adrenergic agents, have also been tried.

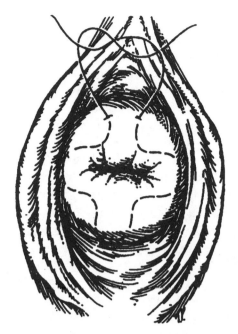

Figure 43.1   McDonald cerclage uses a purse-string suture that is removed before delivery.

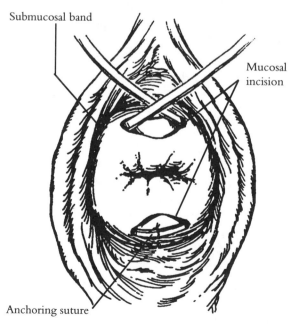

Submucosal band

Mucosal incision

Anchoring suture

Figure 43.2   Shirodkar sutures can remain in place if patient desires another pregnancy.

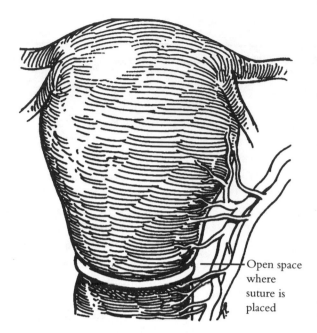

Open space where suture is placed

Figure 43.3   Transabdominal cerclage may be used for damaged cervices.

Success has often been attained, reflecting the difficulty in diagnosis and prediction of outcome without therapy (17).

If the cervix is already dilated, some have reported success using cerclages after replacement of membranes (Figure 43.4) (18, 19). Prophylactic antibiotics may be appropriate in this situation. Bed rest in a Trendelenburg position after confirmation of fetal viability may yield equally as good results as suture placement in the third trimester. However, it is clear that a prophylactic suture placed before cervical dilation and effacement have begun is more effective than one placed afterward.

In one study, overfilling of the urinary bladder successfully reduced bulging membranes in four cases presenting at 21–23 weeks (20). Cerclage could then be placed, and pregnancy was prolonged in these four cases to 24 4/7 weeks (610 g), 27 5/7 weeks (1,050 g), 36 4/7 weeks (1,980 g), and 38 2/7 weeks (3,300 g).

The use of prophylactic cerclage may not be appropriate in patients at risk for preterm delivery but without an obvious diagnosis of incompetent cervix. One study reported no difference in spontaneous pregnancy loss or prematu-

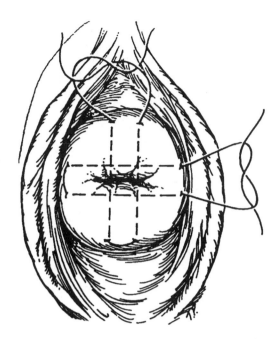

Figure 43.4   Wurm procedure has been successful when the cervix is already dilated.

rity rates between patients at moderate risk treated and not treated with cerclage (21). Investigators noted that those with cerclage were admitted to the hospital and treated with tocolytics more frequently.

In a controlled trial of McDonald cerclage in patients at a high risk for preterm delivery, 194 women with previous midtrimester loss or preterm delivery were randomized to receive a suture or not (22). There was no difference in the prematurity rate in the treated group (34%) versus controls (32%). However, the cerclage group spent more days in the hospital, received more tocolytics, and had a higher risk of puerperal fever.

Complications of cervical suturing may include increased risk of infection, premature rupture of membranes, premature labor, suture displacement, cervical stenosis, and cervical laceration during labor. Ureterovaginal, urethrovaginal, and vesicovaginal fistulas have also been reported. If the patient undergoes spontaneous PROM and elects expectant management, the cervical suture, a nidus for infection, should be removed.

References

1. Hogue CJ, Cates W, Tietze C. The effects of induced abortion on subsequent reproduction. Epidemiol Rev 1982;4:66.
2. Caspi E, Schneider D, Sadovsky G, et al. Diameter of cervical internal os after induction of early abortion by laminaria or rigid dilatation. Am J Obstet Gynecol 1983;146:106.
3. Lieman G, Harrison NA, Rubin A. Pregnancy following conization of the cervix. Complications related to cone size. Am J Obstet Gynecol 1980;136:14.
4. Moinian M, Andersch B. Does cervix conization increase the risk of complications in subsequent pregnancies? Acta Obstet Gynecol Scand 1982;61:101.
5. Larsson G, Grundsell H, Gullberg B, et al. Outcome of pregnancy after conization. Acta Obstet Gynecol Scand 1982;61:461.
6. Zlatnik FJ, Brown RC, Abu-Yousef MM. Radiologic appearance of the upper cervical canal in women with a history of premature delivery. J Reprod Med 1985;30.677.
7. Brook I, Feingold M, Schwartz A, et al. Ultrasonography in the diagnosis of cervical incompetence in pregnancy—a new diagnostic approach. Br J Obstet Gynaecol 1981;88:640.
8. Andersen HF, Ansbacher R. Ultrasound: a new approach to the evaluation of cervical ripening. Semin Perinatol 1991;15:140–8.
9. Feingold M, Brook I, Zakut H. Detection of cervical incompetence by ultrasound. Acta Obstet Gynecol Scand 1984;63:407.
10. Michaels WH, Thompson HO, Schreiber FR, et al. Ultrasound surveillance of the cervix during pregnancy in Diethyl-stilbestrol-exposed offspring. Obstet Gynecol 1989;73:230.
11. Ludmir J, Landon MB, Gabbe SG, et al. Management of the diethylstilbestrol-exposed pregnant patient: a prospective study. Am J Obstet Gynecol 1987;157:665.
12. Novy MJ. Transabdominal cervicoisthmic cerclage for the management of repetitive abortion and premature delivery. Am J Obstet Gynecol 1982;143:44.
13. Herron MA, Parer JT. Transabdominal cerclage for fetal wastage due to cervical incompetence. Obstet Gynecol 1988;71:865.
14. Oster S, Javert CT. Treatment of the incompetent cervix with the Hodge pessary. Obstet Gynecol 1966;28:206.

15. Vitsky M. Simple treatment of the incompetent cervical os. Am J Obstet Gynecol 1961;81:1194.

16. Yosowitz EE, Haufrect F, Kaufman RH, et al. Silicone-plastic cuff for the treatment of the incompetent cervix in pregnancy. Am J Obstet Gynecol 1972;113:233.

17. Harger JH. Comparison of success and morbidity in cervical cerclage procedure. Obstet Gynecol 1980;56:543.

18. Novy MJ, Haymond J, Nichols M. Shirodkar cerclage in a miltifactorial approach to the patient with advanced cervical changes. Am J Obstet Gynecol 1990;162:1412–20.

19. MacDougall J, Siddle N. Emergency cervical cerclage. Br J Obstet Gynaecol 1991;98:1234–38.

20. Scheerer LJ, Lam F, Bartolucci L, et al. A new technique for reduction of prolapsed fetal membranes for emergency cervical cerclage. Obstet Gynecol 1989;74:408.

21. Lazar P, Gueguen S. Multicentered controlled trial of cervical cerclage in women at moderate risk of preterm delivery. Br J Obstet Gynaecol 1984;91:731.

22. Rush RW, McPherson K, Jones L, et al. A randomized controlled trial of cervical cerclage in women at high risk of spontaneous preterm delivery. Br J Obstet Gynaecol 1984;91:724.

44

Preeclampsia-Eclampsia

Baha M. Sibai, M.D.

DESPITE research and practice discoveries, preeclampsia and eclampsia (development of convulsions) remain obstetric enigmas. Preeclampsia is associated with activation of the coagulation system. Findings suggest endothelial injury, enhanced clotting, and increased platelet activation and consumption (1).

Some investigators have speculated that an imbalance in prostaglandin metabolism is central to the pathophysiology of preeclampsia (2). They have cited an observed decrease in prostacyclin production and an increase in the thromboxane A2/prostacyclin ratio. While this hypothesis may explain some hematologic and biochemical peculiarities associated with preeclampsia, it fails to show the primary etiology.

A more basic abnormality of preeclampsia is usually generalized arteriolar constriction and increased vascular sensitivity to pressor peptides and amines. Again, however, it is important to emphasize that vascular pathologic changes seen in the placenta, kidneys, liver, and brain in preeclampsia eclampsia, while characteristic, are not specific to this disease. Although compatible with activation of the coagulation system and vasoconstriction, they are secondary phenomena and do not indicate the primary cause of preeclampsia.

Management Alternatives

The most effective therapy for preeclampsia is delivery of the fetus and placenta. In pregnancies at or near term where the cervix is favorable, labor should be induced. IV MgSO$_4$ should be used both during labor and postpartum to reduce risk of convulsions.

Preeclampsia remote from term presents a much more difficult problem. Disease severity and gestational age usually govern the decision to intervene and deliver a preterm infant, who may require prolonged intensive care, or to institute expectant management.

Mild Preeclampsia

All patients with mild preeclampsia should be hospitalized at the time of diagnosis (Figure 44.1). Allowing them to be up and about later is appropriate in certain situations, espe-

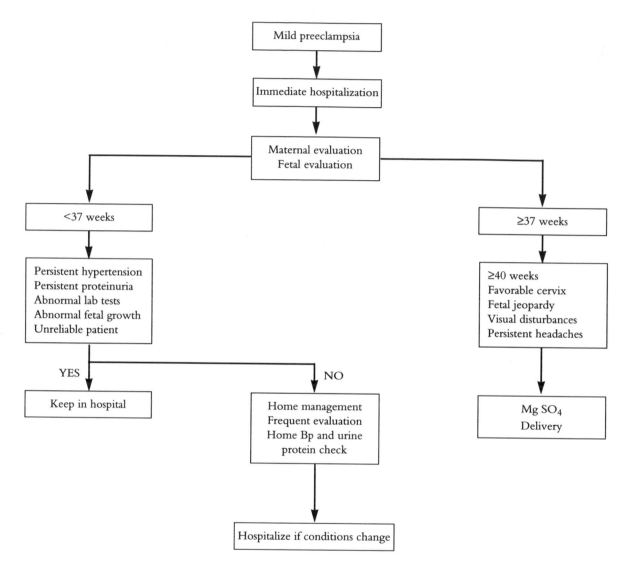

Figure 44.1   Management of mild preeclampsia.

cially in early disease. In such instances, the patient may remain at home but should spend most of the day resting. Blood pressure and urine protein should be measured daily. Maternal and fetal well-being should be evaluated at least twice weekly. Any evidence of disease progression or acute hypertension is an indication for prompt hospitalization.

Once a patient is hospitalized, maternal and fetal mon-

itoring can be instituted. Frequency of testing depends on disease severity. In many cases of mild preeclampsia, disease does not progress, and conservative management is possible until the fetus reaches maturity or the cervix is favorable for induction (see Case 44.1).

During the past eight years, we have hospitalized 2,700 women with mild preeclampsia at 26–38 weeks' gestation. Perinatal mortality was 0.5%, and incidence of fetal growth retardation was only 5%. Patients are usually given regular hospital diets with no salt restriction and allowed to move about as desired. Diuretics and antihypertensive drugs are not prescribed. Our studies indicate that these agents do not improve pregnancy outcome and may increase incidence of fetal growth retardation (3, 4).

During hospitalization, the patient must be monitored continually for vital signs, deep-tendon reflexes, and level of consciousness, and questioned about symptoms of headache, visual disturbances, and epigastric pain. Her weight should be recorded daily, noting any excessive gain or generalized edema.

Laboratory evaluation should include urinalysis, hematocrit, and platelet counts every two days, serum uric acid determination, creatinine, and liver enzyme tests twice weekly, and 24-hour urine examination for creatinine clearance and protein excretion at least once weekly. This evaluation is important since patients may develop thrombocytopenia and abnormal liver enzymes even with minimal blood pressure elevations. Fetal evaluation should include serial ultrasonography to determine fetal growth and amniotic fluid volume, recording of daily fetal movement, and nonstress testing at least twice weekly.

Conservative management is inappropriate if there are signs of progression to severe preeclampsia or if fetal monitoring test results become abnormal. Moreover, since utero-placental blood flow is suboptimal, conservative management of mild disease beyond term is not beneficial to the fetus. After 37 weeks' gestation, labor should be induced as soon as the cervix is favorable.

Severe Preeclampsia

Ample evidence attests to the deleterious effects of severe hypertension in nonpregnant humans and experimental animals. When treating severe preeclampsia, blood pressure should be maintained below 160/110 mm Hg. The goal is to prevent convulsions with $MgSO_4$, control blood pressure within a safe range with hydralazine hydrochloride (apresoline hydrochloride), and then initiate delivery. If the disease develops at or after 34 weeks' gestation, or if there is evidence of fetal lung maturity or fetal or maternal jeopardy before then, delivery is the definitive therapy (Figure 44.2).

For patients having severe preeclampsia at less than 34 weeks with lung maturity absent, management is highly controversial. Some institutions consider delivery mandatory for all cases, irrespective of gestational age, whereas others recommend prolonging pregnancy until the lungs mature.

All such patients should be managed in a tertiary-care center where intensive maternal and neonatal care facilities are available. The patient should be admitted to the labor and delivery area for close observation of maternal and fetal conditions. IV $MgSO_4$ should be administered and blood pressure

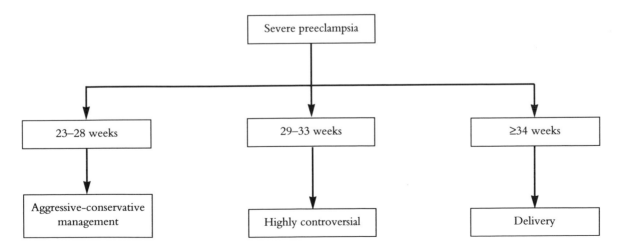

Figure 44.2 Management of severe preeclampsia.

controlled with bolus injections of hydralazine, as indicated.

Women displaying persistent severe hypertension or other signs of maternal or fetal deterioration during observation are usually delivered within 24 hours, regardless of gestational age or fetal lung maturity. Some will have marked diuresis and improvement in blood pressure shortly after hospitalization. If diastolic blood pressure should remain below 100 mm Hg without antihypertensive therapy after 24 hours of observation in labor and delivery, $MgSO_4$ should be discontinued and the patient followed closely in the hospital until fetal lungs mature. Patients' maternal and fetal status should be monitored daily and steroids used to accelerate fetal lung maturity, as indicated.

Occasionally, a patient may develop severe preeclampsia at less than 28 weeks' gestation. These pregnancies are associated with high maternal and perinatal mortality and morbidity (5). If gestation is at or less than 24 weeks, we recommend termination with PGE_2 vaginal suppositories. All such patients will receive IV $MgSO_4$ and have severe hypertension controlled with bolus injections of hydralazine, as needed.

If gestation is more than 24 weeks, the patient should be counselled on risks and benefits of continuing the pregnancy. If she elects conservative management, she should be given IV $MgSO_4$ for 24 hours. Her blood pressure should be controlled aggressively with such antihypertensives as methyldopa or labetalol hydrochloride. In addition, daily intensive evaluation of maternal and fetal status should be initiated, using antepartum fetal heart rate testing and biophysical profiles. The pregnancy should continue until either maternal or fetal jeopardy develops.

HELLP Syndrome

This term describes preeclamptic patients having hemolysis (H), elevated liver enzymes (EL), and low platelets (LP). It has been recognized as a complication of severe preeclampsia-eclampsia for many years. Incidence of the syndrome ranges from 4% to 12% in such pregnancies, and its presence is associated with high maternal and perinatal mortality and morbidity (6).

Approximately 90% of patients with HELLP syndrome are first seen remote from term, complaining of epi-gastric or right upper quadrant pain. About half have nausea or vomiting, and others have nonspecific viral-syndrome-like symptoms. Hypertension or proteinuria may be absent or slight. Thus, some patients may display various signs and symptoms not diagnostic of severe preeclampsia. Consequently, we recommend obtaining for all pregnant wom-en having any of these symptoms a complete blood count and platelet and liver enzyme determinations, irrespective of maternal blood pressure level.

The typical HELLP syndrome patient is white, multiparous, and 25 years of age or older. She is usually heavy and has generalized edema and minimal elevations in blood pressure. Proteinuria may be either absent or significant, depending on duration of signs and symptoms. In some cases, patients may first be seen because of jaundice, GI bleeding, hematuria, or bleeding from the gums. As a result, these patients are often misdiagnosed as having viral hepatitis, gallbladder disease, peptic ulcer, kidney stones, glomerulonephritis, acute fatty liver of pregnancy, idiopathic or thrombotic thrombocytopenic purpura, or hemolytic uremic syndrome. Rarely, presence of HELLP syndrome has been associated with hypoglycemia, leading to coma, severe hyponatremia, cortical blindness, and nephrogenic diabetes insipidus.

Managing HELLP Syndrome

As mentioned above, a number of surgical and medical disorders are associated with the signs and symptoms and hematologic and biochemical abnormalities found in patients with HELLP syndrome. This is particularly true when the syndrome presents during the midtrimester or early third trimester. Management is often complicated by inappropriate treatment and invasive diagnostic procedures, such as bone marrow, liver, renal, and intestinal biopsies and laparotomy, which are associated with significant morbidity. Although various modalities have been used to alleviate or reverse HELLP syndrome, all are controversial (Table 44.1).

Patients with the syndrome should be referred to a tertiary-care center and managed initially as any patient with severe preeclampsia. The first priority is to assess the mother's condition and stabilize it, particularly if she has coagula-

Table 44.1 HELLP Syndrome Treatment

Plasma volume expanders (5% or 25% albumin)

Antithrombotic agents
  Antithrombin III
  Dipyridamole (Persantine)
  Heparin
  Low dose heparin
  Prostacyclin infusions

Steroids

Fresh frozen plasma infusions

Plasmapheresis

HELLP: hemolysis, elevated liver enzymes, low platelets.

tion abnormalities. The next step is to investigate fetal well-being with a nonstress test and biophysical profile. Finally, the decision must be made whether or not immediate delivery is indicated. Amniocentesis may be performed in these patients without risk of bleeding complications, and use of steroids is indicated.

All patients with true HELLP syndrome, irrespective of gestational age, should be delivered. Labor may be initiated with oxytocin infusions, exactly as for routine induction in all patients with a gestational age of 32 weeks or more. In a patient with an unripe cervix and a gestational age of less than 32 weeks, elective cesarean section (CS) is the delivery method of choice.

If maternal analgesia is necessary, intermittent 25- to 50-mg IV doses of meperidine hydrochloride may be used. Local infiltration anesthesia is appropriate for all vaginal delivery cases. The use of prudent block or epidural anesthesia is contraindicated in HELLP syndrome patients because of the risk of bleeding into these areas. General anesthesia should be used for CS.

Platelet transfusions are indicated before or after delivery if the platelet count is less than 20,000/mm³. Correction of thrombocytopenia is particularly important before CS. However, repeated platelet transfusions are contraindicated since consumption occurs rapidly and the effect is transient. Our policy is to transfuse ten units of platelets in all patients having a count of less than 50,000/mm³ before we intubate for CS.

Generalized oozing from the operative site is very common. To minimize risk of hematoma formation, we recommend that a subfascial drain be used, the bladder flap be left open, and the wound left open with sutures in situ from the level of the fascia. All these openings can be closed successfully within 72 hours. Departing from these recommendations will result in a 20% incidence of hematoma formation.

Eclampsia

Eclamptic convulsions are a life-threatening emergency for both mother and fetus. Cardinal steps in management are to prevent maternal injury during the convulsive episode, by such means as inserting a padded tongue blade between the teeth, and to safeguard against potential maternal morbidity afterward.

The most urgent aspect of therapy is to assure maternal oxygenation and minimize risk of aspiration, rather than to stop the convulsive episode. Drugs to shorten or abolish the initial convulsion should not be given but $MgSO_4$ should be started subsequently to prevent further seizures.

After controlling maternal convulsions, arterial blood gas measurements should be obtained to assure presence of normal arterial PO_2 and pH, as well as a chest radiograph to rule out aspiration. Maternal hypoxemia or acidemia may result from aspiration, repeated convulsions, respiratory depression due to the use of multiple anticonvulsive agents, or

Table 44.2 Transitory Changes Associated with Eclamptic Convulsions

Uterine Hyperactivity
Increased frequency
Increased tone
Duration of 2–15 minutes

Fetal Heart Rate Changes
Bradycardia
Compensatory tachycardia
Decreased beat-to-beat
Late decelerations

all of these combined. To avoid toxic side effects, it is necessary to correct hypoxemia and acidemia before administering anesthetic drugs.

Uterine hyperactivity, consisting of increased frequency and tone, and fetal heart rate (FHR) changes usually appear during and after an eclamptic convulsion (Table 44.2). These changes are commonly transient, lasting from three to 15 minutes. Most resolve spontaneously after conclusion of convulsions or correction of maternal hypoxemia and acidosis. An emergency CS should not be performed based on these findings, as this approach might prove detrimental to both the mother and the newborn. If changes persist despite corrective measures, possible placental abruption, fetal distress, or both, may be suspected, especially in the preterm or growth-retarded fetus.

The primary treatment of eclampsia is delivery of the fetus and placenta. Once convulsions and severe hypertension are well-controlled and the patient has been stabilized, delivery preparation should be initiated. FHR and uterine activity must be monitored continuously during labor. If labor is not well established and no fetal presentation or distress is noted, it is possible to use IV oxytocin to induce labor in all patients at 32 weeks' gestation or beyond, irrespective of the extent of cervical dilation or effacement.

A similar approach is appropriate for patients at less than 32 weeks' gestation if the cervix is favorable for induction. Our previous experience of a high incidence of intrapartum complications, such as placental abruption, intrauterine growth retardation, and fetal distress in eclampsia developing before 32 weeks, justifies this method (7).

Maternal analgesia can be provided, if necessary, with intermittent 25- to 50-mg IV doses of meperidine. It is possible to use local infiltration anesthesia with pudendal block in most cases for vaginal delivery. A balanced general or epidural anesthesia is appropriate for abdominal deliveries.

Use of epidural anesthesia for patients having severe preeclampsia-eclampsia is highly controversial. Some authors caution against it in this situation because of the potential for maternal hypotension and reduced uteroplacental blood flow with an already compromised maternal intravascular volume (8, 9). However, others believe that epidural anesthesia not only controls pain but aids in stabilizing blood pressure and improves uterine perfusion. It is important to note that use of an epidural agent requires availability of personnel with special expertise in obstetric anesthesia. In addition, availability of central hemodynamic monitoring is necessary, since precautionary infusions of large amounts of crystalloids or colloids are usually given before an epidural anesthetic is administered. Use of conduction anesthesia is contraindicated if there is fetal distress or coagulopathy, if the platelet count is less than 100 x $10^3/mm^3$, or if bleeding time is prolonged.

All patients must be monitored very closely during labor and delivery. Special attention should be paid to fluid intake and output. Patients with severe preeclampsia-eclampsia are at increased risk for development of pulmonary edema from fluid overload. Urinary output should be monitored every hour, and fluid administration should not exceed 150 mL hourly. If the patient has oliguria (output of less than 100 mL every four hours), the rate of both fluid and magnesium sulfate administration should be reduced accordingly. A pediatrician skilled in neonatal resuscitation should be present in the delivery room.

Prevention or Control of Convulsions

Parenteral magnesium sulfate ($MgSO_4 \cdot 7H_2O$ USP) is the drug of choice for treating convulsions caused by eclampsia. Major advantages include its relative safety for both mother and fetus when used properly. All women diagnosed as having preeclampsia, irrespective of severity, should be given IV $MgSO_4$ during both labor and postpartum.

We administer $MgSO_4$ by controlled continuous IV infusion, with a loading dose of 6 g over 15–20 minutes and maintenance therapy at a rate of 2 g hourly. This regimen provides adequate serum magnesium levels for most patients. If a patient on it develops a convulsion or has recurrent convulsions, it is permissible to give another bolus of 2–4 g over 3–5 minutes. If convulsions recur, a short-acting barbiturate, such as amobarbital sodium, may be given in a dose of up to 250 mg IV over three minutes. An occasional patient will have recurrent seizures even after all these measures, necessitating administration of a paralyzing agent, as well as intubation (10–12).

Patellar reflexes, urine output, and respiratory rate of all patients receiving $MgSO_4$ should be checked hourly.

Because loss of patellar reflexes is the first sign of magnesium intoxication, absent reflexes are an indication for discontinuing magnesium infusion (Table 44.3). It is important to keep at the bedside an ampule containing 1 g of calcium gluconate for IV administration as an antidote in case of magnesium toxicity.

Therapy for Severe Hypertension

The objective of treating severe hypertension is to prevent cerebrovascular accidents and congestive heart failure without compromising uteroplacental blood flow, which is already reduced in severe preeclampsia-eclampsia. Hydralazine is safe and effective for managing severe hypertension during pregnancy. If diastolic blood pressure is 110 mm Hg or greater, 5- to 10-mg bolus doses of hydralazine should be given every 20 minutes to keep it between 90 and 100 mm Hg. This regimen requires monitoring blood pressure every five minutes for at least 30 minutes after giving the drug.

An alternative is to give 20- to 50-mg bolus injections of labetalol. Unlike hydralazine, labetalol does not cause maternal tachycardia, flushing, or headaches (13). Other antihypertensive drugs are rarely needed for management of these patients. Diuretics should be used only when there is pulmonary edema.

Postpartum Care

After delivery, the patient should be monitored in the recovery room for 12–24 hours, including evaluation of reflexes. During this time, maternal vital signs and fluid intake and urine output should be monitored hourly. Because 25% of cases of eclampsia reported occur in the puerperium, vigilance is mandatory (14). Salt should not be restricted, nor diuretics used.

Most patients show evidence of resolution of disease within 24 hours after delivery. Some, however, especially those with severe disease in the second-trimester, HELLP syndrome, or eclampsia, require intensive monitoring for 2–4 days. In such patients, it may be necessary to continue magnesium sulfate for more than 24 hours. These patients are at risk for the development of pulmonary edema from fluid overload and mobilization and compromised renal

Table 44.3 Magnesium Toxicity

Manifestations
Loss of patellar reflex (8–12 mg/dL)
Feeling of warmth, flushing (9–12 mg/dL)
Somnolence (10–12 mg/dL)
Slurred speech (10–12 mg/dL)
Muscular paralysis (15–17 mg/dL)
Respiratory difficulty (15–17 mg/dL)
Cardiac arrest (30–35 mg/dL)

Management
Discontinue $MgSO_4$
Obtain Mg level
Restart or reduce $MgSO_4$ according to Mg level
If Mg level ≥ 15 mg/dL:
Give 1 g calcium gluconate IV
Intubate
Assist ventilation

function (15).

In most cases, patients will be normotensive at time of discharge from the hospital. For these patients, oral contraceptives may be prescribed without anticipating problems.

A few patients will continue to have severe hypertension that can be controlled with either methyldopa or labetalol. Prophylactic anticonvulsive drugs, such as phenobarbital or phenytoin, should not be used.

After discharge, the patient should be seen weekly until her blood pressure is normal without medication. If this change doesn't occur by six weeks postpartum, a workup to assess hypertension should be performed and appropriate therapy instituted.

Conclusion

The crucial components in managing patients with preeclampsia are early detection, prompt hospitalization in an attempt to delay delivery to achieve reasonable fetal maturity, and delivery when appropriate. All patients diagnosed with preeclampsia-eclampsia should receive parenteral $MgSO_4$ during labor, delivery, and postpartum to prevent convulsions.

These pregnancies are at increased risk for complications. Most occur in patients with severe disease who are remote from term and in those with the HELLP syndrome. Consequently, these patients should be cared for at centers with appropriate maternal and neonatal intensive care facilities.

C A S E 4 4 . 1 Induction for Preeclampsia

An 18-year-old white primigravida, at 33 weeks' gestation was found to have a blood pressure of 132/92 mm Hg, 2+ proteinuria, and no edema during a scheduled prenatal care visit. Her course was otherwise uneventful. Two weeks earlier, her blood pressure had been 110/68 mm Hg and urine protein negative.

HOSPITAL FINDINGS

The patient was hospitalized, given regular diet, and salt was not restricted. Evaluation revealed a uric acid of 6.2 mg/dL, a creatinine clearance of 135 mL per minute, and a 24-hour urinary protein excretion of 586 mg. Her platelet count and liver function test results were normal. Ultrasound evaluation showed a fetus appropriate for gestational age, normal amniotic fluid, and a biophysical profile of 10, including a reactive nonstress test.

After hospitalization, the patient had moderate diuresis and lost 4 lb over 48 hours. Her blood pressure ranged between 120–130/76–82 mm Hg without drugs. Reflexes were normal and there were no complaints of headaches or blurred vision.

Repeat renal function tests revealed a clearance of 142 mL per minute, protein excretion of 160 mg every 24 hours, and uric acid of 5.0 mg/dL. All other test results were normal. Diastolic blood pressures remained below 90 mm Hg, and urine dipstick tests were consistently negative. A repeat NST was reactive.

The patient was discharged at a gestational age of 34.5 weeks and directed to report for antepartum testing twice weekly. She was instructed to rest in the left lateral recumbent position and to have her blood pressure and urine protein tested daily.

CERVIX RIPE AT 38.5 WEEKS

At 37 weeks' gestation, she was hospitalized for a blood pressure of 140/100 mm Hg and 1+ urine protein. The cervix wasn't ripe for induction. Maternal and fetal evaluations were normal. She remained in the hospital until 38.5 weeks, at which time her cervix was ripe for induction.

On the morning of induction, a loading dose of 6 g of $MgSO_4$ was administered IV slowly over 15 minutes. Maintenance dosing was then started at 2 g per hour. Hospital personnel inserted a Foley catheter, monitored the intake and output and reflexes hourly, initiated continuous fetal heart rate monitoring and uterine contraction monitoring, and started oxytocin induction.

Once active labor ensued, an epidural agent was given for analgesia. After 9 hours, the patient had spontaneous vaginal delivery under epidural anesthesia. The infant weighed 3,280 g and had good Apgar scores.

$MgSO_4$ therapy was maintained for 14 hours postpartum. The patient's reflexes and urine output, as well as vital signs, were continuously monitored. She was transferred to the floor with a blood pressure of 128/82 mm Hg and negative urine protein. She remained normotensive until discharge 3 days later.

INTERPRETING RESULTS

Initial hospitalization for mild preeclampsia allowed maternal-fetal evaluation and checking of maternal response after hospitalization. This management resulted in maternal improvement and allowed the fetus to reach term.

Outpatient management was possible because the patient was reliable, showed good response in the hospital, and had frequent checkups. Subsequent hospitalization was indicated because of recurrence of hypertension. Such management resulted in vaginal delivery of a healthy term infant.

References

1. Saleh AA, Bottoms SF, Welch RA, et al. Preeclampsia, delivery and the hemostatic system. Am J Obstet Gynecol 1987; 157:331.

2. Makila UM, Viinikka L, Ylikorkala O. Increased thromboxane A2 production but normal prostacyclin by the placenta in hypertensive pregnancies. Prostaglandins 1984;27:87.

3. Sibai BM, Barton JR, Akl S, Sarinoglu C, Mercer BM. A randomized prospective comparison of nifedipine and bed rest versus bed rest alone in the management of preeclampsia remote from term. Am J Obstet Gynecol 1992;167:879.

4. Sibai BM, Gonzalez AR, Mabie WC, et al. A comparison of labetalol plus hospitalization versus hospitalization alone in the management of preeclampsia remote from term. Obstet Gynecol 1987;70:323.

5. Sibai BM, Akl S, Fairlie F, Moretti M. A protocol for managing severe preeclampsia in the second trimester. Am J Obstet Gynecol 1990;163:733.

6. Barton JR, Sibai BM. Care of the pregnancy complicated by HELLP syndrome. Obstet Gynecol Clin N Amer 1991; 18:165.

7. Sibai BM. Eclampsia VI. Maternal-perinatal outcome in 254 consecutive cases. Am J Obstet Gynecol 1990;163:1049.

8. Lindheimer MD, Katz AI. Hypertension in pregnancy. N Engl J Med 1985;313:675.

9. Jones MM, Joyce TH. Anesthesia for the parturient with pregnancy-induced hypertension. Clin Obstet Gynecol 1987; 30:591.

10. Sibai BM, Lipshitz J, Anderson GE, et al. Reassessment of intravenous $MgSO_4$ therapy in preeclampsia–eclampsia. Obstet Gynecol 1981;57:199.

11. Dahmus MA, Barton JR, Sibai BM. Cerebral imaging in eclampsia: Magnetic resonance imaging versus computed tomography. Am J Obstet Gynecol 1992;167:935.

12. Barton JR, Bronstein SJ, Sibai BM. Management of the eclamptic patient. J Mat Fet Med 1992;1:313.

13. Mabie WC, Gonzalez AR, Sibai BM, et al. A comparative trial of labetalol and hydralazine in the acute management of severe hypertension complicating pregnancy. Obstet Gynecol 1987;70:328.

14. Sibai BM, Abdella TN, Spinnato JA, et al. Eclampsia V. The incidence of nonpreventable eclampsia. Am J Obstet Gynecol 1986;154:581.

15. Sibai BM, Mabie BC, Harvey CJ, et al. Pulmonary edema in severe preeclampsia-eclampsia: analysis of 37 consecutive cases. Am J Obstet Gynecol 1987;156:1174.

45

Emergency Care in Pregnancy

Robert H. Hayashi, M.D.

THIS chapter reviews the diagnosis and initial management of emergencies in an obstetric unit. Presentations are arranged to simulate complaints or problems of the obstetric patient. Two illustrative case reports follow.

Difficulty Breathing

Asthma

Acute bronchial asthma complicates fewer than 1% of pregnancies (1, 2). The diagnosis is apparent in a patient with a history of asthma who has varying degrees of bronchospasm and accompanying diffuse inspiratory and expiratory wheezes. Although arterial hypoxemia is present, fetus and mother usually fare well unless the hypoxemia is severe or treatment is inadequate (3).

Asthmatic attacks may be triggered by allergens, pulmonary infections, or emotional factors. Microscopic examination of sputum can give a clue to etiology. Eosinophils are typically found if the attack is triggered by an allergen, and neutrophils are associated with asthma caused by an infection (4, 5).

In outpatients, mild asthmatic attacks can usually be managed with bronchodilators (Table 45.1). A dosage of 250–500 mg of aminophylline in 50 mL of dextrose and water, administered IV over 20 minutes, is often sufficient to terminate a mild asthmatic attack (4). Several doses of epinephrine in a dosage range of 0.2–0.5 mL of a 1:1,000 solution can be administered subcutaneously at 20- to 30-minute intervals if the patient is responding well to treatment (1).

Inhalation of nebulized selective bronchodilator solutions, by either jet nebulizer or metered dose inhaler, has become an established, validated method for treatment of acute bronchospasm (4). Common preparations include 0.2 mL of 0.5 isoproterenol hydrochloride (Isuprel), 0.5% mL of 1% isoetharine (Bronkometer), or 0.83 and 5 mg/mL in 3- and 20-mL containers of albuterol (Proventil, Ventolin). It is safest to use only one adrenergic agent at a time (4).

Another way of managing mild attacks is hydration to prevent thick, stagnant bronchial secretions from becoming inspissated and aggravating bronchospasm. Coughing is also helpful in clearing the airways and should not be suppressed.

The patient should be reassured. Mild sedation is valu-

Table 45.1   Management of Asthma

Mild Attack	Severe Attack or Persisting Mild Attack
Have sputum specimen examined for neutrophils or eosinophils.	Hospitalize.
Reassure patient. Mild sedation may be helpful.	Check arterial blood gases; typically, PO_2 and PCO_2 are both low.
Hydrate.	Give 30%–40% O_2 by mask to keep PO_2 above 70 mm Hg.
Give aminophylline 250–500 mg in 50 mL D_5W IV over 20 minutes.	Administer continuous aminophylline infusion: 20 mg/kg/day total dose.
Administer epinephrine 0.2–0.5 mL of 1:1,000 aqueous solution SC. Repeat in 20–30 minutes, if necessary. You may substitute terbutaline for epinephrine.	Give hydrocortisone 200–300 mg by IV infusion q 4 h.
	Infuse IV fluids. Up to 4 L/day may be necessary.
If infection is suspected, give ampicillin 500 mg PO q 6 h. (If patient is allergic to ampicillin, erythromycin is drug of choice.)	Prescribe antibiotics if infection is suspected.
Encourage coughing.	Clear airways with postural drainage and coughing.
	If PCO_2 is above 45 mm Hg, the patient is potentially very ill. If above 60 mm Hg, have her placed in intensive care unit and see that she receives intubation and mechanical ventilation.

able in treating mild asthmatic attacks, but it must be restricted to small doses of barbiturates in very anxious patients.

If microscopic examination of the sputum reveals neutrophils, antibiotics should be administered. Because *Streptococcus* and *Hemophilus* are the usual organisms responsible for pulmonary infection in asthma, 500 mg of ampicillin given orally every six hours is the drug of choice for pregnant asthmatics (3).

Severe asthmatic attacks or mild attacks that are not relieved promptly by the measures suggested are best managed in the hospital. Have arterial blood gas determinations made on admission. All asthmatics will show varying degrees of hypoxemia and usually a below-normal PCO_2 owing to hyperventilation. Oxygen therapy by mask should be instituted, response to it judged by serial arterial blood gas determinations (3–5). The goal of oxygen therapy is a PO_2 of at least 70–80 mm Hg. A chest x-ray is also necessary.

Continued use of adrenergic agents by aerosol or injection is of no value in treating hospitalized patients (4, 5). However, continuous aminophylline infusion may be extended for a total dose of 20 mg/kg daily (4). A loading dose of 5 mg/kg should be given at 30 minutes, followed by a maintenance infusion of 0.6 mg/kg/h. Because individual aminophylline metabolism varies, blood level determinations should be done frequently early in IV therapy

and the infusion rate adjusted accordingly. Therapeutic levels are 10–20 μg/mL, and toxicity may appear at serum levels above 15 μg/mL (6). Toxicity is commonly manifested by nausea and vomiting but may also cause tachycardia and cardiac dysrhythmias.

Use of corticosteroids IV is appropriate (3–5). Dosages from 200–300 mg of hydrocortisone should be given every four hours for several days. Depending on the patient's status at this time, corticosteroid therapy may be stopped abruptly or continued orally throughout pregnancy without markedly affecting the fetus adversely (7).

Because most asthmatic patients are dehydrated when admitted to the hospital, IV fluid administration of up to 4 L or more daily may be necessary initially. Serial determinations of the patient's weight, hematocrit, and urinary specific gravity are simple ways to monitor fluid replacement. When sputum examination or a chest roentgenogram indicates pulmonary infection, antibiotics should be used parenterally at first and then orally.

Patients may develop life-threatening pulmonary insufficiency. In some asthmatics, the earliest sign of this complication is a rising PCO_2. A PCO_2 above 45 mm Hg indicates noteworthy pulmonary insufficiency; one above 60 mm Hg indicates a condition for which the patient should be in intensive care where she can be intubated, her respiratory drive abolished, and mechanical ventilation performed (5).

Deaths from asthma often result from mucus stagnation. Mobilization of secretions may require postural drainage, endotracheal intubation with suction or bronchoscopy, and some advocate brochoalveolar lavage (3, 4). Tension pneumothorax may occur spontaneously or with mechanical ventilators. Mediastinal emphysema may be auscultated by a crunching sound synchronous with the heartbeat (Hamman's sign) (3).

Newer drugs for asthma treatment are appearing. Terbutaline sulfate (Brethine, Bricanyl) is a synthetic adrenergic agonist that mainly has a B$_2$ action. Effective in relaxing bronchiolar smooth muscle, it may be administered orally in 5-mg doses every six hours (not to exceed 15 mg in 24 hours) or subcutaneously in 0.25-mg doses that may be repeated in 15–30 minutes (not to exceed 0.5 mg in four hours). Terbutaline, which requires the same precautions as other β-agonists, may be used instead of epinephrine but not with other adrenergic drugs because of the risk of possible toxicity.

Cromolyn, a drug for prophylaxis against asthmatic attacks, is of no value in abating an acute attack, and there is little experience with its use for pregnant patients. The Centers for Disease Control recommend that patients with chronic bronchial asthma get yearly influenza immunization and that it be given in the last two trimesters.

Pulmonary Embolus

The most frequent nonobstetric cause of postpartum death is pulmonary embolization (8, 9). Classical findings are sudden onset of dyspnea, pleuritic chest pain, cough, tachypnea, tachycardia, hemoptysis, and cyanosis.

Symptoms and signs from even a large embolus do not always lead to a diagnosis (Table 45.2) (8). Laboratory confirmation is important (Table 45.3) (9). Pulmonary angiography is the most accurate guide to the extent of embolization. A negative angiogram excludes the possibility of a large embolus but not of several small emboli.

Initial treatment is with heparin (Table 45.4). The goal is prevention of thrombus propagation and recurrent embolization. Among contraindications to heparin are severe hypertension, cerebrovascular hemorrhage, hemorrhagic diathesis, or overt bleeding from the gastrointestinal or urinary tract (10).

Although the value of this therapy has been undisputed since 1960, there is still considerable disagreement about the best means of administration and of monitoring effectiveness (11). One can introduce heparin either by intermittent IV bolus or continuous IV infusion. The first method entails giving an IV bolus every 4–6 hours and adjusting dosage to prolong clotting time to two to three times baseline value. The initial dose is usually 5,000– 10,000 U, and

---

Table 45.2 Signs and Symptoms in 90 Patients with Pulmonary Embolization

Tachypnea (88%)

Dyspnea (80%)

Tachycardia (63%)

Anxiety (61%)

Loud pulmonic closure (60%)

Rales (50%)

Hemoptysis (27%)

Pleuritic friction rub (17%)

From Wenger NK, Stein PD, Willis PW III. Massive acute pulmonary embolism: The deceivingly nonspecific manifestations. JAMA 1972;220:843.

Table 45.3 Laboratory Findings in 50 Patients with Pulmonary Embolization

Arterial P$_{O_2}$ <80 mm Hg (100%)

Perfusion defect on lung scan (100%)

Serum LDH >231 Wacker U/mL (83%)

Chest x-ray: abnormal vessel patterns, infiltrates, fluid, or elevated diaphragm (71%)

SGOT <33 Henry U/mL (60%)

Bilirubin > 1.0 mg/dL (21%) Electrocardiogram: right axis shift, S Q$_3$ T$_3$, or new incomplete right bundle branch block (19%)

From Szucs MM Jr, Brooks HL, Grossman W, et al. Diagnostic sensitivity of laboratory findings in acute pulmonary embolism. Ann Intern Med 1971;74:161.

Table 45.4   Management of Pulmonary Embolus

Give 5,000–10,000 units of heparin IV initially and then repeat every 4–6 hours.

Maintain whole blood clotting time at two to three times normal or the activated partial thromboplastin time at one and a half to two times normal.

Constant infusion of approximately 1,000 U of heparin hourly is acceptable. Monitor the same way.

Watch for hemorrhagic complications.

Order O_2 and mild sedation.

If repeated embolization occurs while the patient is on anticoagulant therapy interrupt the inferior vena cava and possibly the left ovarian vein surgically.

---

repeat doses commonly 5,000–7,000 U. Continuous administration uses an initial bolus of 5,000 U, followed by continuous infusion of approximately 1,000 U/h. Some clinicians maintain that this method provides adequate anticoagulation while minimizing risk of hemorrhagic complications (12).

The anticoagulation effects of heparin can be monitored by whole-blood clotting time, activated partial thromboplastin time, or actual plasma heparin level. Generally, whole-blood clotting time should be two or three times the control value. Activated partial thromboplastin time should be one and a half or two times the control value, and plasma heparin concentration about 0.3 U/mL.

Regardless of which monitoring method is used, it is necessary to make repeated hematocrit determinations, examine urine and stools for blood, and check for hemorrhagic complications. One can also treat pulmonary embolization with oxygen. It may be necessary to allay the patient's anxiety with some form of sedation.

Surgical removal is usually reserved for cases in which the pulmonary embolus is large enough to be immediately life-threatening. Interruption of the venous system to prevent embolization may be necessary in patients who have had recurrent emboli while receiving anticoagulant therapy.

Interruption or blockade of the inferior vena cava may be sufficient if the embolus originated in the lower extremities. However, if its source is the pelvis, the left ovarian

vein should also be ligated. Various methods are available for interrupting a vena cava, including complete ligation, Teflon clips, and devices inserted transvenously, such as umbrella and Greenfield filters. Some form of anticoagulation should be maintained for six months after a pulmonary embolus (10). Usually, heparin is given for 10–14 days, followed by warfarin. However, warfarin is contraindicated in pregnant patients, in whom some form of heparin therapy should be continued.

Aspiration Pneumonitis

The most common cause of death from anesthesia among pregnant patients is aspiration pneumonitis. Indeed, aspiration of liquid gastric contents as a cause of respiratory insufficiency was first recognized in obstetric patients (13). Although typically the patient has received a general anesthetic, this syndrome also may accompany heavy sedation with narcotics or barbiturates.

Pathophysiology consists of a chemical pneumonitis caused by the acid of gastric secretion. If liquid with a pH of less than 2.5 is aspirated, the syndrome can occur, although onset may be delayed for several hours (14). Physical examination usually reveals pulmonary rales and ronchi. Chest x-rays commonly show diffuse patchy infiltrates, which may be localized to the most dependent lung area at time of inhalation, usually the right lower lobe (14). Arterial P_{CO_2} is low, and serial hematocrits may rise as plasma enters the lungs.

Successful treatment depends on prompt recognition that aspiration has occurred (Table 45.5). If aspiration is observed, intubation and suctioning of the tracheobronchial

---

Table 45.5   Management of Aspiration Pneumonitis

Perform endotracheal suction if aspiration is noted.

Infuse with hydrocortisone 1 g IV at once and q 4 h.

Give intermittent positive pressure breathing with O_2.

Monitor arterial blood gases (patient may need intubation or tracheostomy).

Give aminophylline 250–500 mg in 50 mL of D_5W over 20 minutes for bronchospasm.

Consider antibiotics to prevent secondary infections.

tree is safe and effective in removing the vomitus (14). Most physicians disapprove of lavage because it can carry vomitus further into the tracheobronchial tree. When aspiration is suspected, massive doses of corticosteroids may be lifesaving. IV infusion of 1 g or more of hydrocortisone should be done at once and repeated every four hours for several days.

Positive pressure administration of 100% O_2 is also of great value in therapy. Monitoring arterial blood gases will assess adequacy of treatment. If it proves inadequate, intubation or tracheostomy may be necessary (14).

Aminophylline (250–500 mg in 50 mL of 5% dextrose in water) infused for 20 minutes may be useful in relieving bronchospasm. The role of antibiotics in preventing possible late infections is uncertain at present.

Prevention includes a magnesium hydroxide or magnesium trisilicate antacid (30 mL orally every 2–3 hours) preoperatively to neutralize gastric acidity. However, if aspirated, the colloidal antacids can themselves cause a chemical pneumonitis. Clear antacids (sodium citrate) may be preferable. Nasogastric suction before induction of general anesthesia can remove surprisingly large volumes of gastric secretions and minimize risk of aspiration syndrome. Use of cuffed endotracheal tubes by skilled anesthesiologists is also very important in preventing aspiration in patients who have been given general anesthesia.

Table 45.6 Management of Pulmonary Edema

Have patient in sitting position.

Administer morphine 5 mg IV or 10–15 mg IM.

Give intermittent positive pressure breathing with O_2.

Infuse furosemide 40 mg IV slowly (may repeat).

Give digoxin 0.5 mg IV, then 0.125 mg IV q 2 h for total of six doses.

Consider phlebotomy.

Give hydralazine 5–10 mg IV, 10 mg IM, or constant IV infusion as needed to keep diastolic pressure between 90 and 110 mm Hg.

Continue medical management if patient has valvular heart disease.

Deliver toxemic patient as soon as she is out of pulmonary edema.

Pulmonary Edema

Patients with acute pulmonary edema present true medical emergencies. Symptoms typically are suffocating dyspnea, tachypnea, apprehension, and labored breathing. Physical examination shows diffuse rales and frothy, possibly blood-tinged, sputum. Chest roentgenograms usually indicate diffuse or peripheral infiltrates in both lung fields.

Pulmonary edema develops in obstetric patients in several ways. Women with underlying cardiac valvular disease may go into left heart failure, causing pressure to rise in the left atrium, and consequently in the pulmonary venous and capillary systems. When intravascular pressure in the lung rises above the colloidal osmotic pressure (COP), free fluid leaves the vessels and enters the alveoli and terminal bronchioles, causing pulmonary edema.

Additionally, pulmonary edema may develop in a patient who has severe preeclampsia, usually superimposed on chronic hypertension, and who experiences heart failure because of the extra work load on the heart. Eclamptic patients with relatively normal cardiac function may also develop pulmonary edema if COP decreases until it is no longer sufficient to overcome normal pulmonary capillary pressure (15). The usual cause of decrease in COP is hypoalbuminemia. Pulmonary edema caused by low COP has also been observed in nonobstetric patients with no evidence of heart failure who have received excessive amounts of IV crystalloid solutions (16).

Treatment of pulmonary edema involves placing the patient in a sitting position, giving morphine (5 mg IV or 10–15 mg IM) to relieve anxiety, and administering oxygen by positive pressure to raise pleural pressure and decrease venous return to the heart (Table 45.6). Furosemide (Lasix), which is of great value in treating acute pulmonary edema, has two distinct actions. First, it decreases venous tone and promotes pooling of blood in the extremities to reduce blood return to the heart (17, 18). Second, it promotes a decrease of blood volume by diuresis. It should be given as a 40-mg, slow IV injection.

Rapid digitalization of the patient with acute pulmonary edema is not judged as important now as formerly, because of the development of powerful diuretics (19). If the patient is not receiving digitalis, digitalization may be achieved with digoxin (Lanoxin), started at 0.5 mg IV. Six additional doses of digoxin (0.125 mg IV) are then given at two-hour intervals (18, 19).

When the clinician believes that severe hypertension is contributing to pulmonary edema, blood pressure should be lowered carefully with hydralazine (Apresoline). One may give this agent as a 5- to 10-mg IV injection, as a 10-mg IM injection, or as a constant IV infusion to lower diastolic pressure to 90–110 mm Hg.

It is also possible to decrease venous return to the heart by phlebotomy. The blood should be saved in blood bank collection bags so that the packed cells can be transfused back to the patient. Rotating of tourniquets, which requires constant attention to avoid compromising the extremities, is thought to be of little value in deceasing cardiac return.

Because furosemide is a potent diuretic, monitoring should include hourly measurement of urinary output and frequent electrolyte level determinations. Arterial blood gas measurements and electrocardiograms should also be monitored. Checking central venous pressure is helpful only in cases where it is elevated. Often, it is within normal limits. If available, flow-directed catheters should be used to observe pulmonary artery wedge pressure. This examination can provide a clue to the pathophysiology of pulmonary edema in a particular patient. An increased pressure (more than 15 mm Hg) may be due to fluid overload, left ventricular failure, or stenotic left ventricular outflow, whereas pressure below 5 mm Hg reflects decreased blood volume, as in preeclampsia.

Measuring plasma COP is valuable for the occasional patient who has pulmonary edema resulting from an abnormally low COP. In this situation, using an albumin infusion along with furosemide might be considered (15).

When the patient is out of danger from pulmonary edema, future management depends on etiology. If valvular heart disease is present, the obstetrician may allow the pregnancy to continue after consultation with a cardiologist. However, an eclamptic patient with acute pulmonary edema should have her pregnancy terminated as soon as possible after the pulmonary edema has improved.

Amniotic Fluid Embolus

Sudden onset of dyspnea accompanied by cyanosis, vomiting, restlessness, shock, coagulopathy, or uterine atony in a patient in active labor or the early puerperium should suggest embolization of amniotic fluid. This catastrophe usually occurs in older parous patients at term or in postdate patients who have hypertonic labors. Frequently, the fetus is large, and meconium may be present in the amniotic fluid, or the fetus may be dead (20).

Because pathophysiology is not completely defined, therapy is empiric (3). We believe that infusion of amniotic fluid into the vascular system has two effects. One is physical plugging of the pulmonary vascular system by debris, which causes acute cor pulmonale with hypoxemia, dyspnea, tachypnea, pulmonary hypertension, tachycardia, and pulmonary edema (20). The second is development of a coagulopathy commonly associated with uterine atony.

Laboratory findings usually show right heart strain on electrocardiogram (ECG) and low PCO_2 and fibrinogen, and the chest x-ray ordinarily reveals diffuse pulmonary infiltrates. Because 80% of cases are fatal (25% within one hour), diagnosis is often made postmortem, when fetal squames, lanugo, fat, and mucin are found in the pulmonary vasculature (20). More recently, diagnosis has been confirmed in surviving patients by a finding of amniotic fluid debris in central venous blood (21).

Treatment is nonspecific and directed at relieving pulmonary vascular spasm and improving oxygenation while combating coagulopathy and uterine atony (Table 45.7). The patient should be sitting and receiving oxygen by intermittent positive pressure. Morphine (5 mg IV or 10–15 mg IM) may help relieve dyspnea and anxiety. Aminophylline (250–500 mg in 50 mL of 5% dextrose in water) infused for 20 minutes can relieve bronchospasm, as well as vascular spasm. Rapid digitalization with 0.5 mg of digoxin IV, followed by 0.125 mg IV every two hours for six does, improves cardiac contractility. IV infusion of 1 g of hydrocortisone should be started and followed by 250 mg every four hours.

There is some disagreement about management of atony and coagulopathy. Typically, patients have uterine atony and are hemorrhaging. However, blood replacement is difficult because of mechanical blockage in the pulmonary vasculature (20). Because aggressive transfusion therapy can worsen acute cor pulmonale, it is wise to try

Table 45.7 Management of Amniotic Fluid Embolus

Have patient in sitting position.

Inject morphine 5–15 mg IM.

Give intermittent positive pressure breathing with O_2.

Give 250–500 mg of aminophylline in 50 mL of D_5W over 20 minutes.

Give digoxin 0.5 mg IV; then 0.125 mg IV q 2 h for six doses.

Order hydrocortisone 1 g IV; follow with 250 mg q 4 h.

Compress uterus to control atony.

Make judicious use of blood transfusion therapy.

Combat coagulopathy with fresh frozen plasma, cryoprecipitate, or both.

---

controlling the atony by manual compression and judicious transfusion. Prostaglandin analogs (15-methyl-prostaglandin $F_{2\alpha}$) may help promote uterine contractility.

Heparin therapy has been advocated in treating coagulopathy (21). However, this approach is controversial, and most prefer to use cryoprecipitate and fresh frozen plasma (22).

Hypotension

Septic Shock

Pregnant women are virtually the only immunologically competent adults under age 40 who develop septic shock (23, 24). Septic abortion was traditionally the most common cause. With the decline of illegal abortions, most cases are now associated with chorioamnionitis, pyelonephritis, or puerperal infections.

Gram-negative organisms are responsible for most cases of septic shock. The immediate effects of gram-negative bacteremia are decreased systemic vascular resistance and central venous pressure and increased cardiac output (25). Onset of shock causes pooling of blood in the venous capacitance bed, which in turn, reduces effective blood volume and decreases cardiac output. Decreased tissue perfusion and oxygenation promote anaerobic metabolism and the rise of blood lactate levels (24).

Typically, septic shock is heralded by a shaking chill and fever. In the early stages, there is hypotension, although the patient's skin is warm and dry and the pulse full (26). Neutropenia and leukopenia are often noted (23). Later, the patient develops leukocytosis, cold skin, weak pulse, pallor or cyanosis, and oliguria. Lactic acid accumulation causes a decline in arterial pH. ECGs may reveal changes in the ST segment and T wave resulting from poor coronary perfusion (23).

Management must start with the correct antibiotic (23). Cultures obtained before starting therapy should come from the suspected source of infection, as well as from blood. Three blood cultures may be taken simultaneously from a single venipuncture site. There is no particular advantage in obtaining blood cultures during a chill or a temperature spike (24).

The initial choice of antibiotic is based on the suspected pathogen. Multiple drug therapy is therefore usually necessary. Penicillin, which may be administered by IV infusion in dosages of 3,000,000–5,000,000 U every four hours, is effective against all gram-positive organisms and anaerobes except *Staphylococcus aureus* and *Bacteroides fragilis*. Kanamycin (Kantrex, Kantrim, Klebcil) or gentamicin (Bristagen, Garamycin) is usually effective against gram-negative enteric organisms (Table 45.8). The first dose of either agent may be given as 7.5 mg/kg of body weight IM every 12 hours for kanamycin or 1–1.7 mg/kg IM every eight hours for gentamicin. Subsequent dosages depend on the patient's renal function, which is often impaired in septic shock.

Table 45.8 Administration of Kanamycin and Gentamicin

	Standard Dose	Route and Frequency
Kanamycin	15 mg/kg/day	7.5 mg/kg q 12 h IM
Gentamicin	3–5 mg/kg/day	1–1.7 mg/kg q 8 h IM

For patients with impaired renal function:

Kanamycin—Multiply serum creatinine concentration (mg/dL) by 9 to obtain time interval (in hours) for injections of 7.5 mg/kg (not more frequently than q 12 h).

Gentamicin—Multiply serum creatinine concentration (mg/dL) by 8 to obtain frequency of injections, or divide total scheduled dose by serum creatinine concentration and repeat this lower dose q 8 h.

Table 45.9 Initial Antibiotic Treatment for Septic Shock

Drug	Dosage	Route	Frequency
Penicillin	3,000,000–5,000,000 units	IV infusion	q 4 h
Kanamycin or	7.5 mg/kg	IM	q 12 h (see Table 45.8)
gentamicin	1–1.7 mg/kg	IM	q 8 h (see Table 45.8)
If *Bacteroides fragilis* is suspected:			
Clindamycin or	600 mg in 100 mL over 20 minutes	IV infusion	q 8 h
Chloramphenicol	12.5 mg/kg	IV infusion	q 6 h, for a total dose of 50 mg/kg/day

Note: Patients allergic to penicillin or with suspected *Staphylococcus aureus* infection may be given clindamycin, but this therapy is ineffective against enterococci. Therefore, vancomycin should be added if enterococci are suspected.

Clindamycin (Cleocin) may be substituted for penicillin when the patient is allergic to penicillin or when *S aureus* or *B fragilis* is suspected (Table 45.9). However, because clindamycin is not effective against enterococci, vancomycin (Vancocin) should be given in dosages of 500 mg IV for 30 minutes every six hours if infection by enterococci is suspected, until cultures are reported. Clindamycin may be given by IV infusion of 600 mg in 100 mL of diluent during a 20-minute period and repeated every eight hours.

Chloramphenicol (Chloromycetin) may also be used for suspected *B Fragilis* infection. Dosage by IV infusion is 12.5 mg/kg every six hours for a total dose of 50 mg/kg/day.

Infusion of IV fluids is the second important treatment modality. Some invasive means of monitoring this therapy is necessary. Catheters in the cardiovascular system allow rapid measurement of the effects of fluid replacement and a more aggressive approach, since as much as 15% of the patient's body weight may need to be replaced with IV fluids.

In the patient without underlying cardiac disease, measurement of central venous pressure can be an adequate guide to fluid replacement. However, central venous catheterization is being replaced by balloon flotation (Swan-Ganz) catheters. These catheters measure pulmonary artery wedge pressure, which is identical to left atrial pressure and can be used to evaluate the heart's ability to handle a fluid load (27). The fluid challenge test, popularized by Weil, is used for patients in shock (Table 45.10) (24, 28, 29).

A collection bag should be used to remove blood by phlebotomy in case of fluid overload. Blood should be given if there is evidence of blood loss. To keep fluid from moving out of the vascular system and into the tissues (including the lungs), colloidal osmotic pressure should be maintained. This may be done by measuring it or by giving one-third to one-half of the IV fluids as colloid solutions.

Table 45.10 Fluid Challenge Test

Initial Central Venous Pressure (cm H$_2$O)	Initial Pulmonary Wedge Pressure (mm Hg)	Infuse in 10 minutes (mL)
<10	<12	200
10–15	12–20	100
>15	>20	50

Evaluation of Fluid Challenge

CVP Rise (cm H$_2$O)	Wedge Pressure Rise (mm Hg)	Action
>5	>7	Stop infusion
2–5	3–7	Wait and reevaluate
<2	<3	Repeat fluid challenge

From Gordon M, Niswander KR, Berendes H, et al. Fetal morbidity following potentially anoxigenic obstetric conditions. VII. Bronchial asthma. Am J Obstet Gynecol 1970;106:421; Grant JA. Bronchial asthma. Texas Med 1978;74:37; and Schatz M, Patterson R, Zeitz S, et al. Corticosteroid therapy for the pregnant asthmatic patient. JAMA 1975;233:804.

Table 45.11 Management of Septic Shock

Take cultures of blood and infected material: uterus, sputum, and pus.

Administer antibiotics: broad-spectrum coverage as per Table 45.9 with the precautions noted in Table 45.8.

Replace fluid using standard monitoring techniques.

Possibly use vasoactive drugs: Isoproterenol 1 mg in 500 mL; give 0.5–5.0 μg/kg/minute. Dopamine 200 mg in 500 mL; start at 2–5 μg/kg/minute.

Monitor CBC, ECG, arterial blood gases, urine output, clotting time, COP, and electrolytes.

Administer O_2 by mask.

Possibly give digoxin 0.5 mg IV, followed by 0.125 mg IV q 2 h for six doses.

Surgery may be necessary to remove or drain source of infection.

COP—colloidal osmotic pressure.

Overly vigorous fluid administration with crystalloids has been reported to decrease COP sufficiently to cause pulmonary edema in patients without heart failure (16).

Corticosteroids are generally not recommended in management of septic shock (Table 45.11). A recent prospective, randomized, double-blind, placebo-controlled trial of 382 patients concluded that the use of high-dose corticosteroids provided no benefit in the treatment of septic shock (30).

Although vasoactive drugs should not be used routinely to treat septic shock, they can be helpful if the measures already discussed have not reversed peripheral vasoconstriction (31). Isoproterenol, a selective β-adrenergic stimulant, increases heart rate, strength of contraction, venous return, and cardiac output, while decreasing peripheral resistance. Although all these effects are beneficial, they also increase the metabolic rate and, if oxygen demands are unmet, can increase lactic acidemia. Isoproterenol is usually given as 1 mg in 500 mL of fluid in a slow IV drip at approximately 0.5–5 μg/kg/min.

Dopamine hydrochloride (Intropin) is a relatively new sympathomimetic amine used to treat shock (32, 33). It has both α- and β-adrenergic effects, which are dose-dependent (31–33). At 1–2 μg/kg/min, it increases urinary output and improves renal and mesenteric blood flow. At 2–1 μg/kg/min, it increases cardiac output with little increas in heart rate. Above 10 μg/kg/min, it may stimulate α adrenergic receptors and produce vasoconstriction.

Initial treatment of shock with dopamine starts wit infusion of 2–5 μg/kg/min. Rates should be increase slowly until the desired effect is attained. Most patien respond well at infusion rates below 20 μg/kg/min (32 33). The infusion should be prepared as 200 mg of dopa mine in 500 mL of saline. The appropriate rate should b maintained once it is achieved.

It may also be necessary to monitor arterial blood gase because some patients with septic shock develop hypox emia that can be resistant to oxygen therapy. In additior digitalization, which may be needed to improve myocardi contractility, can be achieved by using 0.5 mg IV of digoxir followed by 0.125 mg IV every two hours for six doses.

Management of coagulopathy is somewhat controver sial. Replacement of blood loss with fresh whole blood c packed cells and fresh frozen plasma, combined with vigor ous treatment of the infection, will suffice as treatment fc most cases.

Finally, there is a definite role for surgery. If the uteru contains the source of infection, it should be emptied as soo as possible after antibiotic treatment and volume replace ment. If emptying does not suffice, hysterectomy may b necessary. Abscesses should be drained or excised. Manage ment of symptoms with the Trendelenburg position, blar kets, and vasoactive drugs has very limited effectiveness (28).

Conduction Anesthesia

Hypotension induced by conduction anesthesia (spina epidural, or caudal block) is second only to aspiration pneu monitis as a cause of maternal mortality from anesthesi (34). One reason that pregnant women have an exaggerate response to vasomotor blockage is that, during pregnancy vascular tone depends more on sympathetic control. Aortc caval compression by the large gravid uterus when th patient is supine exaggerates peripheral trapping of blooc In addition, the large amount of blood in the gravid uteru adds to peripheral entrapment of blood (35).

Normovolemic hypotension induced by a spinal bloc becomes apparent within five minutes and reaches its max mum during the next 10–12 minutes. Blockage at the T_{10} level is all that is necessary. The patient usually feels uneasy and nauseous and may vomit or lose consciousness. She becomes pale, her systolic pressure drops below 100 mm Hg, and her pulse slows as a result of vagal stimulation associated with markedly reduced venous filling of the heart. Initial fetal tachycardia is followed by bradycardia and fetal death if there is prolonged insufficient placental gas exchange. Onset of symptoms and signs is slower after epidural or caudal block.

Pregnant patients receiving conduction anesthesia should be watched for hypotension. With proper precautions, conduction anesthesia should not produce fatal maternal hypotension. An infusion of 800 mL to 1 L of a balanced salt solution (500 mL over 10 minutes) before placing the anesthetic block will compensate for the volume of blood (16% of total volume) trapped in the lower extremities after the block (Table 45.12).

Because nearly 75% of all pregnant women have impaired venous return in the supine position even without anesthesia, one must displace the uterus laterally after placing the block and before moving the patient into the supine position. Displacement is accomplished either by a mechanical device or by placing a wedge under one hip. If the block is placed just before delivery, the patient should be observed carefully for 15 minutes before the baby is delivered. Hypotension is unlikely to occur after this time.

If placement in the lateral recumbent position or rapid volume expansion with an infusion of balanced salt solution and lateral displacement of the uterus do not prevent or relieve the hypotension after a block, a vasopressor may be used. Most of these decrease placental blood flow by constricting uterine arterioles. Ephedrine, which does not pro-

duce any harmful effects on the fetus, is the vasopressor of choice (36). It should be given IV as a bolus of 12.5–25 mg, repeating the dose every 15–30 minutes until hypotension is relieved.

In addition, the level of anesthesia should be checked in hypotensive patients because the level may be high enough to require respiratory support. With thoughtful preanesthetic management, hypotension secondary to conduction anesthesia should be very uncommon.

Anaphylactic Shock

Even on a busy obstetrics service, anaphylactic shock is relatively rare. However, it can have fatal results. In most cases, anaphylaxis follows parenteral injection of a drug such as penicillin or procaine hydrochloride. Ensuing onset, progression, and duration of symptoms are all highly variable.

The symptom complex includes at least some of the following: conjunctivitis, rhinitis, pilomotor erection, pruritic urticaria, angioedema, various gastrointestinal disturbances (usually diarrhea), laryngeal edema, bronchospasm, hypotension, cardiac arrhythmias, cardiac arrest, and coma. Anaphylaxis may be limited to a single symptom or may rapidly progress to cardiovascular and respiratory collapse and death. In fatal anaphylaxis, laryngeal edema and acute emphysema are the predominant findings (37, 38).

Parenteral injection of antigen may cause a reaction in 5–60 minutes, although most reactions occur within 30 minutes. The reaction may continue for a few minutes or days (39).

The inciting antigen causes the release of IgE antibodies, which attach to the cell membranes of circulating basophils and tissue mast cells, causing release of the two chemical mediators of anaphylaxis, histamine and SRS-A (slow-reacting substance of anaphylaxis), a lipid (38, 40). Both cause bronchiolar constriction and increased capillary permeability, and histamine also causes vasodilation. Although other substances have been implicated in the anaphylactic response, only these two have been proved to cause it (41).

Any sign of an anaphylactic response must be treated promptly and vigorously to prevent respiratory and cardiovascular collapse. The release of the chemical mediators of

---

Table 45.12 Management of Hypotension after Conduction Anesthesia

Displace uterus laterally if patient is supine.

Increase IV infusion of balanced salt solution (>500 mL).

Give ephedrine 12.5–25 mg IV.

Be prepared to support respiration if high spinal level is obtained.

anaphylaxis is an energy-dependent process related to alterations of intracellular 3', 5'-cyclic adenosine monophosphate (cAMP). An increase in intracellular cAMP will inhibit the release of histamine and SRS-A. β-agonists activate the adenylate cyclase system, increasing intracellular cAMP. Epinephrine, an agent that has both α- and β-agonistic activity, is the drug of choice in the treatment of anaphylaxis (Table 45.13). Its beneficial therapeutic effects are related to the α and β effects on the heart, lungs, and peripheral vasculature, as well as to the β effect on the chemical mediator release. However, epinephrine given late in the reaction may be ineffective.

As soon as any sign of anaphylaxis is diagnosed, 0.3–0.4 mL of a 1:1,000 solution of epinephrine should be administered IM and repeated in 5–10 minutes as needed. Should the patient fail to respond, 0.1–0.2 mL of 1:1,000 epinephrine diluted in 10 mL of saline should be given slowly IV, monitoring for cardiac arrhythmias. If the antigen was administered as an IM injection in an extremity, a tourniquet may be placed proximal to the injection site for 15 minutes and then 0.1–0.2 mL of 1:1,000 epinephrine solution may be injected at the same site.

Antihistamines appear to act as competitive inhibitors of histamine at the target cells and not through the cAMP system. These agents can be used in all forms of anaphylaxis. Diphenhydramine hydrochloride (Benadryl) can be given IV in a 60- to 80-mg dose for 3–4 minutes or IM. Although this dose can be repeated in 4–6 hours as needed, it must not exceed a total of 5 mg/kg of body weight daily.

Methylxanthines, such as aminophylline, are potent bronchodilators that act to increase cardiac output through direct action on myocardial contractility. They are also potent vasodilators.

Methylxanthines inhibit phosphodiesterase degradation of cAMP and thus increase cAMP levels. However, because of their unpredictable cardiovascular effects and possible potentiation of hypotension, they are used only when bronchospasm is present and after hypotension has been corrected. Moreover, they are used only if epinephrine has failed to reverse bronchospasm. In these circumstances, aminophylline is administered as a 250- to 500-mg dose in 10–20 mL saline infused IV for five minutes. To shorten the anaphylactic reaction, 100–250 mg of hydrocortisone sodium succinate (Solu-Cortef) should be given in water or IV after epinephrine and antihistamine medications.

During drug administration, the patient's legs should be elevated and an airway established by endotracheal intubation or a tracheostomy to protect against laryngeal edema. Oxygen should be dispensed at a rate of 4–5 L/min.

If epinephrine injections fail to correct hypotension, a balanced salt solution IV may be given to expand intravascular volume. Vasopressors such as levarterenol (Levophed 4 mg/L of dextrose and water) may be given as a continuous titration to help maintain blood pressure.

Table 45.13 Management of Anaphylactic Shock

Give epinephrine (1:1,000 solution) 0.3–0.4 mL IM. Repeat in 5–10 minutes. If no response, give 0.1–0.2 mL (1:1,000 solution) in 10 mL saline *slowly* IV. Watch for cardiac arrhythmia.

Give diphenhydramine hydrochloride 60–80 mg IV for 3–4 minutes or IM to all patients with anaphylaxis.

Elevate legs.

Establish adequate airway and administer oxygen 4–5 L/min.

For bronchospasm without hypotension and unresponsive to epinephrine, give aminophylline 250–500 mg in 10–20 mL saline IV for 5 minutes.

Administer IV fluids to correct hypovolemia.

Give vasopressors to elevate blood pressure (levarterenol 4 mg/L fluid—titrate IV).

Give hydrocortisone sodium succinate 100–250 mg in water or saline IV.

Convulsions

Eclampsia

The two most serious causes of seizures during pregnancy are eclampsia and thrombosis of either the cortical longitudinal venous sinus or its large contributory veins. However, thrombosis is quite rare. A primigravida or chronically hypertensive patient with associated hypertension of pregnancy, proteinuria, and edema who develops monocloni seizures during the late antepartum, intrapartum, or earl postpartum period is presumed to have eclampsia. An accurate history is most important in distinguishing between eclamptic seizures and noneclamptic seizures. If the patient does not show any lateralizing neurologic signs, she should be treated for eclampsia.

Because the seizure activity of eclampsia is related to intense arteriolar vasospasm, magnesium sulfate is the anticonvulsant of choice (Table 45.14). The magnesium ion acts as a neuromuscular blocker by interfering with the release of acetylcholine at the motor end plate (42). However, its antiseizure activity is central, and the mechanism is not yet understood.

After establishing an airway and administering oxygen, a therapeutic blood level of 4–6 mEq/L of $MgSO_4$ should be created quickly and maintained. (This standard procedure comes from Pritchard's successful management of 154 consecutive eclamptic patients (43).) The result is a modest relaxation of arteriolar smooth muscle. More important, IV administration of 20 mL of a 20% $MgSO_4$ solution (4 g) for not less than three minutes achieves ablation of neuromuscular seizure activity. Shortly thereafter, 10 mL of a 50% $MgSO_4$ solution (5 g) should be given IM deep into the upper outer quadrant of each buttock, using a 3-inch, 20-gauge needle.

These maneuvers will quickly establish and maintain a therapeutic blood level of $MgSO_4$ solution for about four hours (44). A repeat maintenance dose of 10 mL of 50% $MgSO_4$ solution (5 g) is given IM every four hours, provided the patient has deep-tendon reflexes and normal respiratory rate and has had a urinary output of at least 100 mL over the previous four hours. The current popular maintenance regimen for $MgSO_4$ is constant IV infusion of 2 g hourly by pump maintained until 24 hours postpartum (45).

If another convulsion occurs within 20 minutes of the initial IV dose of $MgSO_4$, more drug should not be given. If it occurs thereafter, another 20 mL of a 20% $MgSO_4$ solution (4 g) should be given IV over at least three minutes. If the patient is small, only half the dosage should be given. Convulsions that cannot be controlled by this regimen should be treated with 250 mg of sodium amobarbital administered IV over at least three minutes.

If the therapeutic level of $MgSO_4$ is exceeded, respiratory depression can readily occur. The deep-tendon reflexes usually disappear (at 8 mEq/L) before respiration ceases. These depressant effects can be quickly reversed by administering 10 mL of 10% calcium gluconate IV over at least three minutes. Once the eclamptic seizures are controlled and the patient is conscious, the baby can be delivered appropriately.

Epilepsy

Increased frequency of epileptic seizures in late pregnancy can be associated with fluid retention and sudden weight gain. During labor, delivery, and the early puerperium, they can be associated with IM administration of anticonvulsants or withholding of anticonvulsant medication.

Therapeutic blood levels of phenytoin may not be achieved by IM injection because of erratic absorption (46). The IV route is preferred when parenteral administration of anticonvulsants is required.

When an epileptic patient has a succession of monoclonic seizures, prompt IV medication is necessary. After establishing an airway and administering oxygen, the physician can administer IV 150–250 mg of phenytoin (Dilantin) at a rate of 50 mg/min (Table 45.15). Initially, higher dosages are used if the patient has not received maintenance

---

Table 45.14 Management of Eclampsia

Establish airway and give O_2.

Give 20 mL of 20% magnesium sulfate solution (4 g) IV over not less than 3 minutes.*

Inject 20 mL of 50% $MgSO_4$ solution, one half (5 g) into upper outer quadrant of each buttock, using 3-inch, 20-gauge needle. Give a repeat maintenance dose of 10 mL of 50% $MgSO_4$ solution (5 g) IM every 4 hours, if not contraindicated.

If another convulsion occurs within 20 minutes of the first IV dose, do nothing; if it occurs more than 20 minutes after the first IV dose, give 20 mL of 20% $MgSO_4$ solution (4 g) IV over not less than 3 minutes. Give only 2 g of solution if patient is unusually small.

If convulsions persist despite steps above, give sodium amobarbital or phenobarbital up to 250 mg slowly IV.

If respiratory depression develops, give 10 mL of 10% calcium gluconate IV over 3 minutes.

*20 mL of 20% $MgSO_4$ solution can be made by mixing in a syringe 8 mL of 50% $MgSO_4$ solution and 12 mL of sterile distilled water.

recently. If seizure activity persists, 150–400 mg of pheno-barbital or amobarbital IV can be given at a rate of 50 mg/min. These drugs can be lethal if given too rapidly or as overdoses. Therapeutic blood serum levels are 10–25 µg/mL for phenytoin and 15–30 µg/mL for phenobarbital. The total 24-hour dosage for either should not exceed 1 g (46).

Diazepam is also a powerful anticonvulsant. However, the wisdom of using it to treat a pregnant patient about to deliver is debatable. Diazepam crosses the placenta and can cause generalized hypotonia and even respiratory depression in the newborn, who requires several days to metabolize it. If used, diazepam should be given IV, in 5- to 10-mg doses, at a rate of 1–5 mg/min. These amounts can be repeated every 30 minutes to a total dose of 100 mg daily. One must watch for respiratory depression.

Local Anesthetics

The physician administering local anesthetics by either paracervical or pudendal block can produce toxic levels in the central nervous system (CNS) either by inadvertently infiltrating a vessel or, more commonly, by giving more than the recommended maximum dosages (47). When toxic levels of anesthetic drugs are reached, the patient may show the prodromal symptoms and signs of garrulousness, circumoral numbness and tingling, diplopia, and tinnitus. Shortly thereafter, muscular twitching and tremors will herald generalized myoclonic seizures. Cardiovascular and respiratory collapse may then occur.

Any obstetrician administering local anesthetics must be aware of the toxic syndrome and be prepared immediately to use all methods of resuscitation (Table 45.16). The

safest maximum dosage of a single injection of lidocaine (Xylocaine) is 4–7 mg/kg, and of mepivacaine (Carbocaine, Polocaine), 2–3 mg/kg (48). The patient should be aspirated before injecting local anesthetic drugs. Waiting five minutes between injections of a block is also highly recommended (47). Finally, note that patients receiving phenytoin therapy may be more susceptible to a toxic reaction because the drug is protein-bound and competes for binding protein with the local anesthetic (49).

Successful treatment depends on early recognition and prompt initiation of therapy. One must first stop injection of the offending drug and then administer oxygen. If muscular twitching is encountered, 5–10 mg of diazepam (Valium) can be given IV at a rate of 1–5 mg/min or 75–150 mg of thiopental, thiamylal sodium (Surital), or sodium pentobarbital (Nembutal) IV for several minutes. If convulsions appear and continue despite this treatment, 40–60 mg of succinylcholine chloride (Anectine) can be given either IV or IM and the patient intubated. The cardiovascular system can be supported with balanced salt fluids. Vasopressor drugs such as ephedrine (12.5–25 mg IV) can help maintain normal blood pressure. Cardiopulmonary resuscitation may be necessary.

As long as the fetal heart rate is normal and there is no evidence of fetal distress, delivery need not be immediate. In fact, because of the difference of blood volume on each side of the placenta, level of local anesthetic will diffuse

---

Table 45.15 Management of Epilepsy

Establish airway and give O₂.

Give phenytoin 150–250 mg IV at rate of 50 mg/min.

Give phenobarbital or amobarbital 150–400 mg IV at rate of 50 mg/min. With continued seizures, give 50 mg/min until seizure stops or total dose of 1 g is given.

Give diazepam 5–10 mg IV at rate of 1–5 mg/min. Repeat in 30 minutes. Do not exceed total dose of 100 mg/day.

Table 45.16 Management of Toxic Reaction to Local Anesthetics

Stop injection of anesthetic agent with the appearance of any prodrome.

Give O₂ by mask.

If there is muscular twitching or tremors, give diazepam 5–10 mg IV or a rapid-acting barbiturate 75–150 mg IV.

If convulsions persist, start endotracheal intubation with succinylcholine 40–60 mg IV or IM and 100% O₂.

Be prepared to administer cardiopulmonary resuscitation.

Support cardiovascular system with IV fluids and vasopressors, such as ephedrine (12.5–25 mg IV).

back into the maternal side and act as an exchange mechanism for the fetus.

If the toxic reaction occurs when delivery is imminent and it is determined that the fetus is in distress, delivery should proceed. A pediatric team should be prepared to perform exchange infusions to lower neonatal drug level as quickly as possible.

CASE 45.1 Asthmatic Patient

A 28-year-old primigravida had been asthmatic since the age of 18 months and had required corticosteroid therapy to control her asthmatic attacks.

She began experiencing difficulty breathing at 16 weeks' gestation and made numerous visits to physicians and hospital emergency rooms without symptomatic relief. A physician told her she "looked cyanotic" and needed to be hospitalized.

At 20 weeks' gestation, the patient was seen in the emergency room in respiratory distress. She was cyanotic and tachypneic, and her lungs were "tight" and full of wheezes. Fundal height was 20 cm above the symphysis. Arterial blood gases were reported as PO_2 45 mm Hg and PCO_2 55 mm Hg; pH was 7.32.

The patient was hospitalized and treated vigorously with IV aminophylline, IV fluids, and positive pressure oxygen. Three hours later, blood gas tests were repeated, and PCO_2 was 63 mm Hg. She was transferred to the medical intensive care unit, where endotracheal intubation and positive pressure ventilation were accomplished. She was also given IV corticosteroids and ampicillin.

Extubated after two days, she was transferred from the intensive care unit after five days. Therapy for the remainder of her pregnancy consisted of aminophylline and prednisone in a daily dosage of 10 mg. The patient had no more asthmatic attacks and was delivered of a 1,899-g, growth-retarded boy baby at 38 weeks' gestation. ∎

CASE 45.2 Hypertension in a Multipara

A 41-year-old gravida 8, para 7, came for her initial prenatal appointment at 27 weeks' gestation and indicated no complaints. Her history included a cervical conization at another hospital eight years before. Six of her children had been born at home. Her youngest had been delivered at term seven years before in the same hospital where she had had the conization. She denied any complications of that pregnancy.

Important findings on physical examination included blood pressure of 208/110 mm Hg, minimal arteriolar narrowing in the optic fundi, clear lungs, heart rate of 90 beats per minute, fundal height of 27 cm above the symphysis, a fetal heart rate of 140 beats per minute, and 1+ pretibial edema.

She was hospitalized immediately with an impression of elderly grand multiparity, an intrauterine pregnancy at 27 weeks, and chronic hypertension, possibly with preeclampsia. Communication with the other hospital revealed that eight years earlier, while hospitalized for conization, she had had blood pressures of 160/110 mm Hg and 190/130 mm Hg recorded. No treatment was mentioned. One year later, during her "normal delivery," her pressure was 180/108 mm Hg, and she showed 3+ proteinuria. Again, no treatment was mentioned.

Initial laboratory evaluation included hematocrit 37%, chest roentgenogram clear, left ventricular hypertrophy on ECG, urea nitrogen 17 mg/dL, serum creatinine 0.9 mg/dL, creatinine clearance 90 mL/min, and biparietal diameter 6.8 cm (27 weeks).

Antihypertensive treatment was begun with hydralazine and phenobarbital. Her activities were limited to strict bed rest. On the morning of the third hospital day, she seemed to be improving; her blood pressure was lower, she was still asymptomatic, and her hematocrit was 33%.

At 8:30 PM, she complained of shortness of breath. Wheezes and rales were heard throughout both lungs. Her blood pressure was 188/114 mm Hg, her hematocrit had risen to 39%, and chest x-ray showed infiltrates throughout both lungs. Arterial blood gases included a P_{O_2} of 67 mm Hg and a P_{CO_2} of 29 mm Hg. Her central venous pressure was 11 cm H_2O. Diagnosis now was chronic hypertension with superimposed preeclampsia and pulmonary edema.

Treatment was begun at once with furosemide, morphine, positive pressure oxygen, and digoxin. Within three hours her lungs were clear, and arterial blood gases were reported as P_{O_2} 109 mm Hg and P_{CO_2} 30 mm Hg while she was receiving oxygen.

Delivery by cesarean section was performed at 12:30 AM, followed by a tubal ligation. A baby boy weighing 1,050 g was delivered. He remained in the nursery for 55 days and was neurologically normal when seen at eight months of age. The mother had a benign postoperative course and was discharged from the hospital on the seventh postoperative day on antihypertensive therapy. ■

References

1. Kochenour NK, Lavery JP. Managing asthma in the pregnant patient. Contemp Ob/Gyn 1976;7(Jan):27.

2. Gordon M, Niswander KR, Berendes H, et al. Fetal morbidity following potentially anoxigenic obstetric conditions. VII. Bronchial asthma. Am J Obstet Gynecol 1970;106:421.

3. Greenberger PA, Patterson R. Management of asthma during pregnancy. N Engl J Med 1985;312:897.

4. Fanta CH, Rossing TH, MacFadden ER Jr. Treatment of acute asthma: is combination therapy with sympathomimetics and methylxanthines indicated? Am J Med 1986;80:5.

5. Senior RM, Lefrak SS, Korenblat PF. Status asthmaticus. JAMA 1975;231:1277.

6. Grant JA. Bronchial asthma. Texas Med 1978;74:37.

7. Schatz M, Patterson R, Zeitz S, et al. Corticosteroid therapy for the pregnant asthmatic patient. JAMA 1975;233:804.

8. Wenger NK, Stein PD, Willis PW III. Massive acute pulmonary embolism: the deceivingly nonspecific manifestations. JAMA 1972;220:843.

9. Szucs MM Jr, Brooks HL, Grossman W, et al. Diagnostic sensitivity of laboratory findings in acute pulmonary embolism. Ann Intern Med 1971;74:161.

10. Wessler S. Anticoagulant therapy—1974. JAMA 1974;228:757.

11. Barritt DW, Jordan SC. Anticoagulant drugs in the treatment of pulmonary embolism: a controlled trial. Lancet 1960;1:1309.

12. Glazier RL, Crowell EB. Randomized prospective trial of continuous versus intermittent heparin therapy. JAMA 1976;236:1365.

13. Mendelson CL. The aspiration of stomach contents into the lungs during obstetric anesthesia. Am J Obstet Gynecol 1946;52:191.

14. Baggish MS, Hooper S. Aspiration as a cause of maternal death. Obstet Gynecol 1977;127:206.

15. Freund U, French W, Carlson RW, et al. Hemodynamic and metabolic studies of a case of toxemia of pregnancy. Am J Obstet Gynecol 1977;127:206.

16. Stein L, Beraud JJ, Cavanilles J, et al. Pulmonary edema during fluid infusion in the absence of heart failure. JAMA 1974;229:65.

17. Dikshit K, Vyden JK, Forrester JS, et al. Renal and extrarenal hemodynamic effects of furosemide in congestive heart failure after acute myocardial infarction. N Engl J Med 1973;288:1087.

18. Grossman RF, Aberman A. Emergency management of acute pulmonary edema. Ann Intern Med 1976;84:488.

19. Cohn JN. Indications for digitalis therapy: a new look. JAMA 1974;229:1911.

20. Courtney LD. Amniotic fluid embolism. Obstet Gynecol Surv 1974;29:169.

21. Chung AF, Merkatz IR. Survival following amniotic fluid embolism with early heparinization. Obstet Gynecol 1973;42:809.

22. Resnik R, Swartz WH, Plumer MH, et al. Amniotic fluid embolism with survival. Obstet Gynecol 1976;47:295.

23. Weil MN, Shubin H, Biddle M. Shock caused by gram-negative microorganisms. Analysis of 169 cases. Ann Intern Med 1964;60:384.

24. Shubin H, Weil MN. Bacterial shock. JAMA 1976;235:421.

25. Blain CM, Anderson TO, Pietras RJ, et al. Immediate hemodynamic effects of gram-negative versus gram-positive bacteremia in man. Arch Intern Med 1970;126:260.

26. Andriole VT. Bacterial infections: septic abortion and septic shock. In: Burrow GN, Ferris TF, eds. Medical complications during pregnancy. Philadelphia: Saunders, 1975:394.

27. Swan JH. Balloon flotation catheters. Their use in hemodynamic monitoring in clinical practice. JAMA 1975;233:865.

28. Weil MN, Shubin H. The "VIP" approach to the bedside management of shock. JAMA 1969;207:337.

29. Weil MN, Shubin H, Rosoff L. Fluid repletion in circulatory shock. Central venous pressure and other practical guides.

JAMA 1965;192:668.

30. Bone RC, Fisher CJ, Clemmet TP, et al. A controlled clinical trial of high-dose methylprednisolone in the treatment of severe sepsis and septic shock. N Engl J Med 1987;317:653.

31. Weil MN, Shubin H, Carlson R. Treatment of circulatory shock. Use of sympathomimetic and related vasoactive agents. JAMA 1975;231:1280.

32. Dopamine for treatment of shock. Med Lett Drugs Ther 1975;17(4):13.

33. Innes IR, Nickerson M. Norepinephrine, epinephrine and the sympathomimetic amines. In: Goodman LS, Gilman A, eds. The pharmacological basis of therapeutics, ed 5. New York: Macmillan, 1975:494.

34. Hingson RA, Hellman LM. Organization of obstetric anesthesia on a 24-hour basis in a large and a small hospital. Anesthesiology 1951;12:745.

35. Bonica JJ. Principles and practice of obstetric analgesia and anesthesia. Philadelphia: Davis, 1967:690.

36. Marx GF, Cosmi EV, Wollman SB. Biochemical status and clinical condition of mother and infant at cesarean section. Anesth Analg 1969;48:986.

37. Morrow DH, Luther RR. Anaphylaxis: Etiology and guidelines for management. Anesth Analg 1976;55:493.

38. James LP Jr, Austin KF. Fatal systemic anaphylaxis in man. N Engl J Med 1964;270:597.

39. Kelly JF, Patterson R. Anaphylaxis: course, mechanisms and treatment. JAMA 1974;227:1431.

40. Ishizaka K, Ishizaka T, Arbesman CE. Induction of passive cutaneous anaphylaxis in monkeys by human gamma-E antibody. J Allergy 1967;39:254.

41. Lockey RF, Bukantz SC. Allergic emergencies. Med Clin North Am 1976;58:147.

42. Ghoneim MM, Long JP. The interaction between magnesium and other neuromuscular blocking agents. Anesthesiology 1970;32:23.

43. Pritchard JA, Pritchard SA. Standardized treatment of 154 consecutive cases of eclampsia. Am J Obstet Gynecol 1975;123:543.

44. Chesley LC, Tepper I. Plasma levels of magnesium attained sulfate therapy for preeclampsia and eclampsia. Surg Clin North Am 1975;55(2):353.

45. Sibai BM, Lipshitz J, Anderson GD, et al. Reassessment of intravenous MgSO4 therapy in preeclampsia-eclampsia. Obstet Gynecol 1981;57:199.

46. Drugs for epilepsy. Med Lett Drugs Ther 1976;18(6):25.

47. Grimes DA, Cates W Jr. Deaths from paracervical anesthesia used for first trimester abortion, 1972–1975. N Engl J Med 1976;295:1397.

48. Fishburne JI Jr. Local anesthetics in obstetrics. Contemp Ob/Gyn 1975;6(Oct):101.

49. Bonica JJ. Principles and practice of obstetric analgesia and anesthesia. Philadelphia: Davis, 1967:507.

46

Intrauterine Growth Retardation

John T. Queenan, M.D.

A MAJOR clinical condition, intrauterine growth retardation (IUGR) is not a new problem. However, it was only in the 1970s that its clinical importance was recognized.

Regardless of gestational age, newborns weighing less than 2,500 g used to be considered premature. In 1961, Warkany and associates described IUGR as a separate entity (1). Subsequently, other investigators established norms of weight, length, and head circumference for various weeks of gestation. This created the classification by which the low-birthweight infant is designated as premature, growth-retarded, or both (1–4).

During the past decade, clinicians have noted that IUGR increases the risk of perinatal asphyxia and perinatal death by three- to eightfold. In addition to asphyxia, growth-retarded babies are particularly prone to meconium aspiration, polycythemia, hypoglycemia, and long-term problems with growth and development. If IUGR is recognized early, however, its adverse effects can be minimized in many cases.

Specific Perinatal Problems

Although growth retardation may be associated with many unfavorable clinical factors, the following specific ones markedly affect prognosis.

Meconium Aspiration

The growth-retarded fetus has a higher-than-normal incidence of meconium present in the amniotic fluid. During labor and delivery, the increased frequency of fetal distress with IUGR can cause fetal gasping and aspiration of meconium. If meconium descends appreciably into the tracheobronchial tree, the prognosis may be grave.

Asphyxia

The growth-retarded fetus has a three- to fivefold increase in the incidence of distress during labor. Asphyxia is manifested by late decelerations and low cord-blood pH. Although the growth-retarded fetus may also experience increased episodes of antepartum distress, labor appears to cause particular stress.

Acidosis

If fetal distress occurs during labor, acidosis may develop. Furthermore if meconium aspiration occurs during labor and delivery, neonatal acidosis should be anticipated.

Polycythemia

Severely growth-retarded fetuses often have polycythemia during the immediate neonatal period. This must be treated with infusion of IV fluids and, occasionally, phlebotomy.

Hypoglycemia

One of the first organs affected in IUGR is the liver. Because glycogen stores are depleted, the newborn has lost its most important endogenous source of energy. Additionally, these babies have markedly reduced levels of subcutaneous tissue, causing them to have very poor thermostability. Their temperatures begin to fall soon after birth. As part of a compensatory mechanism, their caloric requirements go up and cause hypoglycemia. If the newborn is also premature, the problem may be compounded. Frequently, these babies are poor feeders and need parenteral or gavage supplements.

Impaired Growth and Development

Animal studies have provided some insight into the ravages of IUGR. Winick and Noble have shown that the hyperplasia phase of cellular growth may be irrevocably affected by deprivation in utero (5). The fetal brain in the rat grows by hyperplasia during early and middle pregnancy. During the last portion of pregnancy, it grows by hyperplasia and hypertrophy. After birth, growth is confined to hypertrophy. If an insult affects the fetal rat brain during the hyperplasia phase, the rat is born with a decreased complement of brain cells, as measured by DNA determination. This decreased number of brain cells is a permanent effect, whereas, if the insult occurs later and only the cell size is compromised, recovery is possible with cessation of the insult and restoration of nutritional support.

How closely these data can be applied to humans is difficult to say. True, some severely growth-retarded fetuses are later determined to be mentally retarded. Additionally, some studies indicate that growth-retarded infants require a

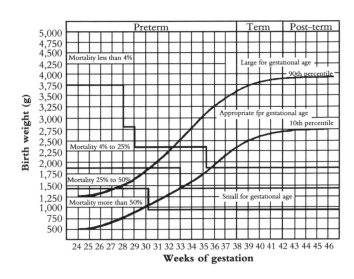

Figure 46.1   Norms of weight for different weeks of gestation. (Adapted from Lubchenco LO, Hansman C, Boyd E. Intrauterine growth in length and head circumference as estimated from live births at gestational ages from 26–42 weeks. Pediatrics 1966;37:403.)

long time to catch up to normal growth and that others never do. Cruise, in a study of growth-retarded infants up to three years of age, showed that these infants maintained retarded growth despite attempts to catch up (6). F. Falkner relates that the Louisville twin study suggests that, in some instances, the growth-retarded twin carries its growth deficiencies through adolescence (personal communication).

Standard Growth Tables

At the University of Colorado, Lubchenco and associates studied normal and abnormal growth at various levels of maturity and expressed their data in tables indicating the percentiles for birthweight, head circumference (HC), and length for each week of gestation from 26 to 42 weeks for each sex (Figure 46.1) (2, 3). If birthweight fell below the tenth percentile, a baby was considered small for gestational age (SGA). If it was above the 90th percentile, the baby was designated large for gestational age. Similar tables for HC and length give the clinician the means for defining the type of growth abnormality.

However, these tables were constructed from observa-

Table 46.1 Differences between IUGR and SGA

Parameter	IUGR	SGA
Growth	Impaired	Impaired or constitutionally small
Size	Usually small	Always small
Condition	Always abnormal	May be abnormal

Table 46.2 Incidence of Low-birthweight Babies According to Commencement of Antenatal Care

When Mother First Sought Care	Low Birthweight (%)
First trimester	6.6
Second trimester	8.7
Third trimester	8.6
Never	21.0

Data from National Center for Health Statistics.

tions of a population of newborns at one mile above sea level. It should be kept in mind that the 10th percentile in Denver could be the third percentile in New York or Los Angeles. Usher and McLean also developed standard measurements of seven dimensions for infants born between 25 and 44 weeks' gestation at sea level (4).

IUGR versus SGA Infants

The terms IUGR and SGA are frequently used interchangeably. Although they often refer to the same situation, they are not truly synonymous (Table 46.1). IUGR means that fetal growth has been impaired, whereas SGA means that the newborn falls below the 10th percentile for birthweight.

A large baby with IUGR may result if the mother has poorly controlled diabetes mellitus with macrosomia and subsequently develops a severe vascular complication caus-ing vascular insufficiency that impairs fetal growth. This newborn, the victim of impaired growth, may be well above the tenth percentile in birthweight, and thus not SGA. Conversely, the normal but quite small newborn falling below the tenth percentile in birthweight may just be constitutionally small. Hence, IUGR should be considered an obstetric term describing a pathologic process, whereas SGA is by definition a neonatal term indicating a small-for-dates baby, including some who are merely constitutionally small (Figure 46.2).

The vast majority of SGA babies result from IUGR. Poor nutrition, vascular insufficiency, preeclampsia, renal disease, infection, and genetic problems are the causes in most cases. However, investigators looking at low birthweight from a broader perspective have added some interesting epidemiologic factors. For example, according to a study by a group at the National Center for Health Statistics, the time at which a patient begins her antenatal care can affect whether she has a low-birthweight baby (Table 46.2). In this study, race also appeared to be a factor: black women had a higher incidence of low-birthweight babies than did white women. Studies from other countries place considerable emphasis on low socioeconomic status in the etiology of low birthweight.

IUGR versus Prematurity

There are many similarities between IUGR and prematurity (Table 46.3), but careful consideration makes it possible to differentiate them. Meconium aspiration, acidosis, and cogenital malformations are associated with IUGR, whereas complications of prematurity include hyaline membrane disease,

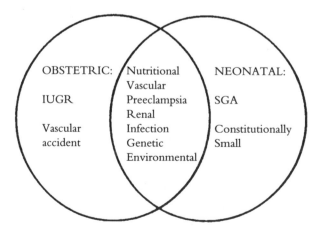

OBSTETRIC:

IUGR

Vascular accident

Nutritional
Vascular
Preeclampsia
Renal
Infection
Genetic
Environmental

NEONATAL:

SGA

Constitutionally Small

Figure 46.2   How various factors produce both IUGR and SGA infants.

Table 46.3 IUGR versus Prematurity

IUGR	Prematurity
Asphyxia	Asphyxia
Temperature instability	Temperature instability
Hypoglycemia	Hypoglycemia
Fetal distress	Hyaline membrane disease
Acidosis	Apnea
Meconium aspiration	Bradycardia
Hypothermia	Feeding difficulty
Polycythemia	Hypocalcemia
Congenital malformations	Hyperbilirubinemia
Impaired growth and development	Intracranial hemorrhage
	Necrotizing enterocolitis

apnea, intracranial hemorrhage, and necrotizing enterocolitis. However, a premature newborn may also have growth retardation, which occurs in about a third of premature births.

Table 46.4 Causes of IUGR

Primary Maternal Disease
(Secondary fetal effect)
Chronic hypertension
Renal disease
Cardiac disease

Maternal and Fetal Disease
Malnutrition
Drugs
Alcohol
Tobacco

Primary Fetal Growth Failure
Congenital malformations
Chromosomal abnormalities
Infection

Placental Dysfunction
Placental insufficiency
Infarction and separation
Anatomic anomalies
Infection
Multiple gestations

Causes of IUGR

One should not regard IUGR as a single disease or condition. On the contrary, the heterogeneity of its causes accurately suggests a broad diversity of prognoses. In general, the causes can be classified as primary maternal (secondary fetal), maternal and fetal, primary fetal, and placental dysfunctional (Table 46.4).

The prognosis is directly related to the variety of growth retardation. For example, if the problem is a fetal one, such as chromosome abnormalities, substrate delivery to the fetus is normal but potential to assimilate substrate is abnormal. When there is a maternal cause, such as pregnancy-induced hypertension (PIH), substrate delivery to the fetus is reduced, but the potential for fetal growth is normal. For these differing forms of IUGR, prognosis, workup, and treatment will vary accordingly (Table 46.5).

Forms of IUGR

Severity of growth retardation depends not only on the cause but also on the length of time the cause has been operational. Even mild nutritional or vascular deprivation will affect the liver. As fetal glycogen stores are rapidly depleted, the liver size is decreased (7). The total body weight will also be decreased as the condition becomes more severe. But head size remains normal, or at least relatively large, even though HC may be smaller than normal. This represents a phenomenon called "head sparing" and accounts for asymmetric IUGR. Approximately 60% of IUGR is asymmetric (Table 46.6). In contrast, when the insult occurs early—as with rubella infection—and is prolonged, HC, body length (L), and weight (Wt) are all

Table 46.5 IUGR: Prognosis versus Cause

Variety	Substrate Delivery to the Fetus	Fetal Potential for Growth
Fetal	Normal	Abnormal
Maternal	Reduced	Normal
Placental	Reduced	Normal

Table 46.6 Patterns of IUGR

Insult	IUGR	Neonatal Parameters
Early and prolonged	Symmetrical	HC = L = Wt (all <10%)
Late	Asymmetrical	HC = L >Wt (Wt <10%)
Subacute	Asymmetrical	HC = L >Wt (all <10%)

affected (symmetric growth retardation).

Because causes and patterns of IUGR vary, different methods of detection must be used. Simply considering gestational age and weight is not enough. HC and abdominal circumference (AC), as well as length, must be evaluated to detect all forms of growth retardation. The origin of the problem and how long it has been operational are also important in determining the type of IUGR. If a problem occurs early in pregnancy, the type of IUGR will most likely be symmetrical and in extreme cases may be detected at 20 weeks' gestation. The best examples are chromosomal abnormalities, malformations, or viral infections (Table 46.7). If the insult occurs later, the IUGR will probably be asymmetrical, as with pregnancy-induced hypertension, placental insufficiency, or idiopathic IUGR. Of course, there are also situations where there is symmetrical or asymmetrical IUGR or both, as in the case of substance abuse.

Importance of Gestational Age

The last normal menstrual period, size of the uterus at the first prenatal exam, and early ultrasound measurements are all used to determine gestational age. Knowing the correct age is imperative because symmetric growth retardation may be missed if gestational age is underestimated.

An ultrasound exam early in pregnancy is very helpful in establishing correct gestational age. From eight to 13 weeks, crown-rump length is very accurate, and from 15 to 26 weeks, HC, biparietal diameter (BPD), and femur length are very accurate.

Accurate dating is also important when growth retardation is asymmetric. Normally, HC exceeds AC before 36 weeks, and after that the reverse is true. Serial scans to check the amount of amniotic fluid and placental texture can help detect asymmetric growth retardation when exact

Table 46.7 Causes of IUGR

Symmetric, Hyperplasia Phase	Asymmetric, Hypertrophy Phase
Chromosome abnormality	Pregnancy-induced hypertension
Congenital malformation	Vascular insufficiency
TORCH infections	Placenta insufficiency
Substance abuse	Substance abuse
Heart disease	Malnutrition
Renal disease	Multiple gestation
Chronic hypertension	

dating is a problem.

Detecting IUGR

Risk Groups

The most common way to detect IUGR is to determine whether a patient belongs to a risk group. Risk factors include poor nutrition, vascular insufficiency, preeclampsia, renal disease, heart disease, infection, genetic abnormalities, multiple gestations, low socioeconomic status, and poor maternal weight gain. Two-thirds of IUGR infants come from these risk groups. Perinatal mortality was found to be higher among members of risk groups (8).

Uterine Growth

Serial measurements of fundal height or abdominal girth indicate whether the uterus is smaller than it should be for particular stages of gestation. Daikoku and co-workers showed that 64% of mothers delivering low-birthweight babies had reduced fundal height (9). Typically, fundi grew less than 2 cm in four weeks. Belizan and co-workers reported that fundal height measurements detected 38 of 44 newborns with birthweights below the 10th percentile (10). They calculate sensitivity to be 86% and specificity 90% for this technique. Although measurement of fundal height does detect many cases of IUGR, it is unlikely to detect the problem very early.

Ultrasound Examination

In contrast to earlier investigations, more recent studies have shown that ultrasound scanning can predict fetal weight accurately (11, 12). It appears to be an ideal screening method for detecting IUGR, as well as a good way to monitor retarded growth once it has been diagnosed.

Initially, in our antenatal testing unit, an ultrasound scan is done for general assessment, and then the following studies are performed systematically.

Biparietal Diameter: Determination is made at the widest transverse portion of the head, usually near the level of the third ventricle or thalami. Serial BPD measurements will detect symmetric IUGR or retardation due to a long-standing insult that has slowed the growth rate (13, 14).

Head Circumference: Using HC compensates for dolichocephaly, brachycephaly, and molding, and hence prevents erroneous diagnosis of IUGR, which could happen if BPD alone were relied on (15). Comparing AC with HC may help identify asymmetric IUGR (Figure 46.3). HC should be taken at the level of the third ventricle. Unfortunately, in 5%–10% of cases, fetal position prevents obtaining accurate measurements.

Abdominal Circumference: A transverse section of the abdomen containing a portion of the stomach and a small section of umbilical vein should be scanned as it traverses the fetal liver. Electronic on-screen tracers are used to determine the circumference. The fetal liver shows effects of growth retardation first because it loses glycogen when deprived of substrate. Thus, reduced AC is the earliest sign of asymmetric growth retardation in a fetus (Figure 46.3).

Head-to-Body Ratio: The ratio obtained from the circumferences normally changes as pregnancy progresses (15). In the second trimester, HC exceeds AC; at about 32–36 weeks', the ratio equals 1; and then AC becomes larger (Figure 46.3). The advantages of using this graph for detecting IUGR are that it differentiates symmetric from asymmetric IUGR and is still useful even if dates are off by a few weeks.

Femur Length: Fetal femur length (FL) provides an early, accurate, and reproducible means of measuring fetal long-bone growth and correlates well with neonatal crown-heel

length. Femur lengths are very valuable in determining gestational age and detecting and monitoring IUGR (16–18).

Obtainable in virtually all cases, FL appears to be as effective as head measurement for detecting symmetric IUGR, and it can be used when head measurements are unobtainable. For long-term follow-up, it should correlate with the height of the child and adolescent. There are two ways to scan the femur: (1) aligning the transducer with the spine and rotating away from the caudal end; (2) placing the transducer at a right angle to the caudal end of the spine

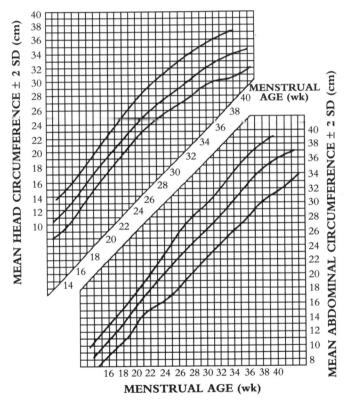

Figure 46.3 Mean head and abdominal circumferences with 5th and 95th percentile confidence limits between 16 and 40 weeks' menstrual age.

(Adapted with permission from Campbell S, Griffin D, Roberts A, et al. Early prenatal diagnosis of abnormalities of the fetal head, spine, limbs, and abdominal organs. In: Orlandi C, Polani PE, Bovicelli L, eds. Recent advances in prenatal diagnosis: proceedings of the first international symposium on recent advances in prenatal diagnosis, Bologna, 15–16 September 1980. New York: John Wiley and Sons, 1980.)

and rotating toward the spine.

The "smoothed" graph shows the mean ultrasound FL (with the 95th plus the 5th percentile limits) from 14 weeks to term (Figure 46.4). The line with dots represents serial ultrasound measurements of the FL from a patient who developed PIH at 25 weeks' gestation. Other ultrasound measurements—BPD, HC, and AC—showed an equivalent decrease in growth rate. Symmetric fetal growth retardation was readily detected.

Placental Morphology: The texture of the growth-retarded placenta may differ from that of a normal placenta of

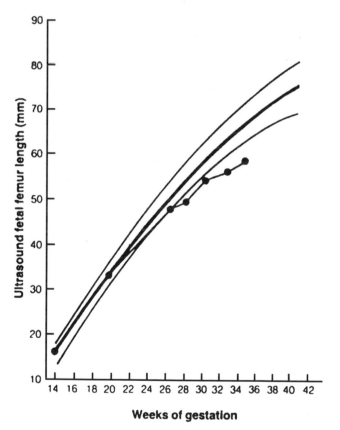

Figure 46.4 Fetal femur length. According to scale of "smoothed" graph, this measurement would put gestational age for a normal fetus at 34–35 weeks. The line with dots shows femur length data for a patient who developed pregnancy-induced hypertension at 25 weeks. Other ultrasound parameters—BPD, and head and abdominal circumference—confirmed symmetric growth retardation.

the same gestational age. Grannum and co-workers developed a scoring system based on texture and architecture ranging from grade zero, with a homogenous texture and no calcifications, up to a mature grade III placenta (19). In a grade I placenta (usually appearing at 31 weeks), there are random echogenic areas of calcification and an undulating pattern of the chorionic plate. In grade II, there are comma-shaped indentations of the chorionic plate and calcifications in the basal layer. In grade III, as distinct cotyledons are visualized, indentations are pronounced; there are echofree "fallout" areas in the cotyledons and irregular densities causing acoustic shadowing.

Premature aging of the placenta may be important, particularly when no accurate dating is available. Acceleration of the placenta-maturation process may occur with IUGR, PIH, or both. Kazzi and co-workers reported that a grade III placenta was followed by delivery of a growth-retarded baby in 59% of cases (20).

Amniotic Fluid Volume: The amniotic fluid index is determined by adding the largest vertical pockets in four quadrants of the uterus (21). If the index is under 5 a diagnosis of oligohydraminos is made. Both polyhydramnios and oligohydramnios may occur with IUGR, but oligohydramnios is much more common.

Manning and co-workers defined oligohydramnios as existing if the widest diameter of AF pockets is less than 1 cm, and AFV is normal if at least one pocket measures 1 cm in its broadest diameter (22). Studying 120 patients referred with suspected IUGR, they found normal AFV in 91, of whom 86 (93.4%) were delivered of a normal fetus. In contrast, qualitative AFV was decreased in 29 patients, of whom 26 (89.9%) were delivered of a fetus with IUGR. These differences were highly significant. Perinatal morbidity was increased tenfold in patients with decreased AFV. Overall, 26 of 31 IUGR fetuses (83.4%) had decreased AFV.

AFV, in association with placental morphology, may help to distinguish the SGA fetus from the one with IUGR, as well as assist in dating, if there is uncertainty. For example, placental aging when there is little AF suggests fetal jeopardy, whereas placental calcifications with normal AFV usually indicate that intervention is unnecessary, provided the fetus continues to grow.

Other Methods

Such determinants as abnormal glucose tolerance curves, indicating maternal hypoglycemia, have been reported to be associated with IUGR. Wald and co-workers showed that patients with elevated maternal serum α-fetoprotein levels (three times the normal median) had a 5.8-fold increase in births before 37 weeks and a 4.7-fold increase of birthweights under 2,500 g, compared with controls (23).

Clinical Assessment

The clinician must first determine the cause of IUGR. If it is due to conditions such as Down or Potter syndrome or anencephaly, clinical management will be entirely different than if the cause is nutritional, vascular, or a multiple gestation. Sonography can determine whether multiple gestations are present and usually can detect congenital malformations. History, physical examination, and such studies as chromosome analysis, TORCH (toxoplasmosis-other-rubella-cytomegalovirus-herpes) titers, and renal function tests help define etiology. A karyotype is absolutely essential. In a study of 458 growth-retarded fetuses, 89 (19%) had chromosome abnormalities (24).

The clinician must then assess the fetus to determine whether it will be better off in the uterus or the neonatal intensive care unit (NICU). Several methods provide valuable information on fetal condition:

1. Biophysical profile, performed weekly or biweekly, provides a particularly appropriate mix of parameters for evaluation of fetal physiology in IUGR.
2. Nonstress testing (NST), performed weekly or biweekly, gives assurance that there is no significant risk in allowing the fetus to remain in utero. If the NST is nonreactive, a contraction stress test (CST) should be done, and other factors, including AFV, placental morphology, and maternally perceived fetal movements, should be carefully evaluated.
3. The CST can potentially elicit an abnormal response when the NST is nonreactive or equivocal. Whenever fetal compromise is suspected, this test is indicated.

(The NST and the CST are important when an underlying vascular or placental defect is causing IUGR. If a genetic defect, such as trisomy, is the cause, they obviously would not be helpful.) Repetitive decelerative electronic fetal monitoring (EFM) patterns correlate with hypoxia. In one study, 15 out of 19 abnormal heart rate patterns were associated with hypoxic and/or acidemic growth-retarded fetuses, as determined by cordocentesis (25). Pulsed Doppler measuring of the aortic mean velocity and common carotid artery pulsatility index can predict asphyxia in the growth-retarded fetus. Another study showed that, when the pulsatility index was abnormal, 89% had an asphyxia index 1 SD above the mean; 60% were 2 SD above the mean, as measured by cordocentesis (26).

4. Clinical parameters in the mother that worsen are highly significant. For example, if the cause of IUGR is chronic maternal hypertension or cyanotic heart disease and the mother's condition begins to deteriorate, the fetus should be delivered as soon as possible.
5. Ultrasound measurements on which the diagnosis of IUGR was based are also critical. In following a fetus with IUGR, it should be noted whether the HC, AC, and FL increase over an appropriate interval. If they do not, the baby may be better off in the NICU than in the uterus.
6. AF studies showing meconium usually indicate fetal compromise. A mature lecithin/sphingomyelin ratio and the presence of phosphatidylglycerol indicate pulmonary maturity.

Treatment

Specific measures for treating a patient with IUGR start with treatment of any underlying condition. Patients should be confined to bed rest in the lateral recumbent position to increase blood flow to the uterus. Mothers who smoke should be encouraged to stop. Maternal nutrition should be carefully evaluated and deficiencies remedied.

With these measures, many patients do well. It is therefore incumbent on us to diagnose IUGR as early as possible so that we can improve the in utero environment.

When this is no longer possible, the best course is to remove the baby from the insult.

Timely delivery is important. It is essential to monitor the fetus closely. Meconium aspiration must be avoided. If necessary, the fetus should be delivered by cesarean section. Finally, the infant will need to be evaluated and treated by skilled neonatologists in the delivery room.

Neonatal Problems

Some problems of the IUGR infant are immediate, and others are remote. Among the most important are meconium aspiration, asphyxia neonatorum, acidosis, polycythemia, hypoglycemia, and impaired future growth and development (Table 46.3). The polycythemia deserves special mention. Recent studies show growth-retarded fetuses have elevated erythropoietin concentrations associated with fetal acidemia and fetal erythroblastosis in response to tissue hypoxia (27).

Growth and Development

From the extensive Louisville study of discordant twin pregnancies, it appears that the IUGR baby has accelerated growth after birth but that some never quite reach the potential of full growth. Cruise's studies on singleton pregnancies also indicate that catch-up growth occurs but that the growth-retarded fetus may never attain the full potential (6). Cruise found that preterm infants whose weight was appropriate for gestational age (AGA) grew faster than SGA infants. At one, two, and three years, the SGA children had the smallest mean measurements of all low-birthweight infants in the study group.

Fancourt and co-workers performed follow-up examinations on 60 children who had serial BPDs in pregnancy and were small for dates at birth (28). The mean age of the children at examination was four years. There were four groups of subjects: 1) those who had cephalometric evidence of growth retardation at or before 26 weeks' gestation; 2) those who had such evidence between 27 and 34 weeks; 3) those who had evidence after 34 weeks; and 4) those who had no cephalometric evidence of IUGR. If BPD growth had decreased before 34 weeks, the child was likely to be below the 10th percentile for weight and height at four years of age. If BPD growth had decreased before 26 weeks, there was slow growth after birth, and these children had a lower developmental quotient according to the Griffiths extended scales when examined at four years. The stage of gestation at which growth retardation occurs thus appears to be very significant.

A more favorable outlook for the growth-retarded fetus has been reported. Vohr and co-workers studied 21 preterm SGA infants sequentially for 2 years (29). The mean birthweight was 1,220 g, and the gestational age was 33.4 ± 2 weeks. Each SGA baby was paired with a birthweight-matched newborn whose weight was AGA (mean birthweight 1,195 g; gestational age 29 ± 2 weeks). Weight, height and HC of the SGA babies had attained the 10th percentile by 6–8 months and were similar to those of the AGA babies. The Bayley scores of infant development of the SGA babies were lower at 18 months, but by 24 months the two groups had similar scores.

This report reflects the good potential these babies have if given excellent neonatal care. Although evaluating growth and development of preterm SGA babies is complex, this well-executed study indicates that they can have a favorable prognosis.

Improving Outcome

Growth retardation is more common than once thought. The keys to preventing mortality and minimizing morbidity are early detection, improving fetal environment, and timely delivery. Methods employed should include determination of patient risk groups, early recognition of insufficient uterine growth, assessment of fetal growth patterns by ultrasound, and thorough clinical assessment to develop a comprehensive approach to treatment.

CASE 46.1

A 21-year-old primigravida had an uneventful pregnancy until 33 weeks' gestation, when her uterus was noted to be smaller than expected. She was certain of the date of her last normal menstrual period. An ultrasound scan revealed little or no amniotic fluid and a fetus with poor tone and no demonstrable kidneys. The fetal bladder did not appear to fill.

A repeat ultrasound scan at 35 weeks' gestation confirmed these findings, and a diagnosis of Potter syndrome was made. The parents were given extensive counselling.

The patient went into spontaneous labor at 39 weeks' gestation. After eight hours, late decelerations and marked variable decelerations were noted. The fetal condition did not respond to the usual corrective measures. Cesarean section was not performed because the fetus had a fatal condition. The female infant weighed 1,500 g and died shortly after birth because her lungs were hypoplastic. Autopsy revealed renal agenesis. ◼

CASE 46.2

A white, 28-year-old gravida 2, para 1, had delivered a growth-retarded infant with her first pregnancy, two years before the second. She had had no history of hypertension or renal disease. The first infant, born at term, weighed 2,250 g.

At 12 weeks into her second pregnancy, her uterus measured 12 weeks' size. Ultrasound scanning revealed a crown-rump length consistent with a 12-week gestation. The pregnancy was uneventful until 32 weeks, when ultrasound revealed an abnormally high head-to-abdomen ratio. The HC and FL were normal. There seemed to be slightly less than the normal amount of amniotic fluid. The fetus appeared normally active. Weekly BPPs were normal; however, the uterus did not seem to be growing.

At 35 weeks' gestation, the HC had grown only slightly and the AC even less, compared with measurements at 32 weeks. The L/S ratio was 2:1, phosphatidylglycerol (PG) was present. The amniotic fluid was clear on amniocentesis and an NST was reactive.

In view of the evidence of IUGR, delivery was scheduled. The cervix was favorable for induction, and oxytocin was administered via infusion pump. When it became possible to rupture the membranes, an internal scalp electrode was inserted. The fetal heart rate (FHR) remained normal throughout labor. At full dilation, slight meconium staining was noted.

To prevent meconium aspiration, the newborn's nose and pharynx were suctioned before delivery of the shoulders. Laryngoscopic examination revealed no meconium below the vocal cords. The male infant weighed 1,850 g and had Apgar scores of 7 at one minute and 9 at five minutes. He had moderate hypoglycemia and polycythemia. In the NICU, he was treated for three days for those conditions and for mild hypocalcemia and hyperbilirubinemia. He regained his birthweight by 12 days and was discharged at three weeks of life, with follow-up procedures planned. ◼

References

1. Warkany J, Monroe BB, Sutherland BS. Intrauterine growth retardation. Am J Dis Child 1961;102:249.
2. Lubchenco LO, Hansman C, Boyd E. Intrauterine growth in length and head circumference as estimated from live births at gestational ages from 26–42 weeks. Pediatrics 1966; 37:403.
3. Battaglia FC, Lubchenco LO. A practical classification of newborn infants by weight and gestational age. J Pediatr 1967; 71:159.

4. Usher R, McLean F. Intrauterine growth of live-born Caucasian infants at sea level: standards obtained from measurements in seven dimensions of infants born between 25 and 44 weeks of gestation. J Pediatr 1969;74:901.

5. Winick M, Noble A. Cellular response in rats during malnutrition at various ages. J Nutr 1966;89:300.

6. Cruise MO. A longitudinal study of the growth of low birthweight infants: I. Velocity and distance growth, birth to 3 years. Pediatrics 1973;51:620.

7. Gruenwald P, Minh HN. Evaluation of body and organ weights in perinatal pathology. Am J Obstet Gynecol 1961; 82:312.

8. Galbraith RS, Karchmar EJ, Piercy WN, et al. The clinical prediction of intrauterine growth retardation. Am J Obstet Gynecol 1979;133:281.

9. Daikoku NH, Johnson JW, Graf C, et al. Patterns of intrauterine growth retardation. Obstet Gynecol 1979;54:211.

10. Belizan JM, Villar J, Nardin JC, et al. Diagnosis of intrauterine growth retardation by a simple clinical method: measurement of uterine height. Am J Obstet Gynecol 1978;131: 643.

11. Sabbagha RE, Minogue J, Iamura RK, et al. Estimation of birthweight by use of ultrasonographic formulas targeted to large-, appropriate-, and small-for-gestational-age fetuses. Am J Obstet Gynecol 1989;160:854.

12. Warsof SL, Wolf P, Coulehan J, et al. Comparison of fetal weight estimation formulas with and without head measurements. Obstet Gynecol 1986;67:569.

13. Campbell S, Dewhurst CJ. Diagnosis of the small-for-dates fetus by serial ultrasound cephalometry. Lancet 1971;2: 1002.

14. Queenan JT, Kubarych SF, Cook LN, et al. Diagnostic ultrasound for detection of intrauterine growth retardation. Am J Obstet Gynecol 1976;124:865.

15. Campbell S. Ultrasound measurement of the fetal head to abdomen circumference ratio in assessment of growth retardation. Br J Obstet Gynaecol 1977;84:165.

16. Queenan JT, O'Brien GD, Campbell S. Ultrasound measurement of fetal limb bones. Am J Obstet Gynecol 1980;138:297.

17. O'Brien GD, Queenan JT. Growth of the ultrasound fetal femur length during normal pregnancy: Part I. Am J Obstet Gynecol 1981;141:833.

18. O'Brien GD, Queenan JT. Ultrasound fetal femur length in relation to intrauterine growth retardation: Part II. Am J Obstet Gynecol 1982;144:35.

19. Grannum PA, Berkowitz RL, Hobbins JC. The ultrasonic changes in the maturing placenta and their relation to fetal pulmonic maturity. Am J Obstet Gynecol 1979;133:915.

20. Kazzi GM, Gross TL, Sokol RJ, et al. Detection of IUGR: a new use for sonographic placental grading. Am J Obstet Gynecol 1983;145:733.

21. Phelan JP, Ahn MO, Smith CV, et al. Amniotic fluid index measurements during pregnancy. J Reprod Med 1987; 32:601.

22. Manning FA, Hill LM, Plat LD. Qualitative amniotic fluid volume determination by ultrasound. Am J Obstet Gynecol 1981;139:254.

23. Wald N, Cuckle H, Stirrat GM, et al. Maternal serum alphafetoprotein and low birthweight. Lancet 1977;2:268.

24. Snijder RJM, Sherrod C, Gosdon CM, et al. Fetal growth retardation: associated malformations and chromosomal abnormalities. Am J Obstet Gynecol 1993;168:547.

25. Visser GH, Sadovsky G, Nicolaides KH. Antepartum heart rate patterns in small-for-gestational-age third-trimester fetuses: correlations with blood gas values obtained at cordocentesis. Am J Obstet Gynecol 1990;162:698.

26. Bilardo CM, Nicolaides KH, Campbell S. Doppler measurements of fetal and uteroplacental circulations: relationship with umbilical venous blood gases measured at cordocentesis. Am J Obstet Gynecol 1990;162:115.

27. Snijder RJM, Abbas A, Melby O, et al. Fetal plasma erythropoietin concentration in severe growth retardation. Am J Obstet Gynecol 1993;168:615.

28. Fancourt R, Campbell S, Harvey DR, et al. Follow-up study of small-for-dates babies. Br Med J 1976;1:1435.

29. Vohr BR, Oh W, Rosenfield AG, et al. The preterm small-for-gestational-age infant: a two-year follow-up study. Am J Obstet Gynecol 1979;133:425.

47

The IUGR Neonate

William Oh, M.D.

WE used to consider all low-birthweight infants premature. In the late 1950s, however, we began to realize that some infants are small because they were unable to grow in utero, not because they were born early. A combination of prematurity and intrauterine growth retardation (IUGR) is, of course, possible; in fact, this group of low-birthweight infants represents a very high risk category because they can have problems relating to prematurity and intrauterine insults leading to IUGR. The terms used over the years to describe these small infants include placental insufficiency or dysfunction, small for gestational age, small for dates, and light for dates, which reflect the heterogeneous nature of the condition.

In some cases, when there is congenital infection, major malformation, or chromosomal abnormality, IUGR is fetal in origin; more frequently, it results from a maternal or placental disorder that decreases the substrate available to the fetus (Table 47.1). In some instances, there is both limited substrate and decreased potential for fetal growth. When a congenital viral infection is present, for example, growth failure could result from viral invasion of the fetal tissue, as well as from disruption of substrate delivery through an infected placenta.

Diagnosing IUGR in a neonate is relatively easy, once the gestational age is determined by obstetric history and by Dubowitz assessment at birth. IUGR is established if the birthweight is below the 10th percentile of the intrauterine growth curve. Often, signs of wasting and decreased subcutaneous tissue are also present, and, at times, there is meconium on the skin and umbilical cord (1).

Head circumference, length and body weight measurements are useful parameters in classifying the IUGR neonates into symmetric or asymmetric type. If head cir-

Table 47.1 IUGR: Prognosis versus Cause

Variety	Substrate Delivery to the Fetus	Fetal Potential for Growth
Fetal	Normal	Abnormal
Maternal	Reduced	Normal
Placental	Reduced	Normal

cumference, length, and body weights are all below the 10th percentile, the IUGR is considered symmetric in variety. In general, this type of IUGR is associated with early onset and longer duration of insults that lead to fetal growth retardation. Examples of this type of IUGR are those due to congenital infection, chromosomal abnormalities, and major congenital malformations. Mothers who smoke heavily or have alcohol or drug abuse early in and throughout pregnancy are also likely to have IUGR neonates who belong to the symmetric variety. Occasionally, symmetric type of IUGR is associated with uneventful pregnancy. These infants may be small proportionally because of constitutional background and tend to have a favorable neonatal course.

In the asymmetric type of IUGR, the infant's body weight is below the 10th percentile, while the head circumference and length are between the 10th and 90th percentile. This variety of IUGR is usually related to a late-onset pathology that led to fetal growth retardation. The best example is in toxemia of pregnancy where the onset of this complication is usually in the late second or early third trimester, at which time the fetus has already attained a certain degree of growth in length and head circumference. Thus, the primary parameter affected with reference to growth retardation is the body weight. In some cases of asymmetric type of IUGR, the head circumference and weight are below the 10th percentile, while the length is above the 10th percentile. This observation generally reflects

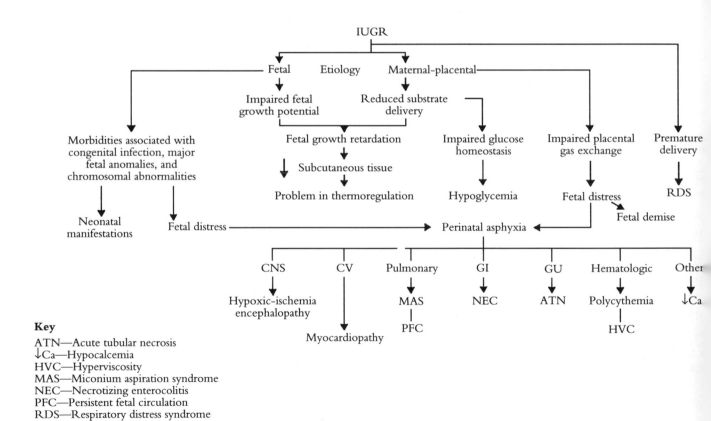

Key
ATN—Acute tubular necrosis
↓Ca—Hypocalcemia
HVC—Hyperviscosity
MAS—Miconium aspiration syndrome
NEC—Necrotizing enterocolitis
PFC—Persistent fetal circulation
RDS—Respiratory distress syndrome

Figure 47.1 Pathophysiology of neonatal morbidities in IUGR.

a late onset of insult without brain sparing. These infants may have a generally less favorable outcome on follow up (2).

As Figure 47.1 shows, IUGR due to congenital anomalies, infection, or chromosomal abnormalities will be associated with morbidities and stigmata relating to the specific cause. Substrate deficiency can lead to hypoglycemia and temperature regulation imbalance: the latter from reduced subcutaneous tissue and increased metabolic rate. Most IUGR-related morbidities result from fetal distress due to placental insufficiency. The illness depends on which organ was affected by hypoxia and ischemia. For instance, if the brain is involved, postasphyxia encephalopathy may occur during the first few days of life.

Immediate Care of IUGR Newborns

The delivery room team should be prepared to resuscitate a growth-retarded baby, because neonatal asphyxia is common. If meconium-stained amniotic fluid has been detected before delivery, meconium should be removed from the upper airway using a combined obstetric-pediatric approach. The nasopharynx of the infant should be aspirated with a suctioning device before delivering the thorax. Immediately after delivery, following further suction of the nasopharynx and oropharynx, the infant's cord can be inspected with a laryngoscope. If meconium is observed, endotracheal suction should be performed (3). This procedure improves the outcome of infants with meconium aspiration syndrome.

In infants who breathe and cry soon after birth and have an Apgar score of greater than 8 at one minute, further suction of nasal and oral cavity to remove any meconium is often all that is necessary. It has recently been shown that attempts to intubate and remove meconium from the trachea of these vigorous and spontaneously breathing infants may produce more harm than benefit (4).

IUGR infants have a high metabolic rate. Maintain their normal body temperatures by having a radiant heat source available in the delivery room during resuscitation. Also, follow their serum glucoses.

These babies also run a high risk of polycythemia because chronic fetal distress may promote erythropoiesis (5). To minimize postnatal placental transfusion, the umbilical cord should be clamped within 10–15 seconds of vaginal delivery of the infant's trunk (6). If cesarean section is used, the cord should be clamped as soon as the baby is delivered.

Specific Problems of IUGR Newborns

Congenital Malformations

Major congenital anomalies, with or without chromosomal aberrations, frequently cause IUGR. If a fetal origin is suspected—for instance, when growth retardation is proportional or when demonstrable maternal and placental factors are absent—a thorough physical examination, looking for congenital anomalies, should be done.

Neonatal Hypoglycemia

This metabolic problem, common in infants with IUGR, generally occurs during the first 12 hours of life. Therefore, it is essential to make blood glucose determinations early. A semiquantitative check, using reagent strips (Dextrostix), can serve as a screen, repeated every 2–3 hours during the first 12 hours. If the strips indicate blood glucose levels below 40 mg/dL, a quantitative test of plasma glucose should be performed. Hypoglycemia is diagnosed when plasma glucose falls below 35 mg/dL in term infants or 25 mg/dL in preterm infants (7). If glucose determinations are done on whole blood, the low limit of normal glucose levels would be 30 mg/dL and 20 mg/dL for term and preterm infants, respectively.

It's important to make the diagnosis early; delay may have serious consequences, because glucose is the major substrate for brain metabolism. With early diagnosis and an immediate continuous IV glucose infusion of 6 mg/kg/minute, the infants will often be symptom free. If the diagnosis is delayed and apnea or seizures develop, a bolus infusion of 25% glucose (0.5 g/kg of body weight) should be given before the continuous infusion. If there are no other cardiopulmonary symptoms, oral feedings should be started as soon as the infant can tolerate them, a practice that may check the hypoglycemia (8). If the hypoglycemia lasts beyond 48–72 hours after birth, a glucocorticoid should be considered. With a few exceptions, however, early diagnosis of low glucose levels and prompt treatment are sufficient.

Respiratory Distress

Meconium aspiration syndrome (MAS), hyaline membrane disease (HMD), or cold stress may cause respiratory problems. Though uncommon in IUGR infants, HMD may occur, particularly in those delivered before 32 weeks; thus, it's important to assess fetal lung maturity when monitoring IUGR pregnancies.

In some cases, the asphyxiated infant, with or without MAS, may have persistent fetal circulation, a condition characterized by pulmonary hypertension with a right-to-left shunt across the foramen ovale, or ductus arteriosus, or both. Usually, the infant will have respiratory distress, with profound hypoxemia: an arterial oxygen tension below 50 mm Hg while breathing 100% oxygen. Arterial pH and PO_2, as well as the chest x-ray, may be normal. If the right-to-left shunt occurs across the ductus arteriosus only, blood from arteries supplying the upper body will have a higher PO_2 than blood from those perfusing the lower body. If blood samples obtained simultaneously from the temporal or right radial artery and the descending aorta reveal differential PO_2 values (20 mm Hg higher in the temporal or right radial artery than in the descending aorta), this may help to establish the diagnosis of persistent fetal circulation. However, this method is not useful when blood is also being shunted through the foramen ovale, because that would make it impossible to obtain a PO_2 differential between the temporal or right radial artery and the descending aorta.

Cyanotic congenital heart disease must be excluded as the cause of profound hypoxemia. Cardiac catheterization in the first few days of life is risky for acutely ill neonates. Fortunately, noninvasive two-dimensional echocardiography can often help make the differential diagnosis. Treatment for the persistent fetal circulation consists of assisted ventilation and a pulmonary vasodilator, tolazoline hydrochloride and inotropic support. Sometimes, a systemic vasoconstrictor, dopamine hydrochloride, is added.

Hypoxic Ischemic Encephalopathy

This frequent complication of IUGR, usually a result of perinatal asphyxia, may begin within a few hours after birth or anytime during the first 24–48 hours. Jittery movements, increased irritability, feeding difficulties, hyper- or hypotonia, and, in some cases, seizures may be evident. Treatment is supportive. For convulsions, the drug of choice is either IV or IM phenobarbital, with a loading dose of 15–20 mg/kg, followed by 2.5 mg/kg every 12 hours. The effectiveness of steroids or a diuretic such as mannitol for treating cerebral edema is undocumented.

Polycythemia and Hyperviscosity

It is well known that IUGR infants are at risk for polycythemia and hyperviscosity (9). Finne has shown that these infants have substantially elevated erythropoietin levels in cord serum (10). This finding suggests prenatal chronic hypoxia, which increases the production of erythropoietin, a hormone that enhances erythropoiesis. Intrapartum hypoxia may also produce intrauterine placental transfusion (11), thus further increasing the infant's blood volume. If placental transfusion continues after birth, the blood volume status could be accentuated. All these events may conspire to increase the blood volume of IUGR infants.

In response to hypervolemia, hemoconcentration, most evident during the first six hours of life, produces polycythemia—venous hematocrit exceeding 65%. In the neonate, hyperviscosity generally results from polycythemia; 90%–95% of polycythemic infants also have hyperviscosity (9). A normal venous hematocrit usually means normal blood viscosity. Hyperviscosity generally means viscosity above 2 SD of the norm. Because polycythemia and hyperviscosity are so closely correlated, hyperviscosity can be assumed when polycythemia is present, particularly if there is no access to a microviscometer.

Polycythemia can be prevented, or its incidence reduced, by recognizing high-risk infants at delivery by quickly clamping the cord after delivering the infant's buttocks. By preventing postnatal placental transfusion one can minimize the risk of polycythemia. Symptomatic polycythemia requires a partial exchange transfusion, with 10%– 15% of the infant's blood volume (80 mL/kg of body weight) removed and replaced with equal volumes of a colloid solution such as Plasmanate. To be more precise, the following formula can be used to calculate the amount of blood to be removed and replaced:

$$\text{Volume (mL)} = \left(\frac{\text{Observed} \quad \text{Desired}}{\text{hematocrit(\%)} - \text{hematocrit(\%)}} \right) \times \begin{array}{c} \text{Blood} \\ \text{volume (80 mL)} \end{array} \times \begin{array}{c} \text{Body} \\ \text{weight (kg)} \end{array}$$

The partial exchange through an umbilical vein requires the same aseptic technique and the same precautions as an exchange transfusion for neonatal hemolytic disease.

How to handle symptom-free infants with polycythemia is controversial. There is a paucity of good data on the potential adverse effects, and it is unclear whether a partial exchange transfusion improves outcome.

Renal Complications

Most renal problems in IUGR infants are associated with asphyxia, with or without hypotension. Actually, any asphyxiated newborn may have renal difficulties. Oliguria and anuria in the first few days after birth may progress to acute renal failure with azotemia and hyperkalemia. Urinalysis, if urine can be obtained, generally reveals cellular elements and casts. Conservative fluid therapy, providing only the allowance for insensible water loss and stool water loss, is in order. In time, most infants with acute renal failure recover, but the condition is often followed by a period of sodium-losing diuresis. When this happens, one must beware of severe hyponatremia. The sodium loss through the kidneys should be quantitated and replaced accordingly.

Neonatal Hypocalcemia

IUGR and appropriately grown infants have a similar incidence of hypocalcemia (12) but the small baby's susceptibility to asphyxia and respiratory distress increases the risk of hypocalcemia. Asphyxia has been associated with high calcitonin levels. In addition, there is a relationship between respiratory distress–induced acidosis and redistribution of calcium ion from the intracellular into the extracellular fluid compartment. When the pH improves because of better respiration (either naturally or through treatment), the calcium ions are mobilized from the extracellular into the intracellular compartment, precipitating a fall in serum calcium level that results in hypocalcemia.

Diagnosis and management of hypocalcemia in IUGR infants is similar to that for appropriately grown neonates. Standard treatment is primarily calcium replacement with IV or oral calcium gluconate. The dose and route of administration will depend on how severe the hypocalcemia is, whether symptoms are present, and if the infant can tolerate oral feeding.

Necrotizing Enterocolitis

Necrotizing enterocolitis (NEC) often appears along with polycythemia and hyperviscosity, probably because of bowel ischemia (13). Since aggressive feeding has been implicated (14) feeding IUGR infants who have polycythemia and hyperviscosity should be done prudently. A reasonable approach is to supplement a conservative oral feeding program with IV glucose to avoid hypoglycemia, another potential complication.

Neurologic and Developmental Outcome

Performance of IUGR infants born in the 1960s and 1970s has been evaluated. Fitzhardinge and associates reported that IUGR infants born with a mean gestational age of 31 weeks had relatively poor neurologic status and developmental performance. The neonatal mortality for this group was also relatively high (15). This suggests that all attempts should be made to avoid delivery of an IUGR fetus before 32 weeks. When the Fitzhardinge group evaluated long-term outcome of IUGR infants born close to term, they found neurologic status to be favorable, although some subtle neurologic and learning deficits were observed (16). Thus, in monitoring an IUGR pregnancy beyond 35–36 weeks, the risk of fetal demise, as well as potential compromise in fetal brain metabolism, should be weighed when considering termination.

Vohr and associates, in a report on IUGR infants born at a mean gestational age of 33.5 weeks, found good neurologic and developmental performance at two years of age. However, at five years of age, although neurologic status was good, four of 9 children had subtle learning deficits

(17). These conflicting results suggest that we don't have enough information to define clearly the optimal timing of delivery of IUGR fetuses beyond 32 weeks' gestation if neurologic and developmental problems are to be avoided.

References

1. Gruenwald P. Fetal deprivation and placental insufficiency. Obstet Gynecol 1971;37:906.

2. Harvey D, Prince H, Bunton J, Parkinson C, Campbell S. Abilities of children who were small-for-gestational-age babies. Pediatrics 1982;69:296–300.

3. Carson BS, Losey RW, Bowes WA, et al. Combined obstetric and pediatric approach to prevent meconium aspiration syndrome. Am J Obstet Gynecol 1976;126:712.

4. Linder N, Aranda JV, Tsur M, Matoth I, Yatsiv I, Mandelberg H, Rottem M, Feigenbaum D, Ezra Y, Tamir I. Need for endotracheal intubation and suction in meconium-stained neonates. J Pediatr 1988;112:613–15.

5. Oh W. Neonatal polycythemia and hyperviscosity. In: The newborn II. Pediat Clin North Am 1986; 33(3):523:532.

6. Yao AC, Lind J. Placental transfusion. Springfield, IL: Charles C Thomas, 1982:146.

7. Cornblath M, Schwartz R. Disorders of carbohydrate metabolism in infancy, 3rd ed. Boston: Blackwell Scientific Publications, 1991.

8. Rabor IF, Oh W, Wu PYK, et al. The effects of early and late feeding of intrauterine fetally malnourished (IUM) infants. Pediatrics 1968;42:261.

9. Hakanson DO, Oh W. Hyperviscosity in the small-for-gestational-age infants. Biol Neonate 1980;37:109.

10. Finne PH. Erythropoietin levels in cord blood as an indicator of intrauterine hypoxia. Acta Paedia Scand 1966;55:478.

11. Oh W, Omori K, Emmanouilides GC, et al. Placental to lamb fetus transfusion in utero during acute hypoxia. Am J Obstet Gynecol 1975;122:316.

12. Tsang RC, Oh W. Neonatal hypocalcemia in low birthweight infants. Pediatrics 1970;45:773.

13. Hakanson DO, Oh W. Necrotizing enterocolitis and hyperviscosity in the newborn infants. J Pediatr 1979;94:779.

14. Kliegman RM, Fanaroff AA. Necrotizing enterocolitis. N Engl J Med 1984;310:1093.

15. Commey JO, Fitzhardinge PM. Handicap in the preterm small for gestational age infants. J. Pediatr 1979;94:779.

16. Fitzhardinge PM, Steven EM. The small for date infant. II. Neurological and intellectual sequelae. Pediatrics 1972; 50:50.

17. Vohr BR, Oh W, Rosenfeld AG, et al. The preterm small-for-gestational age infant: a two-year follow-up study. Am J Obstet Gynecol 1979;133:425.

48

Rh and Other Blood Group Immunizations

John T. Queenan, M.D.

SINCE the advent of Rh immune globulin in 1968, the incidence of Rh immunization has decreased markedly. But because prophylaxis is achieved by passive immunization, protection is short-lived and must be repeated every time the patient is exposed to Rh antigen. Such preventive methods can considerably reduce, but will never eliminate, Rh immunization. Erythroblastosis fetalis (EBF) still accounts for a significant portion of perinatal mortality and morbidity.

Pathophysiology of Rh Immunization

Individuals who lack an Rh antigen on the surface of their erythrocytes are called Rh negative. When such individuals are exposed to the antigen, they may become immunized. Exposure to as little as 0.25 mL of Rh-positive blood may immunize (1). Generally, a clinically significant immunization requires at least two exposures to Rh antigen. The first exposure can result in primary immunization, wherein the patient becomes "sensibilized." The second exposure causes an anamnestic response, characterized by strong, rapid production of antibodies. If the exposure to Rh antigen is large, as when mismatched blood is transfused, the first antigenic stimulus may produce both a primary and an anamnestic response.

The patient who becomes immunized usually first develops IgM (saline-reactive) antibodies: large molecules that do not cross the placenta. These last a variable time but eventually disappear. Shortly after developing IgM antibodies, the patient develops IgG (albumin-reactive) antibodies: small molecules that do cross the placenta. These antibodies are responsible for coating the Rh-positive fetal erythrocytes and causing their hemolysis. If the hemolytic process is extensive, it can cause hydrops fetalis and intrauterine death. If it is milder, the fetus may compensate for the hemolysis by increasing erythrocyte production. In such instances, the baby is born with a positive antiglobulin (Coombs') test of the cord blood. Cord-blood hemoglobin and bilirubin may, however, be normal.

Theoretically, fetal and maternal blood cells do not mix. That is, no erythrocytes or white cells normally cross over from the fetal into the maternal circulation. But, in actuality, small hemorrhages can occur across the placenta in either direction. The Kleihauer-Betke (KB) stain technique provides a unique method of detecting fetal erythrocytes in the maternal circulation (2). The acid elution staining technique detects and measures transplacental hemorrhages (TPH). Numerous studies have shown that the incidence and size of TPH increase as pregnancy progresses (1, 3). At delivery, there may be a large transfer of erythrocytes from the fetus to the mother; indeed, this is the time when most immunizations occur.

Although a mother may be immunized by a dose of Rh antigen as small as 0.25 mL of Rh-positive blood, such an exposure does not always immunize. Numerous factors allow the mother to tolerate Rh antigen during pregnancy, including a high circulating level of corticosteroids and the tendency to immunologic tolerance that characterizes the pregnant state. Also, when the fetus has an ABO blood group antigen that is incompatible with the mother, Rh-positive fetal erythrocytes with the A or B antigen on their surfaces would be destroyed by reacting with the corresponding antibodies in the maternal circulation.

Risks of Immunization

Although TPH is fairly common, it usually does not cause immunization. The risks of Rh immunization in the absence of Rh immune prophylaxis have been carefully determined in numerous studies. If an individual is Rh negative and has never been exposed to Rh antigen, her chances of becoming immunized by an obstetric event are as follows:

Spontaneous Abortion

There is a risk of 3.5%. This study included patients admitted to the hospital with spontaneous incomplete abortion who then had a D&C. Generally, with spontaneous abortion, there is vaginal bleeding, and the fetoplacental circulation has stopped functioning some time before the abortion. (4, 5).

Induced Abortion

There is a 5.5% risk. These studies included patients managed with D&C, suction curettage, and those who had intra-amniotic instillation of hypertonic saline. The procedures were done with the embryo or fetoplacental circulation intact. When the products of conception are disrupted, fetal erythrocytes can enter the maternal circulation through the venous sinuses in the uterus (6).

Third Trimester

There is a risk of 1%–2%. Considering only primigravidas, Bowman (Winnipeg) found a 1.6% incidence of immunization between 28 weeks and delivery. The obvious implication is that these primigravid patients would not be candidates for Rh immune globulin prophylaxis following delivery (7). These data served as the rationale to institute antepartum Rh immune prophylaxis at 28 weeks' gestation.

Term Pregnancies

There is a risk of 14%–17%. In both ABO-compatible and ABO-incompatible pregnancies, if the patient undergoes antibody screening at six weeks and six months postpartum and then is screened in her next pregnancy (following exposure to minute amounts of Rh-positive antigen), the incidence of immunization approximates 17%. This was found in two prospective studies. A full-term pregnancy carries substantial risk of immunization, since most immunizations occur at delivery. Antibodies appear either postpartum or following exposure to Rh antigen in the next pregnancy (1, 8).

Amniocentesis

The risk is between 1% and 2%, depending on the location of the placenta and the skill of the operator (1, 6, 9).

Chorionic Villus Sampling

The risk is still unknown, but it will probably be lower than for genetic amniocentesis.

Ectopic Pregnancy

The risk is less than 1%.

Mismatched Blood Transfusions

There is a 20%–90% chance of immunization.

Rh Immune Prophylaxis

Theobald Smith demonstrated in 1909 that, when an antigen and its corresponding antibodies are injected into a laboratory animal, they do not immunize the animal, provided

TABLE 48.1   Protocols for Protection Against Rh Immunization

Unimmunized Rh–Negative Patient: Two-Dose Regimen (Antepartum and Postpartum)

Initial Visit

Obtain a blood group, Rh type, and indirect antiglobulin (Coombs') antibody screen.

28 Weeks' Gestation

Do an indirect Coombs' test.

If no Rh antibodies are detected, administer 300 μg of Rh immune globulin IM.

At Delivery

Do an anti-D (Rho) titer. A titer of 1:4 or greater probably means the patient is actively immunized and is not a candidate for Rh immune globulin. Lower levels of antibody are due to passively administered Rh immune globulin, and the patient is a candidate for Rh immune globulin.

Obtain a blood group, Rh type, and direct Coombs' test on the cord blood. If the baby is Rh positive, administer 300 μg of Rh immune globulin IM to the mother.

If a large transplacental hemorrhage is suspected, do a Kleihauer-Betke stain to quantitate the size of the fetomaternal hemorrhage.

Give at least 300 μg of Rh immune globulin for each 30 mL of fetal whole blood.

Unimmunized Rh–Negative Patient Undergoing Genetic Amniocentesis

Initial Visit

Obtain a blood group, Rh type, and indirect antiglobulin (Coombs') antibody screen.

15–17 Weeks' Gestation

Following genetic amniocentesis, give 300 μg of Rh immune globulin IM.

Proceed as with "two-dose regimen."

Unimmunized Rh–Negative Patient: Various Clinical Situations

If the patient has a spontaneous or induced abortion or ectopic pregnancy, protect her with 300 μg of Rh immune globin IM.

If the patient is accidentally given an Rh-positive blood transfusion, administer at least 300 μg of Rh immune globulin for each 30 mL of transfused whole blood.

To ensure adequate protection, do an indirect antiglobulin (Coombs') test to demonstrate anti-D (Rho), which indicates an antibody excess.

---

the dose of antibody is in excess (10). In the 1960s, applying this principle, several investigators showed that the administration of Rh immune globulin within 72 hours postpartum would protect against Rh immunization. This prophylactic regimen has become the standard of care in the United States, sharply cutting the incidence of Rh immunization. Because patients have TPHs during pregnancy, approximately 1%–2% become immunized during pregnancy before the postpartum prophylaxis can be ad-

ministered. In an attempt to eliminate these immunizations occurring in the third trimester, 300 μg of Rh immune globulin is now administered at 28 weeks' gestation.

Today the use of Rh immune globulin has been extended to Rh-negative patients who have spontaneous abortions, induced abortions, chorionic villus sampling, amniocenteses, ectopic pregnancies, or mismatched Rh-positive blood transfusions. Theoretically, this system of prophylaxis could be almost 100% effective; in practice, it is not.

The protocols for protection against Rh immunization in various clinical situations are outlined in Table 48.1. Table 48.2 lists the dosages of Rh immune globulin according to indication.

Rh Immune Prophylaxis Failure

Rh immune prophylaxis may not eliminate Rh immunization if:

- Too small a dose is given. The standard dose of Rh immune globulin contains 300 μg of anti-D (Rho) antibody. This is sufficient to protect against a TPH of up to 30 mL of fetal blood. If a TPH was greater, as in abruptio placentae, one ampule may not be adequate to prevent immunization.

  If a question arises about the size of the dose, the laboratory can help by doing an indirect antiglobulin (Coombs') test for anti-D (Rho). If the mother has anti-D (Rho) in her circulation, she has an antibody excess and is protected. Performing a Kleihauer-Betke stain may estimate the amount of fetal cells in the maternal circulation when a large TPH is suspected.

- The protection is administered too late. If the 28-week Rh immune prophylaxis is overlooked, it should be given as soon as possible, provided the patient is not already immunized to the Rh antigen. If the patient goes home postpartum before it is realized that she is a candidate for Rh immune prophylaxis, she should be contacted immediately upon discovery of the omission so she may receive Rh immune globulin.

- The potency of the Rh immune globulin is decreased, either because of a protease or a substandard dose in the vial.

- The patient is already immunized. A mild immunization might escape laboratory detection.

Managing the Rh-Immunized Pregnancy

The patient's blood group, Rh type, and antibody screening should be done on the first prenatal visit. If the patient is Rh negative, screening is performed again at 28 weeks' gestation. If no Rh antibodies are present, Rh immune

Table 48.2 Dosage of Rh Immune Globulin According to Indication

50 μg	300 μg	>300 μg
Chorionic villus sampling	Spontaneous abortion	Large transplacental hemorrhage
	Induced abortion	Mismatched blood transfusion
	Ectopic pregnancy	
	Amniocentesis	
	28 weeks' prophylaxis	
	Premature delivery	
	Term delivery	

globulin is administered according to the protocol for the two-dose regimen outlined in Table 48.1. If antibody is detected, it is identified and a titer is done. The pregnancy is evaluated for EBF.

Today, the Rh-immunized pregnancy may be evaluated by four complimentary modalities:

1. Antibody titers,
2. AF ΔOD_{450},
3. Cordocentesis, and
4. Sonographic evaluation.

In situations where the antibody titer is very low (e.g., 1:4), the outcome is usually favorable because the EBF is mild. In such cases, the following antibody titer is all that is necessary to evaluate the pregnancy. In situations where the titer is higher, the outcome is not predictable and AF ΔOD_{450} and sonography are utilized to determine the fetal condition. In situations where very severe EBF is suspected, cordocentesis is employed to measure the fetal hematocrit. Usually, the operator is prepared to proceed with a fetal transfusion, if it is indicated.

Antibody Titers

Antibody titers may be a source of great misunderstanding. Most laboratories do antibody titers so infrequently that they are not proficient at the technique. In the past, before amniocentesis and amniotic fluid analysis were available, the clinician had to rely on the antibody titer to decide how to manage the pregnancy. In a classic study four decades ago by Allen, Diamond, and Jones, 174 patients had antibody titers of 1:32 or lower, with no history of hydrops fetalis or stillbirth. None of these patients had amniocenteses. Of the 174 patients, 167 (96%) had live fetuses at 37 weeks' gestation. Thus, Allen and colleagues demonstrated that a carefully done antibody titer, along with the patient's history, is an excellent indicator of pregnancy outcome, provided the titer is low (11). If the titer is high, then other parameters like amniotic fluid analysis must be evaluated.

If laboratories can provide accurate and reproducible antibody titers, it will help determine whether amniocentesis is necessary. The first serum for each titer should be frozen so that subsequent titers may be done in duplicate. The laboratory should provide a "critical titer": the antibody titer below which there have been no perinatal deaths from EBF. If, in a first-immunized pregnancy, the antibody titer does not reach the critical level, the patient may be managed without amniocentesis. Once the antibody titer reaches or surpasses the critical level, it no longer provides enough information on the condition of the fetus, and AF ΔOD_{450} must be done.

Amniotic Fluid Analysis

The timing of the initial amniocentesis depends on the patient's history and antibody titer. If the titer is just at the critical level and the patient has not had a baby with EBF, the initial amniocentesis can be done between 28 and 29 weeks' gestation. If the titer or history suggests that the disease may be more severe, the amniocentesis may have to be done as early as 18 weeks' gestation. In this way, a fetus requiring an intrauterine transfusion can be identified.

The amniotic fluid change in optical density at 450 nm (ΔOD) in an Rh-immunized pregnant patient is an almost ideal test of fetal condition. If the clinician fully understands the physiologic properties of amniotic fluid and the pathophysiology of Rh disease, virtually no serious fetal deterioration can be undetected.

Many methods of amniotic fluid analysis have been employed. In the Liley method the AF ΔOD_{450} is placed on a graph, the values fall into one of three zones, which decrease with increasing fetal maturity. These values predict the severity of the fetal condition (12, 13). The graph only dealt with pregnancies 27 weeks and beyond. Many other investigators extended the Liley zones prior to 27 weeks, usually without sufficient data to substantiate the earlier zones.

Whitfield also relied on multiple AF ΔOD_{450}s to see where the trend of values intersected an "action line," indicating when the fetus should be delivered. If the amniotic fluid values are very low, the patient is allowed to go into labor spontaneously (14).

Queenan and Goetschel demonstrated how the trend of values indicates the fetal condition (1, 15). If the trend is falling, the fetus will live. The fetus may be Rh negative and unaffected or Rh positive and mildly or moderately affected, but given proper care, the baby will survive. The only exception to this is when polyhydramnios results in artificially decreasing amniotic fluid bilirubin levels as a result of dilution. A horizontal or rising trend means that the fetus will die in utero if not delivered or given an intrauterine transfusion (Figure 48.1). The clinician must decide whether the fetus is mature enough to be delivered or would do better with intrauterine transfusions.

Ananth and co-workers demonstrated that the AF ΔOD_{450} was also useful before 27 weeks' gestation (16, 17). Two studies of AF ΔOD_{450} 16–20 weeks' gestation show that this window of time provides good information on the outcome of Rh-immunized pregnancies (16, 17). From 16–20 weeks gestation, AF from normal (non-immunized) pregnancies have values that are low but rise gradually throughout this period (16). In a series of Rh-immunized pregnancies, if the AF ΔOD_{450} were 0.09 or lower, the fetus was either Rh-negative (unaffected) or Rh-positive and mildly affected. If the values were greater than 0.15 or if the rising trend of values exceeds 0.15, the fetus always has severe disease and requires intrauterine transfusion. Values between 0.09 and 0.15 require further evaluation of the AF ΔOD_{450} trend to determine the outcome of Rh disease (17).

Current Method

Recently, Queenan and co-workers presented a method

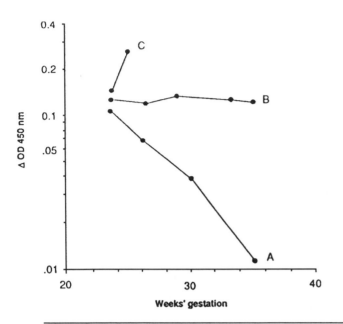

Figure 48.1   Examples of various amniotic fluid bilirubin trend patterns. (A) Decreasing trend, favorable outcome; (B) horizontal or rising trend after 32 weeks indicates need for delivery; (C) rising trend prior to 32 weeks may indicate intrauterine transfusion.

based upon an analysis of 789 single and serial AF ΔOD_{450} values in Rh-immunized pregnancies from 14 to 40 weeks' gestation (18) (Figure 48.2). The advantage of this method is that it is efficacious in both the second and third trimester. In

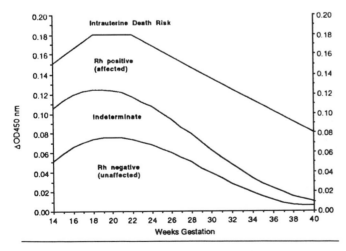

Figure 48.2   Amniotic fluid ΔOD_{450} management zones.

addition, it integrates the complimentary modalities of AF ΔOD_{450}, cordocentesis and sonographic monitoring.

In normal (Rh-negative) pregnancies, the AF ΔOD_{450} values rise until 24 weeks, then they fall until term. In Rh-positive fetuses at risk of dying in utero, the values are higher and the trends rise. This clinical management scheme consists of four zones of increasing severity: Rh-negative (unaffected), Indeterminate, Rh-positive (affected) and Intrauterine Death Risk. By employing this management scheme, Rh-negative fetuses have minimal invasive procedures. Fetuses at risk of death have early cordocentesis for evaluation and therapy. The AF ΔOD_{450} values that fall between these extremes can be separated into two zones based upon the degree of risk.

Clinical Application

If the AF ΔOD_{450} value falls in the "Rh-negative Zone," get a DNA Rh type on the AF. If Rh-negative, deliver at term. If Rh-positive, repeat amniocentesis one time (Table 48.3).

If the AF ΔOD_{450} value falls in the "Indeterminate Zone," get a DNA Rh type. If Rh-positive, repeat amniocentesis every two to four weeks. Decreasing trends generally mean the fetus is Rh-positive with mild or moderate EBF. Rising trends indicate severe EBF. Horizontal trends can be associated with severe EBF.

If the values fall in the "Rh-positive Zone," the fetus has EBF. Repeat the amniocentesis every one to two weeks and do cordocentesis as indicated. Decreasing trends mean moderate EBF. Rising trends indicate severe EBF. Horizontal trends are associated with severe disease and even death if the fetus is not delivered or transfused, depending on gestational age.

Table 48.3   Management

Zone	Action
Rh-Negative	Get DNA Rh type. If Rh positive, repeat amniocentesis × 1
Indeterminate	Get DNA Rh type. If Rh positive, repeat amniocentesis q 2–4 wks
Rh-Positive	Repeat amniocentesis q 1–2 wks; cordocentesis as clinically indicated
Intrauterine Death Risk	Cordocentesis; transfuse as indicated

If the value falls in the "Intrauterine Death Risk Zone," or if the trend of values will cross over into the zone, the fetus is at risk of dying in utero. Cordocentesis should be done to determine fetal condition and, when indicated, to provide access for intrauterine transfusion.

Cordocentesis

Cordocentesis or percutaneous umbilical blood sampling provides a major breakthrough in the evaluation of EBF because it permits a direct measurement of fetal condition. It does not replace the AF ΔOD_{450}, however, because it is a more complex procedure and has a slightly higher risk. Nonetheless, since cordocentesis allows the direct evaluation of fetal blood, it provides such definitive data as the fetal hematocrit and Rh type. Because cordocentesis can cause further maternal immunization, it should be reserved for cases in which severe disease is suspected. The operator is usually prepared to proceed with a direct intravascular transfusion if the EBF has caused a severe fetal anemia. When the cord blood findings indicate that the hematocrit is normal and the fetal blood is Rh-negative, then no EBF exists and subsequent tests are not necessary. This eliminates the need for multiple amniocentesis.

Normal values for fetal hematocrits and hemoglobins have been determined by Forestier et al. (19) according to weeks gestation (Table 48.4).

Sonographic Evaluation

When the fetus is moderately to severely affected with EBF, certain pathophysiologic changes occur. Some of these changes, like cardiomegaly, pericardial effusion, and ascites, are readily detectable by sonography. However, significant

Table 48.4 Normal Blood Values

Week of Gestation	Hematocrit (%)	Hemoglobin (g/dL)
18–20	35.8	11.4
21–22	38.5	12.2
23–25	38.6	12.4
26–30	41.5	13.3

From Forester F, Daffos F, Galacteros F, et al. Hematological values of 163 normal fetuses between 18 and 30 weeks of gestation. Ped Research 1986; 20:342.

EBF can occur without detectable sonographic change. Thus, this modality is not as effective in detecting mild-to-moderate EBF. Sonographic evaluation serves as an excellent safety net because it is accurate, noninvasive, and almost always reveals when a fetus is undergoing serious deterioration due to EBF. Therefore, it is commonly used with antibodies titers and/or AF ΔOD_{450} to check for any undetected fetal deterioration.

Once significant EBF has been established, sonographic evaluation is extremely helpful to monitor fetal condition by following the presence or absence of sonographic features such as ascites and pericardial effusion. Cardiomegaly, pericardial effusions, and ascites can be easily quantitated.

Intrauterine Transfusions

Some fetuses have such severe EBF that they die in utero before they are mature enough to survive extrauterine life. For them, the intrauterine transfusion can be lifesaving.

Intrauterine Intraperitoneal Transfusion

Ever since Liley presented his classic paper describing the intrauterine transfusion (IUT), this technique has become a valuable tool for treating severe fetal anemia and preventing fetal death (20). When first described by Liley in 1963, the procedure was cumbersome and inefficient. He placed paperclips on the maternal abdomen over the area (determined by palpation) that he believed to overlie the target: the lower half of the fetal abdomen. Then an abdominal roentgenogram was obtained. This showed the relationship of the maternal abdominal site to the targeted fetal peritoneal cavity. A Tuohy needle was then inserted through the maternal abdominal wall and the uterus and into the fetal peritoneal cavity. Proper position of the needle tip was ascertained by injecting 10–15 mg of meglumine diazotrizate (Hypaque M 75%) through the needle and taking another abdominal roentgenogram. If the dye was seen on the surface of the fetal bowel, as determined by multiple crescentic opacities, Liley knew the needle was properly placed. Rh-negative, packed red cells were then injected into the fetal peritoneal cavity. These red cells would be absorbed over the next six days via the subdiaphragmatic lymphatics, through the thoracic duct, and into the fetal circulation. In 1963, this was an enormous advance, because it represented the first direct fetal therapy.

Since the introduction of the IUT, many modifications have been made. The first major advance was the use of fluoroscopy in guiding the placement of the needle. Obviously, the use of fluoroscopy was not ideal because of radiation exposure, but it did allow the real-time visualization of the advancing needle and the intraperitoneal injection of the radiopaque dye. The next major advance was the introduction of real-time ultrasound in guiding needle insertion. The operator could watch the placement of the needle in the fetal peritoneal cavity without the risks of ionizing radiation from fluoroscopy.

The intrauterine intraperitoneal transfusion (IUIPT) (Figure 48.3) is self-limited, because the absorption of blood is rather slow, and some of the transfused red cells become hemolyzed. In numerous clinical series, it appeared to save fetuses that would otherwise die in utero from 23 to 32 weeks' gestation. So the severest form of the disease, that in which the fetus would die in utero between 18 and 23 weeks' gestation, was a little out of reach for this therapeutic modality. Despite these limitations, several large series of IUIPTs achieved perinatal survival rates of 75% (21). This was truly remarkable, because the procedure was done only on fetuses that would otherwise die.

Intrauterine Intravascular Transfusion

For two decades, we have been trying to avoid puncturing the umbilical vessels when doing an amniocentesis or intrauterine transfusion. Over the last five years, numerous perinatal centers have been doing direct intravascular fetal transfusions (IUIVT) by placing a sonographically directed needle in the umbilical vein (Figure 48.4). The blood is injected rapidly into the fetal circulation. The IUIVT has several advantages over the IUIPT. First, the blood reaches the fetal circulation immediately instead of over a six-day period. Second, the fetal blood may be sampled before, during, and after the transfusion, yielding valuable data for clinical management. Third, the needle size is smaller (20 gauge) for IUIVT than the sheath required for IUIPT (18 gauge). Fourth, the IUIVT is capable of reversing hydrops fetalis, and, finally, it is able to save fetuses that would die in utero in the 18–23 weeks window during which IUIPT is not effective. Since the fetus never dies due to EBF before 19 weeks' gestation, no matter how severe the EBF, this could potentially salvage even the most severely affected fetus.

It is not always possible to perform an IUIVT, due to technical reasons. When an IUIVT is not feasible, then IUIPT may be done. Some experts prefer to do both proce-

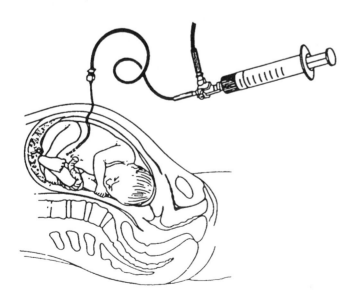

Figure 48.3   Intrauterine fetal peritoneal transfusion.

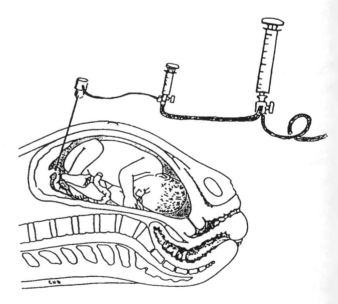

Figure 48.4   Intrauterine intravascular transfusion.

dures, taking advantage of the immediate therapy of IUIVT and the delayed, more physiologic therapy of the IUIPT. In this way, the intervals between transfusions can be prolonged and the total number of transfusions decreased.

Monitoring Fetal Condition

Sonography

Ultrasound scanning gives an accurate means of determining and monitoring fetal condition.

Balancing the risks of extrauterine life due to prematurity with the hostile intrauterine environment is the central problem in managing fetuses with EBF. Monitoring fetal heart size or the progression of ascites is a valuable predictor of fetal condition and the need for immediate delivery.

Heart Size

Erythroblastosis fetalis is characterized by a hemolytic anemia in the fetus. In cases where the hemolysis is severe, the fetus is likely to develop congestive heart failure.

The availability of electronic on-screen digitizers has made measuring fetal heart size considerably easier and more accurate. A transthoracic four-chamber view is obtained. The thorax at this level is almost circular, and ribs may be seen outlining the posterior and lateral chest walls. The circumference of the heart can be measured by the electronic digitizer. It is preferable to do this without the freeze-frame, as the motion of the cardiac muscle makes it easier to delineate the maximum circumference of the heart. In the same view, after employing the freeze-frame, the fetal thoracic circumference can be measured directly. The heart-to-thoracic-circumference ratio can then be calculated. A ratio of 0.5 or less is normal.

Pericardial Effusion

Pericardial effusion is one of the earliest signs of fetal deterioration due to EBF. It is usually easy to detect and is commonly located at the auriculo-ventricular junction of the heart. It may increase or decrease, depending upon the condition of the fetus.

Ascites

Ascites is a definitive indication of fetal deterioration. Very early diagnosis of fetal ascites may be difficult. Pseudo-ascites, which may be seen as an artifact on real-time ultrasound scan, mimics it, and differentiation may be impossible on one examination. Pseudoascites is seen in normal pregnancies and has no significance. We prefer to visualize a section of umbilical vein traversing the falciform ligament in ascitic fluid for a length greater than 2 mm to diagnose ascites.

When early ascites is detected, it is a definitive indication of fetal deterioration secondary to heart failure. Moderate to severe ascites presents very distinctive ultrasound features that would be difficult to overlook.

Hepatosplenomegaly

Hepatic and splenic enlargement result from the markedly increased erythropoieses in the Rh-affected fetus. This may result in a rapidly increasing abdominal circumference.

Umbilical Vein Dilatation

When the fetus develops congestive heart failure, it is reasonable to expect venous distention. Indeed, when there is a combination of venous distention of the umbilical cord and polyhydramnios, the ultrasound scan can produce a striking picture.

The diameter of the umbilical vein can be measured with electronic calipers. The umbilical vein as it traverses the fetal liver can also be distended with severe EBF. But, due to congestion of the liver and accelerated erythropoiesis, the ability of the umbilical vein to distend may be compromised. The best area to measure the umbilical vein is in a loop of cord in the amniotic fluid.

Subcutaneous Edema

When subcutaneous edema, anasarca, is identified, it indicates that the fetus is rapidly deteriorating with hydrops fetalis. Although this usually occurs several days before fetal death, not all fetuses develop this feature before dying in utero. Usually, the fetal scalp is the initial detectable site. Later, the trunk and finally the limbs may be involved.

Placental Changes

With mild EBF, no characteristic placental changes are detected by ultrasound scanning. With moderate or severe

EBF or hydrops fetalis, placental size may increase. The thickness may exceed 50 mm, and the texture may appear to be homogenous, like ground glass. When these findings are detected, other ultrasound signs of severe EBF are almost always present.

Polyhydramnios

Increased amniotic fluid volume is often associated with hyperplacentosis. There are no strict criteria for an ultrasound diagnosis of polyhydramnios; however, an AFI of >24 cm is considered polyhydramnios (see Chapter 50). Although polyhydramnios is a poor prognostic sign because it is usually found with hydrops fetalis, its presence in less severely affected fetuses is inconsistent.

Fetal Movements

Monitoring fetal movements is important. The fetus that dies in utero usually becomes very inactive before death. Fetal movement can be determined by using a system of maternally perceived kicks, such as the Cardiff kick count. Alternatively, fetal movement can be quantitated during a scanning session to provide an estimate of fetal activity that may not be perceived by the mother.

Other Treatment

Administering promethazine hydrochloride to the mother has been suggested to treat severe erythroblastosis fetalis (22). In laboratory animals, this drug effectively inhibits macrophage activity of antibody-coated erythrocytes, thereby lessening hemolysis. However, Stenchever showed that it is not effective in humans (23). In a series of 22 babies born to 21 women treated with promethazine hydrochloride, 150 mg/day, no ameliorating effects of the drug could be demonstrated. Seven of the fetuses required intrauterine transfusions.

In some instances, EBF is so severe that even intrauterine transfusions are not successful. In an attempt to deal with severe disease, Graham-Pole and co-workers have used continuous-flow plasmapheresis (24). They exchanged 24–232 liters of maternal plasma over 7–16 weeks. Seven of the eight patients treated had a fall in antibody concentration, and amniotic fluid bilirubin was lower than in preceding pregnancies. But perinatal outcomes were not much improved. Bowman performed 36 double plasmaphereses plus intrauterine transfusions in one patient in 1967 (25). He did not believe that the plasmaphereses were helpful in improving outcome. It is an enormous undertaking for outcomes no better than most good centers achieve without it and cannot be justified.

A proposed method for treating severe isoimmunization, thus reducing the risk to the fetus, employs the concept of desensitizing the patient to the Rh antigen. Oral desensitization with the use of erythrocyte membrane oral therapy was reported effective for the treatment of Rh disease in patients who had a prior stillbirth (26). Gold and co-workers treated four pregnancies with erythrocyte membrane oral therapy (27). The four pregnancies were in three patients, all of whom had the severest form of Rh immunization as determined by fetal loss due to erythroblastosis fetalis prior to 26 weeks' gestation. In all instances, the study fetuses were markedly hydropic by 27 weeks' gestation. Promethazine was employed in three and intrauterine transfusions in four. No amelioration of the disease process could be determined, therefore this risky method should never be employed.

Delivery

An Rh-immunized mother should usually be delivered by 38 weeks (28). Delivery should be planned, with a neonatal team in the delivery room and blood cross-matched and ready for transfusion into the newborn. If amniotic fluid analysis or fetal evaluation indicates that earlier delivery is desirable, the doctor must exercise clinical judgment. Generally, a vaginal delivery may be accomplished from 36 weeks onward, but the fetus must be carefully monitored during labor. If delivery is to be done between 34 and 35 weeks' gestation, it could be either vaginal or abdominal depending on the condition of the cervix. For all earlier deliveries, however, cesarean section seems more prudent. These fetuses do not tolerate stress well because of their extremely low hemoglobin levels.

It is most important to keep the neonatal team aware of plans so that they are not caught by surprise when the baby is ready for delivery. If the newborn is very severely affected, the first few minutes of life are extremely important; it is therefore essential to have the neonatal team in the delivery room.

Irregular Antibodies

The incidence of irregular antibodies has increased slightly over the past two decades because of greater use of blood transfusions and improved antibody detection techniques. In a large prospective study (29) of more than 18,000 consecutive patients screened by the indirect antiglobulin (Coombs') technique at their initial visit and during the last trimester, 326 (1.7%) had irregular antibodies; 242 has specific and 84 had nonspecific irregular antibodies. Clinically, the presence of irregular antibodies presents a wide spectrum of risk to the fetus. Much depends on whether the antibodies are IgM, which will not cross the placenta, or IgG, which do and cause hemolysis. The strength of the antibody is also important. The Kell antigen, for instance, is potent and capable of eliciting a strong antibody response, usually IgG. If the fetus has the corresponding antigen, hemolysis will occur. The Lewis antigen frequently elicits an IgM antibody, which, since it doesn't cross the placenta, indicates that the fetus is safe. Even if there is an IgG component, the fetus is protected from EBF because the Lewis antigen is not present on the fetal erythrocytes. This antigen is in the fetal plasma and becomes progressively attached to the erythrocytes during the neonatal period.

Managing a patient immunized with an irregular antibody begins with identifying the antibody, followed by determining whether it is IgM, IgG, or both. Next, the antibody titer is determined. If the father is available, his blood should be screened for the antigen. If the mother has become immunized by a blood transfusion and the father does not have the corresponding antigen, the fetus will not have EBF.

If the antibody titer is significant, and the father is known to have the antigen (or there is no information about the father), the pregnancy should be managed with antibody titers and amniotic fluid analysis, the same as for Rh EBF. A scheduled delivery may be crucial because obtaining compatible blood for an exchange transfusion may be extremely difficult.

Should all obstetric patients be screened for irregular antibodies? That depends on the laboratory resources, cost, and money available. If only some patients are screened, it is possible to identify an at-risk group who should always be screened, not only because they have a higher incidence of immunization, but also because they commonly have clinically significant immunizations. Screening all patients who have had induced abortions, cesarean sections, or blood transfusions should identify most of the clinically significant problems (30). If an antibody is so weak that it defies identification, it will usually not cause clinical EBF.

ABO Incompatibility

This form of EBF is generally mild, but the clinician must not be lulled into a false sense of security. If ABO incompatibility is undetected and untreated, it can cause kernicterus. The problem is different from Rh EBF because 50% of cases occur in the first pregnancy. ABO EBF can occur whether the mother's blood group is O, A, or B. It is most common in mothers with O blood because they tend to develop IgG antibodies to A and B antigens.

The various laboratory tests for anti-A and anti-B provide no help in predicting the prognosis in ABO EBF. However, this condition never kills the fetus. Since fetal death is not a threat, amniocentesis should *not* be done to determine the severity of the hemolytic process. Depending on the history of ABO incompatibility, delivery at 38 weeks might be indicated in some cases. In general, babies with ABO EBF are born with normal or slightly decreased hemoglobin. The cord-blood direct antiglobulin (Coombs') test is usually weakly positive. The newborn problem generally is one of mild to moderate hyperbilirubinemia, most often managed with phototherapy. Occasionally, the hyperbilirubinemia is severe, and exchange transfusions are necessary. One word of caution: With the increasing trend to early hospital discharge, vigilance is needed not to let one of these babies escape detection. The consequences could be disastrous.

Summary

Just four decades ago, 50% of Rh-immunized patients lost

their babies. Today, with proper diagnostic and therapeutic management, perinatal mortality should be 1%–2%. Of course, this implies referral of difficult problems to perinatal centers. The perinatal mortality from erythroblastosis fetalis caused by irregular antibodies should be negligible, and there should be no perinatal mortality from ABO incompatibility. With severe Rh EBF, there may be considerable neonatal morbidity. Only skillful neonatal management can ensure a good outcome.

CASE 48.1

The husband of a white, Rh-negative, 29-year-old gravida 2, para 0 was heterozygous for the Rh factor. The patient's first pregnancy had ended with an induced abortion at 12 weeks' gestation 10 years previously. She did not believe that she had received Rh immune prophylaxis.

The patient was seen at six weeks' gestation during her second pregnancy. An indirect antiglobulin (Coombs') test indicated that she was immunized to the Rh factor. The titer was 1:256.

An amniocentesis performed at 24 weeks' gestation revealed a ΔOD_{450} of 0.10. Subsequent amniocenteses performed at 27, 30, and 32 weeks gave values of 0.09, 0.08, and 0.04, respectively. At 36 weeks, the ΔOD was 0.02, and the L/S ratio was 2.4:1.

Labor was induced at 38 weeks' gestation, with the delivery of a 3,250-g Rh-negative male infant. The cord-blood direct antiglobulin (Coombs') test was negative.

A case such as this clearly illustrates the importance of following the trend of amniotic fluid bilirubin values. A decreasing trend indicates that the fetus will survive if appropriate management of pregnancy and neonatal care are provided. With a decreasing trend, the infant may be Rh-negative (unaffected) or mildly to moderately affected with erythroblastosis fetalis. ∎

CASE 48.2

A white, Rh-negative, 24-year-old gravida 4, para 3 (all living) had a husband heterozygous for the Rh factor. She received Rh immune prophylaxis with each pregnancy. The course of her fourth pregnancy was uncomplicated. She received Rh immune globulin at 28 weeks. She desired no further pregnancies and requested sterilization following delivery. She delivered a 3,500-g female infant who was Rh positive, with a negative cord-blood direct antiglobulin (Coombs') test. The patient had a postpartum tubal ligation. She asked her physician whether she should have Rh immune globulin prophylaxis, since she had been sterilized.

Rh immune globulin prophylaxis should be recommended in cases such as the one illustrated here for the following reasons: first, there is a small chance of tubal ligation failure; second, such a young patient may someday desire tubal reanastomosis; and, third, if the patient ever was in need of a blood transfusion under extreme circumstances, Rh-positive blood might be the only available source. ∎

CASE 48.3

A 35-year-old, white, married para 2, gravida 4, immunized Rh-negative woman had a titer of 1:256 when she was seen at six weeks' gestation. Her previous baby was delivered at 37 weeks and is living and well after three exchange and one booster transfusions.

She had a sonographically directed genetic amniocentesis at 17 weeks' gestation. The amniotic ΔOD_{450} was 0.16 at that time. At 17 weeks, cordocentesis was performed, with preparation for an IUIVT if indicated. The fetal cord blood hematocrit was 19%, so an IUIVT was performed, transfusing 20 mL of Rh-negative packed, washed, irradiated red cells. The final hematocrit was 45%. Subsequent IUIVTs were done at 21, 24, 28, and 32 weeks' gestation.

She delivered a 2,900-g Rh-positive female baby at 37 weeks' gestation. The cord hematocrit was 28%. The Kleihauer-Betke showed 80% adult (transfused) red blood cells. The neonatal bilirubin rose slowly but steadily, and an exchange transfusion was necessary on the second day of life. An additional two simple transfusions were necessary for newborn anemia. The baby is living and well. ■

CASE 48.4

A 25 year-old, white, married, para 0, gravida 1, Rh-negative woman had an uneventful antepartum course. Her labor progressed normally until 8 cm of dilatation. Then her contractions increased in intensity and duration. The electronic fetal heart rate pattern revealed slight tachycardia and there was an increased baseline tone between contractions. An increase in bloody vaginal discharge occurred. The obstetrician decided that the mother was experiencing an abruptio placentae. The baby was promptly delivered vaginally and had Apgar's of 7 and 9 at one and five minutes respectively. Because the mother was Rh-negative, the cord blood was sent for cross match for Rh-immune globin. The blood bank indicated that a Kleihauer-Betke stain was necessary because of a large fetomaternal hemorrhage. The K-B stain revealed 40 ml of fetal blood in the maternal circulation. Since the baby was Rh positive, two ampules of Rh immune globulin were administered intramuscularly.

On the second pospartum day, an indirect antiglobulin (Coomb's) test was done revealing an anti-D (Rho) titer of 1:1. This confirmed the presence of an "antibody excess" assuring that the mother was protected from Rh immunization.

In general, the cross-match serves as a determinant of large fetomaternal hemorrhages. A cross-match that shows microagglutination has detected a minor population of Rh-positive fetal erythrocytes. In such cases, it is not enough to give an ampule containing 300 μg of Rh immune globulin. If the laboratory can do a Kleihauer-Betke stain, this is an excellent means of quantitating the size of the fetomaternal

hemorrhage. In general, 300 μg of Rh immune globulin protects against 30 mL of Rh-positive blood. If no fetal erythrocytes are found on the Kleihauer-Betke stain, this by no means indicates that Rh prophylaxis is unnecessary. No fetal erythrocytes are detected in half of those who become immunized. The best test to ensure that adequate Rh immune globulin has been administered is the indirect antiglobulin (Coombs') test. If anti-D (Rh0) can be demonstrated in the maternal serum, "antibody excess" has been achieved. ■

References

1. Queenan JT. Modern management of the Rh problem, 2nd ed. Hagerstown, MD: Harper & Row, 1977.
2. Kleihauer E, Braun H, Betke K. Demonstration von fötalen Hämoglobin in den Erythocyten eines Blutausstrichs, Kin. Wochenschr 1957;35:637.
3. Zipursky, A, Pollock J, Neelands P, et al. The transplacental passage of fetal red blood cells and the pathogenesis of Rh immunization during pregnancy. Lancet 1963; 2:489.
4. Queenan JT, Gadow EC, Lopes AC. Role of spontaneous abortion in Rh immunization. Am J Obstet Gynecol 1971; 110:128.
5. Freda VJ, Gorman JG, Galen RS, et al. Threat of Rh immunization from abortion. Lancet, 1970;2:147.
6. Queenan JT, Shah S, Kubarych SF, et al. Role of induced abortion in rhesus immunization. Lancet 1971;1:815.
7. Bowman JM, Pollock JM. Antenatal prophylaxis of Rh immunization: 28-weeks'-gestation service program. Can Med Assoc 1978;118:627.
8. Ascari WQ, Levine P, Pollock W. Incidence of maternal Rh immunization by ABO compatible and incompatible pregnancies. Br Med J 1969;1:399.
9. Queenan JT, Adams DW. Amniocentesis: a possible immunizing hazard. Obstet Gynecol 1964;24:530.
10. Smith T. Active immunity produced by so-called balanced or neutral mixtures of diptheria toxin and antitoxin. J Exp Med 1909;11:241.
11. Allen FH, Diamond LK, Jones AR. Erythroblastosis fetalis: IX. Problems of stillbirth. N Engl J Med 1954;251:453.
12. Liley AW. Liquor amnii analysis in the management of the pregnancy complicated by rhesus sensitization. Am J Obstet Gynecol 1961;82:1359.
13. Liley AW. Errors in the assessment of haemolytic disease from

amniotic fluid. Am J Obstet Gynecol 1963;86:485.

14. Whitfield CR. A three-year assessment of an action line method of timing intervention in rhesus isoimmunization. Am J Obstet Gynecol 1970;108:1239.

15. Queenan JT, Goetschel E. Amniotic fluid analysis for erythroblastosis fetalis. Obstet Gynecol 1968;32:120.

16. Ananth U, Warsof SL, Coulehan JM, Wolf PH, Queenan JT. Midtrimester amniotic fluid delta optical density at 450 nm in normal pregnancies. Am J Obstet Gynecol 1986;155: 664.

17. Ananth U, Queenan JT. Does midtrimester ΔOD_{450} of amniotic fluid reflect severity of Rh disease? Am J Obstet Gynecol 1989;161:47.

18. Queenan JT, Tomai TP, Ural SH, et al. Amniotic fluid ΔOD_{450} in Rh-immunized pregnancies from 14–40 weeks gestation: A proposal for clinical management. Am J Obstet Gynecol 1993;168:1370.

19. Forestier F, Daffos F, Galacteros F, et al. Hematological values of 163 normal fetuses between 18 and 30 weeks of gestation. Ped Research 1986;20:342.

20. Liley AW. Intrauterine transfusion of foetus in haemolytic disease. Br Med J 1963;2:1107.

21. Queenan JT. Intrauterine transfusion: a cooperative study. Am J Obstet Gynecol 1969;104:397.

22. Gusdon JP Jr, Witherow C. Possible ameliorating effects of erythroblastosis by promethazine hydrochloride. Am J Obstet Gynecol 1973;117:1101.

23. Stenchever MA. Promethazine hydrochloride: use in patients with Rh isoimmunization. Am J Obstet Gynecol 1978; 130:665.

24. Graham-Pole J, Barr W. Willoughby, MLN. Continuous-flow plasmapheresis in management of severe rhesus disease. Br Med J 1977;1:1185.

25. Bowman JM. Intensive antenatal plasmapheresis in severe rhesus isoimmunization. Lancet 1976;1:421.

26. Bierme SJ, Blanc M, Abbal M, et al. Oral Rh treatment for severely immunized mothers. Lancet 1979;1:604.

27. Gold WR, Queenan JT, Woody J, et al. Oral desensitization in Rh disease. Am J Obstet Gynecol 1983;146:980.

28. Queenan JT. Rh immunization. In: Protocols for high-risk pregnancies. Queenan JT, Hobbins JC, eds. Oradell, NJ: Medical Economics Books, 1982.

29. Queenan JT, Smith BD, Haber JM, et al. Irregular antibodies in the obstetric patient. Obstet Gynecol 1969;34:767.

49

Multiple Gestation

J. Patrick O'Grady, M.D.

ALTHOUGH overall perinatal mortality for multiple gestations is at least twice that for singletons, aggressive management can substantially reduce losses. Recent series have reported remarkably low mortality rates for twin gestations (Table 49.1) (1–6). As the number of fetuses rises, so does the risk (7–9). Yet, active attention to detail and serial ultrasonic and biophysical studies produce good results in experienced hands. Success in managing multiple gestations depends on serial fetal monitoring, supportive psychological counselling, and clinical skill (10).

Basic Embryology

Twins arise either by splitting of a single ovum, producing identical (monozygotic) twins, or by multiple ovulation, resulting in fraternal (dizygotic) twins (11). Approximately one of 85 live births is a twin birth. Hellin's law accurately predicts the approximate incidence of spontaneously occurring higher multiples (12). Incidence of triplets is approximately the square of incidence of twins $(1:85)^2$ and for quadruplets, the cube $(1:85)^3$.

One third of twins are monozygotic. The frequency of dizygotic twinning varies with race, being greatest among blacks and lowest in Orientals. Dizygotic twinning also increases with maternal age and parity. In contrast, the frequency of monozygotic twinning is nearly constant. Varying rates for dizygotic twining are believed to be caused by variations in central gonadotropin production. Incidence of multiple gestation is currently much influenced by ovula-

Table 49.1 Perinatal Mortality for Twins

Study	No. deliveries	Rate/1,000
Farooqui MO, et al.,1973 (1)	333	90
Persson PH, et al., 1979 (2)	110	27.3*
Keith L, et al., 1980 (3)	588	66
Chervenak FA, et al., 1984 (4)	362	103
Hartikainen-Sorri AL, 1985 (5)	102	20
Papiernik E, et al., 1985 (6)	197	25.4†

*Gestational age exclusions uncertain.
†Excludes losses <24 weeks.
Modified from O'Grady JP. Clinical management of twins. Contemp Ob/Gyn 1987 (April);29:126.

tion induction. The incidence of twins ranges from 7% to 17% with clomiphene citrate (Clomid, Serophene) and from 20% to 55% with pooled menopausal urinary gonadotropins (13). Prolactin-inhibiting agents do not appear to increase incidence.

Monozygotic twins are genetically identical, but dizygotic twins are no more related than other siblings. In rare cases, dizygotic twins result from matings with two different fathers within the same menstrual cycle. Also different phenotypes or chromosomal complements can occur in monozygotic pairs because of differing environmental influences or spontaneous mutation..

Twins' zygosity is often established by placental and neonatal examination (11, 12). In 20% of deliveries, like sex and a single monochorionic placenta with vascular cross-connections document monozygotic twinning. In an additional 30%, different fetal sex proves dizygosity. Of the remaining pairs, 80% or more are found to be dizygotic by study of blood group markers or human leukocyte antigens.

In dizygotic twinning, a fused placenta is common. Careful examination shows two amnions, two chorions, and no vascular cross-connections. Less frequently, two separate placentas are present.

In single-ovum twins, usually a single-disk placenta with one chorion and two amnions is present. Careful examination or milk injection into placental vessels often reveals vascular cross-connections. Rarely, even in monozygotic twinning, two entirely separate placentas are present. In triplets or other multiples, the placentas can be mono-, di-, or multizygous and may be separate (12).

Fused, multizygous placentas are likely most common, given ovulation induction as a major cause for multifetal pregnancies. In all cases, placentas from multiple gestations should be sent for examination by a pathologist.

Fetal Risks and Complications

Among the most significant risks of multiple gestation is preterm delivery (Table 49.2). The mean gestational age for labor in twins is between 36.5 and 37.5 weeks, with preterm delivery more common in identical than fraternal twins (35% versus 25%) (1, 14). Mean gestation age for delivery in triplets is 33 weeks. Prematurity is of substantial-

ly greater importance in all multiple gestations than are delivery problems. The small percentage (10% or less) of deliveries before 30 weeks accounts for 50% or more of total morbidity and mortality.

Pregnancy-induced hypertension, placental abruption, premature membrane rupture, hydramnios, and uterine overdistention predispose to preterm labor with twins. Hydramnios, due to fetus-to-fetus transfusion, fetal anomalies, or carbohydrate intolerance, is common among multiple pregnancies, especially between monozygotic fetuses.

After 28 to 30 weeks, the fetal weight increases in multiple gestations are uneven, probably owing to varying placentation or vascular cross-connections. Ultrasonic scanning is needed to evaluate the growth of multiple fetuses, as most discrepancies cannot be otherwise detected. Repeating scanning at two- to three-week intervals after 28 weeks' gestation is prudent. At a given gestational age, lung maturity as reflected in the lecithin to sphingomyelin ratio is biochemically comparable between twin and singleton fetuses as well as among twins (15).

Clinically, relative fetal growth is evaluated by com-

Table 49.2 Risks in Multifetal Pregnancy

Fetal
Early fetal loss ("vanishing")
Congenital anomalies
Intrauterine demise
Fetal-fetal transfusion syndrome
Prematurity
Discrepant fetal growth, intrauterine growth retardation
Cord prolapse or entanglement

Maternal
Psychological disorders
Premature labor, delivery
Premature rupture of membranes
Pregnancy-induced hypertension
Antenatal and intrapartum hemorrhage
Hydramnios
Anemia
Glucose intolerance
Dystocia
Operative delivery

From References 1, 3, 4, and 7–21.

parison of BPD, fetal femur length (FL), AC, head circumference, estimated fetal weight (EFW), and amniotic fluid volume at each scanning session (16). Prospectively, the best predictors of abnormal fetal growth are differences in AC and EFW (17).

Intrauterine growth retardation complicates at least 10%–15% of all multiple gestations (16). The most extreme discrepancies arise in the twin–twin transfusion syndrome (15, 17, 18). Hydramnios usually occurs in the recipient twin sac but is seen occasionally in the donor sac, or even in both. Disparity between sac sizes can be extreme, and the risks of intrauterine fetal death, premature labor, premature rupture of membranes, cord prolapse, and placental abruption are high.

The risk of major morbidity to a surviving fetus after death of its sibling, although difficult to estimate accurately, is approximately 15% (18, 19). Similarly, maternal complications from carrying one dead fetus in a multiple gestation are uncommon. Hypofibrinogenemia is rare and is unlikely to develop until the fetus has been dead for four or more weeks.

If intrauterine death of one fetus is documented in the second trimester or later, management depends on both gestational age and fetal monitoring results (18). At less than 34 weeks' gestation, conservative management, involving close observation of the surviving fetus or fetuses and serial testing of maternal coagulation factors, is best (19). After 34 weeks, individualized care and consideration of delivery are recommended, particularly when pulmonic maturity is present. After 37 weeks, little is gained by further delay, and delivery is indicated (18).

Anomalies

The incidence of birth defects in twins is double that for singletons. Monozygotic twins are virtually always concordant for genetic abnormalities, and 2%–10% are concordant for developmental anomalies (16). When amniocentesis is performed for genetic analysis, all sacs should be sampled.

Late separation of the fetal poles in monozygotic pairs results in either conjoined fetuses or a monoamniotic, monochorionic pregnancy. In the latter instance, both fetuses lie within the same amniotic sac and are at a more than 50% risk for fatal cord entanglement.

Conjoined twins occur in approximately one in 40,000 births (11). These twins are monozygotic, same sexed, females in 70% of cases, and have normal chromosomal complements. Most are united facing one another at the thorax.

Another malformation associated with monozygotic twinning that is difficult to diagnose correctly is an acardiac co-twin. Rarely, the second twin produces dystocia. Fetus papyraceus results when a twin dies antenatally and its body is compressed by the growth of its sibling. Other unusual malformations, including fetus-in-fetu and sacrococcygeal teratoma, are presumably caused by an incomplete, attached, or included monozygotic twin.

Diagnostic Criteria

More multiple pregnancies are conceived than carry to viability, and 20% or more are lost (20). Advances in transvaginal ultrasonography permit identification of fetal viability by seven weeks' gestational age. However, a diagnosis of a multiple pregnancy should not be reported in the first trimester unless separate sacs, each with a fetal pole and cardiac activity can be identified. Ideally, the diagnosis of any multiple gestation made before 14 weeks should be reconfirmed by subsequent ultrasonic scan, especially if vaginal bleeding occurs. If a fetus is lost during the first trimester, the prognosis for the remaining fetus or fetuses is good.

Mothers' Problems

Maternal complications of multiple gestation are common. Large placentas predispose to pregnancy-induced hypertension and placental separation. Anemia is also common (21).

Hemodynamic and endocrinologic changes also cause risks (11). Vascular volume expansion is greater than for singleton pregnancies. However, red blood cell mass tends to lag, increasing the physiologic anemia of pregnancy. Also, oral glucose tolerance tests are more likely to be abnormal in women with multiple gestations (16, 22).

Management Considerations

Multiple gestations are more common in older gravidas,

women who have previously been delivered of twins or higher multiples, and patients undergoing ovulation induction. Multiple gestation should be suspected when fundal size exceeds dates, when two or more heart rates can be heard or when preterm labor occurs. A further clue is that virtually all uncomplicated multiple pregnancies have an elevated maternal serum α-fetoprotein level.

Patients carrying several fetuses should stop smoking and avoid drug and alcohol ingestion. Total dietary caloric intake is increased by 1,260 kJ. Iron intake should be at least 60 mg daily and folic acid supplementation of 2 mg daily provided if needed. Optimal maternal weight gain during twin gestation is greater than that for singleton gestation at approximately 44 lb. Ideal weight gain for greater multiples is not established.

Beyond 20 weeks careful attention should be paid to cervical changes, uterine activity, and maternal work habits (Table 49.3) (4, 16, 23). Beyond 28 weeks, when intrauterine growth retardation (IUGR) and preterm stillbirth are the most important causes of perinatal wastage, appropriate antepartum testing and ultrasonic evaluation should be performed (16, 17, 24–26).

Hospitalization may be necessary for early cervical ripening or evidence of preterm labor. Neither routine cerclage nor prophylactic oral betamimetic tocolytics are effective in preventing preterm labor, although the situation is less clear for the higher multiples (13). Similarly, the role for outpatient uterine activity monitoring in multiple gestation is unsettled. For pregnancy in preterm labor, magnesium sulfate remains the preferred parenteral tocolytic.

Effects of multiple gestation on families are profound (10). When presenting diagnosis of first-trimester multiple gestation, the possibility of early fetal loss should be explained to the family. Parents should be prepared for close follow-up in the third trimester and risk of preterm or operative delivery. Management of stress and assistance in planning for the care of two or more possibly premature newborns are additional needs.

It's unclear whether enforced bed rest improves perinatal survival (2, 5, 6, 8, 16, 27). Although mean gestation time is not significantly prolonged by bed rest, incidence of small-for-dates or growth-retarded infants is reduced. Therefore, most clinicians favor resting. Reduced activity at home for women carrying twin gestations, starting arbitrarily at 24 weeks' gestation, is recommended. For twin gestations, hospitalization is reserved for complications. For women carrying three or more fetuses, admission in the early third trimester is advised (17).

Interpretation of the nonstress test (NST) in multiple gestations is the same as in singletons (24, 26). A reactive test indicates fetal well-being. A nonreactive test is ambiguous, calling for induction of uterine contractions, prolonged nonstress testing, acoustic stimulation, obtaining of a fetal biophysical profile (BPP), or all these (Figure 49.1) (16, 24, 25, 27). For triplets and greater multiples, serial monitoring is likely best performed by biophysical testing, combined with serial growth scans (Figure 49.2).

Dilemmas occur when testing suggests possibility of an abnormality in one fetus only. Reevaluation of growth, assessment of amniotic fluid volume Doppler flow studies, a BPP, and determination of pulmonary maturity by amniocentesis may be needed. Management is individualized, and there are no simple rules.

Selective fetal reduction is a possible response to the diagnosis of multiple gestation but is complicated by limited data and both medical and ethical concerns (28). Selective termination has been used in multiple gestations to prevent the birth of abnormal fetuses and, more controversially, to reduce numbers in instances of unintended multiple implantation. Hopefully, future modifications in ovulation induction and in vitro fertilization (IVF)/gamete intrafal-

---

Table 49.3 Antenatal Assessment in Multiple Gestation

Weekly clinical visits from 20 weeks to delivery

Three-hour glucose tolerance test after 26 weeks

Ultrasonography for serial growth every 2–3 weeks from 28 weeks to delivery (twins); 24 weeks to delivery (triplets or greater)

Weekly nonstress test from 28–30 weeks to delivery (twins)

Weekly biophysical profile from 28 weeks to delivery for triplets or greater

Contraction stress test or BPP for nonreactive or equivocal NSTs in twins

Weekly Doppler flow studies if discrepant fetal pairs are observed

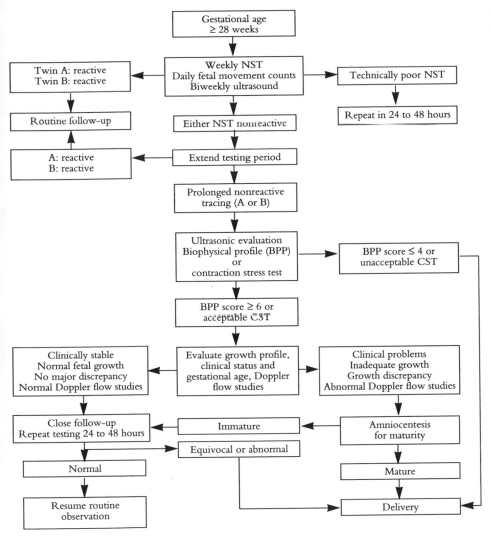

Figure 49.1   Antenatal management of twins.

Delivery Alternatives

If a patient with twins is first seen in labor and the EFW for each twin is less than 1,500 g, operative delivery is probably—although not certainly— desirable (27). In twins weighing more than 1,500 g, delivery mode depends on presentation, facilities, and obstetric skill. Qualified assistants, including a neonatologist or other person capable of assisting with neonatal resuscitation should be available, as

lopian transfer (GIFT) procedures will reduce the likelihood of such multifetal gestation.

well as cross-matched blood, and, if intrapartum version is anticipated, a portable real-time ultrasound machine (Figure 49.3). Gestations of three or more fetuses are best managed by cesarean delivery.

Epidural anesthesia is best for these deliveries. However, the anesthetist should be made aware that there may be a sudden requirement for major operative intervention and possibly general anesthesia.

For twins, scalp-clip monitoring of the leading fetus and Doppler transducer monitoring of the second permit close observation during labor. Real-time ultrasound scanning can be used to document fetal position and estimate

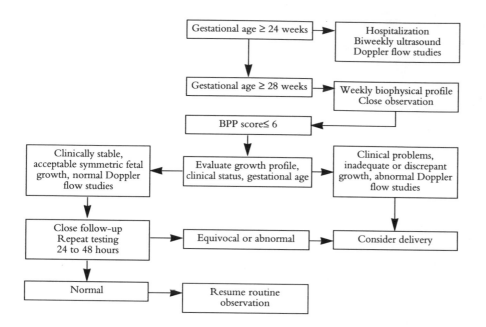

Figure 49.2   Triplets or more: antepartum management.

For triplets and greater multiples, serial monitoring is probably best performed by biophysical testing combined with serial growth scans.

fetal weight. Oxytocin (Pitocin, Syntocinon) may be used in twins as in singleton gestations, but caution must be taken in cases of desultory progress late in the second stage (27).

If the leading twin is breech or transverse, cesarean section is indicated. If it is cephalic, a trial of vaginal delivery is favored. Thereafter, the remaining twin should be regarded as a separate delivery. If the second twin is noncephalic, it becomes necessary to decide whether the moth-

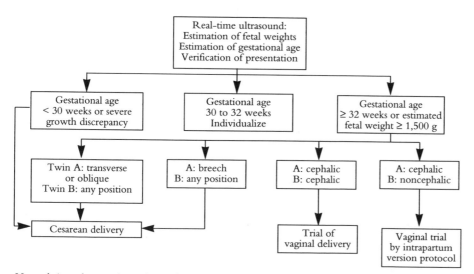

Use real-time ultrasound scanning to document twins' fetal position and estimate fetal weight.

Figure 49.3   Twins: intrapartum management.

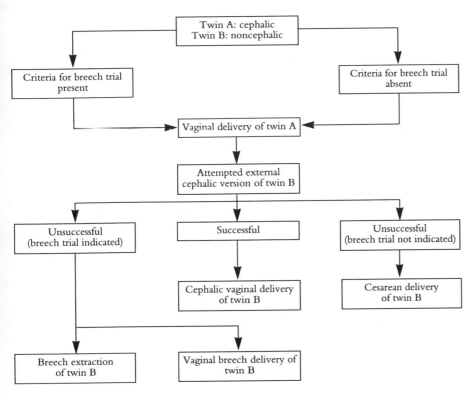

Figure 49.4   Twins: intrapartum version protocol.

If the first twin is cephalic and the second twin noncephalic, it becomes necessary to decide whether the patient is a candidate for spontaneous or breech extraction delivery.

er is a candidate for spontaneous or extracted breech delivery (27, 29). The physician's experience, the patient's preference, and occasionally x-ray pelvimetry, as well as size and attitude of the second fetus, will influence this decision.

If a breech trial is *not* to be done and the clinician has the ability to perform external cephalic version, vaginal delivery of the leading twin and conversion of the second to cephalic presentation may be tried. Should version be unsuccessful or progress with the second attempted cephalic delivery poor, cesarean section (CS) should be performed (27, 28). External version of a noncephalic second twin should be done under real-time ultrasound (29). If fetal bradycardia or cord prolapse occurs before or during version, either CS or breech extraction should be performed (Figure 49.4) (16, 27).

There is no special time interval between delivery of the two infants, and the doctor shouldn't feel compelled to delivery both twins vaginally. In some cases, breech extraction of the second twin can be done safely by skilled—but not by inexperienced—practitioners (1, 16, 27).

The uterine overdistention of multiple pregnancy predisposes to postpartum atony. Obstetricians should be prepared to administer oxytocin, ergonovine maleate (Ergotrate Maleate), or carboprost (Prostin/15 M).

Conclusions

Management of multifetal gestation, with its inherent risks and dilemmas, is a key test of an obstetrician's knowledge, judgment, and skill. To successfully manage such a pregnancy and direct an institution's resources to achieve delivery without harm to mother or infants demonstrates great expertise.

References

1. Farooqui MO, Grossman JH, Shannon RA. A review of twin pregnancy and perinatal mortality. Obstet Gynecol Surv 1973;28(suppl):144.

2. Persson PH, Grennert L, Gennser G, et al. On improved outcome of twin pregnancies. Acta Obstet Gynecol Scand 1979;58:3.

3. Keith L, Ellis R, Berger GS, et al. The Northwestern University multihospital twin study. I. A description of 588 twin pregnancies and associated pregnancy loss, 1971 to 1975. Am J Obstet Gynecol 1980;138:781.

4. Chervenak FA, Youcha S, Johnson RE, et al. Twin gestation: antenatal diagnosis and perinatal outcome in 385 consecutive pregnancies. J Reprod Med 1984;29:727.

5. Hartikainen-Sorri AL. Is routine hospitalization in twin pregnancy necessary? Acta Genet Med Gemellol (Roma) 1985; 34:189.

6. Papiernik E, Mussy MA, Vial M, et al. A low rate of perinatal deaths for twin births. Acta Genet Med Gemellol (Roma) 1985;34:201.

7. Lipitz S, Reichmann B, Paret G, et al. The improving outcome of triplet pregnancies. Am J Obstet Gynecol 1989;161: 1279.

8. Luke B, Keith LG. The contribution of singletons, twins and triplets to low birth mortality and handicap in the United States. J Reprod Med 1992;37:661–6.

9. Syrop CH, Varner MW. Triplet gestation: maternal and neonatal implications. Acta Genet Med Gemellol (Roma) 1985; 34:81.

10. Groothuis JR. Twins and twin families: a practical guide to outpatient management. Clin Perinatol 1982;12:459.

11. Benirschke K, Kim CK. Multiple pregnancy. N Engl J Med 1973;288:1276, 1329.

12. Bardawil WA, Reddy RL, Bardawil LW. Placental considerations in multiple pregnancy. Clin Perinatol 1988;15:13.

13. Dor J, Shalev J, Mashiach S, et al. Elective cervical suture of twin pregnancies diagnosed ultrasonically in the first trimester following induced ovulation. Gynecol Obstet Invest 1982;13:55.

14. Puissant F, Leroy F. A reappraisal of perinatal mortality factors in twins. Acta Genet Med Gemellol (Roma) 1982;31:213.

15. Winn HN, Romero R, Roberts A, Liu H, Hobbins JC. Comparison of fetal lung maturation in preterm singleton and twin pregnancies. Am J Perinat 1992;9:326–8.

16. Ahn MO, Phelan JP. Multiple pregnancy: antepartum management. Clin Perinatol 1988;15:55.

17. Grumbach K, Coleman BG, Arger PH, et al. Twin and singleton growth patterns compared using US. Radiology 1986;158:237.

18. Carlson NJ, Towers CV. Multiple gestation complicated by the death of one fetus. Obstet Gynecol 1989;73:685.

19. Hanna JH, Hill JM. Single intrauterine fetal demise in multiple gestation. Obstet Gynecol 1984;63:126.

20. Landy JH, Weiner S, Corson SL, et al. The "vanishing twin": ultrasonographic assessment of fetal disappearance in the first trimester. Am J Obstet Gynecol 1986;155:14.

21. Spellacy WN, Handler A, Ferre C. A case-controlled study of 1253 twin pregnancies from a 1982–1987 perinatal data base. Obstet Gynecol 1990;75:168.

22. Dwyer PL, Oats JN, Walstab JE, et al. Glucose tolerance in twin pregnancy. Aust N Z J Obstet Gynaecol 1982;22: 131.

23. Ron-El R, Caspi E, Schreyer P, et al. Triplet and quadruplet pregnancies and management. Obstet Gynecol 1981;57: 458.

24. Devoe LD, Azor H, Simultaneous nonstress fetal heart rate testing in twin pregnancy. Obstet Gynecol 1981;58:450.

25. Lodeiro JG, Vintzileos AM, Feinstein SJ, et al. Fetal biophysical profile in twin gestations. Obstet Gynecol 1986;67:824.

26. Knuppel RA, Rattan PK, Scerbo JC, et al. Intrauterine fetal death in twins after 32 weeks of gestation. Obstet Gynecol 1985;65:172.

27. O'Grady JP, Twins and beyond: management guide. Contemp OB/GYN 1991;36:45–63.

28. Selective fetal reduction. Lancet 1988;2:773.

29. Chervenak FA, Johnson RE, Youcha S, et al. Intrapartum management of twin gestation. Obstet Gynecol 1985;65: 119.

50

Polyhydramnios and Oligohydramnios

John T. Queenan, M.D.

ALL that fluid which is contained in the ovum is called by the general name of the waters. The quantity, in proportion to the size of the different parts of the ovum, is greatest by far in early pregnancy. At the time of parturition, in some cases, it amounts to or exceeds four pints. In others, is it scarcely equal to as many ounces. It is usually in the largest quantity when the child has been some time dead, or is born in a weakly state.

It was formerly imagined that the foetus was nourished by this fluid, of which it was said to swallow some part frequently; and it was then asserted that the qualities of the fluid were adapted for its nourishment. But there have been many examples of children born without any passage to the stomach; and a few, of children in which the head was wanting, and which have nevertheless arrived at the full size. These cases fully prove that this opinion is not just, and that there must be some other medium by which the child is nourished, besides the waters.

—T. Denman, *An Introduction to the Practice of Midwifery: 1815*

In 1815, Denman recognized the great variation in amniotic fluid (AF) volume and associated polyhydramnios with congenital malformations, fetal death, or fetal disease. Furthermore, he acknowledged the possibility that the fetus receives some nourishment from swallowed AF (1). Although our knowledge of the intrauterine environment has expanded manyfold, we have not overturned any of Denman's hypotheses.

Polyhydramnios is a pathologic condition characterized by an excessive accumulation of AF: usually greater than 2,000 mL. Although the upper limits of normal can be higher than 2,000 mL from 34 weeks to term, volumes this high are seldom encountered. Using the sodium aminohippurate method of Charles and Jacoby to determine amniotic fluid volumes in normal pregnancies, my associates and I did 187 determinations of AF volume in 115 patients, from 15 to 42 weeks' gestation (2, 3). We found a wide range of values for the various periods of gestation. The mean volumes were 239 mL at 25–26 weeks, 984 mL at 33–34 weeks, 836 mL at term, and 544 mL at 41–42 weeks (Figure 50.1).

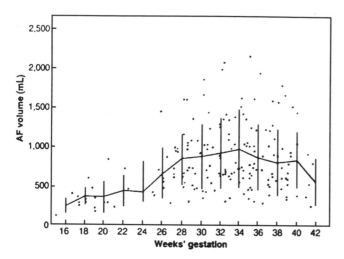

Figure 50.1   Normal amniotic fluid volumes are plotted against weeks of gestation. The mean values ± 1 SD are calculated for each two-week period.

From Queenan JT, Thompson W, Whitfield CR, et al. Amniotic fluid volumes in normal pregnancy. Am J Obstet Gynecol 1972; 114:34.

The mechanisms of AF production and turnover are complex, requiring a delicate balance among mother, fetus, and AF. If the balance of fluid exchange is disturbed, it is easy to imagine how polyhydramnios or oligohydramnios can develop. For instance, if a pathologic condition increased the AF production by 1 oz/day, 1 L of excess fluid may be produced in approximately one month.

Dynamics of AF Turnover

We begin by looking at fetal swallowing. It has long been argued that the fetus must swallow, because earlier investigations had shown epithelial cells, vernix caseosa, and lanugo in the newborn's stomach (4). In 1930, there was x-ray proof of fetal swallowing; in 1963, it was demonstrated on amniography; and it was confirmed in subsequent investigations (4–7).

Fetal Swallowing

The rate at which the fetus swallows has been found to be about 500 mL/day for the term fetus (8, 9). The volume of AF swallowed daily is equivalent to half the total AF vol-

ume, and swallowing is probably the major pathway for its removal.

The effect of swallowing can be seen when we study the pregnancies of patients who go on to deliver infants with tracheoesophageal fistulas. In 228 such cases, 25 fetuses had complete obstruction between the mouth and the stomach, and 19 (76%) of these had polyhydramnios. But in six (24%), there had been no polyhydramnios, even though no AF could reach the fetal GI tract (10).

Anencephaly is also associated with a high incidence of polyhydramnios. Although amniography has demonstrated swallowing in some of these fetuses, it is reasonable to expect at least a decreased ability to swallow. This probably accounts for the pathologic AF accumulation.

In eight anencephalic fetuses and one microcephalic fetus, those with low AF volumes appeared to be swallowing very little fluid, whereas three fetuses with polyhydramnios appeared to swallow normal amounts (11). In light of these findings, it was suggested that presence or absence of swallowing had little effect on the etiology of polyhydramnios in anencephaly.

One investigator suggested that, in anencephaly, transudation from the exposed meninges produced excess AF (12). Others have disagreed, noting that the rudimentary or distorted brain of the anencephalic is almost always covered with a collagen membrane (13). These latter investigators proposed that fetal polyuria may contribute to polyhydramnios because anencephalic fetuses lack antidiuretic hormone. It has also been suggested that polyuria of the anencephalic caused polyhydramnios (14). In 169 cases of polyhydramnios, there were 54 (32%) fetuses unable to swallow (15).

How important fetal swallowing is in controlling AF volume remains undefined. It appears that, when AF volume is normal, swallowing is much less important.

Fetal Micturition

Since Hippocrates' time, physicians have believed that the fetus voids in utero. Today, micturition is accepted as the major source of AF production. When fetal urine flow was studied by inserting indwelling catheters in rhesus monkeys, it was found to be 5 mL/kg/h (16). It is interesting that this rate correlates with the rate of swallowing in Pritchard's studies (9).

Table 50.1 Incidence of Polyhydramnios in Four Studies

	Queenan and Gadow (28)	Jacoby and Charles (29)	Murray (26)	Hill (30)
Total patients	86,301	60,591	12,085	10,214
Incidence of polyhydramnios, %	0.43 (n=358)	0.26	0.7	0.93

In a study of renal function in 255 normal singleton pregnancies between 22 and 41 weeks' gestation and in 133 complicated pregnancies, the hourly fetal urinary production (HFUPR), fetal glomerular filtration rate (GFR), fetal tubular water reabsorption (TWR), and effect of furosemide on fetal micturition were evaluated by ultrasound and by a combination of ultrasound and biochemical tests (17). In normal pregnancies, the HFUPR increased from 2.2 mL/h at 22 weeks to 26.3 mL/h at 40 weeks' gestation. The fetal GFR was 2.66 mL/min at term, and the percentage of TWR was 78%.

In growth-retarded fetuses, the HFUPR was below the tenth percentile in 59% and was above normal in only 6%. The diuretic effect of furosemide was the same in growth-retarded and normal fetuses. In diabetic pregnancies, HFUPR values varied considerably and correlated with the fetal size. In 90% of pregnancies with polyhydramnios, the HFUPR was normal.

Biochemical studies also attest to the important influence of fetal micturition on AF volume. AF is isotonic in early pregnancy, but by term it is hypotonic, compared with fetal and maternal plasma. Lind and associates suggested that the changing concentrations of the AF reflect maturation of fetal renal function (18).

Oligohydramnios has been reported with severe malformation of the fetal urinary system, as in renal agenesis, which is incompatible with urine production. In a review of 295 cases of renal agenesis, in 100 cases, sufficient clinical data were available to indicate oligohydramnios (15). From these data, the investigators inferred that conditions affecting fetal urine production would alter the amount of AF. They also reported a case of renal agenesis and polyhydramnios. Others have reported renal agenesis and normal AF

volume (19–21). Although fetal voiding of urine contributes to AF production, it is not the only source. In fact, even in a blighted ovum, there is some amniotic fluid. Little information is available concerning the volume of urine voided daily by the human fetus. It has been calculated that the term fetus produces 43 mL of urine an hour (8). It has also been suggested that the human fetus swallows and voids similar amounts (500 mL per day) (9).

Respiratory Tract

As early as 1888, investigators believed that the fetus made respiratory movements near term (22). Since then investigators have documented fetal respiratory movements and a fluid-filled respiratory tree.

Fetal respiratory movement can be demonstrated easily with real-time ultrasound. The fetal lamb produces 50–80 mL of tracheal fluid per day (23). The fact that we can gauge fetal lung maturity by measuring the lecithin-to-sphingomyelin (L/S) ratio of AF is evidence of fetal tracheal secretions. But the fetal respiratory tract is not the major source of human AF production.

AF Turnover

The AF is not stagnant. About 500 mL of water leaves and enters the amniotic sac each hour, but this has little effect on the total volume. An average of 3,600 mL of AF is exchanged per hour between mother and fetus, presumably across the chorionic villi of the placenta, where the relatively impermeable amnion is not interposed between the maternal and fetal circulation (24). The transfer of AF from the mother to the fetus must take place in response to osmotic or hydrostatic gradients. It is apparent that the fetus plays a major role in AF volume regulation (25–27).

Table 50.2 Frequency of Incidence of Conditions Associated with Polyhydramnios

Condition	Queenan and Gadow (28) (%) (No.)	Jacoby and Charles (29) (%)	Murray (26) (%)	Hill (30) (%)
Idiopathic	34 (122)	38	40	67
Diabetes mellitus	25 (88)	26	22	14
Congenital malformations	20 (71)	24	22	13
Erythroblastosis fetalis	11 (41)	4	6	1
Multiple gestation	8 (30)	8	10	—
Acute	2 (6)	—	—	—

Polyhydramnios

Polyhydramnios is a pathologic condition characterized by an excessive accumulation of amniotic fluid, usually an amount greater than 2,000 mL. It is generally a problem of the second half of pregnancy, although it can occur in the first half. Although the upper limits of normal can be higher than 2,000 mL, from 34 weeks to term, volumes this high are seldom encountered.

In our review of 358 cases of polyhydramnios, we classified them as either chronic or acute and correlated maternal and fetal conditions with clinical course and pregnancy outcome (28). In the 358 pregnancies, there were 352 cases of chronic polyhydramnios; only six were classified as acute. Table 50.1 shows incidence and Table 50.2 compares the frequency of associated conditions.

Polyhydramnios is not a common obstetric complication. Various authorities state that the incidence varies from 1:150 to 1:280 (26, 27). In a review of all deliveries at the New York Hospital-Cornell Medical Center over a 20-year period, there were 358 cases of polyhydramnios in 86,301 consecutive deliveries: an incidence of 1:240, or 0.43% (28). In another study, the rate was 0.7% among 12,085 patients (29). A third group found a 0.93% incidence among 10,214 patients (30).

In earlier studies, the diagnosis of polyhydramnios was definitive, often being confirmed by actual volume measurement at the time of delivery. In a later study, there was a preponderance of mild polyhydramnios (79%) because of the use of diagnostic ultrasound (30). Therefore, it is not surprising that the incidence of idiopathic polyhydramnios was higher (66.7% versus 34%–40%) in the earlier studies (26–29). The incidence of congenital malformations was also higher in the earlier studies: 20%–24% versus 12.7%. The same was true of the incidence of Rh immunization—4%–11% versus 1%—owing to the widespread use of Rh immune globulin by the time of the later study. The incidence of diabetes mellitus was 14.7%, compared with 22%–26% earlier.

Diagnosis

Polyhydramnios is usually detected clinically during the last trimester. The clinician may note that the uterus is consistently larger than expected for the stage of gestation, or there may be a sudden increase in size. The fetal heart may be difficult to auscultate and the fetal parts difficult to outline. If large quantities of AF are present, it may be possible to ballot the fetus.

In mild cases, there are minimal maternal symptoms, generally consisting of abdominal discomfort and slight dyspnea. In moderate to severe cases (>4,000 mL AF), there is marked respiratory distress—dyspnea and orthopnea—and usually edema of the lower extremities.

The diagnosis of polyhydramnios can be confirmed easily by ultrasound scanning. Adding the largest vertical pock-

Table 50.3 Typical Increases in Amniotic Fluid

Gestation (weeks)	Fluid Volume (mL)
12	50
14	100
16	150
18	200
20	250

ets of amniotic fluid in each of the four quadrants of the uterus determines the amniotic fluid index (31). When this exceeds 24 cm, a diagnosis of polyhydramnios is made (32).

With the advent of ultrasound scanning, the clinician occasionally can see pregnancies in which the amount of AF appears to be increased, suggesting polyhydramnios. This occurs in the second trimester and may or may not develop into true polyhydramnios.

When scanning the pregnant uterus, it is possible to make accurate judgments concerning amniotic fluid volume (AFV). The AFV comprises approximately 50% (early) and 17% (later) of the sonographic view of the pregnant uterus. At 16 weeks' gestation, when genetic amniocentesis would be done, the fetus and placenta each weigh about 100 g, and the AF is 200 mL. Therefore, at this time, the AFV constitutes approximately 50% of the image of the uterus (Table 50.3). At 28 weeks, when the fetus weighs 1,000 g and the placenta weighs 200 g, the AFV is approximately 1,000 mL and takes up approximately 45% of the image of the uterus. At term, when the fetus and placenta weigh 3,300 g and 500 g, respectively, the AFV is approximately 800 mL (Table 50.4) and makes up only about 17% of the image of the uterus. Keeping these guidelines in mind facilitates making a judgment about normalcy of AFV versus oligohydramnios or polyhydramnios.

Further investigation necessitates a comprehensive ultrasound examination to rule out congenital malformations, which investigators have found to account for 20% of cases (33, 34). If all of the known causes of polyhydramnios have been ruled out, the case is considered idiopathic.

The time at which polyhydramnios is detected varies according to the cause. Acute polyhydramnios will be diagnosed very early in pregnancy, the average being 23.4 weeks; the average week of delivery is 26, with an average birthweight of 514 g. Figure 50.2 shows the interval between the diagnosis of polyhydramnios and delivery according to the etiology. The left end of the rectangle indicates the average week of diagnosis; the right end represents the average week of delivery. Birthweight is indicated on the vertical axis. Since the advent of sonography, the diagnosis of polyhydramnios is made much earlier.

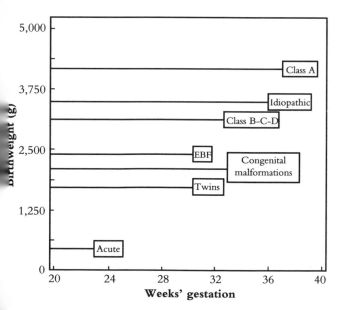

Figure 50.2 Interval between diagnosis of polyhydramnios and delivery varies according to causes.

From Queenan JT, Gadow EC. Polyhydramnios: Chronic versus acute. Am J Obstet Gynecol 1970;108:349.

Table 50.4 Typical Amniotic Fluid Volume

Weeks' Gestation	Fetus (g)	Placenta (g)	Amniotic Fluid (mL)	AF (%)
16	100	100	200	50
28	1,000	200	1,000	45
36	2,500	400	900	24
40	3,300	500	800	17

Table 50.5 Polyhydramnios: Chronic Versus Acute

	Polyhydramnios	
	Chronic	Acute
Week of Diagnosis	28–38	20–24
Height Fundus by 24 Weeks' Gestation by Calipers (cm)	20–26	29–32
Weight Gain per Four-week Interval at Diagnosis (lb)	2–8	10–12
Week of Delivery	32–40	24–27
Outcome	Varies according to cause	Perinatal death
Maternal Symptoms	Mild to severe	Severe

From Queenan JT, Gadow EC. Polyhydramnios: Chronic versus acute. Am J Obstet Gynecol 1970;108:349.

Acute versus Chronic Polyhydramnios

Management and outcome of a pregnancy complicated by polyhydramnios depend on severity. Therefore, it is important to classify the condition as acute or chronic. The differentiation depends on week of onset, rate of uterine growth, and week of delivery (Table 50.5).

Acute polyhydramnios, accounting for fewer than 2% of cases, is characterized by rampant accumulation of AF over a short time (35, 36). The onset is early, before fetal viability, usually during the fourth or fifth month. Maternal symptoms are profound: pain, dyspnea, edema (abdomen, vulva, legs), and nausea and vomiting. If untreated, the patient will go into premature labor, usually before the 28th week. The outcome is guarded because the infant is premature. Acute polyhydramnios is a complication of the second trimester.

Chronic polyhydramnios is characterized by a more gradual increase in AF and, therefore, less maternal discomfort. The condition usually develops after the seventh month and delivery is usually close to term, 32 to 40 weeks. The neonatal outcome varies according to the underlying cause. In multiple malformations or erythroblastosis fetalis, the prognosis is grave; if the polyhydramnios is idiopathic (35%), the prognosis is good. The most serious

risks in idiopathic polyhydramnios are prematurity and malpresentation.

Management

Once polyhydramnios is diagnosed, a systematic maternal workup is necessary to determine the cause. Management is based on treating the underlying cause. During this workup, such conditions as diabetes, erythroblastosis fetalis, and multiple gestation should be ruled out by glucose tolerance testing, antibody screening, and ultrasound, respectively. It is also crucial to do sonography to rule out congenital malformations, which most commonly involve the central nervous system or gastrointestinal tract. These conditions account for 40%–45% of polyhydramnios cases.

Chronic Polyhydramnios

Conservative management is the usual approach. The patient is placed on a high-protein diet. She should have frequent periods of bed rest and, at times, complete bed rest with bathroom privileges. Sedation may be necessary. Diuretics may be considered for symptoms of edema, but they have little effect on the total volume of AF and are discouraged.

When moderate-to-severe polyhydramnios results in pronounced maternal distress, and sonography shows a normal-appearing fetus, then a more aggressive approach becomes necessary. If the fetus is mature, delivery is indicated. Before this decision is made, the patient is hospitalized, placed on complete bed rest, and monitored. In chronic polyhydramnios, where the accumulation of AF is usually slow, amniocentesis is rarely indicated. But if there is maternal dyspnea, orthopnea, or vomiting and the fetus is too small or immature for delivery, amniocentesis is indicated.

If the fetus is found to have major malformations that are incompatible with life, rupturing the membranes with controlled fluid release and delivery should be considered.

Complications

The increased AF volume and overstretched myometrium put the patient with polyhydramnios at increased risk o certain complications. Spontaneous labor with intact membranes usually produces contractions of poor quality because of the excessive uterine size. There is increased incidence of abnormal presentations, and therefore there are more operative deliveries. The sudden decompression of the uterus with spontaneous rupture of the membranes increases the incidence of abruptio placentae and cord prolapse. Therefore, artificial rupture of the membranes must be accomplished slowly and egress of fluid carefully controlled. There is a marked increase in the incidence of postpartum hemorrhage as a result of uterine atony.

In severe polyhydramnios, fetal outcome is guarded. The risk of premature delivery is higher and fetal distress is more likely to occur because of cord prolapse or premature separation of the placenta. The perinatal mortality rate is 50%, half as a result of major malformations. The other causes are prematurity, erythroblastosis fetalis, and the complications of diabetes.

Acute Polyhydramnios

When the clinician is faced with acute polyhydramnios, the diagnostic workup is crucial to determine the underlying cause. Hospitalization is necessary because of severe maternal distress. With the incidence of fetal malformation extremely high, careful investigation to rule out this problem is needed before any aggressive therapy is undertaken. Amniocentesis is always performed with ultrasound guidance.

If no malformation is found to account for the polyhydramnios, therapeutic amniocentesis is the method of management. Amounts of 500–1,000 mL of AF can be removed slowly with continuous aspiration. Reaccumulation will be rapid, and the procedure must be repeated every 2–3 days. Patients can be given a tocolytic agent to decrease uterine contractions.

Hypoproteinemia will be marked, and a high-protein diet must be maintained. Intravenous albumin may be necessary. The use of diuretics is controversial, but they are sometimes given in conjunction with bed rest to relieve symptoms. No antibiotics are given because they may conceal an early amnionitis. This is an extremely stressful situation, and sedation may be part of management.

Oligohydramnios

Oligohydramnios is a pathologic decrease in amniotic fluid volume. Although it can occur in the first half of pregnancy, it is generally a problem of the second half of pregnancy. The time that it occurs has a bearing on the prognosis. When oligohydramnios occurs as early as the second trimester, the prognosis is very poor.

If oligohydramnios is so severe that little or no AF is present, the uterus is usually smaller than expected for dates, and the sonographic image gives a graphic presentation of the condition. Lesser degrees of oligohydramnios are more difficult to ascertain and quantitate. A clinical grading system for oligohydramnios was presented by Manning and co-workers (37). They proposed that the clinician measure the size of vertical AF pockets in the four quadrants of the uterus on sonographic scan. If any of the pockets exceeds 1 cm in the broadest diameter, the volume is considered normal. If the pockets measure less than 1 cm, the volume is coded as decreased and a diagnosis of oligohydramnios is made. The amniotic fluid index is determined by adding the largest vertical pockets in four quadrants of the uterus (31). If the index is under 5, a diagnosis of oligohydramnios is made.

Clinical Significance

Oligohydramnios presents several obvious clinical problems. If the oligohydramnios is severe, the uterus will be smaller than expected for gestational age. This can occur with severe intrauterine growth retardation (IUGR), fetal malformations, premature rupture of the membranes and postdatism to name a few of the potential problems. When oligohydramnios occurs with IUGR, it is usually a poor prognostic sign. Following the AFV sonographically is helpful in monitoring the growth-retarded fetus. The classic example of congenital malformations accompanied by oligohydramnios occurs in Potter syndrome. The fetus usually has renal agenesis, low-set ears, facial deformities, and a variety of malformations. Because of their severe pulmonary hypoplasia, these fetuses never survive.

When premature rupture of the membranes occurs,

the AF continues to leak out through the vagina. The resultant oligohydramnios makes performing an amniocentesis for fetal lung maturity tests difficult because of the decrease in the size of the AF pockets. Keeping the patient in Trendelenburg position prior to amniocentesis may facilitate the collection of AF.

When oligohydramnios occurs in the second trimester, it is associated with a poor prognosis. Mercer and Brown reported on 34 cases of oligohydramnios in the second trimester, diagnosed by ultrasonography (38). Nine of these pregnancies were associated with fetal malformation: Potter syndrome (three), atrioventricular disassociation (two), congenital absence of the thyroid (one), and multiple anomalies (three). There were ten unexplained stillbirths, one demise due to abruptio placentae, eight with perinatal mortality and morbidity after premature labor or abruptio placentae, and six with liveborn term infants. Although oligohydramnios in the second trimester is associated with a marked increase in perinatal morbidity, this finding is not uniformly associated with a poor outcome.

Moore and co-workers demonstrated the reliability and predictive value of a scoring system for oligohydramnios in the second trimester (39). Sixty-two cases of oligohydramnios diagnosed by ultrasound between 13 and 28 weeks' gestation were reviewed, Three experienced ultrasonographers used a subjective scale to rate the oligohydramnios as mild, moderate, severe, or anhydramniotic. Interobserver reliability was excellent (intraclass correlation coefficient, 0.81). The overall perinatal mortality rate was 43%, and the incidence of pulmonary hypoplasia was 33%. One third had lethal congenital anomalies. The frequency of adverse outcome correlated strongly with the most severe degrees of oligohydramnios; 88% of the fetuses with severe oligohydramnios or anhydramnios had lethal outcomes, compared with 11% in the mild/moderate group. The presence of an anuric urinary tract anomaly was associated with the most severe grade of oligohydramnios and was uniformly fatal. Pulmonary hypoplasia was diagnosed in 60% of the severe group versus 6% in the moderate group. The investigators concluded that subjective grading of oligohydramnios by experienced observers is both reliable and predicative of outcome. The finding of severe oligohydramnios in the second trimester is highly predictive of poor fetal outcome and

should stimulate a thorough search for etiology and consideration of intervention. Moderate grades of reduced AF may be managed with relative optimism.

Oligohydramnios occurs with premature rupture of the membranes. In some settings, the decreased amount of AF permits cord compression during uterine contractions. Miyazaki and Taylor have suggested amnioinfusion as a technique for instilling saline into the uterine cavity to restore amniotic fluid volume and allow the fetus to tolerate uterine contractions (40).

When premature rupture of the membranes occurs earlier in pregnancy, the patient may develop oligohydramnios. If keeping the mother on bed rest until the fetus is mature enough to survive extrauterine life is the management plan, the long-term effects of oligohydramnios on the developing fetus must be considered. These are pulmonary hypoplasia and congenital deformations.

In multiple pregnancies, where polyhydramnios and oligohydramnios occur in separate sacs, there is a serious danger to the fetus with oligohydramnios. Chescheir and Seeds reported on seven twin pregnancies with concurrent polyhydramnios and oligohydramnios, resulting in the perinatal mortality rate of 71% (41). The occurrence of the complication before 26 weeks' gestational age resulted in death of all fetuses despite a variety of attempted therapies. They suggested that twin-to-twin transfusion could have caused the disease since all seven of the twins had this syndrome diagnosed antenatally. In this setting, the donor twin becomes anemic and, over time, growth retarded, and develops oligohydramnios. When the oligohydramnios is severe, the fetus becomes immobilized, generally against the uterine wall because of pressure from the sac with polyhydramnios. The fetus does not move despite changing of the maternal position. This has been called the "trapped twin" syndrome.

Conclusion

The AF is a dynamic body of water with many functions in a healthy pregnancy. The extremes of volume—too much and too little—may be associated with an unfavorable prognosis.

When the patient develops polyhydramnios, multiple pregnancies, diabetes mellitus, congenital malformations erythroblastosis fetalis, and other conditions must be ruled out. Polyhydramnios will be idiopathic in over one-half of cases. Management appropriate to the cause will profoundly affect the outcome. If it is idiopathic, the outcome is generally favorable.

Oligohydramnios can be associated with congenital malformations, intrauterine growth retardation, premature rupture of the membranes, postdatism and other causes. It commonly indicates a poor prognosis. When present postdates, it also indicates fetal jeopardy.

References

1. Denman T. An introduction to the practice of midwifery, London: Bliss and White, 1815.

2. Queenan JT, Thompson W, Whitfield CR, et al. Amniotic fluid volumes in normal pregnancy. Am J Obstet Gynecol 1972,114.34.

3. Charles D, Jacoby H. Preliminary data on the use of sodium aminohippurate to determine amniotic fluid volumes. Am J Obstet Gynecol 1966;95:266.

4. Minot CS (1892). Quoted by Becker RF, Windle WF, Barth EE et al. Fetal swallowing, gastrointestinal activity and defecation in utero. Surg Gynecol Obstet 1940;70:603.

5. Menees TO, Miller JD, Hally LE. Amniography. Am J Roentgenol 1930;24:363.

6. McLain CR. Amniography studies of the gastrointestinal motility of the human fetus. Am J Obstet Gynecol 1963;86: 1071.

7. Queenan JT, von Gal H, Kubarych SF. Amniography for clinical evaluation of erythroblastosis fetalis. Am J Obstet Gynecol 1968;102:264.

8. Rosa P. Etude de la circulation du liquide amniotique humain. Gynec et obst 1951;50:463.

9. Pritchard JA. Deglutition by normal and anencephalic fetuses. Obstet Gynecol 1965;25:289.

10. Carter CO. Congenital malformation. Ciba Found Symp Congenital Malformations, 1960:264.

11. Abramovich DR. Fetal factors influencing the volume and composition of liquor amnii. J Obstet Gynaecol Br Commonw 1970;77:865.

12. Gadd RL. Liquor amnii. In: Phillipp EE, Barnes J, Newton M, eds. Scientific foundations of obstetrics and gynaecology. London: Heinemann, 1970.

13. Benirschke K, McKay DG. The anti-diuretic hormone in the fetus and infant. Obstet Gynecol 1953;1:638.

14. Naeye BL, Milic AMB, Blanc W. Fetal endocrine and renal disorders. Am J Obstet Gynecol 1970;108:1251.

15. Jeffcoate TNA, Scott JS. Polyhydramnios and oligohydramnios. Can Med Assoc J 1959;80:77.

16. Chez RA, Smith FG, Hutchinson DL. Renal function in the intrauterine primate fetus. Am J Obstet Gynecol 1964; 90:128.

17. Kurjak A, Kirkinen P, Latin V, et al. Ultrasonic assessment of fetal kidney function in normal and complicated pregnancies. Am J Obstet Gynecol 1981;144:266.

18. Lind T, Billewicz WZ, Cheyne GA. Composition of amniotic fluid and maternal blood through pregnancy. J Obstet Gynaecol Br Commonw 1971;78:505.

19. Schiller W, Toll CM. An inquiry into the cause of oligohydramnios. Am J Obstet Gynecol 1927;12:689.

20. Gowar FJS. Anephrogenesis. J Obstet Gynaecol 1927;12:689.

21. Sylvester PE, Hughes DR. Congenital absence of both kidneys. Br Med J 1954;1:77.

22. Ahlfeld F (1888). Quoted by Farber S, Sweet LK. Amniotic sac contents in the lungs of infants. Am J Dis Child 1931; 42:1372.

23. Goodlin R, Lloyd D. Fetal tracheal excretion of bilirubin. Biol Neonatorum 1968;12:1.

24. Hutchinson DL, Gray MJ, Plentl AA. The role of the fetus in the water exchange of the amniotic fluid of normal and hydramniotic patients. J Clin Invest 1959;38:971.

25. Saunders P, Rhodes P. The origin and circulation of the amniotic fluid. In: Fairweather DVI, Eskes TKAB, eds. Amniotic fluid—research and clinical application. Amsterdam: Excerpta Medica Foundation, 1973.

26. Murray SR. Hydramnios. Am J Obstet Gynecol 1964;88:65.

27. Mueller PF. Acute hydramnios. Am J Obstet Gynecol 1948; 56:1069.

28. Queenan JT, Gadow EC. Polyhydramnios: chronic versus acute. Am J Obstet Gynecol 1970;108:349.

29. Jacoby HE, Charles D. Clinical conditions associated with hydramnios. Am J Obstet Gynecol 1966; 94:910.

30. Hill L, Breckle R, Thomas ML, et al. Polyhydramnios: ultrasonically detected prevalence and neonatal outcome. Obstet Gynecol 1987;69:21.

31. Phelan JP, Ahn MO, Smith CV, et al. Amniotic fluid index measurements during pregnancy. J Reprod Med 1987;32: 601.

32. Moore TR, Cayle JE. The amniotic fluid index in normal human pregnancy. Am J Obstet Gynecol 1990;162:1169.

33. Alexander ES, Spitz HB, Clark RA. Sonography of polyhydramnios. Am J Roentgenol 1982;138:343.

34. Seeds JW, Cefalo RC. Anomalies with hydramnios—diagnostic role of ultrasound. Contemp Ob/Gyn 1984;23(January): 32.

35. Queenan JT. Recurrent polyhydramnios. Am J Obstet Gynecol 1970;106:625

36. Pitkin RM. Acute polyhydramnios recurrent in successive pregnancies. Obstet Gynecol 1976;48:425.

37. Manning FA, Platt LD, Sipos L. Antepartum fetal evaluation: development of a fetal biophysical profile. Am J Obstet Gynecol 1980;136:382. .

38. Mercer LJ, Brown LG. Fetal outcome with oligohydramnios in second trimester. Obstet Gynecol 1986;67:840.

39. Moore TS, Longo J, Leopold GR, et al. The reliability and predictive value of an amniotic fluid scoring system in severe second-trimester oligohydramnios. Obstet Gynecol 1989;73:739.

40. Miyazaki FS, Nevarez F. Saline amnioinfusion for relief of repetitive variable decelerations. Am J Obstet Gynecol 1985;153:301.

41. Chescheir NC, Seeds JW. Polyhydramnios and oligohydramnios in twin gestations. Obstet Gynecol 1988;71:882.

51

Premature Labor

Tom P. Barden, M.D.

THE rate of premature births in the United States has remained relatively constant at approximately 7% of births despite substantial advances in obstetrical care over the last several decades (1). In contrast, the neonatal mortality rate has decreased dramatically, due mainly to increased survival of low-birthweight infants. When compared to other developed countries, the United States continues to rank well down the list of infant mortality rates (2). However, when perinatal mortality rates are calculated to adjust for differences in birthweight, this country consistently has lower rates in each weight increment (3). Unfortunately, the incidence of births with very low birthweights (<1500 g), which have the highest risk of mortality or serious morbidity, has actually increased among blacks in this country (4). The further development of interventions to reduce premature births in our heterogeneous population will certainly require major social, as well as medical, advances.

Definition of Terms

The definition of prematurity has changed over the years. In 1935, the American Academy of Pediatrics defined "premature" as birthweight of 2,500 g or less. In 1961, the World Health Organization defined "premature infants" as those born at 37 weeks' gestation or less, with the term "low birthweight" indicating birthweight of 2,500 g or less. In the current edition of *Williams Obstetrics*, the author suggests that "premature" should be used to describe function, while the terms "preterm" and "low birthweight" should be used in reference to age or weight (5). To complicate the issue further, the terms "intrauterine growth retardation" (IUGR) and "small for gestational age" (SGA) are applied when weight is below the 10th percentile for gestational age. The importance of IUGR is emphasized by reports of follow-up studies that have revealed an increased incidence of mental handicap among individuals with low birthweight and small size for gestational age when compared to others of low birthweight but size appropriate for gestational age (AGA) (6). In contrast, it is also recognized that there is a higher neonatal mortality rate among AGA preterm infants than among SGA infants of the same weight. Thus, the definition of prematurity involves not just the singular determination of weight or gestation, but rather the complex relationship of the two.

Proposed Mechanisms of Labor

Although premature birth may occur from either medically indicated or inappropriate intervention, it usually follows the spontaneous onset of premature labor. Any attempt to prevent or to manage premature labor must include an understanding of the mechanisms of labor onset, as well as various risk factors that may set them in motion. Current concepts of this mechanism primarily focus upon the endocrine and/or paracrine role of progesterone, prostaglandins, and oxytocin as influenced by various risk or mediating factors such as social disadvantage, stress, poor nutrition, infection, or compromised uteroplacental blood flow.

The role of progesterone in the initiation of parturition is most thoroughly understood and documented from studies of the pregnant ewe (7). In that species, the process is initiated by an increase in fetal adrenal secretion of cortisol which acts on placental trophoblasts to increase the activity of steroid 17-α-hydroxylase, causing decreased progesterone secretion and increased estrogen secretion. These events lead to increased prostaglandin formation and sensitization of the uterus to uterotropic agents. Indeed, interruption of the fetal hypothalamic-pituitary-adrenal system in the sheep causes a delay in the onset of labor (7). A similar mechanism may explain delayed onset of parturition in some cases of human fetal anencephaly and fetal adrenal hypoplasia. However, the facts that there is no demonstrable withdrawal of progesterone prior to the onset of labor in women and that cortisol injected into the fetus or mother does not cause labor rather strongly suggest major differences of mechanisms of labor between the two species (8). From observations in humans, it has been suggested that placental production of progesterone during pregnancy serves to stabilize lysosomal phospholipase A_2 (8). Subsequently, a decrease in placental production of progesterone causes the release of phospholipase A_2, which in turn controls the conversion of glycerophospholipids in fetal membranes and decidua to arachidonic acid, the obligatory precursor of prostaglandins. The role of fetal membranes in the mechanism of labor onset has also been suggested by the observation of prostaglandins appearing in amniotic fluid and in maternal blood at the onset of labor

(9) and of high levels of phospholipase A_2 activity in organisms most often involved in perinatal infections, which often are associated with premature labor (10). However, the progesterone withdrawal hypothesis for the onset of human labor seems unlikely when one considers reports of progesterone treatment in humans generally failing to inhibit or arrest the onset of premature labor (11, 12).

The role of oxytocin in the initiation of human parturition continues to be a controversial subject. Most studies have found no changes in blood levels of oxytocin before labor. But the demonstration that oxytocin receptor populations in the human uterus rise markedly at term is strongly suggestive of an important role for oxytocin in the triggering mechanism (13). Also supporting this view were findings of maternal oxytocin levels increasing in early labor, whereas plasma levels of 13, 14-dihydro-15-keto-prostaglandin $F_{2\alpha}$ (PGFM), the principal metabolite of prostaglandin $F_{2\alpha}$ (PGF$_{2\alpha}$), did not increase significantly until relatively late in labor (14). The same studies revealed a consistent increase of PGFM related to spontaneous rupture of membranes and demonstrated that oxytocin induction of labor was successful only when plasma PGFM levels were elevated. These data suggest that both oxytocin and PGF$_{2\alpha}$ are required for adequate stimulation of the human uterus during labor. However, in another study of amniotic fluid prostaglandins during spontaneous or oxytocin-induced labor, there were significantly lower prostaglandin levels in the oxytocin induction group (15). These results suggest that oxytocin may act independent of prostaglandin priming of myometrium.

The mechanism of labor in humans may also include a major contribution by the fetus. It has been clearly demonstrated that the fetal pituitary gland content of oxytocin increases throughout gestation and that there is increased fetal secretion of oxytocin with the onset of spontaneous labor. Another interesting observation was the finding of increased oxytocin content of meconium-stained amniotic fluid compared to clear fluid (17). Perhaps the passage of meconium by the stressed or distressed fetus serves as an escape mechanism from its less-than-optimal uterine environment. If fetal oxytocin is indeed a primary component of the mechanism of labor, some cases of premature labor may occur in response to unrecognized fetal distress.

Epidemiology of Premature Labor

Despite our expanding knowledge of uterine physiology, the factor(s) responsible for premature labor in an individual patient is often obscure. However, among the many conditions that have been implicated in the pathogenesis of premature labor, low socioeconomic status is the most common identifiable risk factor. The rate of premature births among indigent patients is generally found to be as high as 15%–20%, in contrast to about 7% in the general population of the United States (17). Specific factors in the socioeconomically deprived may include the predominance of blacks versus whites, poor nutrition, environmental stress, excessive work, poor hygiene, multiple sexual partners, genitourinary infections, and higher parity. In a review of birth certificate data in the United States for 1983, black women were three times as likely as white women to have a baby with very low birthweight (18). These differences cannot be explained by control of factors such as maternal age, parity, marital status, and education. Premature labor also occurs in association with asymptomatic bacteriuria, acute pyelonephritis, multiple pregnancy, hypertensive disease in pregnancy, smoking and uterine bleeding during pregnancy. The use of cocaine during pregnancy has been associated with lower gestational age at delivery, an increase in preterm labor and delivery, lower birthweights, and delivery of small-for-gestational-age infants (19).

There is considerable evidence suggesting the role of asymptomatic genitourinary infection as a risk factor for premature rupture of membranes and/or premature birth. An elaborate meta-analysis of the relationship between asymptomatic bacteriuria and preterm delivery/low birthweight reached the conclusion that antibiotic treatment is effective in reducing the occurrence of low birthweight (20). Numerous studies have revealed an association of positive amniotic fluid cultures with premature rupture of membranes and/or premature labor (21). Evidence further suggests that most of the bacteria found in perinatal infections have an active phospholipase A_2 system that hydrolyzes the phospholipids in the membranes to produce arachidonic acid, which leads to synthesis of prostaglandins capable of triggering premature labor (22). However, evidence is also gathering that the organisms capable of initiating premature labor may well include species previously considered as normal vaginal flora.

Considering the long list of risk factors for premature labor, it was very logical that a system of predictive scoring be developed. In 1980, Creasy and associates (23) described a risk scoring system for prediction of spontaneous premature birth. It considered 40 factors related to socioeconomic status, past history, daily habits, and current pregnancy problems. Among the most heavily weighed items were history of a previous preterm delivery, multiple pregnancy, abdominal surgery during the pregnancy, uterine anomaly, diethylstilbestrol (DES) exposure, previous second trimester abortion, placenta previa, and hydramnios. Eighty percent of the patients in the study population delivering prior to term had been classified as medium or high risk. However, subsequent studies using the same or a very similar risk assessment tool found that it failed to identify the majority of patients who later experienced premature delivery (24, 25). It has also become apparent that the scoring system is of limited value in primigravid patients; they automatically lack the item relating to a previous preterm delivery that has such strong influence on the predictive power of the score. In a detailed statistical analysis of risk factors in the scoring system, Mueller-Heubach and Guzick (26) reported that the most significant factors, when considered jointly, were prepregnancy weight less than 45.5 kg, black race, single marital status, history of one preterm labor and birth, and history of two or more preterm labors and births.

With the development of a risk scoring system, the next step was to develop a clinical program for prevention of premature delivery. Herron and associates (27) studied 144 high-risk and 1,278 low-risk patients. They conducted an educational program concerning recognition of premature labor for both patients and hospital staff, combined with weekly examinations to detect cervical changes. Patients were admitted to the hospital for tocolytic therapy at the earliest signs of premature labor. The incidence of premature delivery was only 2.4% among all patients studied and only 4.0% in the high-risk group. During the year prior to initiation of the program, their premature delivery rate had been 6.75%. The same program was studied prospectively by Main and associates (28) in a population of poor, inner-city women who previously had a 17% preterm delivery rate. The risk scoring system identified 29% of their patient population to be at high risk for preterm labor who, in turn, accounted for 62% of all preterm births due to preterm labor or preterm rupture of the membranes. Comparing 64 patients followed in their preterm labor prevention clinic, using a program similar to that described by Herron et al (27), to 68 patients randomized to their regular high-risk clinic, they found preterm delivery rates of 17.2% and 16.2%, respectively. They concluded that the risk scoring system and prevention program were of very limited value in a high-risk patient population. However, in another prospective, randomized study of a premature birth prevention program in an indigent patient population, Mueller-Heubach and associates (29) credited the educational program for a significant reduction of preterm births in high-risk and low-risk components of their patient population. The rate of preterm deliveries in their high-risk group declined from 28.6% to 20.2%, while the rate in their total clinic population decreased from 13.8% to 9.3%, which was similar to the 8.5% rate in their private patient population.

Preterm birth prevention programs teach patients to perceive their own uterine contractions. The accuracy of self-detection of contractions by patients was studied by Newman, et al (30) who compared the number of contractions detected by an electronic monitoring device to those perceived by patients. Only 11% of the study group perceived an average of 50% or more of their contractions, and the average patient correctly reported only 15% of her contractions. In 1983, Bell (31) reported a strong correlation between detection of stronger "synchronized" contractions between 20 and 28 weeks and subsequent development of preterm labor compared to other high-risk patients who had less uterine activity and did not develop preterm labor. Subsequently, Katz and associates (32) , using a device developed for assessment of uterine activity in ambulatory patients at home, reported a significant increase in frequency of uterine contractions during the 24 hours preceding the clinical onset of premature labor. Morrison, et al (33), in a prospective randomized study of 67 women at risk for preterm labor, compared the home-monitoring device to patient self-detection of uterine contractions. Subjects in both groups were given instructions regarding early signs and symptoms of premature labor, and they were admitted to the hospital for further evaluation whenever premature labor was suspected. The major difference between the groups was that patients in the control group were in more advanced premature labor upon admission and did not respond as well to tocolytic therapy. Subsequently, 85% of the monitored group and only 55% of the control group reached at least 37 weeks' gestation. Other studies have failed to demonstrate a beneficial effect of home monitoring of uterine activity (34). Iams and associates (35) reported on a prospective controlled trial of 266 patients at high risk of premature labor which compared home monitoring with daily telephone contacts to self-palpation with telephone contacts five days per week. There were no significant differences between the groups for rates of preterm labor (36% versus 34%) or preterm delivery (21% versus 23%). Thus, the role of home monitoring of uterine activity using an electronic device remains of questionable value, pending the results of further studies.

Prevention of Premature Labor

Various pharmacologic interventions have been reported in attempts to reduce the incidence of premature labor and premature births. Among these, the presumed tocolytic effects of progesterone on the gravid uterus have received considerable attention, based upon studies in animal species, such as the rabbit, where the corpus luteum production of progesterone is critical to sustained pregnancy. In a double-blind, placebo-controlled trial, Johnson and associates (36) reported that, in a group of patients at risk of premature labor, there were no instances of labor prior to 36 weeks' gestation among those who received weekly injections of 17-α-hydroxyprogesterone, but, in contrast, 41% of those who received a placebo injection developed premature labor. However, in a subsequent extension of the study, which started treatment only after 16 weeks' gestation to avoid possible teratogenic effects, no significant differences in the incidence of premature delivery were found between the same two groups (37). The use of betamimetic drugs in attempts to prevent premature delivery has been studied by Briscoe (38), who failed to demonstrate a beneficial effect of oral isoxsuprine in a placebo-controlled trial, and Gummerus and Halonen (39), who found no difference in outcome between patients with multiple pregnancy given oral salbutamol versus a placebo. In a randomized controlled trial of oral magnesium supplementation during pregnancy, Sibai and associates (40) found no effect on the incidence of preterm labor or birthweight. The role of infection in the pathogenesis of premature labor was further suggested by the report of McGregor and associates (41), who, in a prospective randomized double-blind study, compared erythromycin therapy to placebo in a group of patients receiving tocolytic therapy for clinical premature labor. In those with cervical dilatation of 1 cm or less at the initiation of therapy, they found a beneficial effect by prolongation of pregnancy by 32.5 days in the antibiotic-treated group versus 22.4 days in the placebo group. Morales et al. (42) reported on a similar study of adjunctive use of antibiotics during tocolytic therapy, but in patients with cervical dilation of 1 cm or more. They compared ampicillin or erythromycin to controls. In patients with similar gestational age and cervical dilation, the use of antibiotic therapy was associated with delay from admission to delivery of 30 days versus 17 days for controls. In a thorough review of this subject, Gibbs and associates (43) conclude that antibiotic trials allow no definite conclusion as to the efficacy of antibiotics in prolonging pregnancy in patients with either preterm labor or preterm premature rupture of membranes, but suggest the need for randomized trials in selected groups of patients at high risk for preterm delivery. Unfortunately, risk scoring indices generated on the basis of historic and current pregnancy factors have positive predictive values for preterm delivery of only 15% to 30%, which are not adequate to warrant most interventions (44). However, there may prove to be a very beneficial effect from a simple manipulation of diet during pregnancy. Villar and Repke (45) have reported a significant reduction in preterm delivery among a group of teenage pregnant patienets who had taken 2.0 gm of calcium as calcium carbonate each day as compared to a similar group of patients who ingested placebo. The incidence of spontaneous labor and preterm delivery was 6.4% and 17.9% in the two groups, respectively.

Diagnosis of Premature Labor

The diagnosis of premature labor is suspected when a pa-

tient presents prior to term complaining of laborlike uterine contractions. The estimation of gestational age is based upon menstrual history, physical examination findings during prenatal care, and sonographic evidence. The presence of regular contractions may be confirmed by either physical examination or by electronic monitoring using an abdominal wall tocotransducer. The diagnosis of premature labor is established only when the initial vaginal examination reveals advanced cervical dilation or when the same examiner finds progressive cervical changes on serial examinations. Of course, vaginal digital examination may be contraindicated by suspected premature rupture of membranes or placenta previa. Not infrequently, labor progress stops during the period of observation which may be due to the enforced bed rest and enhanced uteroplacental blood flow. There is also growing evidence that intravenous hydration is beneficial in management of early premature labor (46). A possible mechanism is decreased secretion of oxytocin and vasopressin by the neurohypophysis.

Management Decisions

The decision to initiate pharmacologic tocolysis should be based upon a thorough evaluation of the clinical circumstances. For example, the diagnosis of fetal intrauterine growth retardation is a relative contraindication to inhibiting premature labor, because the chronic fetal compromise may have been responsible for triggering labor. However, even the growth-retarded fetus may be deprived of developmental potential if delivered too early. When the fetus is small but possibly mature, one might consider temporary inhibition of labor, followed by amniocentesis for evaluation of fetal maturity indices, and then make a decision as to timing of delivery. It is generally acknowledged that tocolytic therapy is usually ineffective and even risky due to newborn side effects when cervical effacement is advanced or dilation has progressed beyond 4 cm. Other contraindications to inhibiting premature labor include intrauterine infection, a major separation of the placenta, a lethal fetal malformation, or fetal death. In the presence of ruptured membranes, delay of labor may permit time for maternal administration of a glucocorticoid to enhance fetal pulmonary maturation, but such a delay also provides an opportunity for development of intrauterine infection. The management of premature labor in a pregnancy complicated by diabetes mellitus, hypertensive disease, or other placental insufficiency states should be based on a judgment of the method that offers the least potential risk to the mother and fetus. After patients with contraindications to inhibition of labor are excluded, there remains a group of potential candidates for pharmacologic treatment.

Use of Tocolytic Drugs

The ideal treatment of established premature labor would include an effective tocolytic agent with no maternal or fetal adverse side effects. Such an agent has yet to be identified despite the many years of intense interest in this subject. Historically, the most popular drugs used to treat premature labor have been various hormones, psycholeptics, sedatives, vasodilators, and neuromuscular agents. For example, the inhalation of amyl nitrite or injection of a few minims of epinephrine solution may produce brief relaxation of the uterus; however, neither is suitable for inhibition of labor because of their ineffectiveness and undesirable side effects. Although administration of progesterone may be of some value in sustaining early pregnancy complicated by threatened abortion, it has not proven to be an effective inhibitor of premature labor in more advanced pregnancy. Also, various biological formulations prepared from mammalian ovaries have been reputed to relax the human uterus, but none has been subjected to controlled studies that might establish efficacy and safety for clinical use. Sedatives and analgesic drugs have a clinical reputation as uterine relaxants, but quantitative studies of some have actually revealed an associated increase of uterine activity.

Aminophylline, a dimethylxanthine derivative used for its bronchial relaxant effect, also acts to inhibit uterine contractions. The uterine action is apparently mediated through its blocking action on the intracellular degradation of cyclic adenosine monophosphate. Although there have been several reports of its inhibitory effect on labor, there have been no properly controlled studies of aminophylline or related drugs for management of premature labor.

Diazoxide, a potent vasodilator used for its antihypertensive properties, can also inhibit premature labor (47). Its mode of action on the uterus has not been fully elucidated. However, from studies in pregnant baboons, Wilson and associates (48) reported that diazoxide, but not several β-adrenergic agents, inhibited prostaglandin $F_{2\alpha}$-induced uterine activity. In view of the importance of prostaglandins in the mechanism of labor, diazoxide deserves further evaluation for treatment of premature labor.

Ethanol, administered by intravenous infusion, became one of the most popular methods for treatment of premature labor in the United States during the early 1970s after animal studies suggested that it interferes with release of oxytocin from the pituitary. In a placebo-controlled study of 42 patients in premature labor, Zlatnik and Fuchs (49) reported that delivery was delayed by at least three days in 81% of the ethanol-treated group and in only 38% of the control group. Maternal side effects usually consist of nausea, vomiting, headache, diuresis, and restlessness. Although animal studies with ethanol have revealed decreased uterine blood flow and fetal asphyxia, there has been no clear evidence in humans of adverse effects on the fetus or neonate. In general, the use of intravenous ethanol for treatment of premature labor has fallen into disrepute due to the frequency of annoying maternal side effects.

Indomethacin and several other nonsteroidal antiinflammatory drugs that inhibit prostaglandin synthesis have been used to treat premature labor. Studies in several species of animals gave evidence that administration of these drugs during pregnancy was followed by a delay in the onset of labor. From Israel, Zuckerman and associates (50) reported that indomethacin successfully inhibited premature labor in 40 of 50 patients. This report stimulated widespread clinical use of indomethacin for treatment of premature labor in the United States. However, it soon became apparent from animal studies and observations in humans that antiprostaglandin compounds such as indomethacin may promote premature closure of the fetal ductus arteriosus, with resultant pulmonary hypertension, congestive heart failure, and death in utero. Despite these concerns, cautious studies in human premature labor generally failed to document evidence of fetal ductus arteriosus closure (51, 52). But, in a study specifically designed to examine the effects of indomethacin on the human fetus, Moise and associates (53) reported echocardiographic evidence of transient constriction of the ductus arteriosus in seven of 14 fetuses, even after short-term use. In other studies (54, 55), indomethacin has been shown to reduce fetal urine output and effectively control the development of hydramnios in twin pregnancies. Considering the available evidence, indomethacin should be used only with extreme caution in carefully controlled studies until its efficacy and relative safety have been more clearly elucidated.

Nifedipine, verapamil, and other calcium-entry blocking agents have been reported as potent tocolytic agents in sheep (56), rats (57), and rabbits (58). However, these and other studies (59, 60) have also revealed evidence of decreased uteroplacental blood flow and decreased fetal oxygenation during maternal intravenous infusion of these agents. Despite these potential dangers, others (61) have reported preliminary studies of nifedipine in human pregnancy with no indication of significant side effects. These drugs should be considered experimental and potentially very dangerous until further well-designed studies are reported that establish their efficacy and safety.

An oxytocin antagonist, 1-deamine-[D-Tyr(Oethyl)^2, Thr^4,Orn^8] vasotocin, yet to be named, has been reported to antagonize effectively the action of oxytocin in pregnant guinea pig uterus in vitro and in vivo and induce a dose-dependent delay of ongoing labor in rats (62). Akerlund and associates (63) reported a pilot study of this agent administered intravenously to 13 patients in premature labor. In all cases, there was a reduction in uterine activity and there were no detectable maternal or fetal side effects. This drug clearly deserves further study.

Magnesium sulfate, the preeminent drug in treatment of severe preeclampsia and eclampsia, has also become one of the most widely used tocolytic agents. Its action is probably due to a modulating effect on calcium uptake and binding in myometrial cells. In a randomized trial, Steer and Petrie (64) reported magnesium sulfate to be more effective than intravenous ethanol for control of premature labor. However, their study involved relatively few patients. Subsequently, Spisso and co-workers (65) reported on 192 patients in premature labor who were treated with magnesium sulfate. Delay of delivery for 48 hours or more was achieved in 71% of patients with intact membranes and 60% of patients with ruptured membranes. These authors reported no significant side effects of the drug. Elliott and colleagues (66), however, reported on two patients who developed acute pulmonary edema during combined treatment with magnesium sulfate and beta-methasone. Subsequently, Elliott (67) reported on a series of 355 patients treated for premature labor with intravenous magnesium sulfate. In singleton pregnancies with intact membranes, the treatment was successful in preventing delivery for 48 hours or more in 87% (150/173) of the patients with cervical dilatation of 2 cm or less and in 62% (53/85) with cervical dilatation of 3–5 cm. Side effects occurred in 24 patients (7%) and necessitated stopping the drug in only seven (2%). The dosage of intravenous magnesium sulfate in this study and in most subsequent clinical experience was a 4-g bolus, followed by 2 g/h. Generally, patients have been switched to oral terbutaline or ritodrine therapy by 12–24 hours. Dudley and associates (68) reported on a series of 22 patients who received intravenous magnesium sulfate for 10 days or longer, compared to 60 patients who were treated for three or fewer days. Although side effects such as ileus, visual blurring, and headache were more common in the long-term group, no life-threatening complications were seen. In a well-designed prospective, randomized trial comparing treatment of premature labor with intravenous magnesium sulfate versus intravenous ritodrine, Hollander and associates (69) reported similar efficacy, with delay of delivery for a week or more in 75% and 72% of cases, respectively. Side effects were considered less alarming in the magnesium sulfate treated patients, with a predominance of lethargy compared to nervousness and palpitations with ritodrine. The authors suggested that magnesium sulfate should be used as the first line of tocolytic therapy, with ritodrine hydrochloride as its pharmacologic backup. Martin and co-workers (70) reported on a study comparing oral ritodrine and magnesium gluconate for ambulatory tocolysis. Using a dosage of 1 g of oral magnesium gluconate every 2–4 hours or 10 mg of ritodrine every 2–4 hours, they found a similar number of patients progressing to 37 weeks or more (21 of 25 versus 19 of 25). They also noted a trend toward more side effects during use of oral ritodrine (40%), compared to oral magnesium gluconate (16%). The use of intravenous magnesium sulfate as a primary or secondary drug for treatment of premature labor has gained widespread acceptance and appears to be relatively free of serious side effects.

Various β-sympathomimetic amines have been the most widely used tocolytic agents in the United States, and throughout the world since the late 1970s. They are a series of related drugs structurally resembling epinephrine, which act through β-adrenergic receptors of smooth muscle cells to trigger activation of adenylate cylcase, the enzyme that catalyzes the intracellular conversion of adenosine triphosphate to cyclic adenosine monophosphate (cAMP). Increased cAMP in myometrial cells activates protein kinases which move calcium to sequestration sites and relax the muscle cell. However, in addition to their uterine-relaxing effects, these agents relax smooth muscle of the bronchial tree and arterioles, increase cardiac rate and force of contraction, and produce glycogenolysis and lipolysis. Thus, the effects of various β-mimetic drugs on uterine blood flow depend on their relative cardiac versus peripheral vascular effects.

Prior to late 1980, the only β-mimetic drugs generally available in the United States suitable for parenteral administration were isoproterenol, isoxsuprine, and terbutaline. Although none of these drugs was (or is currently) FDA-approved for treatment of premature labor, by 1980, isoxsuprine and terbutaline had become the most commonly used tocolytic drugs in the United States. They were administered by intravenous infusion for 12–24 hours, followed by oral therapy. Their most common side effects were maternal tachycardia, palpitations, and widened pulse pressure. Significant hypotension was a rare complication. From placebo-controlled studies (71, 72), these drugs were effective in managing premature labor in more than 80% of patients receiving active drug, compared with approximately 30% of those given placebo.

Ritodrine hydrochloride was identified through animal studies as another β-mimetic drug with a more favorable balance of tocolytic to cardiovascular effects than its predecessors. From an early double-blind, placebo-controlled European study of ritodrine in the treatment of human premature labor, Wesselius-de Casparis and associates (73) reported that delivery was delayed at least seven days in 80% of the ritodrine-treated group and in only 48% of the placebo group. Lauersen and colleagues (74) reported a randomized trial of ritodrine versus ethanol in treatment of

premature labor conducted at three medical centers in the United States. Among the patients who received ethanol, 73% were delayed by 72 hours or more, and 54% delivered after 36 weeks' gestation. In contrast, in the group treated by ritodrine, 90% were delayed at least 72 hours, and 72% delivered after 36 weeks. These data showed statistically significant differences in favor of greater efficacy of ritodrine. In 1980, a large U.S. collaborative study was reported (75, 76) which involved 13 investigators at 11 medical centers who had studied 366 women presenting in premature labor using three treatment protocols involving administration of ritodrine, ethanol, and placebo. When ethanol and placebo treatment were designated as controls, and considering only the subgroup of patients who had labor onset prior to 33 weeks' gestation, the mean time gained in utero for infants of the ritodrine group was 40.9 days, as compared with 24.4 days for the controls. In the same subgroup, the incidence of newborn respiratory distress syndrome was 13% in the ritodrine group and 29% in the controls, while the incidence of neonatal death was 8% in the ritodrine group and 24% in the controls. All of these differences between the ritodrine and control groups were statistically significant. With this and other evidence of the relative safety and efficacy of ritodrine, the FDA in late 1980 approved its use for treatment of premature labor. The initial intravenous infusion is started at 0.1 mg/min and increased by 0.05 mg/min every 10 min until labor ceases, significant side effects develop, or upon reaching the 0.35-mg/min level. The infusion is continued for at least 12 hours after contractions cease before switching to oral maintenance. The oral dosage is 10 mg every two hours during the first 24 hours, followed by 10–20 mg every four hours. Subsequent reports of Caritis and associates (77, 78) have recommended lowering the intravenous dosage to the lowest effective dosage after contractions cease and substantially increasing only the oral dosage.

From widespread experience, ritodrine was found to be reasonably well tolerated, with minor side effects similar to other β-mimetic agents. But, there also were reports of serious cardiovascular complications during tocolytic therapy with β-mimetics, as well as magnesium sulfate (74–82). Among these were cases of maternal pulmonary edema, myocardial ischemia, cardiac arrhythmia, and cerebral vasospasms. In general, the apparent risk factors associated with pulmonary edema have been recognized as maternal anemia, fluid overload, multiple pregnancy, and maternal infection. Although the concomitant use of corticosteroids has been implicated in the development of pulmonary edema, the evidence is not entirely convincing. Most authors agree that pulmonary edema is best avoided during tocolytic therapy by limiting total fluids to 125 mL/h during intravenous drug therapy. Although rare, cardiac arrhythmias with and without evidence of myocardial ischemia have also been encountered during treatment with β-mimetic drugs. There is a consensus that a history of organic heart disease is an absolute contraindication for the use of these drugs. In addition to their cardiovascular actions, β-mimetic drugs also produce several metabolic effects, including hyperglycemia, hyperinsulinemia, hypokalemia, and hyperlactacidemia (83–85). These metabolic effects tend to resolve spontaneously as the intravenous infusion continues. However, such changes can be of considerable clinical significance in women with diabetes, renal disease, or heart disease.

Terbutaline, although not FDA approved for this indication, has been widely used in management of premature labor. Most authors have described its efficacy and side effects as very similar to ritodrine (86, 87). Others have reported lack of effectiveness (88) or excessive side effects (89). Ingemarsson and Bengtsson (86) described a dosage regimen as follows: an initial intravenous infusion of 0.01 mg/min, increased by 0.005 mg/min every 10–20 min until contractions stopped, or a maximum rate of 0.025 was reached. When inhibition of contractions was obtained, the infusion was continued for one hour and then reduced by .005 mg/min every 30 min to reach the lowest effective maintenance dosage. This dosage was then maintained for eight hours or more. Next, patients received subcutaneous injections of terbutaline 0.25 mg four times daily for three days, and then were continued with oral treatment with 5 mg three times daily. Stubblefield and Heyl (90) described a dosage regimen of terbutaline for management of premature labor in which initial therapy was 0.25 mg subcutaneous, repeated hourly until contractions stopped. They reported efficacy similar to most other studies, but with minimal side effects. Lam and associates (91) described a

small series of patients treated with subcutaneous terbutaline administered by a portable infusion pump which proved to be effective tocolysis at exceptionally low dosage levels. This approach, although very expensive, may prove to be more effective than the usual oral dosage used for maintenance therapy.

In a 1988 review of both published and some unpublished data from randomized controlled trials of beta-mimetic treatment of preterm labor subjected to meta-analysis, King and associates (92) reported that although ritodrine treatment delayed delivery for 24 hours, it did not significantly modify the ultimate perinatal outcome. More recently, a large placebo-controlled study of intravenous ritodrine treatment of preterm labor was reported by the Canadian Preterm Labor Investigators Group (93). This study consisted of 708 patients with a diagnosis of preterm labor at six hospitals who received either intravenous ritodrine or a placebo. Ritodrine was found to be more effective than placebo in delaying delivery for up to 48 hours, but it had no significant beneficial effect on perinatal mortality or birth weight. However, it may be of significance that cerebral palsy was subsequently diagnosed once in the ritodrine group (n = 352) and five times in the placebo group (n = 356).

The use of a combination of tocolytic agents with different foci of action is theoretically attractive. One would hope to improve the effectiveness of tocolysis, while reducing side effects by using lower dosage regimens than necessary with single agent therapy. Ferguson and associates (94) reported significantly more cardiovascular side effects among patients receiving simultaneous ritodrine and magnesium sulfate than in those receiving only ritodrine. In contrast, Hatjis and associates (95) reported improved efficacy and no excess of side effects in a group of patients given ritodrine plus magnesium sulfate versus a group who received only ritodrine. The most obvious difference in these two conflicting studies was a lower dosage of magnesium sulfate in the Hatjis study.

An exciting new approach to tocolytic therapy of premature labor involves the use of oxytocin analogues. These synthetic peptides are thought to block the action of endogenous oxytocin by effectively competing for the finite number of myometrial cell oxytocin receptors. Akerlund and associates (96) initially reported on the use of one of these compounds in 13 patients with established preterm labor. In addition to effective inhibition of uterine contractions, there were no apparent maternal or fetal side effects of the drug. Further studies of these compounds continue.

Clinical Results

Despite the widespread use of tocolytic drugs during the past 15–20 years, the incidence of premature birth has not changed appreciably (97). However, there has been a continuing decline in perinatal mortality rates during the same period. To what extent our efforts at tocolytic therapy has contributed remains obscure. Goldenberg and associates (98) reviewed the results of 13 published articles on perinatal mortality statistics and concluded that the major benefits in survival occur between 24 and 27 weeks' gestation. The biggest change in survival free of major morbidity was found at 25–26 weeks' gestational age, with an improvement of about 30% per week, or about 4% per day. On the other hand, there are clinical situations, such as severe preeclampsia or placenta previa with severe hemorrhage, where further delay of delivery by tocolysis would be life-threatening to the fetus and mother. In fact, Tejani and Verma (99) found that only 13.8% of patients in premature labor at their institution were candidates for tocolytic therapy. The major reasons for not giving a tocolytic drug were premature rupture of membranes, chorioamnionitis, severe maternal disease, labor too advanced, second-/third-trimester bleeding, fetal growth retardation, and fetal demise or anomaly. These authors concluded that the availability of tocolytic agents should not be expected to lower the overall low-birthweight rate, but their appropriate use will benefit individual patients. Finally, we must certainly recognize that the cost of tocolytic therapy is very substantial. Korenbrot and associates (100) compared the costs of maternal and neonatal medical care associated with beta-adrenergic drug therapy and delay of delivery to the cost of care of a premature infant at the same gestational age. Between 20 and 25 weeks' gestation, the expected costs per surviving infant were $39,000 lower with tocolytic therapy. After 33 weeks, there was no substantial difference in expected costs with or without tocolytic treatment. Unfortunately, much of the literature related to tocolytic therapy involves patients in the more advanced gestational age group where success is almost predestined.

Conclusions

The evaluation of various clinical approaches to prevention and/or treatment of premature labor is confused by the inherent difficulty in diagnosis of premature labor versus false labor, the many variables that influence the onset of labor prior to term, the still unknown mechanism of labor onset, the confusing literature on drug trials, and the definition of success or failure. Our continued quest for reasonable solutions to these and other puzzles related to premature labor and delivery will likely keep it at the investigative forefront of our specialty for many years to come.

References

1. US Department of Health and Human Services, Public Health Service. Vital Statistics of the United States. 1982. Vol. 1 (Natality). Hyattsville, MD: National Center for Health Statistics, 1986.

2. Wegman ME. Annual summary of vital statistics—1987. Pediatrics 1988;82:817.

3. NIH Week, Vol. 2, No. 19, April 14, 1982.

4. Kleinman JC, Kessel SS. Racial differences in low birthweight. N Engl J Med 1987;317:749.

5. Williams Obstetrics, 18th ed. Cunningham FG, MacDonald PC, Gant NF, eds. Norwalk, CT: Appleton and Lange, 1989.

6. Fitzhardinge PM, Steven EM. The small-for-date infant. I. Neurological and intellectual sequelae. Pediatrics 1972; 50:50.

7. Liggins GC, Fairclough RJ, Grienes SA, Forster CS, Knox BS. Parturition in the sheep. In: Knight J, O'Connor M, eds. The fetus and birth (Ciba Foundation Symposium) North Holland, Amsterdam: Elsevier, 1977.

8. MacDonald PC, Porter JC, Schwarz BE, Johnson JM. Initiation of parturition in the human female. Semin Perinatol 1978; 2:273.

9. Karim SMM. Appearance of prostaglandin $F_{2\alpha}$ in human blood during labor. Br Med J 1968;4:618.

10. Bejar R, Curbelo V, Davis C, et al. Premature labor. II. Bacterial sources of phospholipase. Obstet Gynecol 1981; 57:479.

11. Fuchs F, Stakemann G. Treatment of premature labor with large doses of progesterone. Am J Obstet Gynecol 1960; 79:173.

12. Hauth JC, Gilstrap LC, Brekken AL, Hauth JM. The effect of 17 hydroxyprogesterone caproate on pregnancy outcome in an active-duty military population. Am J Obstet Gynecol 1983;146:187.

13. Fuchs AR, Fuchs F, Husslein P, Soloff MS, Fernstrom MJ. Oxytocin receptor and human parturition: a dual role for oxytocin in the initiation of labor. Science 1982;215:1396.

14. Fuchs AR, Goeschen K, Husslein P, Rasmussen AB, Fuchs F. Oxytocin and the initiation of human parturition. III. Plasma concentrations of oxytocin and 13,14–dihydro-15-keto-prostaglandin $F_{2\alpha}$ in spontaneous and oxytocin-induced labor at term. Am J Obstet Gynecol 1983;147: 497.

15. Padayachi T, Norman RJ, Reddi K, Shweni PM, Philpott RH, Joubert SM. Changes in amniotic fluid prostaglandins with oxytocin-induced labor. Obstet Gynecol 1986;68: 610.

16. Khan-Dawood FS, Dawood MY. Oxytocin content of human fetal pituitary glands. Am J Obstet Gynecol 1984;148:420.

17. Abramowicz M, Kass EA. Pathogenesis and prognosis of prematurity. N Engl J Med 1966;275:878.

18. Kleinman JC, Kessel SS. Racial differences in low birthweight. Trends and risk factors. N Engl J Med 1987;317: 749.

19. MacGregor SN, Keith LG, Chasnoff JJ, Rosner MA, Chisum GM, Shaw P, Minogue JP. Cocaine use during pregnancy: adverse perinatal outcome. Am J Obstet Gynecol 1987, 157:686.

20. Romero R, Oyarzun E, Mazor M, Sirtori M, Hobbins JC, Bracken M. Meta-analysis of the relationship between asymptomatic bacteriuria and preterm delivery/low birthweight. Obstet Gynecol 1989;73:576.

21. Romero R, Mazor M. Infection and preterm labor. Clin Obstet Gynecol 1988;31:553.

22. Bejar R, Curbelo V, Davis C, Gluck L. Premature labor. II. Bacterial sources of phospholipase. Obstet Gynecol 1981; 57:479.

23. Creasy RK, Gummer BA, Liggins GC. System for predicting spontaneous preterm birth. Obstet Gynecol 1980;55:692.

24. Main DM, Richardson D, Gabbe SG, Strong S, Weller SC. Prospective evaluation of a risk scoring system for predicting preterm delivery in black inner city women. Obstet Gynecol 1987;69:61.

25. Konte JM, Creasy RK, Laros RK. California North Coast preterm birth prevention project. Obstet Gynecol 1988; 71:727.

26. Mueller-Heubach E, Guzick DS. Evaluation of risk scoring in a preterm birth prevention study of indigent patients. Am J.

Obstet Gynecol 1989;160:829.

27. Herron MA, Katz M, Creasy RK. Evaluation of a preterm birth prevention program: preliminary report. Obstet Gynecol 1982;59:452.

28. Main DM, Gabbe SG, Richardson D, Strong S. Can preterm deliveries be prevented? Am J Obstet Gynecol 1985; 151: 892.

29. Mueller-Heubach E, Reddick D, Barnett B, Bente R. Preterm birth prevention: evaluation of a prospective controlled randomized trial. Am J Obstet Gynecol 1989; 160: 1172.

30. Newman RB, Gill PJ, Wittreich P, Katz M. Maternal perception of prelabor uterine activity. Obstet Gynecol 1986; 68:765.

31. Bell R. The prediction of preterm labour by recording spontaneous antenatal uterine activity. Br J Obstet Gynaecol 1983;90:884.

32. Katz M, Gill PJ, Newman RB. Detection of preterm labor by ambulatory monitoring of uterine activity: a preliminary report. Obstet Gynecol 1986;68:773–8.

33. Morrison JC, Martin JN, Martin RW, Gookin KS, Wiser WL. Prevention of preterm birth by ambulatory assessment of uterine activity: a randomized study. Am J Obstet Gynecol 1987;156:536.

34. Grimes DA, Schulz KF. Randomized controlled trials of home uterine activity monitoring: a review and critique. Obstet Gynecol 1992;79:137.

35. Iams JD, Johnson FF, O'Shaughnessy RW. A prospective random trial of home uterine activity monitoring in pregnancies at increased risk of preterm labor. Am J Obstet Gynecol 1988;159:595.

36. Johnson JWC, Austin KL, Jones GS, et al. Efficacy of 17α-hydroxyprogesterone caproate in the prevention of premature labor. N Engl J Med 1975;293:675.

37. Johnson JWC, Lee PA, Zachary AS, et al. High-risk prematurity: progestin treatment and steroid studies. Obstet Gynecol 1979;54:412.

38. Briscoe CC. Failure of oral isoxsuprine to prevent prematurity. Am J Obstet Gynecol 1966;95:885.

39. Gummerus M, Halonen O. Prophylactic long-term oral tocolysis of multiple pregnancies. Br J Obstet Gynaecol 1987; 94:249.

40. Sibai BM, Villar MA, Bray E. Magnesium supplementation during pregnancy: a double-blind randomized controlled clinical trial. Am J Obstet Gynecol 1989;161:115.

41. McGregor JA, French JI, Reller LB, Todd JK, Makowski EL. Adjunctive erythromycin treatment for idiopathic preterm

labor: results of a randomized, double-blinded, placebo-controlled trial. Am J Obstet Gynecol 1986;154:98.

42. Morales WJ, Angel JL, O'Brian WF, Knuppel RA, Finazzo M. A randomized study of antibiotic therapy in idiopathic preterm labor. Obstet Gynecol 1988;72:829.

43. Gibbs RS, Romero R, Hiller SL, et al. A review of premature birth and subclinical infection. Am J Obstet Gynecol 1992; 155:1515.

44. Creasy RK. Preterm birth prevention: where are we? Am J Obstet Gynecol 1993;168:1223.

45. Villar J, Repke JT. Calcium supplementation during pregancy may reduce preterm delivery in high risk populations. Am J Obstet Gynecol 1990;163:1124.

46. Valenzuela G, Cline S, Hayashi RH. Followup of hydration and sedation in the pretherapy of premature labor. Am J Obstet Gynecol 1983;147:396.

47. Adamsons K, Wallach RC. Treating preterm labor with diazoxide. Contemp Ob/Gyn 1988;31:161.

48. Wilson KH, Laverson NH, Raghavan KS, et al. Effects of diazoxide and beta adrenergic drugs on spontaneous and induced uterine activity in the pregnant baboon. Am J Obstet Gynecol 1974;118:499.

49. Zlatnick FJ, Fuchs F. A controlled study of ethanol in threatened premature labor. Am J Obstet Gynecol 1972;112:610.

50. Zuckerman H, Reiss U, Rubinstein I. Inhibition of human premature labor by indomethacin. Am J Obstet Gynecol 1974;44:787.

51. Niebyl JR, Blake DA, White RD, et al. The inhibition of premature labor with indomethacin. Am J Obstet Gynecol 1980;136:1014.

52. Niebyl JR, Witter FR. Neonatal outcome after indomethacin treatment for preterm labor. Am J Obstet Gynecol 1986; 155:747.

53. Moise KJ, Huhta JC, Sharif DS, et al. Indomethacin in the treatment of premature labor: effects on the fetal ductus arteriosus. N Engl J Med 1988;319:327.

54. Kirshon B, Moise KJ, Wasserstrum N, et al. Influence of short-term indomethacin therapy on fetal urine output. Obstet Gynecol 1988;72:51.

55. Lange IR, Harmon CR, Manning FA, et al. Twins with hydramnios: treating premature labor at source. Am J Obstet Gynecol 1989;160:552.

56. Golichowski AM, Hathaway DR, Fineberg N, et al. Tocolytic and hemodynamic effects of nifedipine in the ewe. Am J Obstet Gynecol 1985;151:1134.

57. Hahn DW, McGuire JL, Vanderhoof M, et al. Evaluation of drugs for arrest of premature labor in a new animal model. Am J Obstet Gynecol 1984;148:775.

58. Holbrook RH, Lirette M, Katz M. Cardiovascular and tocolytic effects of nicardipine HCl in the pregnant rabbit: comparison with ritodrine HCl. Obstet Gynecol 1987; 69:83.

59. Lirette M, Holbrook H, Katz M. Cardiovascular and uterine blood flow changes during nicardipine HCl tocolysis in the rabbit. Obstet Gynecol 1987;69:79.

60. Harake B, Gilbert RD, Ashwal S, et al. Nifedipine: effects on fetal and maternal hemodynamics in pregnant sheep. Am J Obstet Gynecol 1987;157:1003.

61. Read MD, Wellby DE. The use of a calcium antagonist (nifedipine) to suppress preterm labor. Br J Obstet Gynaecol 1986;93:933.

62. Hahn DW, Demarest KT, Ericson E, et al. Evaluation of 1-deamine-[D-Tyr(Oethyl)^2,Thr^4,Orn^8] vasotocin, an oxytocin antagonist, in animal models of uterine contractility and preterm labor: a new tocolytic agent. Am J Obstet Gynecol 1987;157:977.

63. Akerlund M, Stromberg P, Hauksson A, et al. Inhibition of uterine contractions of premature labour with an oxytocin analogue. Results from a pilot study. Br J Obstet Gynaecol 1987;94:1040.

64. Steer CM, Petrie RH. A comparison of magnesium sulfate and alcohol for the prevention of premature labor. Am J Obstet Gynecol 1977;129:1.

65. Spisso KR, Harbert GM, Thiayarajah S. The use of magnesium sulfate as the primary tocolytic agent to prevent premature delivery. Am J Obstet Gynecol 1982;142:840.

66. Elliott JP, O'Keefe DF, Greenberg P, et al. Pulmonary edema associated with magnesium sulfate and betamethasone administration. Am J Obstet Gynecol 1979;134:717.

67. Elliott JP. Magnesium sulfate as a tocolytic agent. Am J Obstet Gynecol 1983;147:277.

68. Dudley D, Gagnon D, Varner M. Long-term tocolysis with intravenous magnesium sulfate. Obstet Gynecol 1989;73:373.

69. Hollander DI, Nagey DA, Pupkin MJ. Magnesium sulfate and ritodrine hydrochloride: a randomized comparison. Am J Obstet Gynecol 1987;156:631.

70. Martin RW, Martin JN Jr, Pryor JA, et al. Comparison of oral ritodrine and magnesium gluconate for ambulatory tocolysis. Am J Obstet Gynecol 1988;158:1440.

71. Csapo AI, Herczeg J. Arrest of premature labor by isoxsuprine. Am J Obstet Gynecol 1977;129:482.

72. Ingemarsson I. Effect of terbutaline on premature labor: a double-blind placebo-controlled study. Am J Obstet Gyne-

col 1976;125:520.

73. Wesselius-de Casparis A, Thiery M, Yo le Sian A, et al. Result of double-blind, multicentre study with ritodrine in premature labour. Br Med J 1971;3:144.

74. Lauersen NH, Merkatz IR, Tejani N, et al. Inhibition of premature labor: a multicenter comparison of ritodrine and ethanol. Am J Obstet Gynecol 1977;127:837.

75. Barden TP, Peter JB, Merkatz IR. Ritodrine hydrochloride: a betamimetic agent for use in preterm labor. I. Pharmacology, clinical history, administration, side effects, and safety. Obstet Gynecol 1980;56:1.

76. Merkatz IR, Peter JB, Barden TP. Ritodrine hydrochloride: a betamimetic agent for use in preterm labor. II. Evidence of efficacy. Obstet Gynecol 1980;56:7.

77. Caritis SN. A pharmacologic approach to the infusion of ritodrine. Am J Obstet Gynecol 1988;158:380.

78. Caritis SN. Venkataramanan R, Cotroneo M, et al. Pharmacokinetics of orally administered ritodrine. Am J Obstet Gynecol 1989;161:32.

79. Jacobs MM, Knight AB, Arias F. Maternal pulmonary edema resulting from betamimetic and glucocorticoid therapy. Obstet Gynecol 1980;56:56.

80. Katz M, Robertson PA, Creasy RK. Cardiovascular complications associated with terbutaline treatment for preterm labor. Am J Obstet Gynecol 1981;139:605.

81. Benedetti TJ. Maternal complications of parenteral β-sympathomimetic therapy for premature labor. Am J Obstet Gynecol 1983;145:1.

82. Hatjis CG, Swain M. Systemic tocolysis for premature labor is associated with an increased incidence of pulmonary edema in the presence of maternal infection. Am J Obstet Gynecol 1988;159:723.

83. Gross TL, Sokol RJ. Severe hypokalemia and acidosis: a potential complication of beta-adrenergic treatment. Am J Obstet Gynecol 1980;38:1225.

84. Young DC, Toofanian A, Levene KJ. Potassium and glucose concentrations without treatment during ritodrine tocolysis. Am J Obstet Gynecol 1983;145:105.

85. Richards SR, Chang EE, Stempel LE. Hyperlactacidemia associated with acute ritodrine infusion. Am J Obstet Gynecol 1983;146:1.

86. Ingemarsson I, Bengtsson B. A five-year experience with terbutaline for preterm labor: low rate of severe side effects.

Obstet Gynecol 1985;66:176.

87. Caritis SN, Toig G, Heddinger LA, et al. A double-blind study comparing ritodrine and terbutaline in the treatment of preterm labor. Am J Obstet Gynecol 1984;150:7.

88. Cotton DB, Strassmer HT, Hill LM, et al. Comparison of magnesium sulfate, terbutaline and a placebo for inhibition of preterm labor: a randomized study. J Repro Med 1984;29:92.

89. Beall MH, Edgar BW, Paul RH, et al. A comparison of ritodrine, terbutaline, and magnesium sulfate for the suppression of preterm labor. Am J Obstet Gynecol 1985;153:854.

90. Stubblefield PG, Heyl PS. Treatment of premature labor with subcutaneous terbutaline. Obstet Gynecol 1982;59:457.

91. Lam F, Bill P, Smith M, et al. Use of the subcutaneous terbutaline pump for long-term tocolysis. Obstet Gynecol 1988;72:810.

92. King JF, Gant A, Keirse MJNC, et al. Beta-mimetics in preterm labour: an overview of the randomized controlled trials. Br J Obstet Gynaecol 1988;85:211.

93. The Canadian Preterm Labor Investigators Group Treatment of preterm labor with the beta-adrenergic agonist ritodrine. N Engl J Med 1992;327:308.

94. Ferguson JE, Hensleigh PA, Kredensten D. Adjunctive use of magnesium sulfate with ritodrine for preterm labor tocolysis. Am J Obstet Gynecol 1984;148:166.

95. Hatjis CG, Swain M, Nelson CH, et al. Efficacy of combined administration of magnesium sulfate and ritodrine in the treatment of preterm labor. Obstet Gynecol 1987;69:317.

96. Akerlund M, Stromberg P, Hauksson A, et al. Inhibition of uterine contractions of premature labour with an oxytocin analogue. Results from a pilot study. Br J Obstet Gynaecol 1987;94:1040.

97. Leveno KJ, Little BB, Cunningham FG. The national impact of ritodrine hydrochloride for inhibition of preterm labor. Obstet Gynecol 1990;76:12.

98. Goldenberg RL, Nelson KG, Davis RO, et al. Delay in delivery: influence of gestational age and the duration of delay on perinatal outcome. Obstet Gynecol 1984;64:480.

99. Tejani NA, Verma UL. Effect of tocolysis on incidence of low birthweight. Obstet Gynecol 1983;61:556.

100. Korenbrot CC, Aalto LH, Laros RK. The cost effectiveness of stopping preterm labor with beta-adrenergic treatment. N Engl J Med 1984;310:691.

52

Prematurity: Prevention and Treatment

Jay D. Iams, M.D.

Pathogenesis and Epidemiology

In developed nations, approximately 7% of births occur before 37 weeks' gestation. Complications related to prematurity are the leading cause of perinatal mortality and morbidity in nonanomalous infants. The large majority (70%–80%) of these births occur following just two related diagnoses: preterm labor and preterm prematurely ruptured membranes. These are termed *spontaneous* preterm births. The remaining 20%–30% of births before 37 weeks are called *indicated* and follow diseases producing maternal or fetal compromise, e.g., acute or chronic hypertension, diabetes mellitus, placenta previa, intrauterine growth retardation, and others (Figure 52.1).

There has been steady progress in elucidating the pathophysiology of spontaneous preterm birth over the past decade. Premature activation of the same mechanism that produces labor at term appears to precede most spontaneous preterm deliveries. Although incomplete, the current understanding of the genesis of labor at term is that the fetal membranes and decidua are the site of labor initiation in response to a fetal signal excreted in the fetal urine and mediated across the membranes. The membranes and decidua contain abundant prostaglandin precursors which, when activated by the fetal signal, act to ripen the cervix and produce uterine contractions. This normal system may

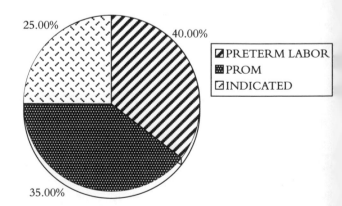

Figure 52.1   Schematic of underlying causes of birth <37 weeks.

(Data from Iams JD, ed. Symposium on preterm labor. Clin Obstet Gynecol 1988;31:519–670 and Main DM. Epidemiology of preterm birth. Clin Obstet Gynecol 1988;31:521–32.)

Table 52.1 Risk Factors for Preterm Birth

Historical	Current Pregnancy
Prior preterm birth	Multiple gestation
Cervical abnormality Incompetence Cone biopsy Diethylstilbestrol (DES)progeny	Bleeding after 1st trimester Smoking ≥10/day Urinary tract infection
Uterine anomaly	Anemia (hematocrit <34%)
>1 2nd trimester abortion	Premature cervical dilation (>1 cm) or effacement (<1 cm length) before 32 weeks' gestation
History of sexually transmitted disease	

be prematurely activated by any stimulus that triggers an inflammatory response. Microorganisms ascending through the cervix and systemic or local tissue hypoxia may lead to sufficient inflammation to trigger either preterm labor or preterm amniorrhexis (1). These observations fit well with the epidemiology of spontaneous preterm birth (2), as summarized in Table 52.1. Increased rates (20%–30%) of preterm birth are noted in populations in which either the opportunity for cervicovaginal inflammation is increased (e.g., a history of sexually transmitted diseases such as vaginosis, chlamydia, mycoplasma, ureaplasma, group B streptococcus, urinary tract infection) or the host resistance or response to infection may be compromised (e.g., abnormal cervical effacement or dilation, anemia, cigarette smoking) or, more likely, both. A history of previous preterm birth confers a 15%–30% risk of subsequent preterm delivery, with even higher rates if there have been multiple prior preterm deliveries. Some patients who deliver preterm have none of these risk factors, but may have others related to uterine overdistention (e.g., multifetal gestation or polyhydramnios) or excessive uterine contractions (e.g., degenerating uterine fibroid).

There are racial differences in the prevalence of prematurity that remain unexplained. Black women have the highest rate of preterm delivery, even when corrected for socioeconomic risk factors. In contrast, Hispanics have a lower rate of preterm birth than other ethnic groups, with rates for the Anglo and Asian populations in between. The reason for these differences are not clear.

Prevention of Preterm Birth

The prevention of preterm birth has become an increasingly important goal of antenatal care, as prematurity-related problems have been identified as the primary source of perinatal mortality and morbidity (3). Various scoring systems have been developed to identify women at risk of preterm birth, but have fallen into disuse because of low positive predictive value (~25%) and low sensitivity (~50%). The majority of preterm deliveries occur in women who are not identified by these systems. A knowledge of the major risk factors described in Table 52.1, coupled with a general awareness of the importance of prematurity, is more useful than a numerical score to the obstetrician who wishes to prevent prematurity.

Obstetricians may act to prevent preterm births both before and during pregnancy. Primary prevention occurs when women receive medical care aimed at eliminating or reducing preventable risk factors for prematurity. The best opportunity for such care precedes conception. For example, maternal cigarette smoking has been estimated to contribute significantly to the overall rate of preterm births, with an attributable risk of 20% in one series (4). Reduction of the prevalence of cigarette smoking among reproductive-age females could then be expected to have an effect similar to the effect on highway mortality statistics seen when speed limits were reduced to 55 mph. There are other preventive strategies for prevention of prematurity that may also be effective for populations more than for individuals. Prepregnancy prevention and treatment of sexually transmitted diseases, urinary tract infections, and anemia in reproductive-age women may act indirectly to reduce overall risk of preterm birth. The role of the cervix in protecting microbial access to the uterus is also seen as an important defense against preterm delivery. Injury to the cervix as a result of conization, unrepaired obstetrical laceration, or traumatic dilation may therefore have subsequent obstetric consequences, especially for women who are heavily colonized with the microorganisms associated with prematurity. Increased attention to care of the cervix during obstetrical and gynecological procedures might then be expected to aid in preventing prematurity.

Access to routine obstetrical care is associated with a lower rate of preterm birth, even when sociodemographic risks are considered (5). Perhaps the salutary effect of prenatal care on prematurity rates address the risk factors cited in the previous paragraph. Regardless of the method by which prenatal care affects preterm birth rate, obstetricians can collectively reduce prematurity by working to improve access to early and regular prenatal care for all women.

Some risks for preterm birth, such as multiple gestation or bleeding in pregnancy, are recognizable but cannot be entirely prevented. Modification of physical and sexual activity and attention to other avoidable risks for these patients may be of some use, but has not been definitively established in controlled trials. Use of prophylactic medication to suppress uterine activity in high-risk patients also lacks a basis in the literature, yet drugs such as terbutaline are often prescribed by physicians for this purpose. This is unfortunate for several reasons. Our best understanding of the genesis of preterm labor does not include spontaneous uterine muscle contraction as a primary event, but rather as the end result of a pathologic process that begins with untimely activation of the membranes and decidua. Strategically, preventive use of tocolytic agents therefore makes little sense. Prophylactic use of β-mimetic agents is aimed at suppressing uterine muscle contractions without in any way addressing the underlying stimulus to uterine activity. Prophylactic tocolysis is therefore analogous to applying the brake of an automobile without removing one's foot from the accelerator. Another reason to avoid β-mimetic drugs given as prophylaxis is the tachyphylaxis that invariably occurs after 2–3 weeks of use. This requires an increasing dose, with increasing side effects, and limits the effectiveness of this class of drugs should actual preterm labor occur. Beta-mimetic agents also have significant potential for metabolic and cardiovascular side effects. Glucose intolerance induced by β-mimetic medication is especially common and carries the same morbidity as for any other gestational diabetics. Cardiac side effects are unpleasant and may even be life threatening for the woman with unrecognized heart disease. Such risks are not justified in the absence of strong evidence of benefit. Other tocolytics, such as magnesium, indomethacin, and calcium channel blockers, also

have no supporting literature for prophylactic use. There are conflicting data regarding the efficacy of prophylactic administration of progesterone supplements to women at risk of preterm birth.

Prematurity prevention programs, in which women at risk were identified and taught the early warning signs of preterm labor, were enthusiastically greeted by physicians in the 1980s after promising reports from France and San Francisco (6, 7). Unfortunately, the success seen in these initial efforts was not uniformly reproduced in other locations (8), leading many to abandon, or even deride, this approach. In light of what is now known about the pathogenesis of spontaneous prematurity, it may be useful to review the features of the successful programs. The French experience (6) was aimed at the elimination or modification of population risks, as well as at early use of tocolytics for women with preterm labor. American translations (7–9) of the French experience focused much more on the early use of tocolytics and did not emphasize the prevention of risk. The American literature is not uniformly dismal on this subject, however. Reports of successful prematurity prevention projects have come from North Carolina (10), New York (11), Minnesota (12), and Ohio (13). These programs, like the French one, have emphasized avoidance of risk, as well as early tocolysis. The reported experience with programs using ambulatory monitoring of uterine activity has also indicated that frequent contact with a supportive and knowledgeable nurse can reduce the rate of preterm delivery in high-risk subjects (13).

Home Uterine Activity Monitoring

Ambulatory monitoring of uterine activity in women at increased risk of premature delivery has been proposed as a method of early detection of preterm labor. The underlying rationales for this approach are that the symptoms of preterm labor may be subtle and that contractions that produce cervical change may not be detected by the patient until advanced cervical effacement or dilation has occurred. Initial trials comparing women using a home monitor to a control group showed a decline in the frequency of preterm birth (14, 15). Later trials comparing patients who received daily contact with a prematurity prevention nurse to those using the monitor showed that the data generated by the monitor provided no additional benefit, especially for patients with singleton gestations (13, 16) (Figure 52.2). The report by Dyson et al. (16) suggested some benefit for women with twins. This study observation is interesting because multiple gestation is one of the few conditions predisposing to prematurity in which uterine distention (and therefore contractility, rather than decidual inflammation) may be the primary initiator of preterm labor. The use of home monitoring is still controversial (17, 18) and requires further study. Its use has not been approved by the American College of Obstetricians and Gynecologists.

Premature Labor

Diagnosis of Preterm Labor

The diagnosis of preterm labor is traditionally made when contractions occur prior to 37 weeks at a frequency of 6–8 per hour, are persistent despite rest and hydration, and result in cervical change (19) (Table 52.2). The initial goal of the diagnostic evaluation of a patient with possible preterm labor is sensitivity. Women with possible signs or symptoms should be urged to come in for additional evaluation. Symptoms of preterm labor are nonspecific and include both painful and painless contractions, pelvic pressure, increase in vaginal discharge, backache, and menstruallike cramps (20). Many women with these symptoms do not have labor, yet those in preterm labor often dismiss them as

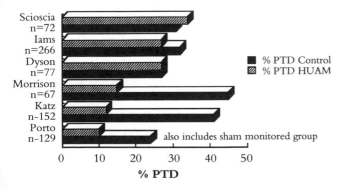

Figure 52.2 Data from six prospective random trials of ambulatory monitoring.

(From References 13–18.)

Table 52.2 Diagnostic Criteria for Preterm Labor

1. Gestational age ≥20 weeks and <37 weeks.

2. If the cervix is less than 2 cm dilated *and* less than 50% effaced, then additional cervical change is required to make a diagnosis of PTL.

3. If the cervix is already ≥2 cm dilated or >50% effaced, then the diagnosis may be made on the basis of a contraction frequency of four in 20 min or eight in 60 min, without waiting for additional change.

"normal" in pregnancy. Signs of preterm labor in addition to contractions include vaginal spotting or fluid leakage and "documented" cervical change. Digital examination of the cervix is expected to identify subtle changes in the cervical effacement or consistency, but has not been reliable except at the extremes of dilation and effacement (21).

Traditional obstetric wisdom is that early institution of drug treatment is necessary in order to assure successful tocolysis. This strategy has, as a necessary by-product, the treatment of some women with persistent contractions who do not in fact have preterm labor. Utter et al. (22) studied 209 women with preterm labor. They found that, when the cervix was less than 2 cm dilated at the initial examination, waiting for obvious cervical change was not associated with any increase in adverse perinatal outcome. This study is reassuring regarding the second goal of the evaluation of the patient with possible preterm labor: specificity. Great care in selecting patients is necessary to avoid overzealous treatment. The diagnosis of preterm labor at present is not an easy algorithm. Recently suggested techniques to improve diagnostic accuracy include sonographic assessment of fetal breathing and of cervical length, and markers such as oncofetal fibronectin in vaginal secretions and maternal serum C reactive protein.

Despite the widespread use of tocolytic drugs, their efficacy is controversial. King et al. (23) reported a meta-analysis of trials of β-mimetic treatment of preterm labor. They found benefit in prolonging pregnancy by 24–48 hours and, in some studies, a reduction in the prevalence of births before 37 weeks. However, there was no advantage noted in this review for neonatal end points such as mortality, low birthweight, or severe respiratory distress. A randomized trial of ritodrine treatment in Canada reached a similar conclusion (24). The controversy surrounding the advantages of treatment, the difficulty in accurate diagnosis, and the risks of tocolytic medication underscore the need for great care in choosing patients for treatment with tocolytics.

Once a diagnosis of preterm labor has been made, consideration of maternal and fetal contraindications to tocolysis is appropriate (see Table 52.3). Tocolytic agents in current use are reviewed in Table 52.4. Although each class of agents has distinct advantages and disadvantages, the choice of tocolytics is often a matter of local custom. Magnesium and the β mimetics are the most commonly used agents. All have some potential for adverse effect, so protocols for administration are advisable (25). Combination therapy with agents of different classes has been suggested, with mixed results. Some authors have found an increase in side effects without improved efficacy, while others have found the opposite. Combined use of magnesium and a β mimetic makes some pharmacologic sense, but the potential for increased complications is worrisome. Magnesium should not be combined with a calcium channel blocker. The prostaglandin synthetase inhibitor indomethacin appears to be an effective tocolytic with few maternal side effects. Concern about its safety has arisen because of the reported effect on flow through the fetal ductus arteriosus

and the decrease in fetal urine output seen when this agent is used. Despite these concerns, there have been several series attesting to safe use when treatment is limited to 48–72 hours in patients ≤32 weeks' gestation. The calcium channel blockers are popular in some centers and also appear to be effective tocolytics. These drugs are also well tolerated by the mother, but concern about maternal hypotension and reduced uterine blood flow has limited their use.

Complications of Tocolysis

Tocolytic drugs are potent agents with significant potential for adverse side effects (25). The relative youth and good health of most women with preterm labor allow them to tolerate these drugs in most instances, but complaints of side effects should never be ignored. Complications of tocolytic treatment are more common in the following situations:

1. Multiple gestation,
2. Occult amnionitis,
3. Occult abruptio placenta,
4. Significant maternal anemia (hemoglobin < 9 g),
5. Maternal heart disease,
6. Prolonged (≥24 hour) infusion of parenteral tocolytics,
7. Concomitant administration of steroids, and
8. Maternal age >30 years.

Careful attention to fluid balance is required. A pretreatment electrocardiogram is a reasonable precaution, especially for the patient over 30 years of age. Pulmonary edema may first present in the preterm labor patient as a dry cough, with later development of rales. An amniocentesis for gram stain and fluid culture should be considered whenever a patient treated with tocolytics develops pulmonary edema.

The clinical situation should be fully reassessed if contractions are not successfully arrested (success = ≤4 per hour) with standard doses of tocolytic agents within 4–6 hours or if parenteral tocolytics are required for more than 24 hours. The criteria for the original diagnosis should be reconsidered and the potential for complications such as amnionitis or abruption reviewed. Again, an amniocentesis may be helpful in this setting. When no underlying problems are found in the patient with persistent contractions, the original diagnosis of preterm labor may be questioned. The most appropriate care at this point is often cessation of

Table 52.3 Contraindications to Tocolysis

Maternal Contraindications

Significant hypertension
Cardiac disease
Significant bleeding
Hyperthyroidism
Any condition in which there is a maternal indication for delivery
Cervical dilation ≥5 cm

Fetal Contraindications

Fetal demise or lethal anomaly
Intrauterine infection
A hostile intrauterine environment, evidenced by:
    Fetal distress
    Intrauterine growth retardation
Gestational age >37 weeks

tocolytic treatment and additional observation.

Steroid treatment should be considered when premature delivery seems likely despite initially successful tocolysis. The patient with advanced cervical effacement (≥80%) or a high (>0.8) admission C reactive protein is a good candidate for steroid therapy because the likelihood of delivery within seven days is high.

Follow-up of Successful Tocolysis

The duration of hospitalization after an episode of preterm labor is governed by the status of the cervix, the need to treat associated complications (e.g., urinary tract infection,

Table 52.4 Tocolytic Choices

Agent	Dose and Route of Administration	Side Effects/Comments
Ritodrine	50–350 μg/min IV	Only Food and Drug Administration (FDA)-approved agent
		Maternal Side Effects
	Start at 50 μg/min	Tachycardia: decrease rate if maternal pulse is 120–130
	Increase by 50 μg/min every 20 min, until labor stops or side effects, to a maximum of 350 μg/min.	Arrhythmia: decrease rate and get electrocardiogram (ECG), serum potassium
	Once contractions cease, hold infusion rate for 60 min, then decrease by 50 μg/min until lowest effective dose.	Chest pain: stop infusion and check ECG and serum potassium
	Sustain this rate for 12 h.	Hyperglycemia: usually requires no treatment in nondiabetics
	Oral ritodrine, 20 μg q 2 h × 24 h, then q 4 h	Hypokalemia: no treatment unless arrhythmia is present
		Pulmonary edema: see text
		Neonatal Side Effects
		Rare unless intravenous (IV) infusion continued to within few hours of delivery; hypoglycemia, hypocalcemia, ileus
Terbutaline	0.25 mg subcutaneously q 1–3 h	Maternal and neonatal side effects same as for ritodrine
	Useful prior to transfer to tertiary center. Oral dose, 2.5–5.0 mg q 2–4 h	Not FDA approved but has abundant support in literature
Magnesium sulfate	Loading dose of 4–6 g, followed by infusion of 2 to 4 g/h	Can use larger doses than for preeclampsia with relative safety because preterm labor PTL patients rarely have impaired renal function
	Intravenous magnesium sulfate is usually followed by oral β-mimetic, but some favor oral magnesium gluconate, 1 g P.O. q 4 h	Maternal side effects: nausea, vomiting, flushing, respiratory depression, pulmonary edema; diarrhea with oral magnesium. Neonatal side effects: hypotonia, respiratory depression, hypocalcemia
Indomethacin	25–50 mg P.O. or as rectal suppository q 6 h for 48 h	Maternal side effects: minimal and limited to gastrointestinal upset. Fetal side effects: constriction of the fetal ductus arteriosus and diminished urine output leading to oligohydramnios

From Quilligan EJ, Zuspan FP. Current therapy in obstetrics and gynecology. Philadelphia: WB Saunders Co., 1990.

anemia), the gestational age, and the patient's home environment. Maternal serum C reactive protein determined at the time of admission may assist in making this decision. A C reactive protein value of ≤0.8 ng/mL has been associated with an 80% rate of continuation of the pregnancy for >7 days after a preterm labor episode. A value of >0.8, in contrast, has been found (26) to produce delivery within seven days in 80% of women treated for preterm labor. Women with a CRP of >0.8 should remain in the hospital for at least 5–7 days.

Women with preterm labor should be taught to recognize the symptoms of preterm labor and to appreciate the importance of painless as well as painful contractions. The role of home uterine monitoring after an episode of preterm labor is unsettled. There are only two reported studies in this population, with opposite conclusions (27, 28). Adjunctive antibiotic treatment of women with preterm labor is also controversial. The original report by McGregor and associates (29) of benefit for patients with preterm labor treated with erythromycin has prompted two additional prospective randomized trials. One showed benefit (30), and the other did not (31). Certainly, treatment of urinary tract infection and eradication of known pathogens such as group B streptococcus and chlamydia is appropriate, but routine adjunctive antibiotic prophylaxis is not an established therapy.

A subcutaneous terbutaline infusion pump has been marketed as an adjunct for care of patients with refractory preterm labor. The premise for this method of administration is that the lower doses used can minimize both the side effects and the tachyphylaxis commonly seen with oral terbutaline treatment. There are no trials demonstrating a decrease in the rate of preterm birth for women using this device compared to those using oral or no therapy. We have found the device to be helpful in the care of the relatively uncommon patient whose preterm labor treatment is complicated by insulin-dependent diabetes mellitus. Compared to oral terbutaline, the small doses infused with the pump approach have minimal effect on maternal glucose control.

Preterm Premature Rupture of Membranes

Premature rupture of membranes (PROM) defined as rupture prior to the onset of labor, occurs in 5%–10% of all pregnancies and precedes 30%–40% of all preterm births. The etiology is thought in most cases to relate to inflammation of the membranes, secondary to infectious or hypoxic insult. The current theory holds that preterm PROM occurs as a result of a synthesis of inflammatory and host response factors, in which microorganisms gain access to the membranes in an ascending fashion through the cervix (32). Enzymes produced by microorganisms may damage membrane integrity and, together with the inflammatory host immune response, lead to weakening and eventual rupture of the sac. The number of organisms invading the endocervical canal may be influenced by other factors that are linked epidemiologically to preterm PROM, such as cervical length and dilation, coital frequency, and the pathogenicity of the organisms themselves. Maternal nutrition and smoking history may influence the host response to infection or the strength of the membrane collagen (33). Direct prevention of preterm PROM is not possible without additional understanding of the exact sequence of events, but perhaps population-based strategies as described previously can have an impact on prevalence.

Diagnosis of Preterm PROM

The diagnosis of preterm PROM is established when a vaginal pool of fluid with pH ≥7 displays a fern pattern when dried. The diagnosis is obvious is such cases but may be less clear in others. The patient who complains of perineal wetness or spotting should always be suspected of having ruptured membranes. Ultrasound assessment of amniotic fluid volume and repeated sterile speculum examination are often helpful in excluding or making a diagnosis in difficult cases.

Management of Preterm PROM

The most urgent task after diagnosis is an estimate of the gestational age, fetal weight, and expected consequences for mother and fetus of immediate delivery or continued observation. These estimates will vary considerably according to the sociodemographic characteristics of the population. The most common result of preterm PROM is labor, occurring within 48 hours in 50% and within seven days in 80% of women with PROM between 26 and 34 weeks' gestation. Most perinatal morbidity and mortality seen in infants born after preterm PROM relates to prematurity, but infectious complications cannot be underestimated, especially in indigent patients. Several studies have correlated the risk of both labor and infection to the amount of amniotic fluid remaining in the uterus after rupture occurs (34,35). Both labor and infection are reportedly more common in women whose largest residual pocket of amniotic fluid is ≤1 cm (Table 52.5). Such patients may be candidates for antibiotic treatment and prompt delivery, while those with larger residual fluid pockets may be better candidates for conservative observation. These observations have been challenged by others (37).

Additional morbidity in the patient with preterm PROM may occur secondary to cord compression or prolapse, placental abruption, or fetal pulmonary hypoplasia. Prolonged lack of amniotic fluid, especially if the onset is prior to 26 weeks, is associated with a 10%–50% risk of pulmonary hypoplasia in the neonate (38). The effect of the duration of ruptured membranes on the functional maturity of the newborn lung is controversial. Some authors have reported a decrease in hyaline membrane disease if membranes are ruptured for more than 18–24 hours before birth, while an equal number of studies have reported no such effect.

Management Strategies

Many obstetricians choose to delivery any patient with preterm PROM for whom pulmonary maturity can be demonstrated. Indigent patients have a higher rate of infection and, in many studies, a lower rate of neonatal respiratory morbidity than do other populations. Immediate delivery may therefore be a logical strategy for indigent patients when ultrasound indicates a fetal weight or gestational age compatible with minimal risk of neonatal morbidity, usually ≥32 weeks or 1,500 g (Table 52.6) (39). This strategy may lead to unacceptable morbidity in patients with a lower risk of infection and a higher risk of respiratory complications. Routine induction of labor for women with PROM at any gestational age has been associated with a significantly higher rate of cesarean delivery compared to expectant management.

When observation and continuation of the pregnancy is elected, it is necessary to assess risk of infection and fetal well-being on a regular basis. Routine surveillance for infection includes frequent physical examination of the uterus for tenderness and measurement of maternal temperature and fetal heart rate. The ideal end point, or gold standard, for the diagnosis of infection in these patients has not been established. Studies of the subject have used a clinical diagnosis of amnionitis, a positive amniotic fluid culture, histologic evidence of membrane infection, and/or various indicators of neonatal sepsis. An early diagnosis of infection is important because there is a two- to fourfold increase in perinatal mortality, intraventricular hemorrhage, and neonatal sepsis in infants born after a diagnosis of maternal amnionitis has been made (40) (Table 52.7). This risk can be reduced by antepartum antibiotic treatment. Ohlsson and Wang (Table 52.8) reviewed methods of detecting infection in pregnancies complicated by preterm PROM (41). They found no perfect method for detecting infection in all cases. A combined approach using clinical examination, maternal white blood cell count and C reactive protein, and culture and Gram's stain of amniotic fluid was recommended. Measurement of amniotic fluid leukocyte esterase (positive) and glucose concentration (low) may also

Table 52.5 Ultrasound Assessment of Residual Volume

Author	End Point	N	Sens	Spec	PVP	PVN
Gonik (35)	Amnionitis	39	73	68	47	86
	Neonatal sepsis	39	50	57	17	86
Vintzeleos (41)	Amnionitis	90	56	86	17	90
	Neonatal sepsis and possible sepsis	90	61	89	58	90

Reduced = <1 cm pocket of fluid remaining

Table 52.6 Considerations for Delivery if Mature and PROM

47 patients with mature pulmonary indices
indigent women with mean gestational age of 32 weeks
random assignment to delivery versus expectant
no change in neonatal outcome
may not apply to other populations

From Spinnato JA, et al. Preterm PROM with fetal maturity present: A prospective study. Obstet Gynecol. 1987;69:196–201.

Table 52.7 Does Early Diagnosis of Infection Really Matter?

Author	N	Neonatal Sepsis Intrapartum Treatment (%)	Neonatal Sepsis Postpartum Treatment (%)
Sperling	257	2.8	19.6
Gilstrap	273	1.5	5.7
Gibbs	45	0	21.0

Note: Two- to fourfold increase in perinatal morbidity, intraventricular hemorrhage, neonatal sepsis with amnionitis. Antepartum treatment of amnionitis *decreases* neonatal sepsis.

indicate infection, but these studies are preliminary. Several authors (42, 43) have promoted the biophysical profile (BPP) as a good method of surveillance for infection in preterm PROM, but Miller, et al. found no improvement in outcome in 47 women managed with biophysical profiles compared to controls (44). The differences in study results are largely due to differing definitions of infection in mothers and neonates.

Interventions to Improve Outcome in Preterm PROM

Frustration with inadequate surveillance techniques and the high rate of delivery within seven days in preterm PROM

Table 52.8 Diagnosis of Infection

Maternal White Blood Count and Clinical or Histologic Amnionitis
Sens 23%–80%; Spec 60%–95%; PVP 50%–75%; PVN 40%–90%
C Reactive Protein and Clinical or Histologic Amnionitis
Sens 37%–100%; Spec 44%–100%; PVP 10%–100%; PVN 50%–100%
Amniocentesis (possible in ~45%–90% of patients)
Culture + →65%–85% sen, 85% spec, 67% PVP, and 85%–95% PVN for clinical chorioamnionitis; AF glucose may be a rapid screen
Gram's Stain and Positive Culture Result
Sens 36%–80%; Spec 83%–97%; PVP 77%–86%; PVN 55%–92%

From Ohlsson A, Wang E. An analysis of antenatal tests to detect infection in preterm PROM. Am J Obstet Gynecol 1990;162:809.

has led many physicians to attempt interventions designed to improve outcome for these patients. Administration of steroids, tocolytics, and antibiotics have all been reported. There have been several prospective trials of steroids given to women with preterm PROM, with conflicting but largely negative results (Figure 52.3). These studies have been subjected to meta-analysis by Ohlsson (45), who concluded that steroids, antibiotics, and tocolytics are all "of unproven benefit and should not be used for premature PROM outside of randomized controlled trials." The strongest evidence of benefit for steroids was reported in a trial in which the rate of respiratory distress in the control group was 50%, substantially greater than is found in most centers (46). Absent that study, Ohlsson's analysis indicates minimal benefit to this approach.

Treatment with prophylactic tocolytic agents is similarly controversial. There are two prospective random trials of this approach (47, 48) (Table 52.9). Both trials were limited to patients who did not receive steroids, and neither showed any benefit in treated subjects. Weiner et al. (47) suggested a possible benefit for patients less than 26 weeks,

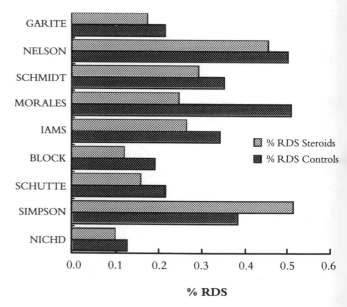

Figure 52.3 Data from nine prospective random trials of corticosteroids in pregnancies complicated by preterm PROM.

(From Ohlsson A. Treatment for preterm premature rupture of the membrane. Am J Obstet Gynecol 1989; 160:890.)

Table 52.9 Data from Two Prospective Random Trials of Tocolytic Treatment of Women with Preterm PROM*

	Weiner	Garite
Prospective	Yes	Yes
Randomized	Yes	Yes
Steroids	No	No
Digital exams	1	0
Change in		
Birthweight	No	No
Latency	No (?<26 w)	No
Amnionitis	No	> in tocolysis group
Perinatal Mortality	No	No

*There are other trials in which tocolytics were used, but no other random trials that tested only the efficacy of tocolytic therapy.

From Weiner CP, et al. Tocolysis vs. bedrest in PROM less than 34 weeks gestation. Am J Obstet Gynecol 1988;159:216 and Garite TJ, et al. A randomized trial of ritodrine tocolysis vs. expectant management in patients with preterm PROM at 25 to 30 weeks. Am J Obstet Gynecol 1987; 157:388.

but Garite et al. (48) found no such advantage for these patients and also noted an increase in infection in treated subjects.

Prophylactic use of antibiotic medication has been found to be beneficial in two prospective trials of women with preterm PROM (49, 50), but a third trial found no benefit (51). Current recommendations for the management of preterm PROM are summarized in Table 52.10.

References

1. Iams JD, ed. Symposium on preterm labor. Clinical Obstet Gynecol 1988;31:519–670.

2. Main DM. Epidemiology of preterm birth. Clin Obstet Gynecol 1988;31:521–32.

3. Iams JD, Peaceman AM, Creasy RK. Prevention of prematurity. Seminars in Perinatol 1988,12:280–91.

4. Guyer B, Wallach LA, Rosen SL. Birthweight standardized neonatal mortality rates and the prevention of low birthweight. N Engl J Med 1982;306:1230–3.

5. Leveno KJ, Cunningham FG, Roark ML, et al. Prenatal care and the low birthweight infant. Obstet Gynecol 1985; 66:599–605.

6. Papiernik E, et al. Prevention of premature births: a perinatal study in Haguenau, France. Pediatrics 1985;76:154–8.

7. Herron M, Katz M, Creasy RK. Evaluation of a preterm birth prevention program: preliminary report. Obstet Gynecol 1982;59:452–6.

8. Main DM, Gabbe SG, Richardson D, Strong S. Can preterm births be prevented? Am J Obstet Gynecol 1985;151: 892–8.

9. Goldenberg RL, Davis RO, Copper RL, Corliss DK, Andrews JB, Carpenter AH. The Alabama preterm birth prevention project. Obstet Gynecol 1990;75:933–9.

10. Meis PJ, et al. Regional program for prevention of premature birth in northwestern North Carolina. Am J Obstet Gynecol 1987;157:550–6.

11. Anderson HF, Freda MC, Brustman L, et al. Decreased incidence of low birthweight for pregnant women participating in the PROPP preterm prevention educational program. (Abstr 72) Eighth Annual Meeting of the Society of Perinatal Obstetricians, Feb 5, 1988.

Table 52.10 Recommendations for PPROM Management

Known rates of RDS and infection for *your* population

Admission evaluation of the patient with PPROM

  Complete blood count, diff, CRP, vaginal cultures for Group B Steptococcus (GBS), GC

  Ultrasound for amniotic fluid (AF) volume, biophysical profile (BPP)

  Collect AF for maturity studies, culture, Gram stain, and glucose

  Nonstress test (NST)

Deliver if mature lungs and >90% survival by estimated weight

Interventions:

  Steroids? No

  Tocolytics? No

  Antibiotics? Yes until admission GBS is known

Surveillance

  Daily: Exam, temperature, white blood count, NST for decelerations, contractions

  p.r.n.: BPP

Twice weekly: Ultrasound for AF volume

12. Yawn BP, Yawn RA. Preterm birth prevention in a rural practice. JAMA 1989;262:230–3.

13. Iams JD, Johnson FF, O'Shaughnessy RW. A prospective random trial of home uterine activity monitoring in pregnancies at increased risk of preterm labor, part II. Am J Obstet Gynecol 1988;159:595–603.

14. Katz M, Gill PJ, Newman RB. Detection of preterm labor by ambulatory monitoring of uterine activity: a preliminary report. Obstet Gynecol 1986;68:773–8.

15. Morrison JC, Martin JM, Martin RW, et al. Prevention of preterm birth by ambulatory assessment of uterine activity: a randomized study. Am J Obstet Gynecol 1987;156:536–43.

16. Dyson DC, Crites YM, Ray DA, Armstrong MA. Prevention of preterm birth in high risk patients: the role of education and provider contact versus home uterine monitoring. Am J Obstet Gynecol 1991;164:756–62.

17. Sachs BP, Hellerstein S, Freeman R, Frigoletto F, Hauth JC. Home monitoring of uterine activity. N Engl J Med 1991;325:1374–7.

18. Grimes DA, Schultz KF. Randomized controlled trials of home uterine activity monitoring: a review and critique. Obstet Gynecol 1992;79:137–42.

19. Gonik B, Creasy RK. Preterm labor: its diagnosis and management. Am J Obstet Gynecol 1986;154:3–8.

20. Iams JD, Stilson R, Johnson FF, Williams RA, Rice R. Symptoms that precede preterm labor and preterm premature rupture of the membranes. Am J Obstet Gynecol 1990;162:486–90.

21. Holcomb WL, Smeltzer JS. Cervical effacement: variation in belief among clinicians. Obstet Gynecol 1991;73:43–5.

22. Utter GO, Dooley SL, Tamura RK, Socol ML. Awaiting cervical change for the diagnosis of preterm labor does not compromise the efficacy of ritodrine tocolysis. Am J Obstet Gynecol 1990;163:882–6.

23. King JF, Grant A, Keirse MJNC, Chalmers I. Beta-mimetics in preterm labor: an overview of the randomized clinical trials. Br J Obstet Gynaecol 1988;95:211–22.

24. The Canadian Preterm Labor Investigators Group. Treatment of preterm labor with the beta-adrenergic agonist ritodrine. N Engl J Med 1992;327:308–12.

25. Caritis SN, Darby MJ, Chan L. Pharmacologic treatment of preterm labor. Clinical Obstet Gynecol 1988;31:635–51.

26. Benedetti T. Maternal complications of parenteral betasympathomimetic therapy for premature labor. Am J Obstet Gynecol 1983;145:1–6.

27. Dodds WG, Iams JD. Maternal C-reactive protein and preterm labor. J Repro Med 1987;32:527.

28. Katz M, Gill PJ, Newman RB. Detection of preterm labor by ambulatory monitoring of uterine activity for the management of oral tocolysis. Am J Obstet Gynecol 1986;154:1253–6.

29. Iams JD, Johnson FF, O'Shaughnessy RW. Ambulatory uterine activity monitoring in the post-hospital care of patients with preterm labor. Am J Perinatol 1990;7:170–3.

30. McGregor JA, French JI, Reller LB, et al. Adjunctive erythromycin treatment for idiopathic preterm labor: results of a randomized double blinded placebo controlled trial. Am J Obstet Gynecol 1986;154:98–103.

31. Morales W, Angel JL, O'Brien WF, Knuppel RA, Finazzo M. A randomized study of antibiotic therapy in idiopathic preterm labor. Obstet Gynecol 1988;72:829–33.

32. Newton ER, Dinsmoor MJ, Gibbs RS. A randomized, blinded, placebo-controlled trial of antibiotics in idiopathic preterm labor. Obstet Gynecol 1989;74:562–6.

33. McGregor JA. Prevention of preterm births: new initiatives bases on microbial host interactions. Ob Gyn Survey 1988;43:1–14.

34. Harger JH, et al. Risk factors for preterm PROM: a multicenter case study. Am J Obstet Gynecol 1990;163:130–7.

35. Silver RK, et al. Impact of residual amniotic fluid volume in patients receiving parenteral tocolysis after premature rupture of the membranes. Am J Obstet Gynecol 1989;161:784–7.

36. Gonik B, et al. Amniotic fluid volume as a risk factor in preterm PROM. Obstet Gynecol 1985;65:456–9.

37. Balaskas TN, Ottman E, Spinnato JA. Is oligohydramnios predictive of pregnancy outcome in preterm premature rupture of membranes? Am J Obstet Gynecol 1993;168:378.

38. Rotschild A, et al. Neonatal outcome after prolonged preterm rupture of the membranes. Am J Obstet Gynecol 1990;162:46–52.

39. Spinnato JA, et al. Preterm PROM with fetal pulmonary maturity present: a prospective study. Obstet Gynecol 1987;69:196–201.

40. Gibbs RS, et al. A randomized trial of intrapartum versus immediate postpartum treatment of women with intraamniotic infection. Obstet Gynecol 1988;72:823–8.

41. Ohlsson A, Wang E. An analysis of antenatal tests to detect infection in preterm PROM. Am J Obstet Gynecol 1990;162:809–18.

42. Goldstein I, Romero R, Merrill S, et al. Fetal body and

breathing movements as predictors of intraamniotic infection in preterm premature rupture of membranes. Am J Obstet Gynecol 1988;159:363–8.

43. Vintzeleos AM, Campbell WA, Nochimson DJ, Weinbaum PJ, Mirochnick MH, Escoto DT. Fetal biophysical profile versus amniocentesis in predicting infection in preterm premature rupture of the membranes. Obstet Gynecol 1986; 68:488–94.

44. Miller JM, et al. Clinical chorioamnionitis is not predicted by an ultrasonic biophysical profile in patients with premature rupture of membranes. Obstet Gynecol 1990;76:1051–4.

45. Ohlsson A. Treatments for preterm premature rupture of the membranes. Am J Obstet Gynecol 1989;160:890.

46. Morales W, Deibel D, Lazar A, Zadrosny D. The effect of antenatal dexamethasone administration on the prevention of respiratory distress syndrome in preterm gestations with premature rupture of membranes. Am J Obstet Gynecol 1986;154:591–5.

47. Weiner CP, et al. Tocolysis vs. bedrest in PROM less than 34 weeks gestation. Am J Obstet Gynecol 1988;159:216.

48. Garite TJ, et al. A randomized trial of ritodrine tocolysis vs. expectant management in patients with preterm PROM at 25 to 30 weeks. Am J Obstet Gynecol 1987;157:388.

49. Amon E, Lewis SV, Sibai BM, Villar MA, Arheart KL. Ampicillin prophylaxis in preterm premature rupture of the membranes: a prospective randomized study. Am J Obstet Gynecol 1988;159:539–43.

50. Johnston MM, Sanchez-Ramos L, Vaughn AJ, Todd MW, Benrubi GI. Antibiotic therapy in preterm premature rupture of membranes: a randomized prospective double blind trial. Am J Obstet Gynecol 1990;163:743–7.

51. Blanco J, Iams J, Artal R, et al. Multicenter double-blind prospective random trial of ceftizoxime vs. placebo in women with preterm prematurely ruptured membranes. Am J Obstet Gynecol 1993;168:378.

53

Infection in Premature Rupture of the Membranes

Kyung Seo, M.D.
James A. McGregor, M.D., C.M.
Janice I. French, C.N.M, M.S.

Premature Rupture of the Membranes and Preterm Birth

Preterm birth remains a paramount problem in health care worldwide. In the United States, approximately 6%–10% of births occur preterm. Gestational age at birth is the most important determinant of infant mortality. Preterm infants account for approximately 75% of neonatal deaths (1), as well as incalculable direct and indirect financial costs and morbidity. Cost of premature infant care may be astronomical.

Preterm premature rupture of membranes (PROM) remains an important cause of preterm births. Approximately one-third of preterm births occur after PROM. The pathogenesis of PROM remains uncertain. Infection has long been recognized as a complication of PROM for both the newborn and mother, putatively due to ascent of cervicovaginal flora through the cervix. Infection with inflammation of the chorioamnion and lower uterine segment has been proposed as an important factor in the pathogenesis of PROM and/or preterm labor.

Infection as a Cause of PROM

There is probably no single cause of PROM. Diverse risk factors, including chorioamnionitis, multiple gestation, polyhydramnios, incompetent cervix, cervical operations, trauma, maternal smoking, nutritional factors, coitus, and barometric pressure changes, have been reported to be associated with PROM. These risk factors are not present in the majority of mothers with PROM.

Supporting evidence includes epidemiologic, histologic, microbiologic and other laboratory information, suggesting that focal infection and inflammation may play primary or secondary roles in the pathogenesis of PROM. Limited epidemiologic data suggest an association between uteroplacental infection and PROM and/or preterm labor. Similar demographic risk factors, such as young age and unmarried or low socioeconomic status have been associated with both PROM and an increased incidence of sexually transmitted diseases (STDs). Seasonal variations in both STDs and also coital frequency parallel variations in the diagnosis of amniotic fluid infection and perinatal mortality.

After preterm delivery, endometrial infections develop more frequently. A rise in C-reactive protein (CRP), an acute-phase reaction of hepatic origin, has been reported with preterm labor, with or without PROM. Those with preterm labor and elevated CRP are more refractory to tocolysis. Elevated CRP is significantly associated with chorioamnionitis with PROM.

Preterm newborns have an increased risk of neonatal infections. This may be due to the increased susceptibility of the premature to infection. Many neonatal infections are diagnosed within 48 hours after delivery, suggesting that antepartum infection might have occurred. Immunoglobulin concentrations in cord blood revealed an increase in IgA and/or IgM after PROM (2). Clinical and immunologic evidence of one peak of infection 1–12 hours after PROM and another 72 hours after PROM suggests that some were infected before PROM.

Histologic examination of placenta and fetal membranes demonstrates that histologic evidence of chorioamnionitis is more common in women with preterm PROM and preterm labor (3). Positive cultures of amniotic fluid or placenta and histologic evidence of chorioamnionitis commonly coexist. Inflammatory changes in the fetal membranes has been noted adjacent to the site of membrane rupture.

Studies comparing the microbiologic flora of the cervix and vagina in patients with PROM demonstrate inconsistent findings. This may be partially due to the great variety of microorganisms involved and also to the possibility of rupture of membranes altering the microbiologic flora. Possible lower genital tract pathogens linked with preterm labor and delivery and PROM include *Neisseria gonorrheae*, Group B streptococci, *Chlamydia trachomatis, Mycoplasma hominis, Ureaplasma urealyticum, Trichomonas vaginalis*, and other aerobic and anaerobic organisms consistent with bacterial vaginosis.

Microbiologic studies of amniotic fluid (4) have demonstrated that intraamniotic infection is associated with PROM and preterm labor. Women with preterm labor and intact membranes frequently had positive amniotic fluid cultures, even in the absence of clinical evidence of infection. Those with positive amniotic fluid cultures were more likely to subsequently develop chorioamnionitis, be refractory to tocolysis, and rupture their membranes prematurely than were women with negative amniotic fluid cultures.

Cultures obtained between amnion and chorion demonstrated increased recovery of *Ureaplasma urealyticum*, as well as aerobic and anaerobic microorganisms associated with bacterial vaginosis after preterm delivery (5). Greater recovery of cervicovaginal microorganisms within fetal membranes than in amniotic fluid suggests that cervicovaginal microorganisms associated with preterm birth ascend through the cervix into the lower uterine segment where they can infect membranes and decidua without causing amniotic fluid infection. Microbes, microbial products, and cells and substrates involved in host defenses may enter the uterus and mediate PROM or preterm labor by the following routes: 1) transcervical passage into amniochorion and amniotic fluid; 2) transcervical passage to the decidua/chorion junction of the low uterine segment; 3) direct penetration into cervical tissue; 4) hematogenous spread to the placenta and membranes; and 5) hematogenous spread to myometrium (Figure 53.1). Some of these pathways suggest that ascending infection may be important in the pathogenesis of intrauterine infections. Supporting evidence includes: 1) microorganisms isolated between amnion and chorion are more frequent after preterm delivery, with higher concentrations than in amniotic fluid; 2) histologic chorioamnionitis is more prevalent in the first-born twin than in the second; and 3) histologic evidence of chorioamnionitis is more intense at the rupture site.

Host Defense Mechanisms versus Ascending Cervicovaginal Microorganisms

IgA secretory immunogloblin (IgA) present in cervical and vaginal fluid is important in defending mucous membranes against infection. Production of IgA specific protease may be an important feature of pathogenic strains of *Neisseria gonorrhea*. IgA protease production has been demonstrated in Ureaplasma urealyticum and other aerobic and anaerobic lower genital tract microorganisms. We have demonstrated that many other aerobic and anaerobic lower genital tract microorganisms also produce IgA protease and IgG protease (7). Cervical mucus also contains other antimicrobial factors, including lysozyme.

Cervical mucus serves as a physical barrier during pregnancy. Some low genital tract microorganism have muci-

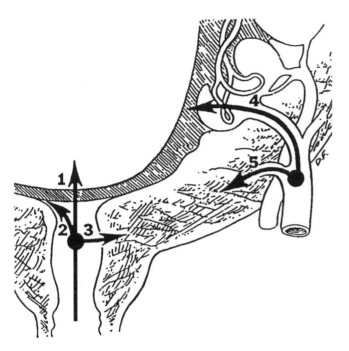

Figure 53.1   Possible routes whereby microbes or their products may enter the uterus include: 1) transcervical passage into amniochorion and amniotic fluid, 2) transcervical passage into decidua/chorion junction of the low uterine segment, 3) direct penetration into cervical tissue, 4) hematogenous spread to the placenta and membranes, and 5) hematogenous spread to myometrium.

(Modified from McGregor JA: Preventing preterm birth caused by infection. Contemp Obstet Gynecol 29:33, 1987.)

nase activities. It is possible that mucinase–producing cervicovaginal microorganisms impair the host defense function of the cervical mucus in pregnancy. Bacterial mucolytic action may further impair local cervical defense mechanisms if cervical mucus is displaced by uterine contractions, cervical ripening, or iatrogenic digital examination.

Amniotic fluid inhibits the growth of several aerobic and anaerobic bacteria. Antimicrobial activity of amniotic fluid is highest at approximately 36–40 weeks' gestation. Several antibacterial factors, including lysozyme, B-lysin, transferrin, spermine, immunoglobulin, peroxidase, fatty acids, steroids, metal-mediated systems, cationic peptide, and phosphate-sensitive bacterial inhibitors, have been detected in human amniotic fluid (8). These antibacterial factors may play important roles in defending against amniotic fluid infection. Marked reduction of the amniotic fluid vol-

ume after PROM may be associated with increased risk of amnionitis and postpartum endometritis. Amniotic fluid from patients with intraamniotic infection and preterm birth demonstrates less antimicrobial activity than amniotic fluid from women delivering at term (9).

Proposed Mechanisms of Microbial Involvement in PROM

Infection and inflammation may mediate PROM by inducing increased uterine contractions and/or focal weakening of fetal membranes. Infection and inflammation may initiate uterine contractions and preterm birth. Numerous cervicovaginal microorganisms produce phospholipases (A_2 and C) (10, 11) which may increase local concentrations of arachidonic acid, leading to subsequent release of PGE_2 and PGF_2 alpha. Inflammatory mediators, e.g., IL-1 and TNF alpha, play important roles in local inflammatory response which may lead to local release of factors important in mediating uterine contractions. Fetal membranes behave as viscoelastic materials with both tensile strength and elasticity. Repeated stretching of the fetal membranes during contractions may progressively weaken these structures and predispose to rupture. Membrane weakening would be most likely to occur at the cervix, where membranes are less well supported.

Focal weakening or alterations of the chorioamniotic membranes is another possible mechanism whereby infection/inflammation may cause PROM. Bacterial enzymes and/or host products secreted in response to infection may lead to weakening and rupture of the membranes. Elevated levels of nonspecific protease in vaginal washing has been associated with preterm PROM. Many commensual and pathogenic cervicovaginal flora have the ability to produce protease (12) and collagenase which significantly reduce the tensile strength of membranes (13). There is decreased membrane collagen after preterm PROM, specifically in levels of type III collagen (14). Human polymorphonuclear leukocyte elastase specifically cleaves human type III collagen. This suggests that leukocyte infiltration of the fetal membranes due to bacterial colonization or infection may lead to depletion of type III collagen and PROM. Other hydrolytic enzymes, including cathepsin B, cathepsin N, and collagenase produced in neutrophils and macrophages, appear to weaken fetal membranes. Human inflammatory cells also elaborate plasminogen activator (PA) which converts plasminogen into plasmin, potentially leading to PROM. Trypsin activity in amniotic fluid was found to be higher after PROM than without PROM. In another study, PROM was not associated with generalized changes of protease activity in fetal membranes and amniotic fluid, suggesting that localized alteration of protease activity may play a role in the pathogenesis of PROM.

Various protease inhibitors have been found in human serum and amniotic fluid (15). Alpha-1-antitrypsin, which comprises 70% of antitryptic activity of human serum, was found in amniotic fluid. The concentration of alpha-1-antitrypsin was found to be significantly lower in amniotic fluid from the women with PROM. Some portion of the protease inhibitors in amniotic fluid is supposed to originate from fetal urine or lung. Fetal contributions to protease inhibitors may play a role in protecting the membranes from proteolytic destruction.

Fetal membranes, placenta, and decidual macrophages are known to possess peroxidase activities. Peroxidase-hydrogen peroxide halide antimicrobial system by phagocytosis of bacteria was also reported to cause protein hydrolysis in the membranes, lowering the bursting pressure (16). Proposed mechanisms of PROM have been summarized in Figure 53.2.

The result of antibiotic prophylaxis to prevent the

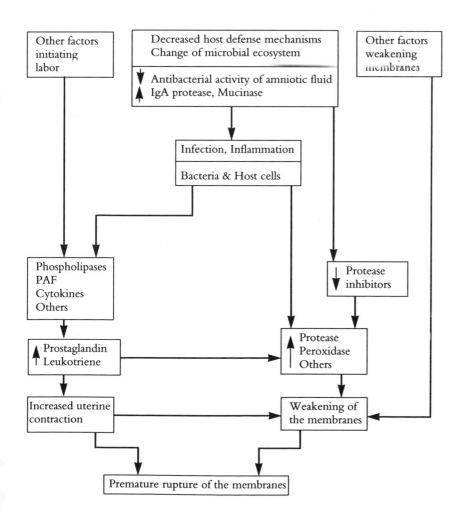

Figure 53.2   Proposed mechanisms for premature rupture of the membranes.

development of PROM has been inconsistent. This might be due to differing effects and antimicrobial coverage of various antibiotics used in those trials. Erythromycin treatment has been consistently associated with significant prolongation of time to delivery, whereas ampicillin treatment has not.

Infection as a Complication of PROM

Historically, once membranes have been ruptured, maternal/fetal infection becomes an important concern. Obstetric management of term PROM has been to deliver the baby within as short an interval as possible. The management goal of preterm PROM has been a compromise between the risk of infection and the viability of the neonate. Reported incidence (17) of maternal/fetal infection after PROM varies according to different diagnostic criteria of infection and the composition of study populations. Chorioamnionitis occurred in 5.2%–21.9% of mothers with preterm PROM. Maternal endometritis developed in 3%–14% of patients with PROM. Incidence of neonatal infection increased significantly with decreasing gestational age. The reported rate of neonatal sepsis following PROM varied from 0.2% of culture-proven sepsis to 19.7% of clinical sepsis. Possible risk factors for maternal and perinatal infection include the latent period, duration of rupture of membranes, number of pelvic examinations, interval from first vaginal examination, and volume of amniotic fluid.

Study of Intraamniotic Infection

Whether infection is a cause or a sequela of PROM, prompt diagnosis and vigorous treatment can improve the outcome of the neonate and mother. Diagnosis of intraamniotic infection/chorioamnionitis is difficult because its clinical and laboratory criteria are not specific (18). Classical symptoms and signs are fever, maternal and fetal tachycardia, uterine tenderness and foul odor of the amniotic fluid. Although fever is a strong clinical sign of infection, it usually develops several hours after infection is histologically apparent. Evaluation of a febrile woman must include a search for other causes of fever, such as urinary tract infection or dehydration. Maternal and fetal tachycardia may be

an early signal of infection. However, dehydration, medications, anxiety, prematurity, hypoxia, and heart disease also produce similar tachycardia. Uterine tenderness appeared to be nonspecific, and malodorous amniotic fluid may not occur with infection. Laboratory criteria of intraamniotic infections include leukocytosis, increased erythrocyte sedimentation rate (ESR), CRP, and measurement of serum complement level. Normal pregnancy is also associated with increased leukocytes and ESR. Changes in laboratory findings are not pathognomonic of intraamniotic infection. Blood culture from women with fever is more specific. However, bacteremia was detected only in 12%. Ultrasonographic examination has been suggested as a useful diagnostic tool in predicting impending fetal infection in PROM. Its diagnostic validity remains to be confirmed.

Direct examination of amniotic fluid is more specific in the diagnosis of intraamniotic infection. Amniocentesis under ultrasonographic guidance has been successful in obtaining amniotic fluid after PROM. Leukocyte counts and Gram staining of bacteria to diagnose intraamniotic infection have been contradictory. Detection of organic metabolites of pathogenic bacteria using gas liquid chromatography has been proposed to detect intraamniotic infection. Amniotic fluid culture for aerobic and anaerobic microorganisms appeared to be most specific in the diagnosis of intraamniotic infection. Positive culture rates from amniotic fluid of the patient with preterm PROM were between 20% and 30%. Bacteria are often cultured from the amniotic fluid without clinical evidence of infection. There is no consensus regarding the significance of bacteria in the amniotic fluid without clinical evidence of infection. Although infection has been strongly suspected as a cause of PROM, it remains to be proven that all bacteria found in amniotic fluid have some pathogenic role in infection and/or initiation of PROM or preterm labor. The situation is more complex if subclinical infection initiates the process of PROM, and the initial infection then subsides. Consequently, the intraamniotic infection may not be found at the diagnosis of PROM, even though the infection was the instigator. Positive culture of amniotic fluid is found to be associated with clinical infection, although some discrepancies exist. Analysis of amniotic fluid and umbilical cord serum for immunoglobulin may also aid in the diagnosis of intraamniotic infection.

Histologic examination of the placenta and umbilical cord has also been controversial in the diagnosis of intraamniotic infection. Prevalence of placental inflammation was usually more frequent than clinical chorioamnionitis. There are two possible explanations for these discrepancies: 1) subclinical chorioamnionitis was more frequent; and 2) placental inflammation may originate, not only from intraamniotic infection, but also from other nonspecific stimuli.

Management of PROM as a Compromise between the Risk of Prematurity and Infection

Management of PROM at term is primarily aimed at delivery as soon as safely possible. When spontaneous labor does not occur after 24 hours, labor is usually induced. Some studies suggest that expectant management of term PROM, particularly with an unfavorable cervix, would decrease the cesarean section rate. One study showed that increased perinatal mortality is directly related to the duration of the waiting period after PROM at term.

Management of PROM at preterm requires assessment of the risk of prematurity versus infection. Although infection may be an important cause of PROM, expectant management is currently favored because perinatal deaths from prematurity exceed those from infection. The principle of expectant management of preterm PROM is to provide time until lung maturity is verified or infection is evident. Additional management options include the use of: 1) antibiotics to prevent infection and suppress the progress of PROM; 2) corticosteroids to accelerate lung maturity; and 3) tocolytics to prolong pregnancy.

Administration of antibiotics before clinical signs of infection appear should be reappraised as a treatment option. This may prevent maternal and fetal infection after PROM and eradicate or delay subclinical infection that could lead to PROM and preterm labor. Results of prophylactic antibiotic to prevent maternal and fetal infections have not been consistent. Many favor the use of antibiotics after PROM in women receiving steroids, undergoing cesarean section, or having positive cultures of Group B streptococci. Women with obvious intraamniotic infection should be treated as soon as possible, prior to delivery. Infusion of antibiotics dissolved in physiologic saline through a cervical indwelling catheter has been reported with some success in decreasing positive cultures of amniotic fluid (19).

Administration of corticosteroids to reduce the incidence of respiratory distress syndrome (RDS) in patients with preterm PROM has shown contradictory results. Some studies reported an adverse effect of corticosteroids with an increased incidence of maternal endometritis. Use of tocolytic agents to prolong the pregnancy in patients with preterm PROM has been considered as an additional management option since the main concern is prematurity. Efficacy of tocolytic agents to prolong the pregnancy in patients with PROM is inconsistent. Furthermore, the effects of tocolytic agents on the incidence of lung maturity have been confusing. Increased risk of infection should always be considered in prolonging pregnancy after PROM. Exclusion of active infection is essential before use of tocolytics.

Promising New Treatment of PROM

Antibiotic treatment for PROM may have untoward or unexpected effects. Beta-lactam antibiotics, such as ampicillin, may disrupt bacterial cell walls and further provoke host inflammation responses. Bacteriostatic antimicrobials "shut-down" bacteria and appear more effective in prolonging delivery (21, 22).

Erythromycin has been used in placebo-controlled trials to reduce the occurrence of PROM and to increase birthweight (22). Such antibiotics may work in ways other than simple killing of bacteria. Effects of different concentrations of various antibiotics on bacterial protease production by cervicovaginal microorganisms were studied. Antibiotic concentrations above minimal inhibitory concentrations (MICs) reliably decreased protease production. Antibiotics also reversed the bacterial effects of weakening membranes. Some protein-synthesis-inhibiting antibiotics, including erythromycin and clindamycin, reliably curtail the protease release at concentrations well below MICs. Some microbial antibiotics combinations have resulted in increased protease release, which might be caused by a transient increase of microbial factors from killing the microorganism. Theoretically, short-term tocolytic treatment could reduce uterine contractions while initiating factors are being eradicated. Promising new treatment regimens include antimicrobials, antiinflammatory agents, antiprotease, antiphospholipase, antiprostaglandin synthetase, platelet activating factor antagonists, and tocolytic agents.

References

1. McCormick MC. The contribution of low birthweight to infant mortality and childhood morbidity. N Engl J Med 1985;312:82.

2. Cederqvist LL, Zervoudakis IA, Ewool LC, Litwin SD. The relationship between prematurely ruptured membranes and fetal immunoglobulin production. Am J Obstet Gynecol 1979;134:784.

3. Guzick DS, Winn K. The association of chorioamnionitis and preterm delivery. Obstet Gynecol 1985;65:11.

4. Romero R, Major M. Infection and preterm labor. Clin Obstet Gynecol 1988;31:553.

5. Kundsin RB, Driscoll SG, Monson RR, et al. Association of ureaplasma urealyticum in the placenta with perinatal morbidity and mortality. N Engl J Med 1984;310:941.

6. McGregor JA. Preventing preterm birth caused by infection. Contemp Obstet Gynecol 1987;29:33.

7. McGregor JA, Lawellin D, Schroeter U, et al. IgG protease activity in microorganisms associated with upper genital tract infection determined by ELISA. Abstracts #157P, Society for Gynecologic Investigation Scientific Program and Abstracts, Toronto, Canada, March 19–22, 1986:111.

8. Schlievert P, Johnson W, Galask RP. Amniotic fluid antibacterial mechanism: newer concepts. Semin Perinatol 1977; 1:59.

9. Blanco JD, Gibbs RS, Krebs LK, Castaneda YS. The association between the absence of amniotic fluid inhibitory activity and intra-amniotic infection. Am J Obstet Gynecol 1982;143:749.

10. Bejar R, Curbelo V, Davis C, Gluck L. Premature labor: bacterial sources of phospholipase. Obstet Gynecol 1981; 57:479.

11. McGregor JA, Lawellin DW, Franco-Buff A, Todd JK. Phospholipase C production by lower genital tract microorganisms. Am J Obstet Gynecol 1991;164:682–6.

12. McGregor JA, Lawellin D, Franco-Buff A. Protease production by microorganism associated with reproductive tract infection. Am J Obstet Gynecol 1986;154:109.

13. McGregor JA, French JI, Lawellin D, et al. In vitro study of bacterial protease-induced reduction of chorioamnionitis membrane strength and elasticity. Obstet Gynecol 1987; 69:167.

14. Mainardi CL, Hasty DL, Seyer JM, et al. Specific cleavage of human type III collagen by human polymorphonuclear leukocyte elastase. J Biol Chem 1980;255:12006.

15. Bhat AR, Issac V, Pattabiraman TN. Protease inhibitors in serum and amniotic fluid during pregnancy. Br J Obstet Gynaecol 1979;86:222.

16. Sbarra AJ, Selvaraj RJ, Cetrulo CL, et al. Infection and phagocytosis as possible mechanism of rupture in premature rupture of the membrane. Am J Obstet Gynecol 1985;153:38.

17. Blackmon LR, Alger LS, Crenshaw C. Fetal and neonatal outcomes associated with premature rupture of the membranes. Clin Obstet Gynecol 1986;29:779.

18. Gibbs RS. Diagnosis of intra-amniotic infection. Semin Perinatol 1977;1:71.

19. Ogita S, Mizuno M, Takeda Y, et al. Clinical effectiveness of a new cervical indwelling catheter in the management of premature rupture of the membranes: a Japanese collaborative study. Am J Obstet Gynecol 1988;159:336.

20. McGregor J, French JI, Seo K. Antimicrobial therapy in preterm premature rupture of membranes: results of a prospective, double blind, placebo-controlled trial of erythromycin. Am J Obstet Gynecol 1991;165:632–40.

21. Mercer B, Moretti M, Rogers R, Sibai B. Erythromycin therapy in preterm premature rupture of the membranes: prospective randomized trial of 220 patients. Am J Obstet Gynecol 1992;166:794–802.

22. McGregor JA. Prevention of preterm birth: new initiative based on microbial-host interactions. Obstet Gynecol Surv 1988;43:1–14.

54

Placenta Previa and Related Disorders

Charles J. Lockwood, M.D.

PLACENTAL tissue overlying or proximate to the internal cervical os complicates between 3.5 and 6 of every 1,000 pregnancies after 20 weeks' gestation (1–3). The disorder may be complete, partial, or marginal, or consist of a low-lying placenta (Table 54.1, Figure 54.1).

Risk increases substantially with increasing parity, the number of previous cesarean sections (CS), and the number of curettages for spontaneous (nonelective) abortion (1–4). These risk factors suggest that extensive endometrial scarring promotes either trophoblastic nidation or subsequent migration of trophoblast into the relatively unscarred lower uterine segment.

Additional risk factors include smoking, residence at higher altitudes, a male fetus, and multiple gestation (1, 3, 5). All of these factors suggest that the increased placental surface area compensates for reduced uteroplacental oxygen delivery or that increased fetal nutritional requirements promote previa formation.

The characteristic clinical sign of placenta previa is painless vaginal bleeding, which occurs in 70%–80% of cases (1, 6). An additional 10%–20% of patients are first seen for uterine contractions associated with bleeding, while less than 10% have their condition incidentally detected by ultrasound and remain asymptomatic.

Mean gestational age at presentation is 30 weeks, with delivery at 35 weeks (2). Approximately one-third of pregnancies complicated by placenta previa develop bleeding before 31 weeks' gestation. This group of patients requires a greater number of blood transfusions and carries a greater risk of preterm delivery and perinatal mortality (1, 2, 6). An

---

Table 54.1 Previa Types

Complete: Placental tissue completely overlies the internal cervical os (can be central or noncentral, depending on whether or not the placenta's center is directly over the os).

Partial: Placental tissue is situated over part of the os but doesn't completely overlie it.

Marginal: Placental tissue approaches the edge of the os but doesn't overlie any part of it.

Low-lying: Placental tissue is implanted in the lower uterine segment but doesn't reach the edge of the os.

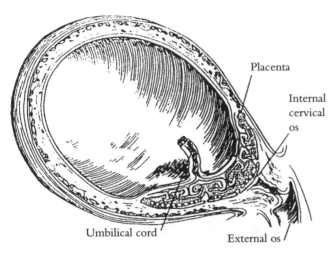

Figure 54.1   Complete central placenta previa. In this variety, placental tissue completely overlies the internal cervical os, with the placenta's center situated directly over the os.

additional third develop symptoms between 31 and 36 weeks, while the remaining third are seen after 36 weeks.

Preterm Delivery

The perinatal mortality rate in pregnancies complicated by

placenta previa has been reduced over the past 20 years, principally because of improved neonatal care, but also because of the introduction of conservative obstetric management. Nonetheless, current perinatal mortality rates remain elevated at 40–80 per 1,000 live births (2, 6).

The chief cause of excess perinatal mortality is preterm delivery and not fetal anemia or hypoxia (1, 2). The earlier in gestation that bleeding develops, the higher the probability of a preterm delivery.

In contrast, it does not appear that the type of previa significantly influences perinatal outcome (1). However, it is possible that investigators may have underestimated the prevalence and exaggerated the pathogenic importance of marginal previas and low-lying placentas. Indeed, patients affected with these conditions are more likely to remain free of symptoms until term and to lose less blood (1, 6).

Other Clinical Features

Additional obstetric complications in patients with placenta previa include malpresentations in approximately 30% of cases and a twofold increase in the rate of congenital anomalies (1, 2, 6). An excess of fetuses affected with intrauterine

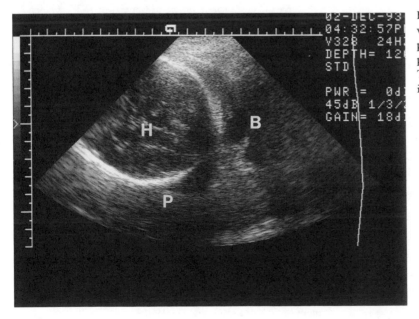

Figure 54.2   Transabdominal sonography at 31 weeks gestation. Fetal head (H) overlying a posterior placenta (arrow). The relationship between the placenta (P) and the cervix is impossible to ascertain. The maternal bladder (B) is on the right side of the image.

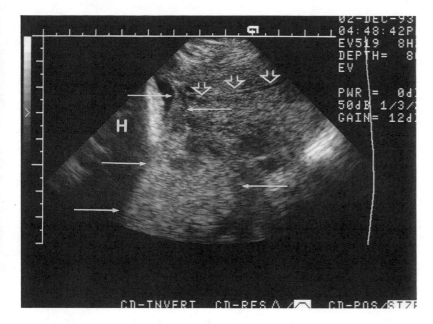

Figure 54.3   Same patient as in Figure 54.2 evaluated with transvaginal sonography. The precise relationship of the cervical·canal (open arrow-heads) to the placenta (arrows) is clearly appreciated and the presence of a posterior previa noted. The fetal head (H) is on the left side of the image.

growth retardation has been reported by some—but not all—investigators (2, 3, 7, 8). Premature rupture of membranes (prevalence: 11%) has also been reported as more common in these patients (1).

While bleeding in placenta previa patients by definition involves some degree of placental separation, true abruption with retroplacental hematoma formation is also possible and can compromise the fetus. The reported recurrence risk for placenta previa is 2.3% (1).

Diagnosis

Sagittal, parasagittal, and transverse views of the relationship between the placenta and the cervix are needed with abdominal sonography to make the diagnosis of placenta previa (Figure 54.2).

However, an anterior previa can be mistakenly produced by an overdistended bladder. Therefore, it is essential to obtain confirmation in postvoid views. In contrast, a posterior previa can be missed near term if the fetal head is low in the pelvis, since the fetal calvarium may obscure placental location by acoustic shadowing (Figure 54.3). In this instance, transvaginal ultrasound is required to determine the precise relationship of the cervical canal to the placenta (Figure 54.3).

A complete central previa is readily apparent since placental tissue is imaged anterior and posterior to the cervix. Complete noncentral previas, particularly when lateral, are more difficult to confirm. Transverse views at and above the internal cervical os should permit a precise diagnosis.

Vaginal sonography appears to be a safe and efficacious approach to the diagnosis of placenta previa (9). The sensitivity of this approach is approximately 90% (10). Vaginal sonography is particularly useful in differentiating marginal from partial previas.

The overall effectiveness of abdominal and vaginal sonographic diagnosis of placenta previa at term is difficult to determine. Low-lying and marginal previas may be missed without untoward clinical consequences. Alternatively, it may be impossible to confirm the diagnosis of complete and partial previas at cesarean section if there is marked blood loss or operative placental disruption. False-negative diagnoses occur in fewer than 10% of cases (10). However, inaccurate characterization of previa type may be more common (11).

Ultrasound evidence indicates that placenta previa is ten times more common before 20 weeks' gestation than during the third trimester. Approximately 4%–26% of all pregnant patients display sonographic evidence of a complete, partial, or marginal previa between 16 and 20 weeks (12–16). Fortunately, 90% of these early previas "convert," or appear to move away from the internal os, by the third trimester (12, 14–17). Precise location of the previa with respect to the os may correlate with the probability of conversion. Complete previas are much less likely to convert (0%–10%) than are partial and marginal ones (91%–98%) (12, 18).

A low placental implantation in the second trimester appears to increase the risk of bleeding and fetal loss (7, 17). Despite this, the vast majority of these patients will experience no symptoms and have a normally implanted placenta by 28 weeks' gestation. Thus, it appears unreasonable to restrict a patient's activities unless a repeat ultrasound evaluation confirms continued placenta previa after 28 weeks.

Two theories have attempted to explain placental conversion. The first holds that, as the lower uterine segment develops, it moves the stationary lower edge of the placenta away from the internal cervical os. The second postulates that there is progressive growth of trophoblastic tissue toward the fundus within the relatively stationary uterus. However, not all investigators have confirmed the high prevalence of sonographically identified placenta previa at midgestation (19). Therefore, the theory of placental conversion remains unproven.

Magnetic resonance imaging (MRI) may provide a more precise method of placental localization. MRI aids in the detection of posterior placenta previa since the fetal calvarium does not obscure placental imaging (20). This modality is well suited for assessing placental–cervical relationships because the two tissues have differing magnetic resonance characteristics. However, the biological safety of MRI has yet to be confirmed and the advent of vaginal sonography may obviate its need.

When using ultrasound to evaluate a possible placenta previa, it is important to identify the umbilical cord's insertion into the placenta's chorionic surface. If there is no central insertion, splaying of the vessels at the placenta's periphery suggests a velamentous insertion.

Velamentous cords contain a single umbilical artery in 12.5% of cases (21). Therefore, if a two-vessel cord is visible, a velamentous insertion may be suspected. Velamentous vessels over the internal os indicate a vasa previa. By repositioning the mother, it may be possible to differentiate a vasa previa from a simple funic presentation (22). We have found Doppler color flow analysis can be useful for visualizing these vessels.

Management Alternatives

Once placenta previa is confirmed, fetal anatomic malformations must be ruled out and fetal weight estimated after 24 weeks even if the patient has no symptoms. During the third trimester, the patient should be advised to avoid coitus. The patient should notify the obstetrician of any uterine contractions or vaginal spotting, and seek immediate medical attention with the onset of vaginal bleeding. Cervical examinations should be avoided, but serial ultrasound evaluations are indicated every 3–4 weeks to assess placental location and fetal growth.

In patients with placenta previa who are beyond 23 weeks' gestation, any vaginal bleeding necessitates hospitalization and acute care (see Case 54.1). Should such care result in cessation of active bleeding before delivery, the patient may be transferred to the antepartum unit for conservative management (see Case 54.2).

The aim of conservative management is to prevent premature delivery—the primary cause of excess morbidity and mortality in placenta previa—by maximizing the duration of pregnancy without risking fetal compromise. Cotton and co-workers have reported that delivery may be deferred and conservative management initiated in 75% of patients with a symptomatic placenta previa (1). Indeed, they noted that one-half of patients with an initial hemorrhagic episode exceeding 500 mL did not require immediate delivery and that the mean prolongation of pregnancy in this group was 16.8 days. According to Silver and co-workers, conservative management can prolong pregnancy by at least four weeks in 50% of patients with a symptomatic previa (6).

It is unclear whether outpatient management of patients with placenta previa is effective. D'Angelo and Irwin who compared patient management in a retrospective non-randomized study, noted a longer duration of pregnancy (35.3 weeks versus 32.4 weeks), higher mean birthweight (2,442 g versus 1,824 g), and lower overall maternal-neonatal hospital costs for inpatients (23).

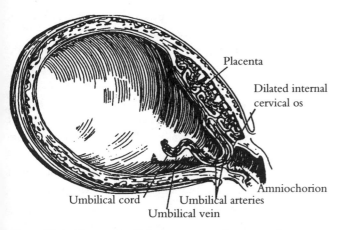

Figure 54.4 Vasa previa. Velamentous vessels traverse the membranes in the lower uterine segment in advance of the fetal head and insert marginally at the edge of the placenta.

Vasa Previa

The incidence of velamentous (membranous) insertion of the umbilical vessels—a condition associated with placenta previa—is 0.2%–1.2% in singleton gestations but up to 10% in twins and greater than 50% in triplets (24). Vasa previa occurs when velamentous vessels traverse the membranes in the lower uterine segment in advance of the fetal head (Figure 54.4).

Rupture of these vessels can occur with or without rupture of the membranes and results in fetal exsanguination. Velamentous vessels need not be present over the os to rupture, and they need not rupture to cause fetal distress or death. Simple compression of the vessels by the descending fetal presenting part may result in death.

The perinatal mortality rate from vasa previa with intact membranes is 50%–60%, while the fetal loss rate exceeds 75% when membranes rupture (25). In twin gestations, perinatal mortality approaches 100% for first twins with vasa previa. In addition, 55% of second twins die because of placental vascular anastomoses.

The association of velamentous cord insertions with placenta previa and multiple gestations has led to the theory that relatively greater trophoblastic growth toward the well-vascularized uterine fundus (trophotropism) is responsible for this condition (21). It is postulated that an initially cen-tral cord insertion has the tendency to become progressively more peripheral as one pole of the placenta actively proliferates while the other remains quiescent or involutes.

Vasa previa should be suspected in the setting of vaginal bleeding immediately after rupture of membranes occurs. The concomitant finding of fetal heart rate abnormalities, particularly a sinusoidal pattern, is highly suggestive of vasa previa. An Apt or Kleihauer-Betke test can determine the origin of the vaginal bleeding. If results confirm a vasa previa, an immediate abdominal delivery should be performed.

The incidence of vasa previa appears to be one in every 5,000 pregnancies (21). Associated fetal anomalies are present in up to 25% of cases of velamentous cord insertion. However, ascertainment biases may exaggerate this association.

Placenta Accreta

Another condition found with placenta previa is placenta accreta, or invasion of the trophoblastic myometrium. Placenta accreta is caused by absence of an adequate decidua basalis. Invasion into the myometrium is called placenta increta, and invasion through it is termed placenta percreta.

Some form of placenta accreta complicates 5%–10% of pregnancies with placenta previa (1, 26). Prevalence, which appears to be increasing, is closely correlated with the number of times that the patient has undergone CS (27). Clark and co-workers noted that 5% of previa patients without previous CS developed placenta accreta, with 58% requiring hysterectomy (26). In contrast, one-quarter of previa patients with one previous CS and at least half of those patients with two or more previous CS operations developed placenta accreta, and 82% required hysterectomy. For this reason, placenta previa and one or more uterine CS scars place a patient at an extremely high risk for placenta accreta and create the need for cesarean hysterectomy.

Conclusion

Placenta previa is often associated with endometrial scarring and increased placental mass. The excess perinatal mortality in affected pregnancies is primarily a consequence of premature delivery and is correlated with gestational age at the onset of symptoms.

Although a diagnosis of placenta previa before 20 weeks' gestation is common, more than 90% of cases will spontaneously resolve by the third trimester. The diagnosis of an asymptomatic placenta previa after 28 weeks requires education of the patient, pelvic rest, and serial sonographic assessment of placental location and fetal growth. Patients with symptomatic previas of longer than 24 weeks' duration require hospitalization with conservative management to prolong gestation. In rare cases, outpatient management can be used with reliable, currently asymptomatic patients.

Delivery is mandated by refractory maternal hemorrhage at any gestational age, fetal distress after 23 weeks' gestation, and attainment of fetal pulmonary maturity at or after 36 weeks' gestation. When delivery is indicated, the abdominal route is mandatory in cases of sonographically diagnosed complete and partial previas and for most cases of marginal previa. It is also important to rule out coexistent vasa previa or placenta accreta.

C A S E   5 4 . 1   Acute Care for Symptomatic Placenta Previa

1. Admit the actively bleeding placenta previa patient at between 24 and 36 weeks' gestation to the labor and delivery area.
2. Establish IV access with two 16-gauge IV lines and administer crystalloid infusion adequate to maintain hemodynamic stability and urine output.
3. Precisely monitor vaginal blood loss by weighing perineal pads. Assess whether blood is maternal or fetal by either an Apt test or Kleihauer-Betke analysis if vasaprevia is suspected.
4. Evaluate urine output hourly with a Foley catheter and collecting device. Intermittently obtain urine-specific gravity. Assess serum electrolytes and renal func-

tion indices every eight hours (more frequently if significant transfusion are required).

5. Check maternal pulse and blood pressure every 15 minutes to one hour depending on the degree of blood loss. Use a maternal ECG monitor and automated blood pressure cuff, if available.
6. If the patient is hemodynamically unstable despite apparently adequate fluid replacement or has underlying cardiac, pulmonary, or renal disease, place a triple-lumen Swan-Ganz catheter for assessment of central venous pressure, pulmonary capillary wedge pressure, and cardiac output.
7. Evaluate hematocrit every 30 minutes to eight hours, depending on the degree of blood loss. Have the patient typed and cross-matched for four units of packed red blood cells and transfused to maintain hemodynamic stability.
8. Check the maternal coagulation profile (fibrinogen, platelet count, prothrombin time, and partial thromboplastin time) every 1–8 hours, depending on the degree of blood loss or if there is any suspicion of coexistent abruption. Development of disseminated intravascular coagulation is an indication for delivery.
9. Continuously monitor the FHR. An unexplained loss of reactivity and long-term variability or development of fetal tachycardia, recurrent late decelerations, or a sinusoidal pattern is evidence of fetal distress from either hypoxia or anemia.
10. Tocolysis doesn't appear to be indicated in an actively bleeding patient with a placenta previa.
11. Delivery is mandated by fetal distress unresponsive to maternal oxygen therapy, left-sided positioning, or intravascular volume replacement, and is also indicated for refractory or life-threatening maternal hemorrhage. Abdominal delivery is mandated except when the fetus is dead or before 24 weeks' gestation and when the mother is hemodynamically stable.
12. In cases of marginal placental previa where there is advanced cervical dilation and fetal descent without excessive hemorrhage or fetal distress, you may perform a "double set-up exam" in the operative suite. This procedure entails full preparation for an emergent CS. With the patient prepped and draped in the dors

lithotomy position, do a careful sterile vaginal examination. If you palpate placental tissue through the vaginal fornix, do a CS. If no placental tissue is found, place a finger carefully into the cervix and gently palpate 360 degrees around the internal os. If no placental tissue is noted, a vaginal delivery can be allowed. At any point, if placental tissue is suspected over the internal os or if excessive vaginal bleeding is encountered, proceed to an immediate CS. ∎

CASE 54.2 Conservative Management of Placenta Previa

Conservative management is appropriate for the hospitalized but currently asymptomatic or minimally symptomatic placenta previa patient who is between 24 and 36 weeks' gestation and has had bleeding.

1. Prescribe bed rest with bathroom privileges. Use stool softeners and a high-fiber diet to minimize constipation and avoid excess staining.

2. Daily maternal hematocrits are not required in the absence of active bleeding unless there is a chronic bloody vaginal discharge or evidence of a retroplacental hematoma. In stabile patients, only periodic assessment of maternal hematocrit is necessary.

3. Initiate therapy with 300 mg of ferrous gluconate orally three to four times daily. Vitamin C may be given to improve intestinal iron absorption.

4. Always have a maternal blood sample available in the blood bank for immediate type and cross-match to provide 2–4 units of packed red blood cells. "Prophylactic" transfusions to maintain maternal hematocrit above 30% in anticipation of future blood loss are of dubious value. However, in patients experiencing continuous low-grade vaginal bleeding, resulting in a falling hematocrit despite iron therapy, use transfusions to maintain hematocrit above 21%.

   An alternative to possible homologous transfusions is the use of autologous blood storage (28, 29). Although autologous donation appears safe for mother and fetus, a minimum hematocrit of 34% is generally required to donate one unit, a requirement that will exclude many placenta previa patients.

5. Give the mother betamethasone (Celestone) or dexamethasone (Aeroseb-Dex, Decaderm, Decadron Tablets, Elixir) at least once between 26 and 32 weeks' gestation to enhance fetal pulmonary maturity.

6. The value of frequent fetal heart rate monitoring in an asymptomatic placenta previa patient who is without evidence of fetal growth retardation is unclear. However, a weekly nonstress test or biophysical profile appears prudent. When there is fetal growth retardation, do fetal testing every other day. With intermittent moderate vaginal bleeding, do daily or twice daily fetal testing.

7. Carry out ultrasound evaluation of fetal growth, amniotic fluid volume, and placental localization every 2–3 weeks. The cessation of fetal growth over a two- to three-week interval may be an indication for delivery. Doppler-flow analysis may be a useful adjunct for assessment of fetal risk. Barr and co-workers noted that a ratio of the maximum systolic and minimum diastolic umbilical artery velocities greater than 3.0 was associated with adverse pregnancy outcomes, even in the absence of fetal growth retardation (8).

8. Tocolysis has been used by a number of centers to eliminate uterine contractions, which theoretically exacerbate placental detachment and bleeding (1, 2). The usefulness of tocolysis in placenta previa patients hasn't been confirmed by adequately sized, randomized, placebo-controlled trials.

9. If preterm PROM occurs in a patient with a placenta previa, manage the obstetric condition independently. Labor or chorioamnionitis is an indication for delivery.

10. Carry out amniocentesis at 36 weeks to assess pulmonary maturity. If immature indices are present, repeat the procedure weekly until the lungs are mature. Carry out elective abdominal delivery with confirmation of maturity since the risk of fetal anemia is approximately tenfold higher (28% versus 2.8%) with

emergent than with elective delivery (1).

11. Abdominal delivery is always indicated with sonographic evidence of a complete or partial placenta previa. Occasionally, you can do a "double set-up examination" (described in Case 54.1) if there is uncertainty in the asymptomatic term patient between a diagnosis of posterior marginal previa and low-lying placenta previa. However, vaginal ultrasound will obviate the need for double setup examination in most cases.

Have 2–4 units of packed red blood cells available for the delivery. Have surgical instruments ready to carry out a cesarean hysterectomy, since there is a 5%–10% risk of placenta accreta (1, 2, 26).

Before abdominal delivery, find the placental outline by ultrasound and try not to disrupt it when entering the uterus. If there is an anterior-lateral previa, make a vertical incision in the lower uterine segment on the opposite side. Also, a transverse incision can occasionally be carried out above a low-lying anterior previa. Ultrasound may also reveal evidence of placenta accreta including loss of normal hypoechoic retroplacental myometrial zone, abnormal uterine serosa-bladder interface, and exophytic masses adjacent to the serosa (30).

We have used intraoperative ultrasound to precisely delineate the placental outline. This procedure, as described to the author by John C. Hobbins, MD, of the University of Colorado School of Medicine, requires that the transducer be placed in a sterile plastic bag and sheath. On entry into the abdominal cavity, place sterile sonographic media on the uterus and directly image the placenta. Using this approach, we can tailor the uterine incision to spare the placenta and at the same time avoid a classic incision scar.

12. Outpatient management has been used in selected patients with placenta previa if asymptomatic for more than one week and without evidence of fetal growth retardation or fetal distress if they 1) lived within 15 minutes of the hospital, 2) had an adult companion available 24 hours a day who could immediately transport them to the hospital, 3) were reliable and could maintain strict bed rest at home, and 4) understood the risks entailed by outpatient management. ∎

References

1. Cotton DB, Read JA, Paul RH, et al. The conservative aggressive management of placenta previa. Am J Obstet Gynecol 1980;137:687.
2. McShane PM, Heyl PS, Epstein MF. Maternal and perinatal morbidity resulting from placenta previa. Obstet Gynecol 1985;65:176.
3. Brenner WE, Edelman DA, Hendricks CH. Characteristics of patients with placenta previa and results of "expectant management." Am J Obstet Gynecol 1978;132:180.
4. Rose GL, Chapman MG. Aetiological factors in placenta praevia—a case-controlled study. Br J Obstet Gynaecol 1986; 93:586.
5. Williams MA, Mittendorf FR, Lieberman E, Monson RR, Schoenbaum SC, Genest DR. Cigarette smoking during pregnancy in relation to placenta previa. Am J Obstet Gynecol 1991;165:28–32.
6. Silver R, Depp R, Sabbagha RE, et al. Placenta previa: aggressive expectant management. Am J Obstet Gynecol 1984; 150:15.
7. Varma TR. Fetal growth and placental function in patients with placenta previa. Br J Obstet Gynaecol 1973;80:311.
8. Brar HS, Platt LD, DeVore GR, et al. Fetal umbilical velocimetry for the surveillance of pregnancies complicated by placenta previa. J Reprod Med 1988;33:741.
9. Farine D, Fox HE, Jakobson S, Timor-Tritsch IE. Vaginal ultrasound for diagnosis of placenta previa. Am J Obstet Gynecol 1988;159:566–9.
10. Leerentveld RA, Gilberts ECAM, Arnold MJCWJ, Wladimiroff JW. Accuracy and safety of transvaginal sonographic placental localization. Obstet Gynecol 1990;76: 759–62.
11. Gorodeski IG, Neri A, Haimovich L, et al. Placenta previa: the ultrasonographic placental localization and its influence on the mode of delivery. J Reprod Med 1982;27:655.
12. Gallagher P, Fagan CJ, Bedi DG, et al. Potential placenta previa: definition, frequency, and significance. AJR 1987; 149:1013.
13. Townsend RR, Laing FC, Nyberg DA, et al. Technical factors responsible for "placental migration": sonographic assessment. Radiology 1986;160:105.
14. Wexler P, Gottesfeld KR. Early diagnosis of placenta previa. Obstet Gynecol 1979;54:231.
15. Zanke S. Die ultrasonographische Frühdiagnose der Placenta Praevia und ihr klinischer Stellenwert. Geburtshilfe Frauenheilkd 1985;45:710.

16. Rizos N, Doran TA, Miskin M, et al. Natural history of placenta previa ascertained by diagnostic ultrasound. Am J Obstet Gynecol 1979;133:287.

17. Newton ER, Barss V, Cetrulo CL. The epidemiology and clinical history of asymptomatic midtrimester placenta previa. Am J Obstet Gynecol 1984;148:743.

18. Schmidt W, Boos R, Hendrik HJ, et al. Pathologischer Placentasitz nach der 20. Schwangerschaftswoche: Bedeutung für den Schwangerschafts und Gerburtsverlauf. Geburtshilfe Frauenheilkd 1986;46:206.

19. Artis AA, Bowie JD, Rosenberg ER, et al. The fallacy of placental migration: effect of sonographic techniques. AJR 1985;144:79.

20. Powell MC, Buckley J, Price H, et al. Magnetic resonance imaging and placenta previa. Am J Obstet Gynecol 1986; 154:565.

21. Kouyoumdjian A. Velamentous insertion of the umbilical cord. Obstet Gynecol 1980;56:737.

22. Gianopoulos J, Carver T, Tomich PG, et al. Diagnosis of vasa previa with ultrasonography. Obstet Gynecol 1987;69:488.

23. D'Angelo LJ, Irwin LF. Conservative management of placenta previa: a cost-benefit analysis. Am J Obstet Gynecol 1984; 149:320.

24. VanDrie DM, Kammeraad LA. Vasa previa: case report. Review and presentation of a new diagnostic method. J Reprod Med 1981;26:577.

25. Antoine C, Young BK, Silverman F, et al. Sinusoidal fetal heart rate pattern with vasa previa in twin pregnancy. J Reprod Med 1982;27:295.

26. Clark SL, Koonings PP, Phelan JP. Placenta previa/accreta and prior cesarean section. Obstet Gynecol 1987;66:89.

27. Weckstein LN, Masserman JSH, Garite TJ. Placenta accreta: a problem of increasing clinical significance. Obstet Gynecol 1987;69:480.

28. Herbert WN, Owen HG, Collins ML. Autologous blood storage in obstetrics. Obstet Gynecol 1988;72:166.

29. Kruskall MS, Leonard S, Klapholz H. Autologous blood donation during pregnancy: analysis of safety and blood use. Obstet Gynecol 1987;70:938.

30. Finberg HJ, Williams JW. Placenta accreta: prospective sonographic diagnosis in patients with placental previa and prior cesarian section. J Ultrasound Med 1992;11:333–43.

55

Placental Abruption

Steven L. Clark, M.D.

PREMATURE complete or partial separation of a normally implanted placenta constitutes placental abruption (1). Incidence of this condition varies between 1 in 50 and 1 in 500 pregnancies, depending on the diagnostic criteria used. Undoubtedly, many cases of minor intrapartum bleeding arise from clinically unimportant placental abruption (2, 3).

Causes of Abruption

The most important risk factor for an abruption is chronic or pregnancy-induced maternal hypertension. Although the incidence of hypertension does not appear to be increased in women with placental abruption as a whole, it is five times more common in those having severe abruption (4). Other factors implicated in the genesis of placental abruption include an unusually short umbilical cord, maternal trauma, sudden uterine decompression (as with delivery of a first twin or too vigorous therapeutic amniocentesis), and high parity (4, 5). In women with a previous placental abruption, reported recurrence ranges from 5% –15% (2, 4). Recently, cocaine use has become a significant cause of placental abruption (6, 7).

Clinical Course

The initiating event in placental abruption is hemorrhage into the decidua basalis with subsequent hematoma formation. This clot further separates the basal plate from the decidua and causes additional bleeding. Abruption may thus become self-sustaining.

In severe cases, the process damages and disrupts placental vessels and casts thromboplastin-rich decidual debris into the mother's bloodstream. Disseminated intravascular coagulopathy occurs in roughly 30% of cases, so severe as to kill the fetus.

Sher, in a study of 79 abruptions, observed that clinical uterine hypertonus correlated with presence of a placental clot exceeding 150 mL (8). Fetal death was usually associated with a retroplacental clot of 500 mL or more, and clinical hemorrhage due to consumptive coagulopathy did not occur until the clot exceeded 1,000 mL.

In general, abruption with separation of more than 50% of the total placental area results in fetal death unless

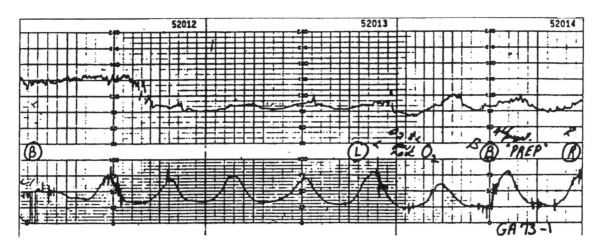

Figure 55.1 Contraction patterns. Increased baseline uterine tonus and tachysystole characteristic of placental abruption. (From Paul RH, Petrie RH. Fetal intensive care. North Haven, CT: William Mack Co, 1979:1–5.)

delivery is immediate. Rarely, the combination of severe hemorrhage, hypotension, and intravascular coagulation may lead to maternal acute tubular or cortical necrosis.

Placental abruption classically is first noted as painful vaginal bleeding or bleeding with uterine contractions. The pain may be related directly to placental separation, but often it is a result of forceful uterine contractions initiated by hemorrhage into the decidua. Such contractions are often frequent and intense, and baseline uterine tonus may be increased (Figure 55.1) (9). Uterine tenderness may also be present.

Although vaginal bleeding is evident in 80% of patients with abruption, absence of bleeding does not exclude an abruption. This diagnosis must be considered in any patient seen with abdominal pain in late pregnancy. Prolonged observation may be necessary, especially in patients who have sustained blunt abdominal trauma. Abruption and fetal distress may not be clinically evident until 24–48 hours after the injury (10–12).

Unlike placenta previa, in which ultrasound by itself is usually sufficient, the diagnosis of placental abruption requires clinical presentation and tests, which are occasionally supportive but not diagnostic. Placental abruption can be documented sonographically, but it is not possible to exclude an abruption on the basis of ultrasound alone (13). False-positive diagnoses are also common (14, 15).

History, physical examination, and the observation of uterine contraction pattern and fetal response, as assessed by electronic fetal heart rate (FHR) monitoring, will assist in the diagnosis or exclusion of placental abruption. Occasionally, laboratory documentation of coagulation abnormalities are helpful in making the diagnosis. However, in most cases, diagnosis is clinically obvious if abruption is severe enough to have initiated disseminated intravascular coagulation (16, 17).

Recently, magnetic resonance imaging has been used to diagnose placenta previa (18). However, its superiority to more readily available ultrasound is doubtful. Older radiologic methods of placental localization, such as amniography, are no longer appropriate.

If a placenta previa has been ruled out, third-trimester bleeding, regardless of etiology, is unlikely to be of immediate danger to the mother's life. The next step, therefore, is to evaluate the fetus. External electronic FHR monitoring should be instituted and continued until conditions harmful to the fetus, including placental abruption and vasa previa, have been clinically excluded.

Should it prove that neither mother nor fetus are in immediate danger, and placenta previa has been excluded, speculum examination may rule out vaginal or cervical lesions as the source of bleeding. This measure may be carried out simultaneously with fetal assessment.

Finally, placental abruption must be excluded. Both false-positive and false-negative rates of sonographically identified retroplacental hemorrhage are high. Therefore, it must be emphasized that the principal purpose of an ultrasound scan for vaginal bleeding is to rule out placenta previa, not to diagnose abruption. Rather, the diagnosis or exclusion of placental abruption must be based principally on clinical findings.

Symptoms of abdominal or back pain and signs such as tender uterus, labor (especially with uterine tachysystole or hypertonus), hypotension, anemia, or fetal distress all suggest placental abruption. In many cases, the proper diagnosis requires an extensive period of fetal and maternal monitoring. Frequently, an initially reassuring FHR tracing will deteriorate over hours as abruption progresses or will deteriorate abruptly during the observation period. Only after all symptoms and signs have abated and fetal well-being is documented by nonstress or contraction stress test criteria or biophysical profile can such monitoring be discontinued. In some cases, minor peripheral placental separation will cause transient bleeding that has no clinical consequence (19).

Management Considerations

Gestational age determines the management of clinically diagnosed placental abruption. If it is compatible with extrauterine life, delivery is generally indicated. Most patients with placental abruption will be in spontaneous labor. In such cases, cesarean delivery is not invariably necessary. If careful electronic FHR monitoring is instituted, up to 48% of these patients may be delivered vaginally without evidence of fetal distress (16).

However, the FHR tracing may change abruptly from a reassuring to an ominous pattern. Since the goal of such monitoring is to delivery an infant *before* it is compromised, it is important to intervene if rapid deterioration is likely. If bleeding is heavy and cervical dilation is not advanced, timely cesarean section (CS) may obviate later need for an emergency procedure.

In the previable or extremely premature fetus, a more conservative approach may be appropriate. Bleeding and cramping may be substantial at times, yet may spontaneously subside, allowing the fetus to remain in utero and achieve extrauterine viability.

With the clinical diagnosis of placental abruption, tocolytic agents are not generally recommended. Such therapy has no proven value in patients with abruption. Further, sympathomimetic agents may have profound and potentially harmful hemodynamic effects on a heavily bleeding patient (20).

However, in a patient in preterm labor who exhibits only minimal bleeding, tocolysis is not necessarily contraindicated, even though some degree of placental separation cannot be excluded. In such cases, magnesium sulfate is often the agent of choice (21).

Because of the possibility of abruption-associated coagulopathy, assessing the fibrinogen level, prothrombin and partial thromboplastin times (PT and PPT), and platelet count is sometimes helpful when abruption is suspected. Since such abnormalities are extremely unlikely with a live fetus, these costly studies may not be necessary in the patient whose labor is progressing rapidly, whose bleeding is minimal, and whose FHR tracing shows fetal well-being. In such cases, observation of clot formation in a glass tube within 4–8 minutes may be sufficient to exclude a clinically important coagulopathy.

If coagulopathy is present, delivery must be expedited. Replacement of clotting factors with fresh frozen plasma will usually be sufficient. A fibrinogen level below 100 mg/dL in a bleeding patient indicates replacement therapy. Prolongation of the PT and activated PPT are not seen until 50% or more of the clotting factors have been consumed. Therefore, such a finding represents substantial consumption.

Because a coagulopathy is rarely encountered with a live fetus, oxytocin induction or augmentation of labor to achieve vaginal delivery is generally appropriate. Low-dose heparin infusion (between 5,000 and 10,000 units every 12 hours) may be helpful in rare cases of severe coagulopathy with a dead fetus while delivery is being effected (21, 22). Full anticoagulant doses are no more effective than low-dose therapy and are associated with additional side effects.

Rarely, subserosal extravasation of blood associated with placental abruption may lead to the so-called Couvelaire uterus. In such cases, uterine atony may be encountered. However, such atony usually responds well to standard therapy, including oxytocin and 15-methyl prostaglandin F, and is not, by itself, an indication for hysterectomy (23).

CASE 55.1 A Chronic Hypertensive

A 28-year-old chronic hypertensive patient was admitted to the hospital at 38 weeks' gestation with contractions and vaginal bleeding of sudden onset. On admission, fetal heart tones were absent. Blood pressure was 150/105 mm Hg, and urine protein was 3+. Laboratory evaluation revealed a hematocrit of 26%, a serum fibrinogen level of 60 mg/100 mL, a prothrombin time of 17 seconds (control 12 seconds), a partial thromboplastin time of 42 seconds (control 28 seconds), and a platelet count of 85,000/mL. Pulse was 112 bpm. The abdomen was tense and tender in all quadrants. Uterine contractions were occurring every minute. The cervix was dilated 4 cm. Real-time ultrasound examination revealed a posterior placenta that did not encroach on the cervical os. A retroplacental lucency suggested possible placental abruption.

The membranes were ruptured, revealing bloody, meconium-stained amniotic fluid. An IV line was started. The patient's blood was typed and cross-matched for four units of packed red blood cells and four units of fresh frozen plasma. A strict intake and output record was initiated. The patient received two units of fresh frozen plasma and two units of red blood cells (RBC). At this time, the hematocrit had fallen to 25%, the fibrinogen level to 50 mm/dL, and the platelet count was 65,000/mL. Two additional units of fresh frozen plasma were infused, followed by two units of packed RBCs.

The infant was delivered as the second unit of packed cells was being infused. The placenta delivered spontaneously immediately thereafter, confirming the presence of a complete placental abruption.

After delivery, massive uterine atony was encountered.

This was controlled by bimanual compression and IM injection of four units (1 mg) of carboprost tromethamine (Hemabate). Total blood loss was estimated at 2,000 mL. However, fluid and component replacement prevented the patient from becoming hypotensive, and urine output remained good.

Thirty minutes after infusion of the second unit of packed cells, the patient was clinically stable without bleeding. Platelet count was 33,000/mL, serum fibrinogen 37 mg/dL, and hematocrit 21%. At that time, bleeding from the IV sites was noted. In addition, although uterine atony had been corrected, continued moderate vaginal bleeding was observed. The patient was then transfused successfully with 10 units of platelets, an additional four units of fresh frozen plasma, and four units of packed RBCs.

Four hours after delivery, hematocrit was 28%, fibrinogen level 110 mg/dL, platelet count 92,000/mL, and all clinical bleeding had subsided. No additional blood components were infused, and laboratory evaluations obtained eight hours later showed continued improvement in platelet count and fibrinogen level, with return of PT and PPT to normal. The patient required transfusion of an additional two units of packed red blood cells and was discharged from the hospital on day 4.

CASE 55.2 An Accident Victim

A 22-year-old woman was involved in an automobile accident at 32 weeks' gestation. She was not wearing a seat belt, and her abdomen struck the steering wheel. She was brought for evaluation to the emergency room and sent to labor and delivery. She complained only of mild abdominal tenderness without uterine contractions. Physical examination results were unremarkable except for slight tenderness reported over the mid- to upper abdomen. No bruising was visible. The patient's vital signs were stable, and a fetal heart rate tracing showed a baseline rate of 145 bpm, with frequent accelerations and no periodic decelerations. The patient was admitted to the hospital for observation with continuous electronic FHR monitoring.

Fourteen hours after admission, the FHR pattern no longer showed accelerations. The patient was having irregular uterine contractions at the rate of one to two per hour, and late decelerations were noted following two sequential contractions. The patient then underwent cesarean section. A 2,200-g baby boy was delivered with Apgar scores of 5 and 9. A 20% placental abruption was noted. Cord gases showed an umbilical artery pH of 7.18.

The child required ventilatory support but subsequently did well and was discharged in good condition. Laboratory analysis of the mother's blood revealed no evidence of clotting abnormalities. ■

References

1. Pritchard JA, MacDonald PC, Gant NF. Williams Obstetrics. Norwalk, CT: Appleton-Century-Crofts, 1985:395.
2. Patterson MEL. The aetiology and outcome of abruptio placentae. Acta Obstet Gynecol Scand 1979;58:31.
3. Abdella TN, Sibai BM, Harp JM, et al. Perinatal outcome in abruptio placentae. Obstet Gynecol 1984;63:365.
4. Pritchard JA, Mason R, Corley M, et al. Genesis of severe placental abruption. Am J Obstet Gynecol 1970;108:22.
5. Marbury MC, Linn S, Monson R, et al. The association of alcohol consumption with outcome of pregnancy. Am J Public Health 1983;73:1165.
6. Hoskins IA, Friedman DM, Frieden FJ, et al. Relationship between antepartum cocaine abuse, abnormal umbilical artery doppler velocimetry and placental abruption. Obstet Gynecol 1991;78:279.
7. Slutsker L. Risks associated with cocaine use during pregnancy. Obstet Gynecol 1992;79:778.
8. Sher G. A rational basis for the management of abruptio placentae. J Reprod Med 1978;21:123.
9. Paul RH, Petrie RH. Fetal intensive care. North Haven, CT: William Mack Co, 1979:1–5.
10. Lavin JP, Miodornick M. Delayed abruption after maternal trauma as a result of an automobile accident. J Reprod Med 1981;26:261.
11. Rothenberger D, Quattlebaum FW, Perry JF, et al. Blunt maternal trauma: a review of 103 cases. J Trauma 1978; 18:173.
12. Higgins SD, Garite TJ. Later abruptio placentae in trauma patients: implications for monitoring. Obstet Gynecol 1984;63:105.
13. Nyberg DA, Mack LA, Benedetti TJ, et al. Placental abruption and placental hemorrhage: correlation of sonographic findings with fetal outcome. Radiology 1987;164:357.
14. Jaffe MH, Schoen WC, Silver TM, et al. Sonography of abruptio placentae. AJR 1979;133:877.
15. Spirit BA, Kagan EH, Rozanski RM. Abruptio placentae: sonographic and pathologic correlation. AJR 1979;133: 877.
16. Hurd WW, Miodornik M, Hertzberg V, et al. Selective management of abruptio placentae: a prospective study. Obstet Gynecol 1983;61:467.
17. Hovatta O, Lipasti A, Rapola J, et al. Causes of stillbirth: a clinicopathologic study of 243 patients. Acta Obstet Gynecol Scand 1983;90:691.
18. Powell MC, Buckley J, Price H, et al. Magnetic resonance imaging and placenta previa. Am J Obstet Gynecol 1986; 154:565.
19. Harris BA. Peripheral placental separation: a review. Obstet Gynecol Surv 1988;43:577.
20. Beall MH, Edgar BW, Paul RH, et al. A comparison of ritodrine, terbutaline and magnesium sulfate for the suppression of preterm labor. Am J Obstet Gynecol 1985;153:854.
21. Romero R, Duffe JP, Berkowitz RL, et al. The use of heparin to prolong a preterm gestation complicated by maternal DIC due to death of a single twin in utero. N Engl J Med 1984;310:772.
22. Weiner CP. The obstetric patient and disseminated intravascular coagulation. Clin Perinatol 1986;13:705.
23. Clark SL, Phelan JP. Surgical control of obstetric hemorrhage. Contemp Ob/Gyn 1984;24(Aug):70.

PART SEVEN Complications of Labor and Delivery

56

Prolonged Pregnancy

Jeffrey C. King, M.D.

THE decisions associated with the management of prolonged pregnancy make this relatively common obstetric problem a difficult one. The specific clinical dilemmas are: 1) identification of the at-risk fetus, 2) establishment of a prospective management plan, and 3) determination as to whether vaginal or cesarean delivery is appropriate. Clearly, the safety of both the mother and the fetus must be considered, along with patient expectations, cost assessment, and the medicolegal environment of contemporary obstetrical practice.

In order for a management plan to be most effective in reducing both physician and parental anxiety, the exact gestational age should be confirmed in early pregnancy, and the at-risk fetus must be monitored appropriately (Figure 56.1). It is critical that the patient be brought into the decision-making process during the development of her individual management plan. Lastly, the patient and her physician must always be reminded that the assessment techniques for postterm pregnancy are limited in safeguarding against unpredictable events that may jeopardize outcome.

Duration of Pregnancy

The mean duration of human pregnancy calculated from the first day of the last menstrual period (LMP) is 280 days, with a standard deviation of 14 days. It is critical to remember that the clinician will measure age in terms of menstrual weeks (not conceptual weeks), based on an assumption of ovulation and conception occurring on day 14 of a 28-day cycle. Women whose menstrual cycles are not 28 days or who do not ovulate on day 14 will have more difficulty in establishing accurate pregnancy dating.

The most often used definition for a postterm pregnancy is one that persists beyond 42 weeks (294 days) of confirmed gestational age. Approximately 50% of patients deliver by their due date, with an additional 35%–40% delivering within the following two weeks. The remaining patients extend their pregnancy beyond the start of the 43rd week. The exact incidence of postterm pregnancy is uncertain, but it has been reported to be between 3.5% and 14% (1–3). Generally, the higher percentages are seen in prospective studies of this problem (2). Fortunately, only 4%–7.3% of pregnancies extend beyond 43 weeks (4). The

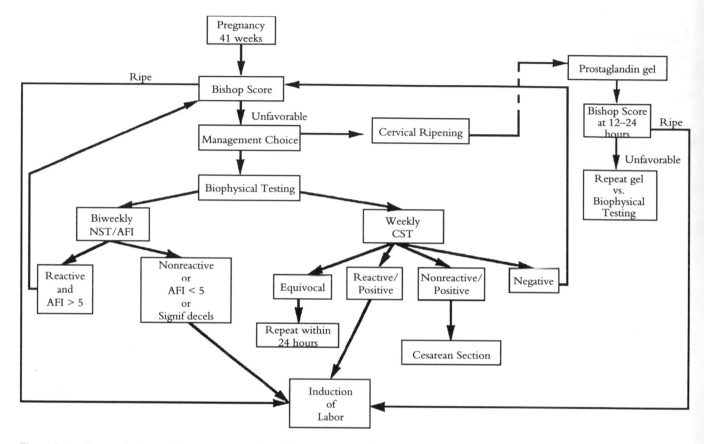

Figure 56.1   Proposed scheme for management of postdate pregnancy. This flow diagram describes the variety of clinical decision steps and the potential interventions.

term postmaturity syndrome or dysmaturity should be reserved for that subset of postterm infants who exhibit either overt growth retardation or fetal malnutrition. Only 5%–40% of postterm pregnancies result in postmaturity syndrome (1, 5–7).

The most frequent cause of apparently prolonged gestation is error in determining the time of ovulation and conception according to the time of the last menstrual period. There can be little doubt that menstrual data cannot be blindly accepted as reliable. Using ultrasound to determine gestational age, Dewhurst (8) showed that it was impossible to assign reliable dates using menstrual data alone in up to 22% of gravid women. The uncertain timing of ovulation and fertilization, along with its resultant impact on menstrual regularity, must always be considered. There have been two significant studies that have established the ovula-

tion-to-delivery interval as 276–280 days (9, 10). Using the ovulation-to-delivery interval resulted in a 41% reduction in the incidence of postterm pregnancy, from 15.5% to 9.1% (9, 10). Early prenatal examination and ultrasound confirmation allow accurate gestational age estimation and lower the incidence of prolonged pregnancy (6).

Definition of Terms

The term "prolonged" or "postterm" pregnancy should be used to refer to a gestation in which there is firm, objective evidence to support a menstrual (gestational) age of at least 42 weeks (294 days from the onset of the last menstrual period). The less specific term of "postdate" pregnancy refers to a gestation that extends beyond the due date based on menstrual history. The difficulty for the clinician is to separate truly prolonged pregnancy from those that are only postdate. For a small but significant number of fetuses, prolonged pregnancy increases the risk for chronic intrauterine asphyxia, meconium aspiration, long-term neurologic sequela, and occasionally death.

Etiology of Prolonged Pregnancy

The most frequent cause of an apparently prolonged gestation is an error in determining the time of ovulation and conception in relation to the first day of the last menstrual period (10). While there have been various theories advanced to explain the pathogenesis of the prolonged pregnancy (11, 12), the actual physiologic mechanism responsible has not been identified. When a postterm pregnancy actually exists, the cause is usually unknown. Until the mechanism for the initiation and maintenance of labor is more clearly defined, the exact etiology of the postterm pregnancy will remain obscure.

However, there are clinical conditions or associations that have been found to predispose the parturient to this problem. Fetal anencephaly has frequently been associated with postterm pregnancy. The delay in the onset of labor is believed to be due to pituitary-adrenal insufficiency. The potential role of this fetal pituitary-adrenal axis is supported by the work of Naeye (13) in which 56% of postterm fetuses whose deaths were attributed to congenital malformations had evidence of marked adrenal gland hypoplasia. This concept is further supported by the work of Nwosu (12), who reported that labor began soon after intraamniotic injection of glucocorticoids in a group of postterm women.

Rare fetal conditions associated with prolonged pregnancy include placental sulfatase deficiency and advanced extrauterine pregnancy. The former is an X-linked recessive disorder characterized by both low estriols and prolonged pregnancy. Since both urinary and serum estriols are no longer used to monitor pregnancy, the diagnosis of this disorder has become rather difficult.

The exact relationship between extrauterine pregnancy and prolonged pregnancy is unknown. While some feel that the removal of the uterine factor is explanatory, others maintain that the pituitary-adrenal axis becomes affected. Fortunately, the utilization of ultrasound and various screening tests, such as maternal serum alpha-fetoprotein testing, will place both anencephaly and extrauterine pregnancy in the historical association category.

There is no association between either advancing maternal age or parity and the development of postterm pregnancy. Similarly, ethnic extraction has no specific impact on the incidence of prolonged pregnancy. However, a woman's socioeconomic status does appear to play a role in whether she will go postterm. The incidence of prolonged pregnancy seems to be related to the gravida's socioeconomic status and education (12). However, this information must be evaluated carefully since patients of lower socioeconomic status and education may have delayed access to prenatal care, making confirmation of gestational age through either early clinical landmarks or ultrasound assessment impossible.

The occurrence of threatened abortion or vaginal bleeding early in pregnancy may lead to inaccurate assignment of an estimated delivery date. With these complications, the clinician should recognize the need to confirm not only fetal viability but also gestational age. Eden (14) has shown that women who deliver postterm infants weigh significantly more than those women who deliver at term. However, his findings do not allow a prediction of exactly which patients will become postdates. The maternal weights at delivery had considerable overlap for both the postterm and term infants (167.6 ± 27.5 and 161.4 ± 25.9 pounds, respectively).

A history of a prior prolonged pregnancy results in a woman having a 50% recurrence risk. This high risk for recurrence suggests either a genetic basis or a mechanism operating through the fetus (4).

Morbidity and Mortality

Previously, one accepted management for a prolonged pregnancy was to advise induction of labor for all patients when they reached 42 weeks. Other clinicians did not feel that prolonged pregnancy required such active management. Maternal complications from postterm pregnancy do not usually result in major physical problems, but the emotional and physiologic impact may be substantial. These include the anxiety and frustration that patients frequently develop after passing an estimated date of confinement (EDC) that has been their central focus for weeks or months. In addition, the inconvenience, expense, and risk associated with the various forms of antepartum testing make postterm pregnancy a major problem. The attendant risks associated with the management of these pregnancies, plus the considerations of labor and the potential for operative delivery, must also be considered. The primary maternal risk is cesarean section, with its associated risks of postpartum infection, hemorrhage, wound complications, and pulmonary emboli. Eden (14) showed that the rate of cesarean section doubled when passing 42 weeks, as compared to gestations at 38–40 weeks. The contemporary approach to this problem is to attempt to identify that subset of prolonged pregnancies that are at significant risk for uteroplacental insufficiency.

Most studies show a significant increase in perinatal morbidity and mortality as a pregnancy extends beyond 42 weeks of gestation due to four principal problems:

1. *Oligohydramnios*. The volume of amniotic fluid reaches a peak at 34–36 weeks (1000 mL), followed by a gradual loss. At term, the mean volume is 800 mL, but, at 42 weeks, it has declined to 250–300 mL. The rate of further decrease is variable and unpredictable. Oligohydramnios has traditionally been associated with the increased risk of meconium staining, fetal distress, fetal acidosis, umbilical cord compression, and low Apgar scores. Prior to the widespread use of ultrasound, the diagnosis of oligohydramnios was rarely made prior to rupture of membranes. Currently, assessment of amniotic fluid volume (AFV) has become a routine part of antepartum testing (15). Unfortunately, the development of oligohydramnios can occur without warning, often prior to the onset of labor. Additionally, the timing of its development is not predictable by the results of antepartum testing.

2. *Meconium*. The event of meconium passage appears to be due to either function of a more mature, active vagal reflex within the fetal gastrointestinal tract or increased hypoxic stimulation to the parasympathetic system. While meconium is rarely found prior to 32 weeks, the frequency increases progressively with ges-

tational age. Meconium is found in 10%–15% of normal pregnancies at term and in 25%–30% of pregnancies at 42 weeks (14). As the amniotic fluid volume declines, there is very little dilution of the meconium by the amniotic fluid. This results in the meconium becoming thicker and more problematic for delivery management. While in utero aspiration of meconium-stained fluid may occur, the most common time for aspiration is during the delivery process. Thick meconium may cause obstruction to the respiratory bronchioles, with resultant neonatal respiratory distress. Meconium aspiration may result in a severe chemical reaction that can cause persistent fetal circulation, hypoxia, and even death.

3. *Macrosomia*. In most postterm pregnancies, the fetal size is appropriate. However, with adequate placental function, the fetus will continue to grow. About 25%–30% of postterm neonates weigh more than 4,000 g, a percentage that is three times greater than that of term newborns (14, 16). A fetus whose weight is in excess of 4,500 g should be considered macrosomic (17). The overall incidence of macrosomia in postterm pregnancy is 2.5%–10%. (18, 19). The principal risk of macrosomia is maternal and/or fetal trauma from delivery. Large infants frequently undergo prolonged labors and difficult deliveries. Vaginal sidewall lacerations, cervical tears, or fourth-degree extensions, plus the risks of operative delivery, such as fistula formation, must be considered. Dystocia from impaction of the fetal shoulders may result in death or neurologic and orthopedic injury While this usually occurs in the larger-size infants, it may occur with any size. The incidence of shoulder dystocia for the macrosomic infant is 1.9 times that of average-size infants (14). Knowledge of the estimated fetal weight, using ultrasound measurements, may be very helpful in the decision-making process regarding the management of protracted labor or arrest of descent. In the postdate patient with abnormalities of labor, cesarean delivery may be more appropriate than additional pitocin or attempted operative vaginal delivery.

4. *Dysmaturity*. The tertiary villus structure of the placenta has reached 11-m^2 surface area for exchange by 37

weeks of gestation (20). Since there is no further growth, the placental function may decrease. Maternal conditions such as hypertension or advanced diabetes may accelerate the placental maturation process, which can further jeopardize placental function and lead to a loss of placental reserve. Postmaturity syndrome, as described by Clifford (21), is characterized by skin changes, loss of subcutaneous fat and muscle mass, and meconium staining. This occurs when the placenta is unable to support the fetus adequately and leads to placental insufficiency (1). First, the placenta deprives the fetus of support for anabolic processes. Fetal weight is compromised as the fetus uses energy stored in its adipose tissue and liver. Second, diminished fetal plasma volume eventually leads to oligohydramnios. The antepartum detection of the postmaturity syndrome is extremely difficult even with the use of ultrasound, fetal movement assessment, and fetal heart rate testing.

Gestational Age Assessment

The accurate determination of the time of conception is critically important in order to reduce the false diagnosis of postterm pregnancy and to help identify the point at which risk does increase. There can be no doubt that the EDC is most reliably and accurately determined in early pregnancy. Many prolonged pregnancies could be eliminated if accurate assignment of gestational age were possible. However, postterm pregnancies determined by accurate gestational age assessment are more likely to suffer the previously noted complications.

Consistency between historical and physical data is important in establishing the reliability of pregnancy dating. The length and regularity of the last normal menstrual cycle, along with the first day of the last spontaneous menses, should be recorded. Confirming the work of Dewhurst (8), Anderson (22) found that the last menstrual period was the best clinical predictor of gestational age. Seventy-one percent of his patients could recall the exact date of their last period, 25% an approximate date, with only 4% recalling no date. An EDC can be calculated by subtracting three months from the first day of the last menses and adding seven days (Naegele's rule). Basal body temperature

would be extremely helpful in eliminating a large percentage of postterm pregnancy, but it is often unavailable. In cases of assisted reproductive technologies, including artificial insemination or embryo transfer, the incidence of postdate pregnancy will be reduced because the exact date of fertilization will be known.

Since it is impossible to predict which woman will be undelivered by 42 weeks' gestation, all prenatal patients must be dated accurately. Patients should be encouraged to seek early prenatal care in order to facilitate clinical correlations. The menstrual history must include the range of menstrual cycles and the recent use of oral contraceptives. At least 10% of women with a history of regular cycles do not resume regular cycles within three months of discontinuation of oral contraceptives. However, even the most skilled clinician cannot always equate physical estimation of uterine size with gestational age. Additional factors such as obesity, patient anxiety, uterine leiomyomata, multiple gestation, or multiparity frequently make this correlation difficult, if not impossible.

The determination of fundal height using a centimeter-marked tape should be 20 centimeters above the symphysis at 20 weeks. This usually corresponds to the umbilicus. Additional clinical parameters that may be helpful in determining gestational age include the date of first positive pregnancy test, the patient's initial perception of fetal movement (quickening) at about 16–18 weeks, and the time when the fetal heart is first heard (10–12 weeks with Doppler and 19–20 weeks with fetoscope).

Inconsistencies or specific concern about the accuracy of fetal age dating necessitates further assessment by ultrasound. Ultrasound has become the gold standard for the determination of gestational age. The accuracy of ultrasound estimation of fetal age is inversely related to the gestational age at the time of the ultrasound examination. The most useful measurement during the first trimester is the fetal crown-rump length, while, during the second trimester, the clinician uses the biparietal diameter (BPD), head circumference, and femur length. Based on crown-rump length measurements, the 90% confidence limits are ±3 days. Biparietal diameters prior to 20 weeks yield a 90% confidence limit of ±8 days, but, between 18 and 24 weeks, it is ±12 days. Femur lengths are generally obtainable by 14 weeks, and, when used prior to 20 weeks, their accuracy is ±7 days. In contrast, measurements of the BPD and femur obtained in the 3rd trimester yield an accuracy of ±21 days and ±16 days, respectively (23). The most cost-effective time for ultrasound confirmation of gestational age and for developmental survey seems to be between 16 and 20 weeks.

If the sonographic age differs by two or more weeks from the menstrual age or there are risk factors for uteroplacental insufficiency, a second ultrasound scan at 31–33 weeks may help establish both a "growth-adjusted sonographic age" and a cephalic percentile growth pattern (24). Subsequent serial ultrasound assessment at two- to three-week intervals will determine if cephalic and abdominal growth is appropriate. Additionally, determination of abdominal circumference allows an estimation of fetal weight using standard tables and may help in diagnosing symmetrical versus asymmetrical growth retardation. The use of ultrasound measurement may be helpful in identifying the fetus who has or will develop the postmaturity syndrome when intrauterine growth retardation or fetal malnutrition is accompanied by the finding of oligohydramnios.

The prudent clinician must determine early in gestation if the assigned EDC is relatively firm and therefore reliable or suspect, requiring additional confirmation. Once the EDC is confirmed, it must not be changed. Because of the previously noted problems of irregular cycles, delayed ovulation, bleeding in early pregnancy, and the inaccuracies of clinical parameters, a relatively large group of patients deserve consideration for early sonography. It must be remembered that, because of the variability of bone growth during the third trimester, a late pregnancy sonogram should never be used to "confirm" an EDC or disprove a postterm pregnancy.

Estimating Fetal Morbidity

Approximately 10% of postterm fetuses will experience morbidity, which may include cesarean section for distress, low Apgar scores, malnutrition, or meconium aspiration syndrome. The number of fetuses placed at these risks may be lower than 10% if aggressive, early gestational age assessment is employed, along with a carefully followed protocol for the management of postterm pregnancy. Complications

such as persistent fetal circulation or seizures are fortunately very infrequent, occurring in 1% or less. However, long-term poor outcome probably occurs in less than 5% of prolonged pregnancy cases in spite of the active management.

Antepartum Management

If the gestational age is well established, there is no proven need for induction of labor prior to 42 weeks unless other complications develop. Serial assessment by Bishop scoring may begin as early as 40 weeks in an attempt to identify the favorable cervix. If the patient has developed preeclampsia, growth retardation, or has preexisting hypertension or diabetes, earlier delivery would be appropriate. Unfortunately, the cervix is seldom favorable in true postterm pregnancy. Harris (25) found that only 8.2% of pregnancies at 42 weeks had a ripe cervix, as defined by a Bishop score above 7. If the cervix is favorable for delivery at 41–42 weeks, induction of labor should be seriously considered. There are two major reasons for induction of labor when the cervix is ripe. First is that the fetus may continue to grow, risking the development of macrosomia. Second is that antenatal surveillance is not perfect, with fetal monitoring failing to predict a poor outcome in 1/1,000 patients (26). With confirmed dates and an unripe cervix, there are two possible approaches to management. The most established is to initiate antepartum fetal surveillance while awaiting spontaneous labor (27) and/or attempts at cervical ripening. The other approach is to administer prostaglandin gel for cervical ripening prior to attempts at induction of labor (28).

Cervical ripening agents such as laminaria, breast stimulation, low-dose oxytocin, and prostaglandin gel (29) have been used. Antepartum fetal assessment has been developed to detect fetal compromise or oligohydramnios in these patients. Current assessment tools include the biophysical profile, fetal heart rate monitoring, and ultrasound.

Although prostaglandin gel ripening of the cervix has not been extensively studied in postdate pregnancy, the reported studies do indicate some shortcomings. Dyson (28) found that 50% of patients in whom the cervix was not ripened by gel administration required cesarean delivery. Additionally, prostaglandin gel may result in uterine hyperstimulation, suggesting that its use in patients with worrisome antenatal tests is questionable. However, prostaglandin E2 gel applied locally to the cervix does produce softening, dilatation, and shortening. Dyson (28) used both 3.0-mg intravaginal and 0.5-mg intracervical doses in managing his postterm pregnancies. The gel group delivered earlier and had less meconium, dysmaturity, and fetal distress.

The protocol for prostaglandin ripening may be employed in patients with an unripe cervix at 41 weeks' gestation. The gel is administered during the afternoon or evening prior to a scheduled induction of labor. Prior to application of the gel, a reassuring fetal heart rate pattern should be obtained. If there are baseline fetal heart rate abnormalities, decreased variability, or frequent or prolonged uterine contractions, prostaglandin gel would not be an appropriate choice for ripening. If all parameters for use of the prostaglandin gel are fulfilled, the patient should be observed on a fetal monitor for at least two hours after the gel has been administered or until uterine activity has subsided. Approximately 15% of patients will begin spontaneous labor subsequent to the gel application and do not require oxytocin induction. If the cervix does not sufficiently ripen, a second application may be considered.

The most frequently used tests to assess fetal well-being include some type of fetal heart rate monitoring (30). However, there is no agreement as to the best method or time to initiate testing. Either the nonstress test (NST) or the contraction stress test (CST) or both can be used for evaluation of fetal health in the postterm gestation. The general trend in the United States is to begin some form of testing during the 41st week of gestation. Although several testing protocols have evolved, none has proven superior to the CST for antenatal surveillance. It is still regarded as the most reliable method for antenatal evaluation and remains the "gold standard" (27). The CST stresses the fetus by the intermittent cessation of blood flow to the uteroplacental bed during uterine contraction. This stress will unveil the fetus whose reserves have been depleted because of maternal disease or deficient placental function. When uteroplacental insufficiency is present, the changes in placental blood flow that occur during contractions will result in the development of repetitive late decelerations.

A prospective evaluation of 679 postdate infants by Freeman (16) using the CST reported no perinatal deaths.

The major benefit of the CST is that negative results predict fetal well-being for seven days. Weekly CSTs are effective in preventing stillbirth and have a false-negative rate of only 0.71/1,000 (26). In the postterm group of patients, there is the expected increased risk for intrapartum distress, meconium, macrosomia, and cesarean section for either arrested progress of labor or fetal distress, compared to the normal control term group. There is a high incidence of abnormal CST results (38.9%), but the vast majority of the abnormals are equivocal rather than true positive. Importantly, the patients with equivocal results are at significant risk for subsequent intrapartum distress (16). The disadvantage of the CST is the time required to perform the test and the high incidence of abnormal results necessitating further evaluation. However, the low rate of perinatal mortality and morbidity using this testing protocol suggests that it is a reliable indicator of fetal health. Nipple stimulation techniques have significantly reduced the testing time without sacrificing accuracy (31). If the CST is reactive but positive, an attempt at a trial of labor is indicated since up to 66% of such patients will deliver vaginally (26). Should the CST be nonreactive and positive, the patient should be continuously monitored while preparing for cesarean section (26).

Recently, the most widely advocated and used method for antepartum testing of the postdate pregnancy has become the NST (32, 33). It is noninvasive, simple, inexpensive, requires significantly less time to perform, and is easy to interpret. The NST results in few equivocal results, and interventions are rarely necessary. Weekly NSTs have a false-negative rate of 6.1/1,000, which is defined as stillbirth within one week of a reactive test (34). However, when applied to the postterm group, there have been reports of poor outcome following a weekly NST protocol (35). This is probably related to the simplistic interpretation of the test as reactive or nonreactive on the basis of fetal heart accelerations alone. The tracing should be evaluated for baseline fetal heart rate, long- and short-term variability, and the presence of any decelerations. Spontaneous decelerations are associated with nonreactive tests, oligohydramnios, fetal heart rate (FHR) abnormalities in labor, low Apgar scores, the need for neonatal resuscitation, and perinatal morbidity (36, 37). Boehm (34) has shown that the frequency of testing may be critical. He was able to reduce the false-negative rate from 6.1 to 1.9/1,000 by the implementation of a twice-weekly testing protocol. Eden (36) studied 583 postdate pregnancies and compared various testing schemes, each using the NST. His study showed that twice-weekly NST plus amniotic fluid assessment was comparable to the results of CST testing alone. Both these testing protocols had minimal morbidity and mortality, but there was a high frequency of both intervention and cesarean delivery.

The use of real-time ultrasound has allowed the development of the fetal biophysical profile (BPP) (38), which provides a further approach to the evaluation of the postdate fetus. The BPP evaluates fetal breathing, gross fetal movements, fetal tone, amniotic fluid volume, and incorporates the NST. The fetal central nervous system is responsible for the complex integration of the mechanisms necessary for the initiation and regulation of all fetal activity. When affected by hypoxia, the fetus loses normal fetal breathing, fetal movements, and fetal tone (39). Fortunately, AFV is not affected by changes in the fetal central nervous system. Rather, the finding of oligohyramnios results in part from the hypoxia-induced reflex redistribution of fetal cardiac output to preserve cerebral blood flow by the preferential shunting of blood away from the lungs, kidneys, and splanchnic circulation (40). Weekly testing yields results similar to those of the weekly NST, with false-negative rates of approximately 7/1,000 (38). Johnson (41) showed that there was improved efficacy by twice-weekly BPP testing, with aggressive intervention if oligohydramnios is discovered.

The significance of oligohydramnios and spontaneous FHR decelerations during antepartum testing of postdate pregnancy has been evaluated by Phelan and Small (42). The discovery of decreased AFV or the occurrence of FHR decelerations during testing necessitates hospitalization and careful consideration for prompt delivery. Fetuses with decreased AFV are at high risk for both cord compression and in utero fetal death (39, 43). The previous work by Eden (36) was confirmed by Clark (44) who showed that the use of twice-weekly NSTs in conjunction with twice-weekly amniotic fluid assessments has a low risk for the occurrence of an antepartum stillbirth.

The development of the four-quadrant assessment of AFV may be beneficial in characterizing borderline oligohydramnios (45, 46). The ultrasound criteria for oligohydramnios have been modified since the initial report of Manning (38) which regarded a pocket of fluid < 1 cm in vertical diameter as abnormal. This was liberalized to 2 cm by Chamberlain(43) and further expanded to a vertical diameter of 3 cm by Crowley (47). The four-quadrant approach divides the uterine cavity into four sections. The sum of the maximum vertical measurement of the largest amniotic fluid pocket in each of the four quadrants results in a calculation referred to as the amniotic fluid index (AFI). Using this AFI tool, 330 patients were evaluated, and an adverse perinatal outcome occurred only when the AFI was less than 5 cm (46). Apparently the four-quadrant technique is more sensitive than single-pocket assessment in the postdate pregnancy. This evaluation is easy to perform and can be taught to residents, nurses and technicians who may have limited ultrasound experience.

The clinical utility of acoustic stimulation remains questionable. The use of the external auditory larynx results in a 48% reduction in nonreactive NSTs (48). In addition, total testing time may be reduced. The combination of NST, acoustic stimulation, and AFV assessment twice weekly appears to be logical. The routine use of noninvasive Doppler blood flow has not been proven to be clinically useful in the management of postdate pregnancy. However, if fetal malnutrition is suspected, the finding of absent end diastolic flow or reversal of flow is strongly suggestive of critical fetal status. At this time, it is unlikely that Doppler will provide any diagnostic advantage in an otherwise uncomplicated postterm gestation.

If a patient remains undelivered by 43 weeks of confirmed gestation, an attempt at labor induction is advised. The use of cervical ripening agents and intensive fetal surveillance should be considered. However, there are no confirmatory data that this approach will improve perinatal outcome.

Intrapartum Management

It is well established that the perinatal mortality increases dramatically following 42 completed weeks of gestation. The rate is doubled at 42 weeks, tripled at 42 1/2 weeks, quadrupled at 43 weeks, and more than quintupled at 44 weeks (49). Therefore, as a pregnancy is approaching postterm status, a prospective management plan must be established.

As mentioned previously, induction of labor at 41–42 weeks is reasonable in the face of a favorable cervix. If the cervix is unfavorable, the patient should participate in the decision to continue the pregnancy and institute frequent antepartum testing or to end the pregnancy by induction of labor. There are four critical conditions that must always be considered during the management of a postterm gestation.

1. *Fetal hypoxia*. Fetal heart rates must be watched closely for evidence of fetal intolerance or distress. Interpretation of these fetal heart rate patterns remains the basis for the determination of fetal well-being. Continuous fetal monitoring is the standard of care for the intrapartum assessment of the postterm pregnancy. The incidence of cesarean section for fetal distress increases from 5.4%–13.1% in postterm patients with oligohydramnios (50).

2. *Variable decelerations*. Variable decelerations may signal cord compression. These changes are frequently the result of oligohydramnios. If oligohydramnios is discovered, the use of saline amnioinfusion (51) has been found to be beneficial in eliminating variable decelerations when maternal position change is not helpful.

3. *Macrosomia*. The route for delivery should be considered after an assessment for fetal weight. There is no question that fetal size estimates using ultrasound are possible, but the accuracy of prediction is variable. Ultrasound weight estimates generally fall within 20% of the actual birthweight (52). Injuries due to fetal size may include brachial plexus injuries, phrenic nerve palsies, and fractures of the humerus or clavicle. While some have advocated cesarean delivery when the estimated weight is greater than 4500 g, a fetal weight estimate of 5000 g or more would make abdominal delivery a prudent choice (53). Particularly when managing a postterm pregnancy, the clinician must be familiar with the maneuvers for managing shoulder dystocia since it is an unpredictable occurrence. Benedetti and Gabbe noted that the risk of shoulder dystocia was increased from 0.16 to 4.57% in patients with

a prolonged second state of labor who undergo mid-pelvic delivery of a macrosomic infant (54). Although cesarean section is not always appropriate when the estimated fetal weight is greater than 4000 g, this knowledge should impact the consideration for the performance of an operative vaginal delivery, particularly when failure of descent is noted.

4. *Thick meconium*. Thick meconium presents a significant risk for the fetus and newborn. The use of a DeLee trap with wall suction is critical for clearing the infant's airway after the head emerges from the vagina or the abdominal incision. This will help remove the meconium before it can be aspirated into the airways of the newborn, thereby preventing the chemical irritation. If there is neonatal depression, immediate intubation and suction must be performed (55). However, if the oropharyngeal aspirate is clear and the infant is vigorous with normal respiration and cry, the value of direct visualization of the trachea with a laryngoscope is of questionable benefit. In spite of this aggressive approach, some infants will suffer from meconium aspiration syndrome due to in utero aspiration of meconium prior to labor or delivery (56).

Labor Management

There is no question that the true postterm fetus is at substantial risk and that continuous fetal heart monitoring during labor is essential. As mentioned previously, the postterm and postmature fetus may have significantly diminished placental respiratory reserve. In the past, external fetal monitoring was unable to provide the critical information of beat-to-beat variability. However, current fetal monitor technology is able to provide accurate representation of heart rate variability from either external or direct fetal heart signals. Based on this advancement in technology, the indication for the performance of artificial rupture of membranes and placement of a spiral electrode is less clear. However, rupture of membranes does allow evaluation of the amniotic fluid for the presence of meconium. Outcomes are worse in patients who initially had clear fluid but subsequently passed meconium compared to patients without meconium, patients with meconium noted at rupture of membranes, and patients with meconium present only at delivery. When meconium is found only at delivery, these infants had a poorer outcome than the nonmeconium group. The type of meconium may also provide some assistance in deciding on management. The finding of thick, particulate meconium should warn the clinician of the possibility of oligohydramnios. Thin-meconium or no-meconium patients do significantly better than those with the thick, particulate type of meconium. There is no significant difference in outcome between patients with thin meconium and those with clear amniotic fluid (57). These clinical outcomes were confirmed by Meis (58) who found a significantly poorer outcome when there was early, heavy passage of meconium either at the time of membrane rupture or later. In addition, he noted that fresh meconium observed in late labor was associated with a higher frequency of depressed infants and meconium aspiration syndrome. Amnioinfusion in one study diluted meconium, improved Apgar scores, and decreased the number of infants with meconium below their cords (59).

Careful and continuous attention to the fetal heart tracing is necessary. As previously mentioned, the incidence of cesarean section specifically for fetal distress rises from 5.4% to 13.1% in postterm patients who also have oligohydramnios (50). Cord compression is more frequently seen in postterm pregnancy since oligohydramnios and a thin, easily compressible umbilical cord often coexist (60). Saline amnioinfusion is frequently helpful in reducing the incidence and severity of variable fetal heart rate decelerations secondary to oligohydramnios (50).

The finding of a variable deceleration pattern does not require immediate delivery as long as the fetal heart variability and baseline remain normal. While variable decelerations are due to cord compression, not hypoxia, this pattern must be watched for signs of evolving hypoxia. These signs include a slow return to baseline, decreasing variability, blunting of the shape of the deceleration, overshooting, and worsening depth or prolonged duration of the deceleration.

Late decelerations are more characteristically associated with fetal hypoxia and distress. When late decelerations are intermittent, they should be managed conservatively by changing maternal position, oxygen administration, intravenous fluid infusion, and discontinuation of oxytocin. If these maneuvers fail to eliminate the decelerations and vaginal delivery is not imminent, strong consideration should be given to performing a cesarean section. When persistent late decelerations are associated with decreased variability and a rising fetal heart rate baseline, emergency delivery is indicated. The choice of anesthesia in the face of suspected fetal distress is difficult. Since maternal hypotension may further jeopardize fetal status, strong consideration of general anesthesia is advised.

Assessment of fetal well-being may be possible by using either fetal scalp stimulation or pH sampling (61). While actual fetal scalp blood sampling has been advocated to provide direct assessment of fetal acid-base status, numerous factors may make interpretation difficult. Clark (62) has shown that, for those fetuses whose heart rate rises in response to scalp stimulation during vaginal examination, there is a virtual absence of acidosis. This simple test frequently precludes the need for the more complex procedure of fetal scalp blood sampling.

Induction or augmentation of labor frequently becomes necessary in the management of prolonged pregnancy. It is essential that contraindications to labor be ruled out. The exact indication for and method of induction or augmentation of labor should be documented in the patient record. The clinician must be familiar with the pharmacokinetics of oxytocin. Recent data suggest that it takes 40–60 minutes to reach a steady-state plasma concentration after initiating or altering the infusion rate (63). The actual uterine response to a particular level of oxytocin infusion is dependent on preexisting uterine activity, uterine sensitivity, and cervical status. These are related to individual differences and gestational age. It is known that the uterine response to oxytocin increases slowly from 20–30 weeks of gestation and then is unchanged from 34 weeks until term. At that time, the uterine sensitivity increases rapidly (64).

Regardless of whether labor is induced or augmented, it is critical that certain principles be followed. Oxytocin is diluted (10 U USP) in 1,000 mL of a balanced salt solution and is administered via a controlled infusion pump. In order to prevent accidental bolus infusion, the oxytocin solution should be piggybacked into the primary intravenous line near the venous puncture site. The goal of therapy is to produce uterine activity that is sufficient to result in cervical change and fetal descent while avoiding fetal distress and uterine hyperstimulation.

The infusion rates and amounts of oxytocin that are necessary for induction of labor are often significantly greater than those required for augmentation (65). The clinical utility of an intrauterine pressure catheter may be extremely helpful when managing oxytocin-stimulated uterine activity. Current dry pressure catheters have the transducer at the distal tip, making calibration simple. In addition, the fluid-filled system has been eliminated as a possible contamination route. The fluid-filled pressure catheter system made concurrent amnioinfusion difficult. Either a second infusion catheter was necessary or the evaluation of baseline uterine tone was hampered due to the need for a piggyback setup. Contemporary dry intrauterine pressure catheters almost always have a second port for the performance of saline amnioinfusion when necessary.

Adequate labor, resulting in cervical change, may be present with a wide range of uterine activity. The actual effective dose for oxytocin induction or augmentation of labor is also variable. Generally, oxytocin is begun at 0.5–1 mU/min and increased at 1–2 mU/min increments (66). As mentioned previously, the incremental time intervals may be as long as 40–60 minutes.

Delivery Room Considerations

It is the responsibility of the delivering physician to insure that all necessary precautions have been taken and that all anticipated personnel and equipment are available. Assessment of fetal size should preclude operative vaginal delivery of a fetus whose labor has been prolonged or complicated by failure of descent. Similarly, the known presence of meconium will allow dilution by amnioinfusion and aggressive suctioning at delivery. Strong consideration of obtaining umbilical venous and arterial cord blood gases at delivery is advised. The documentation of fetal acid-base status at the time of delivery may be critical if childhood performance is suboptimal.

Summary

Proper management of this complex clinical problem is dif-ficult. While many opinions exist, there are a variety of acceptable testing protocols for the identification of the at-risk fetus. The critical factors are accurate, early pregnancy dating and the development of a prospective, individualized management plan. The patient must be informed of the risks and involved in the management choices. If induction of labor is chosen, attention to fetal heart rate and labor progress is essential. If serial antepartum evaluation is elected, twice weekly assessment of AFV and fetal heart rate reactivity has been proven to be effective. Once the cervix becomes favorable, induction of labor should be considered. Unfortunately, in spite of the marked improvement in outcome, no protocol has yet been developed to guarantee avoidance of all maternal and neonatal morbidity/mortality.

References

1. Vorherr H. Placental insufficiency in relation to postterm pregnancy and fetal postmaturity. Evaluation of fetoplacental function; management of the postterm gravida. Am J Obstet Gynecol 1975;123:67–103.
2. Beischer NA, Evans JH, Townsend L. Studies in prolonged pregnancy. I. The incidence of prolonged pregnancy. Am J Obstet Gynecol 1969;103:476–82.
3. Rayburn WF, Chang FE. Management of the uncomplicated postdate pregnancy. J Repro Med 1981;26:93–5.
4. Zwerdling MA. Factors pertaining to prolonged pregnancy and its outcome. Pediatrics 1967;40:202–12.
5. Homburg R, Ludomirski A, Insler V. Detection of fetal risk in postmaturity. Br J Obstet Gynaecol 1979;86:759–64.
6. Rayburn WF, Motley ME, Stemple LE, Gendreau M. Antepartum predition of the postmature infant. Obstet Gynecol 1982;60:148–53.
7. Yeh SY, Read JA. Management of postterm pregnancy in a large obstetrical population. Obstet Gynecol 1982;60:282–7.
8. Dewhurst CJ, Beazley JM, Campbell S. Assessment of fetal maturity and dysmaturity. Am J Obstet Gynecol 1972;113:141–9.
9. Boyce A, Mayaux M, Schwartz D. Classical and "true" gestational postmaturity. Am J Obstet Gynecol 1976;125:911–14.
10. Saito M, Yazawa K, Hashiguchi A, Kumasaka T, Nishi N, Kato K. Time of ovulation and prolonged pregnancy. Am J Obstet Gynecol 1972;112:31–8.
11. Csapo AL. The "seesaw" theory of parturition. Ciba Found

Symp 1977;47:159–210.

12. Nwosu U, Wallach EE, Bolognese RJ. Initiation of labor by intraamniotic cortisol instillation in prolonged human pregnancy. Obstet Gynecol 1976;47:137–42.

13. Naeye RL. Causes of perinatal mortality excess in prolonged gestations. Am J Epidemiol 1978;108:429–33.

14. Eden RD, Seifert LS, Winegar A, Spellacy WM. Perinatal characteristics of uncomplicated postdate pregnancies. Obstet Gynecol 1987;69:296–9.

15. Phelan JP. Antepartum fetal assessment. Newer techniques. Semin Perinat 1988;12:57–65.

16. Freeman RK, Garite TJ, Modanlow H, Dorchester W, Rommal C, Devaney M. Postdate pregnancy utilization of the contraction stress test for primary fetal surveillance. Am J Obstet Gynecol 1981;140:128–35.

17. American College of Obstetricians and Gynecologists. Fetal macrosomia. Technical Bulletin 159. Washington, DC: ACOG, 1991.

18. Wible JL, Petrie RH, Koons A, Perez A. The clinical use of umbilical cord acid-base determinations in perinatal surveillance and management. Clin Perinatol 1982;9:387–97.

19. Spellacy WM, Miller S, Winegar A., Peterson PQ. Macrosomia—maternal characteristics and infant complications. Obstet Gynecol 1985;66:158–61.

20. Ahearne W, Dunnill MS. Morphometry of the human placenta. Br Med Bull 1966;22:5–8.

21. Clifford SH. Postmaturity—with placental dysfunction. J Pediatr 1954;44:1–13.

22. Anderson HF, Johnson TRB, Flora JD, Barclay ML. Gestational age assessment. II. Prediction from combined clinical observations. Am J Obstet Gynecol 1981;140:770–4.

23. Romero R, Jeantry P. Obstetrical ultrasound. New York: McGraw Hill, 1984.

24. Saggagha R, Barton B, Barton F, Klingas E, Orgill J, Turner JH. Sonar biparietal diameter. II. Predictive of three fetal growth patterns leading to a closer assessment of gestational age and neonatal weight. Am J Obstet Gynecol 1976;126: 485–90.

25. Harris BA Jr, Huddleston JF, Sutliff G, Perlis HW. The unfavorable cervix in prolonged pregnancy. Obstet Gynecol 1983;62:171–4.

26. Lagrew DC, Freeman RK. Contraction stress test in assessment and care of the fetus. In: Eden RD, Boehm FH, eds. Assessment and care of the fetus: physiologic, clinical and medicolegal principles. East Norwalk, CT:. Appleton & Lange, 1990.

27. Lagrew DC, Freeman RK. Management of postdate pregnancy. Am J Obstet Gynecol 1986;154:8–13.

28. Dyson DC, Miller PD, Armstrong MA. Management of prolonged pregnancy: induction of labor versus antepartum fetal testing. Am J Obstet Gynecol 1987;156:928–34.

29. Roberts WE, North DH, Speed JE, et al. Comparative study of prostaglandin, laminaria, and minidose oxytocin for ripening of the unfavorable cervix prior to induction of labor. J Perinatol 1986;6:16–19.

30. Thornton YS, Yeh SY, Petrie RH. Antepartum fetal heart rate resting and the post-term gestation. J Perinat Med 1982;10:196–202.

31. Huddleston JF, Sutliff G, Robinson D. Contraction stress test by intermittent nipple stimulation.Obstet Gynecol 1984; 63:669–673.

32. Rochard F, Schifrin BS, Goupil F, Legrand H, Blottiere J, Sureau C. Nonstressed fetal heart rate monitoring in the antepartum period. Am J Obstet Gynecol 1976;126:699–706.

33. Visser GHA, Redman CWG, Huisjes HJ, Turnbull AC. Nonstressed antepartum heart rate monitoring: implications of decelerations after spontaneous contractions. Am J Obstet Gynecol 1980;138:429–35.

34. Boehm FH, Salyer S, Shah DM, Vaughn WK. Improved outcome of twice weekly nonstress testing. Obstet Gynecol 1986;67:566–8.

35. Miyazaki FS, Miyazaki BA. False reactive nonstress tests in post-term pregnancies. Am J Obstet Gynecol 1981;140: 269–76.

36. Eden RD, Gergely RZ, Schifrin BS, Wade ME. Comparison of antepartum testing schemes for the management of the postdate pregnancy. Am J Obstet Gynecol 1982;144: 683–92.

37. Phelan JP, Platt LD, Yeh SY, Tmjilla M, Paul RH. Continuing role of the NST in the management of postdates pregnancy. Obstet Gynecol 1984;64:624–8.

38. Manning FA, Platt LD, Sipos L. Antepartum fetal evaluation development of a fetal biophysical profile. Am J Obstet Gynecol 1980;136:787–95.

39. Vintzileos AM, Campbell WA, Ingardia CJ, Nochimson DJ. The fetal biophysical profile and its predictive value. Obstet Gynecol 1983;62:271–8.

40. Seeds AE. Current concepts of amniotic fluid dynamics. Am J Obstet Gynecol 1980;138:575–86.

41. Johnson JM, Harman CR, Lange IR, Manning FA. Biophysical profile scoring in the management of the postterm pregnancy: an analysis of 307 patients. Am J Obstet Gyne-

col 1986;154:269–73.

42. Small ML, Phelan JP, Smith CV, Paul RH. An active management approach to the postdate fetus with a reactive non-stress test and fetal heart rate decelerations. Obstet Gynecol 1987;70:636–40.

43. Chamberlain PE, Manning FA, Morrison I, Harman CR, Lange IR. Ultrasound evaluation of amniotic fluid volume. I. The relationship of marginal and decreased amniotic fluid volumes to perinatal outcome. Am J Obstet Gynecol 1984; 150:245–54.

44. Clark SL, Sabey P, Jolley K. Nonstress testing with acoustic stimulation and amniotic fluid volume assessment: 5973 tests without unexpected fetal death. Am J Obstet Gynecol 1989;160:694–7.

45. Phelan JP, Smith CV, Broussard P, Small M. Amniotic fluid volume assessment with the four-quadrant technique at 36–42 weeks' gestation. J Reprod Med 1987;32:540–2.

46. Rutherford SE, Phelan JP, Smith CV, Jacobs N. The four-quadrant assessment of amniotic fluid volume: an adjunct to antepartum fetal heart rate testing. Obstet Gynecol 1987; 70:353–6.

47. Crowley P. Non quantitative estimation of amniotic fluid volume in suspected prolonged pregnancy. J Perinat Med 1980;8:249–51.

48. Smith CV, Phelan JP, Platt LD, Broussard P, Paul RH. Fetal acoustic stimulation testing. II. A randomized clinical comparison with the nonstress test. Am J Obstet Gynecol 1986; 155:131–4.

49. Browne JCM. Postmaturity. Am J Obstet Gynecol 1963; 85:573–82.

50. Leveno KJ, Quirk, JG, Cunnigham FG, Nelson SD, Santos-Ramos R, Toofanian A, DePalma R. Prolonged pregnancy: observations concerning the causes of fetal distress. Am J Obstet Gynecol 1984;150:465–73.

51. Miyazaki FS, Taylor NA. Saline amnioinfusion for relief of variable or prolonged decelerations: a preliminary report. Am J Obstet Gynecol 1983;146:670–8.

52. Shepard MJ, Richards VA, Berkowitz RL, Warsof SL, Hobbins JC. An evaluation of two equations for predicting fetal weight by ultrasound. Am J Obstet Gynecol 1982; 142:47–54.

53. American College of Obstetricians and Gynecologists. Diagnosis and management of postterm pregnancy. Technical Bulletin 130. Washington, DC: ACOG, 1989.

54. Benedetti TJ, Gabbe SG. Shoulder dystocia: a complication of fetal macrosomia and prolonged second stage of labor with midpelvic delivery. Obstet Gynecol 1978;52:526–9.

55. Carson BS, Losey RW, Bowes WA Jr, Simmons MA. Combined obstetric and pediatric approach to prevent meconium aspiration syndrome. Am J Obstet Gynecol 1976; 126:712–15.

56. Davis RO, Phillips JB III, Harris BA Jr, Wilson ER, Huddleston JF. Fatal meconium aspiration syndrome occurring despite airway management considered appropriate. Am J Obstet Gynecol 1985;151:731–6.

57. Miller FC, Sacks DA, Yeh SY, Paul RH, Shiffrin BS, Martin CB, Hon EH. Significance of meconium during labor. Am J Obstet Gynecol 1975;122:573–80.

58. Meis PJ, Hall M III, Marshall JR, Hobel CJ. Meconium passage: a new classification for risk assessment during labor. Am J Obstet Gynecol 1978;131:509–13.

59. Wenstrom KD, Parsons MT. The prevention of meconium aspiration in labor using amnioinfusion. Obstet Gynecol 1989;73:647–51.

60. Silver RK, Dooley SL, Tamura RK, Depp R. Umbilical cord size and amniotic fluid volume in prolonged pregnancy. Am J Obstet Gynecol 1987;157:716–20.

61. Clark SL, Gimovsky ML, Miller FC. Fetal heart rate response to scalp blood sampling. Am J Obstet Gynecol 1982;144: 706–8.

62. Clark SL, Gimovsky ML, Miller FC. The scalp stimulation test: an alternative to fetal scalp blood sampling. Am J Obstet Gynecol 1984;148:274–80.

63. Seitchik J, Castillo M. Oxytocin augmentation of dysfunctional labor. II. Uterine activity data. Am J Obstet Gynecol 1983;145:526–9.

64. Carderyo-Barcia R, Poseiro JJ. Physiology of the uterine contraction. Clin Obstet Gynecol 1960;3:386–408.

65. Hauth JC, Hankins GDV, Gilstrap LC, Strickland DM, Vance P. Uterine contraction pressures with oxytocin induction/augmentation. Obstet Gynecol 1986;68:305–9.

66. American College of Obstetricians and Gynecologists. Induction and augmentation of labor. Technical Bulletin 157. Washington, DC: ACOG, 1991.

57

Failure to Progress in Labor

Emanuel A. Friedman, M.D., Sc.D.

ASSESSING failure to progress in labor requires differentiating several unrelated disorders. Reversing it requires managing these disorders according to guidelines derived from studies of patterns of cervical dilation and fetal descent. The results of these studies have not only elucidated the physiology of labor but also clearly defined normal limits for diagnosis and management (1, 2).

Using graphs to plot variations in cervical dilation and descent of the fetal presenting part against time simplifies interpreting the dynamic changes of labor. This approach replaces the more subjective concept that progression in uterine contractility associated with any changing cervical dilation and fetal descent is adequate and therefore normal. Using graphs also supersedes applying the arbitrary limits for duration that were once commonly used to define abnormal labor. Many serious disorders must be detected as they arise, before any such arbitrary time limits are exceeded, so that the physician can more expeditiously undertake meaningful evaluation and specific therapy.

Graphing the Progress of Labor

Any square-ruled graph paper can be used to construct labor curves. A standard form provides a vertical scale on the left, numbered in ascending order from 0 to 10 cm of cervical dilation (Figure 57.1). The vertical scale on the right side can be keyed in descending order to denote the station of the fetal presenting part in centimeters above (minus values) or below (plus values) the plane of the ischial spines, designated as zero station. The horizontal scale represents the number of hours spent in labor, with onset of labor defined as the starting time of regular uterine contractions as perceived by the patient. Each point on the graph represents an estimate of cervical dilation and fetal station obtained at consecutive rectal or vaginal examinations.

By convention, estimates of cervical dilation are indicated by a small circle and those of station by an X. Each observation is joined to the preceding one by a straight line. A graphic representation can thus be quickly traced to furnish a simple visual pattern.

The pattern of cervical dilation seen in all normal labor is S-shaped. Each patient evolves a unique dilation pattern, providing a reliable means for following the course

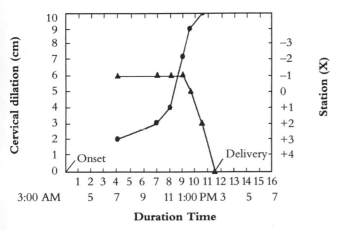

Figure 57.1   Graphic labor record. Estimates of cervical dilation plotted against time elapsed during labor yield the sigmoid curve characteristic of the normal dilation pattern. Similarly, estimates of station yield the hyperbolic curve of descent characteristic of a normal pattern.

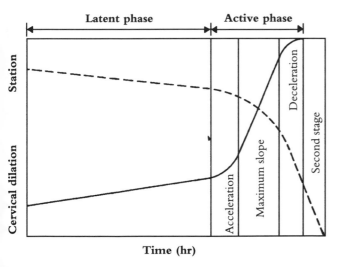

Figure 57.2   Dilation and descent. The standard relationship between dilation and descent patterns during labor is shown by plotting composite cervical dilation and fetal station against time and subdividing the resulting curves, according to functional distinctions, into latent and active phases and second stage. The active phase of dilation is further subdivided into a linear midportion phase of maximum slope, an initial acceleration phase, and a terminal deceleration phase.

of normal labor and for distinguishing it objectively from dysfunctional labor (3–5).

The descent pattern characteristically forms a hyperbolic curve in which the onset of fetal descent is usually concurrent with the time when the cervical dilation rate reaches its peak (the phase of maximum slope). The fetal descent proceeds to its maximum rate of progression just before the end of the first stage of labor and continues thereafter without any further change until the fetal presenting part reaches the perineum.

The S-shaped dilation curve can be divided into two major components: a latent phase and an active phase (Figure 57.2). The latent phase involves the initial arm of the curve, beginning at the onset of regular perceived uterine contractions and ending at the upswing of the dilation pattern.

The active phase, which includes the remainder of the first stage, may be subdivided into an acceleration phase, a phase of maximum slope, and a deceleration phase. The phase of maximum slope is the linear midportion of the active phase and represents an important, practical, and clinically useful way to assess the efficiency of the labor forces in accomplishing dilation.

Defining Disorders of Labor

Phases of the dilation and descent curves have been analyzed separately, and normal values have been derived from the study of data on large numbers of cases. It has been determined, for example, that the latent phase under normal circumstances seldom exceeds 20 hours in nulliparas or 14 hours in multiparas. A latent phase that exceeds these limits is defined as a prolonged latent phase (Figure 57.3). The maximum slope of dilation is normally greater than 1.2 cm/hour for nulliparas and 1.5 cm/hour for multiparas. Dilation in the active phase that proceeds more slowly than these limits reflects a protracted active-phase dilation pattern, also called protracted dilation. The deceleration phase should not normally last for more than three house for nulliparas, or one hour for multiparas. If it is longer in either case, the resulting disorder is called prolonged deceleration phase (Figure 57.4). The slope of descent is normally greater than 1 cm/hour in nulliparas and 2 cm/hour in multiparas. A slope under these limits characterizes labor with protracted descent.

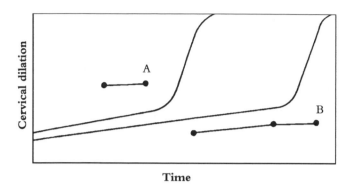

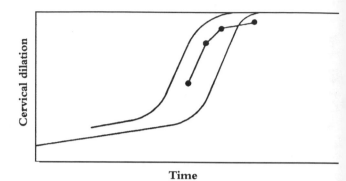

Figure 57.3   Prolonged latent phase. The mean nulliparous dilation pattern (*curve at left*) is contrasted with the pattern of a prolonged latent phase (*curve at right*), exceeding 20 hours (14 hours in multiparas). Interval of observation (*A*) probably represents a normal latent phase in a patient with some degree of dilation at onset of labor, often confused with secondary arrest of dilation. Dilation pattern (*B*) is readily diagnosed as prolonged latent phase.

Three additional disorders of the progression of labor are recognizable: 1) cessation of progressive dilation during the active phase before full dilation (secondary arrest of dilation, Figure 57.5); 2) cessation of the progressive linear descent in the second stage (arrest of descent, Figure 57.6); and 3) failure of descent (descent that does not begin at or after the beginning of the deceleration phase of dilation).

At least two hours of arrest is usually required before the diagnosis of secondary arrest of dilation can be confirmed. One hour is ordinarily sufficient to diagnose arrest of descent.

Figure 57.4   Prolonged deceleration phase. Mean nulliparous dilation pattern (*curve at right*) is contrasted with composite curve (*at left*) and a specific example of prolonged deceleration phase (*curve with points*).

Differential diagnosis can now be made in patients who fail to progress in labor. These patients are not a homogeneous group. Their symptoms may include any of several distinct labor aberrations, including prolonged latent phase, a secondary arrest of dilation, arrest or failure of descent, and prolonged deceleration phase.

Moreover, patients seen in the course of a normal latent phase, particularly those who began labor with some degree of cervical dilation, may sometimes be mistakenly considered to have failure of progress because they are indeed not progressing (see Case 57.1). The error arises because the attendant does not recognize that this situation normally occurs during the latent phase, when active dila-

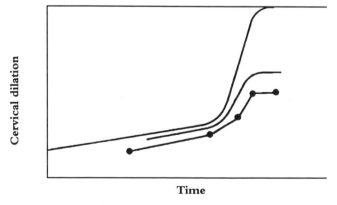

Figure 57.5   Secondary arrest of dilation. A composite dilation pattern (*center curve*) and a specific example of an abnormal pattern of secondary arrest of dilation (*curve with points*) are compared with the mean nulliparous dilation pattern (*curve at left*).

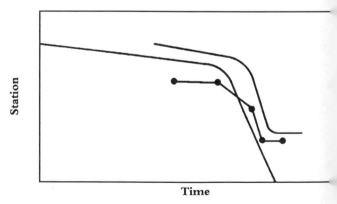

Figure 57.6   Arrest of descent. The mean nulliparous curve of descent (*longest curve*) is contrasted with the composite curve for arrest of descent (*curve at top*) and a specific example of arrest of labor progression (*curve with points*).

tion and descent have not yet begun.

These conditions are specific and discrete in etiologic factors, response to therapy, and prognosis. A specific management program must therefore be selected for each type.

Causes and Contributory Factors

The latent phase is particularly sensitive to excessive narcotic-analgesic-sedative medication and is readily prolonged by administration of these agents, which inhibit uterine contractility. This sensitivity is exhibited, not with any specific agent or dosage, but by effects on the sensorium and on myometrial function.

Women who begin labor with a cervix characterized as unripe usually experience a prolonged latent phase because of the amount of time required for the cervix to be prepared for active dilation. The cervix is long, uneffaced, closed, and rigid. Since false labor cannot be distinguished from true labor by any available physiologic measurements, this diagnosis of false labor tends to be made only in hindsight. Patients whose contractions continue beyond the critical limits should therefore be considered to have a prolonged latent phase and should be managed accordingly.

The most important factor contributing to the arrest patterns discussed above is cephalopelvic disproportion. About half of patients who develop one of the arrest disorders have insurmountable degrees of disproportion. It is this relationship that makes an arrest pattern so much more ominous than a prolonged latent phase.

Conduction anesthesia, such as peridural block, can also cause an arrest pattern, but only if administered improperly. To avoid this complication, anesthesia should not be induced before the active phase has been entered, and the level of anesthesia should be kept below dermatome T10. It is also advisable not to use peridural anesthesia in patients suspected of having fetopelvic disproportion, those to whom excessive analgesia has been given, or those who already demonstrate one of the protraction disorders. The latter are patients with abnormally slow rates of dilation in the active phase (less than 1.2 cm/hour in nulliparas or less than 1.5 cm/hour in multiparas) or slow rates of descent in the second stage (less than 1 or 2 cm/hour in nulliparas and multiparas, respectively).

Fetal malpositions are commonly associated with arrest patterns, specifically occiput transverse and occiput posterior positions with deflexion attitudes. These are probably the result of the labor aberration rather than its cause. Similarly, excessive sedation is commonly encountered with arrest patterns. Despite this, however, the normally progressive active phase is relatively insensitive and can be diverted from its extrapolated pathway only with great difficulty. If excessive sedation does cause arrest, some other deleterious factor—disproportion, a protraction disorder, or inappropriately administered conduction anesthesia, for example—is usually present as well.

Once a specific disorder of labor has been diagnosed, it must be determined whether one or more of the factors known to be associated with or causative of that aberrant pattern is operating. Of critical importance in patients with a documented arrest disorder is a thorough evaluation of the cephalopelvic relationships by careful digital examination (see Case 57.2). Since x-ray pelvimetry is no longer widely available or relied upon as accurate, special pains should be taken to determine whether there is ample available space for the fetal presenting part to be accommodated in its descent through the pelvis.

An internal examination carried out during a contraction, with additional fundal pressure applied, will often prove to be a satisfactory way to evaluate whether the fetal head is fixed or is capable of descending further if labor is allowed to continue. Oxytocin (Pitocin) must not be given before it can be confirmed that no disproportion exists. If uterotonic stimulation is initated in the face of disproportion, both mother and fetus may sustain substantial trauma and irreparable damage.

Management

The principles of management differ according to the type of labor disorder encountered. The recommended management of a prolonged latent phase is inappropriate for arrest patterns, and vice versa. Patients who experience a prolonged latent phase tend to become exhausted and are often discouraged by their lack of progress.

The recommended regimen for a prolonged latent phase includes a period of rest induced by use of morphine or another narcotic agent given in sufficient amounts to stop uterine contractions temporarily. Depending on the patient's weight, an initial dose of 15–20 mg of morphine sulfate is given IM; after 20 minutes, an additional 10- to 15-mg dose may be given if uterine contractions persist, active dilation has not yet occurred, and respiration is not depressed.

Expect the patient to benefit from six or more hours of rest. After this time, she will demonstrate one of three conditions:

1. She may be out of labor, establishing the diagnosis of false labor. Such a patient can be allowed to return home as soon as she can walk alone easily.
2. Most often, however, the patient will have entered the active phase; if so, further progressive dilation can be expected. Such patients are not, of course, immune to other labor aberrations but are not necessarily susceptible to them, either. If all continues well, vaginal delivery can be anticipated.
3. About 5% will awaken to find that the original problem is recurring and continuing unrelentingly. Since such patients have benefited from a well-deserved rest, they may be stimulated with an infusion of oxytocin, provided that no contraindication exists.

Therapeutic rest for patients with prolonged latent phase is particularly effective and should be considered as a first treatment. If a delay is clinically inappropriate, however, due to an urgent problem such as amnionitis or severe preeclampsia, that warrants delivery, oxytocin infusion may be substituted as the primary form of therapy. Such instances are rare.

For patients demonstrating one of the arrest patterns, pelvimetry is essential. As stated earlier, digital examination should confirm or clearly rule out cephalopelvic disproportion. Unless disproportion can be ruled out definitively, cesarean section is mandatory in the presence of a documented arrest pattern. This strong statement is based on the finding that patients with disproportion who manifest arrest of dilation or descent, failure of descent, or prolonged deceleration phase in labor will almost invariably (98.8%) require cesarean section ultimately, regardless of what means are used to promote progress in labor. The prognosis

for a patient and fetus allowed to continue in labor with this combination of disproportion and arrest is poor.

For patients with an arrest disorder in whom disproportion can be ruled out, support should be offered when needed. Most such patients benefit greatly from oxytocin, particularly if it is administered cautiously and in doses sufficient to simulate strong normal labor.

Most patients managed in this way do well. Unfortunately, however, errors in the assessment of cephalopelvic relationships are possible. The most serious problem is the situation in which disproportion appears to have been ruled out but is actually present and unrecognized. An important sign suggesting this potentially tragic situation is seen in the clinical response to oxytocin stimulation, which can be measured by comparing the postarrest slope of dilation or descent with the preceding prearrest slope. In the absence of disproportion, the postarrest slope is usually as great as or greater than the prearrest slope. That is, progression after uterotonic stimulation has begun should be at least as rapid as it was before arrest occurred. Any postarrest response of lesser magnitude carries an ominous portent that disproportion may actually exist. Reevaluation of the fetopelvic relationships under these circumstances is vital, and cesarean section is likely to be indicated.

A patient in the latent phase of an otherwise normal labor may be diagnosed incorrectly as showing a failure to progress. Before it was widely recognized that no progress need be expected in the normal latent phase, this erroneous diagnosis was common. Patients were subsequently subjected to either superfluous uterotonic stimulation or inappropriate cesarean section. An interval of observation should reveal the true nature of the patient's condition; the expected acceleration in cervical dilation will occur as the active phase is entered, provided that progress is not being delayed by analgesic agents.

Differential diagnosis tends to be more difficult if the patient began labor with some degree of cervical dilation, so that "arrest" appears to have occurred in the active phase presumably after the unobserved interval of progressive dilation. Without documentation that the active phase has begun and subsequent arrest has take place, it is difficult to differentiate between a normal latent phase and a secondary arrest of dilation. Similarly, if only a relatively short period of unobserved labor preceded the interval of "arrest," true arrest is very unlikely; this is so particularly if the uterine contraction pattern has been more or less progressive and uninterrupted. Although this latter sign is not uniformly reliable, true arrest of progress, particularly in association with secondary arrest of dilation or of descent, is often preceded by an apparent diminution in strength of contractions.

Regarding fetal prognosis, babies delivered spontaneously and vaginally do well after normal labor or after a prolonged latent phase treated as recommended. After arrest patterns have occurred, however, fetal prognosis is less optimistic. Those who delivered spontaneously as well as those delivered by cesarean section tend to do well. Prognosis for the fetus is considerably worsened if a potentially traumatic operative vaginal delivery is superimposed on preexistent risk factors related to the labor. Midforceps operations are particularly hazardous, posing the risk of long-term neurologic and developmental defects and even fetal death. It is clear that the only rational options are easy vaginal delivery and cesarean section (6).

A graphic portrayal of labor progression is a useful approach to diagnosing abnormal patterns of dilation and descent. Such a depiction enables the recognition of several specific disorders comprising failure to progress in labor as they arise. It is then possible to quickly seek and evaluate causes and initiate a program of management that is most likely to yield good results for both mother and infant.

CASE 57.1   No Documented Disproportion

A 19-year-old woman in her first pregnancy was admitted at term in labor with no antepartum care after an apparently uneventful pregnancy. Uterine contractions, begun 10 hours earlier and now recurring at five- to six-minute intervals, were moderately intense and lasted for 35–45 seconds. The patient was 4 feet, 11 inches tall and weighed 96 lb. Her contractions caused intermittent distress.

The uterus extended to the xiphoid process. Estimated fetal weight was 3,000 g. Vaginal examination revealed a small gynecoid pelvis. The cervix was dilated 4 cm and completely effaced. Membranes were intact. The fetus was in vertex presentation, position not determined, at station -2. Because of the patient's discomfort and the presumed likelihood that she was in active labor, she was given 100 g of meperidine hydrochloride (Demerol).

MEDICATION MUDDLES THE ISSUE

Three hours later, conditions were unchanged. Failure to progress was correctly deemed a critical concern, but the differential diagnosis could not be made because the medication had confused the clinical picture. On one hand, cephalopelvic disproportion was considered possible because of the patient's small stature and small pelvis as well as a rather large baby at high station. These conditions might have resulted in secondary arrest of dilation. On the other hand, she might have begun labor with advanced cervical dilation and now been merely in a normal latent phase, perhaps inhibited by sedatives. Accordingly, the pelvis was reevaluated more critically. Contrary to expectations, the pelvic dimensions appeared adequate to accommodate the fetus. During a contraction with fundal pressure applied by a nurse, vaginal examination showed the fetal head thrusting caudad.

HAPPY ENDING

Sedation was allowed to abate over the next four hours. The contractile pattern improved and cervical dilation began to advance. The membranes were ruptured for purposes of applying a fetal scalp electrode for monitoring. Six hours later (19 hours after onset of labor) the cervix was fully dilated and the vertex, now left occiput anterior, was at station +2. The second stage progressed normally, and the patient was delivered spontaneously of a 3,300-g boy over a mediolateral episiotomy with pudendal block anesthesia. The baby was alert and healthy and had good Apgar scores.

OVERVIEW

In this case the failure to progress in labor was merely a reflection of the nonprogressive preparation for later active dilation that one should expect during a normal latent phase. The attendant physicians had been properly alerted to the possibility of cephalopelvic disproportion and therefore realized that secondary arrest of dilation might occur. When labor failed to advance, they had to pursue the differential diagnosis vigorously. If disproportion had been documented, the risks of further trial of labor, in the face of possible secondary arrest, would have been too great to accept and cesarean section would have been indicated. In the absence of disproportion, allowing labor to proceed—and stimulating it with infusion of oxytocin, if necessary—was the right decision.

CASE 57.2 The Treacherous Multipara

A 26-year-old woman, gravida 4, para 3, was admitted at term in advanced labor. Her largest baby, the most recent, had weighed 4,150 g at birth. The woman's antepartum course had been complicated only by mild hypertension. Her weight was 210 lb, 45 of which she had gained during this pregnancy.

NO PROBLEMS ENVISIONED

The uterus was pendulous. Estimated fetal weight was 4,100 g. The pelvis was deemed ample for childbirth, based on history and examination. The cervix was soft, dilated 9 cm, and about 10 mm thick (75% effaced). Contractions, which had begun six hours earlier, were 3–4 minutes apart, lasting 50–60 seconds each. The uterus could be indented easily. The vertex was in direct occiput posterior position at station zero. Membranes had ruptured two hours earlier.

The patient refused medication for pain and was al-lowed to labor. When she was examined an hour later, nothing had changed except that only the anterior lip of the cervix was palpable. After another hour, conditions remained the same.

DIFFICULTY RECOGNIZED

Belatedly, it became clear that labor had failed to progress adequately. Because of the patient's good past performance and rapid current labor, no consideration had been given to the possibility that her pelvis might not be adequate for a larger baby. At the second examination, the physicians should have become aware that the deceleration phase was already abnormally prolonged and that cephalopelvic disproportion might exist. To have ascribed the delay to positional dystocia—a reasonable possibility in view of the occiput posterior position and its usual accompanying deflexion—would have been unduly optimistic. Disproportion had to be ruled out.

A dynamic test of cephalopelvic relations, consisting of Kristeller pressure applied during a contraction, revealed the fetal head tightly wedged in the midpelvis. Evaluation occupied another hour, during which labor progressed no further. A cesarean section was undertaken under epidural anesthesia. The lower uterine segment was markedly attenuated. A healthy 4,775-g girl was delivered.

DISASTER AVERTED

This obstetric patient was a classic "treacherous multipara." Her pelvis was presumed adequate because of past obstetric achievements. The subtle labor disorder—readily diagnosed, but only if the pattern of dilation is traced—was the first evidence of the serious obstruction that existed. Recognizing the disproportion in time prevented major adverse consequences: a ruptured uterus, for example, or even fetal death.

References

1. Friedman EA. Labor: Clinical evaluation and management, ed 2. New York: Appleton-Century-Crofts, 1978: chap 8–11.

2. Friedman EA. Patterns of labor as indicators of risk. Clin Obstet Gynecol 1973;16:172.

3. Friedman EA, Sachtleben MR, Bresky PA. Dysfunctional labor: XII. Long-term effects on the infant. Am J Obstet Gynecol 1977;127:779.

4. Friedman EA, Acker DB, Sachs BP, eds. Obstetrical decision making, ed 2. St. Louis: CV Mosby, 1987:234–43.

5. Cohen WR, Acker DB, Friedman EA, eds. Management of labor, ed 2. Rockville, MD: Aspen, 1989: chaps 1 and 16.

6. Friedman EA, Neff RK. Labor and delivery: impact on offspring. Littleton, MA: PSG Publishing, 1987: chaps 10–14.

58

Cesarean Section: Modern Perspectives

Edward J. Quilligan, M.D.

IN the years between 1970 and 1978, the operative delivery rate rose from 5.5% to 15.2% (1). Recently, the rate seems to have leveled off to a national average of about 24%. During the past decade, perinatal mortality has decreased and, although perinatal morbidity figures are more difficult to obtain than those on mortality, there appears to be less morbidity as well. It is true that some of the reductions in morbidity and mortality have been the result of more liberal use of cesarean section (CS). However, many other factors have contributed to the improvement, including better prenatal care, fetal monitoring, and advances in newborn care.

If we assume there is some benefit to CS, why all the furor when some hospitals report a 30% rate? The reason is that every CS does increase the risk of maternal morbidity and mortality, and it increases the costs of the medical care system as well. In places such as level III centers, where case loads include a substantial proportion of high-risk patients, such a high rate may be legitimate. In other institutions, however, CS may occasionally represent an avenue of escape from medicolegal problems, an easy way out of a difficult delivery, even a way to increase an obstetrician's personal income.

The mother's risk of dying during the operation is slight in terms of real numbers. In California, in 1975, for example, the maternal death rate associated with vaginal delivery was 9.6/100,00 live births. With CS, it was 19.4/100,000 (2). Thus, a woman delivered operatively had a 100% greater chance of dying than if she delivered vaginally. In Georgia, cesarean section increases the risk of death ten times; in Rhode Island, 25 times (3). Such comparisons may be somewhat biased in that the inherent risks of the two populations, those delivered by CS and those delivered vaginally, may differ. In the Georgia study eliminating patients whose illness may have contributed to their demise left the increase in maternal death after CS six times higher.

The increased maternal morbidity associated with operative delivery is primarily the result of postpartum endometritis, with urinary tract infection the next leading reason for morbidity. The varying frequency of puerperal morbidity, from 12% to 50%, is usually attributed to population differences. Generally, indigent patients have a higher rate of puerperal morbidity after cesarean section. Table 58.1 com-

Table 58.1 Complications of Childbirth

Complication	Cesarean Section (%)	Vaginal Delivery (%)
Endometritis	16.11	1.40
Urinary tract infection	6.74	0.95
Wound infection	3.16	0.10

From Obstetrical Statistical Cooperative 1973–1977. In: Cesarean childbirth. US Department of Health and Human Services Publication No. (NIH) 82–2067, October 1981.

pares the incidence of CS and vaginal delivery for three common complications (4). Table 58.2 compares costs of vaginal and cesarean deliveries in the U.S. The higher risks and costs seem to justify examining the most frequent indications to see if there are safe alternatives.

Indications

Has the philosophy of managing labor changed? And, if it has, is the change justified?

Cesarean section is now ordered much earlier in labor than was the case previously. One reason is that fewer assisted vaginal deliveries are being performed, apparently because of Friedman's studies showing increased perinatal mortality and decreased IQ in infants born after difficult midforceps deliveries (5).

Failure to Progress

The most common indication for primary CS is failure to progress in labor. It accounts for roughly a third of the increase in CS rates. Since the increase must involve the power (uterine activity), the passenger (fetus), or the passage, it is legitimate to ask if there has been an actual change in one of these. There is no evidence that maternal pelves or uterine activity have changed over the past 20 years. As for the fetus, the number of infants born weighing more than 4,000 g, over a 10-year period at Los Angeles County/University of Southern California (LAC/USC) Medical Center, has remained steady at about 8%.

To reduce the cesarean section rate for failure to progress, the diagnosis should be prompt and it should be complete. We consider that the patient is failing to progress if

she deviates from the Friedman curve for one or two hours at the most. The diagnosis must include the degree of uterine activity, usually determined by an intrauterine catheter and the fetal position (occiput anterior or occiput posterior).

After a firm diagnosis, the treatment should be adequate in both time and amount. It is important to give enough oxytocin (Pitocin, Syntocinon) to achieve at least three contractions in 10 minutes, each with an intensity of 50 mm Hg. When the fetal heart rate is normal, a trial of 6–8 hours without progress is adequate in the latent phase. In the active phase, a two-hour trial with the fetus in an anterior position and 3–4 hours in a posterior position seems reasonable. The longer times apply to primigravidas. If a true arrest of dilation or descent occurs, as determined by the Friedman curve, the child should be delivered by cesarean section.

Friedman's findings are not definitive, but they do indicate that true arrest disorders have a higher perinatal mortality (6). Using these criteria, we can anticipate a section rate for failure to progress of 2%–4%. A substantially higher rate may require examination of individual cases by a peer review committee.

Repeat Sections

In the past, when a classic CS was the usual procedure, rupture of a uterine scar during a subsequent delivery resulted in high maternal (up to 5%) and fetal (about 50%) mortality (6–8). Widespread use of the low transverse incision reduced the risk to both mother and fetus. Maternal mortality from a ruptured uterine scar is now rare. In the United Kingdom, between 1961 and 1969, five cases were reported, and most of these patients seem to have had poor obstet-

Table 58.2 Delivery Costs: U.S. Averages (1991)

	Cesarean Section	Vaginal Delivery
Physician's Fee	$2,235	$1,625
Hospital Charges	$5,590	$3,095
Total	$7,825	$4,720

From Health Insurance Association of America. The cost of maternity care and childbirth in the United States: 1991 surgical prevailing healthcare charges system

ric management (9). The rate of fetal loss associated with uterine rupture of a low transverse scar is low, and, in those studies of trials of labor where continuous fetal heart rate (FHR) monitoring was done, no fetal deaths have been reported (7, 10).

Recent British figures on fetal and maternal mortality led Shy and colleagues to estimate an excess maternal mortality of 0.7/10,000 births and perinatal mortality of 39/10,000 births when elective repeat CS is done rather than a trial of labor (11). It is true that the excess perinatal mortality is the result primarily of iatrogenic prematurity, which should not happen when the lecithin/sphingomyelin (L/S) ratio is used properly. Unfortunately, even today, premature infants are being delivered electively by repeat CS.

Case 58.1 describes the guidelines outlined by the American College of Obstetricians and Gynecologists for trial of labor after cesarean section (2). Obstetricians used to feel that only patients whose previous sections had been for nonrecurrent indications were candidates for a trial of labor. Recently, Seitchik and Rao showed that 70% of patients previously sectioned for failure to progress delivered vaginally after a trial of labor (12).

Other Indications

Since failure to progress and elective repeat CS are the major indications for the high section rate, these are the areas most amenable to reduction of the overall rate. However, the following two indications, breech presentation and fetal distress, deserve comment.

In 3%–4% of laboring patients, the fetus is a breech. Current practice calls for delivery by CS, except in specific circumstances (13). This philosophy leads to a cephalic version. Some obstetricians use external cephalic version, but this method has never been popular because of the potential for such difficulties as cord entanglement, placental abruption, fetomaternal transfusion, and ruptured uterus. These problems seem to be more theoretic than real. Ranney reported no such problem in over 1,000 versions (14). Furthermore, his incidence of breech presentation in labor was 1.1%.

A problem with the timing of the version, as practiced by Ranney, is the 33% rate of spontaneous reversion to breech. This difficulty has been substantially overcome by doing the version after 37 weeks' gestation. External cephal-

ic version after 37 weeks would have been hazardous and difficult before good tocolytic agents were available.

There are several reports of 70% success rates in performing external cephalic version when patients were given 100 to 150 µg/min of IV ritodrine for 30 minutes (15, 16). The reversion-to-breech rate was less than 1%, and fetal problems were minimal. Van Dorsten and colleagues reported that one fetus in 25 had sufficient bradycardia to indicate induction of labor, which proceeded uneventfully to vaginal delivery of a normal baby (16). Even this small degree of fetal distress could be eliminated by observing the fetal heart constantly with real-time ultrasound during the version. If bradycardia occurs, the version should be stopped for observation; if it persists, the fetus should be turned back to a breech. To assure safety, do version only in the hospital. This technique could cut the CS rate for breech presentation in half.

With regard to fetal distress, most prospective studies that have compared continuous FHR monitoring with intermittent auscultation showed increased section rates in the monitored groups (17–20). Not all fetuses with ominous FHR patterns are truly in distress; scalp blood sampling is the only way to detect which fetus with an ominous pattern is truly in distress. At LAC/USC, our section rate for fetal distress was about 1.5%, compared with the 2.5%–3% it would have been without scalp sampling (21). Many feel that the technique is difficult to perform under any circumstances and impossible in hospitals that lack a micro-blood-gas laboratory. The latter problem has been overcome by the development of testing equipment that can be used on any delivery floor (22). A somewhat simpler test is to stimulate the fetal scalp or apply a sound stimulus (artificial larynx) to the maternal abdomen (22–24). If the FHR accelerates by 15 beats per minute, the pH will be above 7.20, and labor may continue.

Conclusion

If a hospital were to pursue a conservative policy on CS for the usual obstetric population, what rate should it expect? This question is hard to answer, because hospital obstetric populations differ so markedly. However, hospital staff should examine their CS rates frequently, indication by indication.

Table 58.3 Ideal Cesarean Section Rates

Indication	Percentage
Failure to progress	4–6
Repeat cesarean section	2–3
Breech and abnormal lie	2–3
Fetal distress	2–3
Third-trimester bleeding	1

From Rubin GL, Peterson HB, Rochat RW, et al. Maternal death after cesarean section in Georgia. Am J Obstet Gynecol 1981;139:681.

Purely as a guide, Table 58.3 lists values obtainable in a level I or level II hospital. Using the Georgia figures and based on 3 million deliveries a year overall, the conservative approach would result in about 140 fewer maternal deaths a year in the United States (4). This would reduce our maternal mortality by 50%, a goal worth working toward if it can be accomplished with safety for the fetus.

CASE 58.1 Guidelines for Trial of Labor after CS

The concept of routine repeat cesarean birth should be replaced by a specific indication for a subsequent abdominal delivery. In the absence of a contraindication, a woman who has had one CS with a low transverse incision should be counselled and encouraged to attempt labor in her current pregnancy.

A woman who has had two or more previous CSs with low transverse incisions who wishes to attempt vaginal birth should not be discouraged from doing so, provided there are no contraindications.

When specific data on risk are lacking, the question of whether to allow a trial of labor must be assessed on an individual basis.

A previous classic uterine incision is a contraindication to labor.

Professional and institutional resources must have the capacity to respond to acute intrapartum obstetric emergencies, such as performing CS within 30 minutes from the time the decision is made until the surgical procedure is begun, as is standard for any obstetric patient in labor.

A physician who is capable of evaluating labor and performing a cesarean delivery should be readily available.

Normal activity should be encouraged during the latent phase of labor; there is no need for restriction to a labor bed before actual labor has begun (25). ∎

References

1. Placek PJ, Taffel SM, Kleinman JC. Trends and variations in cesarean section delivery. In: Heath United States. US Department of Health and Human Services, Publication No. (PHS) 81-1232, 1980:73–6.

2. Petitti D, Olson RO, Williams RL. Cesarean section in California 1960 through 1975. Am J Obstet Gynecol 1979;133:391.

3. Rubin GL, Peterson HB, Rochat RW, et al. Maternal death after cesarean section in Georgia. Am J Obstet Gynecol 1981;139:681.

4. Obstetric Statistical Cooperative 1973–1977. In: Cesarean Childbirth. US Department of Health and Human Services Publication No. (NIH) 82-2067, October 1981.

5. Friedman EA, Sachtleben MR, Bresky PA. Dysfunctional labor: XII. Long-term effects on the infant. Am J Obstet Gynecol 1977;127:779.

6. Cragin EB. Conservatism in obstetrics. NY Med J 1916;104:1.

7. Dewhurst CJ. The ruptured cesarean section scar. J Obstet Gynaecol Br Emp 1957;64:113.

8. Cunningham EG, MacDonald PC, Gant NF, Leveno KJ, Gilstrap LC III. Williams obstetrics, ed 19. New York: Appleton-Century-Crofts, 1993:546.

9. British Maternal Mortality Survey, 1961–1969.

10. Gibbs CE. Planned vaginal delivery following cesarean section. Clin Obstet Gynecol 1980;23:507.

11. Shy KK, LoGerfo JP, Karp LE. Evaluation of elective repeat cesarean section as a standard of care: an application of decision analysis. Am J Obstet Gynecol 1981;139:123.

12. Seitchik J, Rao VR. Cesarean delivery in nulliparous women for failed oxytocin-augmented labors: route of delivery in subsequent pregnancy. Am J Obstet Gynecol 1982;143:393.

13. Collea JV, Chein C, Quilligan EJ. The randomized manage-

ment of term frank breech presentation: a study of 208 cases. Am J Obstet Gynecol 1980;137:235.

14. Ranney B. The gentle art of external cephalic version. Am J Obstet Gynecol 1973;116:239.

15. Saling E, Muller-Holve W. External cephalic version under tocolysis. J Perinat Med 1975;3:115.

16. Van Dorsten JP, Schifrin BS, Wallace RL. Randomized control trial of external cephalic version with tocolysis in late pregnancy. Am J Obstet Gynecol 1981;141:417.

17. Haverkamp AD, Thompson HE, McFee JG, et al. The evaluation of continuous fetal heart rate monitoring in high-risk pregnancy. Am J Obstet Gynecol 1976;125:310.

18. Renou P, Chang A, Anderson I, et al. Controlled trial of fetal intensive care. Am J Obstet Gynecol 1976;126:470.

19. Kelso IM, Parsons RJ, Lawrence GF, et al. An assessment of continuous fetal heart rate monitoring in labor: a randomized trial. Am J Obstet Gynecol 1978;131:526.

20. Haverkamp AD, Orleans M, Langendoerfer S, et al. A controlled trial of the differential effects of intrapartum fetal monitoring. Am J Obstet Gynecol 1979;134:399.

21. Zalar RW Jr, Quilligan EJ. The influence of scalp sampling on the cesarean section rate for fetal distress. Am J Obstet Gynecol 1979;135:239.

22. Pearse KE, Paul RH. Comparison of fetal scalp blood pH measurement with an automated blood microprocessor and a clinical blood gas laboratory. Am J Obstet Gynecol 1982; 144:40.

23. Clark SL, Gimovsky ML, Miller FC. The scalp stimulation test: a clinical alternative to fetal scalp blood. Am J Obstet Gynecol 1984;148:274.

24. Smith CV, Nguyen HN, Phelan JP, et al. Intrapartum assessment of fetal well-being: a comparison of fetal acoustic stimulation with acid-base determinations. Am J Obstet Gynecol 1986;155:726.

25. American College of Obstetricians and Gynecologists: Guidelines for vaginal delivery after a previous cesarean section. ACOG Committee Opinion No. 64, October, 1988.

59

Breech Delivery

Martin L. Gimovsky, M.D.
Roy H. Petrie, M.D.

BECAUSE breech infants are in far greater danger of morbidity and mortality than vertex ones, many practitioners now virtually exclude a trial of labor and vaginal delivery, citing various authorities to justify routine cesarean section (CS) (1–4). Simultaneously, external cephalic version has regained some advocates. The overwhelming concern of earlier practitioners was maternal safety. Before introduction of blood banking, antibiotics, and safe anesthetic techniques, routine vaginal delivery was reasonable. Inability to support the premature infant (breech presentation being four to ten times more frequent in labor before 37 completed weeks) or materially to improve outcome for newborns with a major congenital anomaly (three to five times more common among breech fetuses of all gestational ages) further justified this approach. The notable exceptions allowing CS involved severe maternal problems, such as bleeding, hypertension, and sepsis.

Liberalization of indications for CS followed development of relatively safe operative procedures. As cesarean section became a more useful tool, its application in breech delivery increased dramatically (Figure 59.1). In 1959, Wright stated that any patient of more than 35 weeks' gestation who entered labor with a living baby in breech pre-

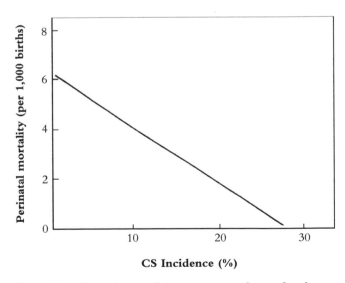

Figure 59.1 CS use increased. Statistics accumulating after about 1940 led many to conclude that, to eliminate preventable breech deaths, one should always resort to cesarean section. Graph based on term infant breech series of the 1940s.

sentation should be delivered by CS, provided no maternal disease contraindicated abdominal delivery (1). Hall and Kohl, after analyzing 11,456 breech presentations delivered at seven hospitals in the early 1950s, concluded that cesarean delivery produced the lowest mortality, without implying that it should be used in all breech deliveries (2).

Examining data from that era, we compared breech deaths of term infants (potentially directly attributable to effects of labor and vaginal delivery) with the rate of cesareans performed (5). In contrast with Wright and his followers, we concluded that a CS rate of about 30%—rather than 100%—appears sufficient virtually to eliminate any *preventable* breech deaths. Elsewhere, the "correct" CS rate for breeches is still debated (6–11).

Current Situation

Development of obstetrics since Wright's investigation has favored his position rather than ours. Introduction of continuous electronic fetal monitoring (EFM), ability to perform emergency CS within minutes, and availability of neonatal intensive care units, all making childbirth much safer, have impacted on breech delivery. In the United States, CS rates for breech presentation rose sharply from between 5% and 20% in the 1950s to 80% and higher in 1980. However, we must still ask: Is such a trend justified?

Testifying to its efficacy are many recent reports confirming a corrected perinatal mortality rate of zero for the term breech infant delivered by CS. Infants who die after sectioning for this indication invariably are either congenitally malformed or premature. The rare exception is a normal infant compromised by cord prolapse. (Of course, intrapartum death from the same causes occurs with other fetal presentations.)

However, poorly performed breech extraction at CS results in injuries similar to those sustained during vaginal delivery, namely, brachial plexus injuries, bone fractures, and lacerations (6–13). In one study, these injuries occurred at cesarean breech delivery in virtually the identical manner seen at vaginal breech delivery (12). Moreover, CS results in far more maternal morbidity and mortality than vaginal delivery (6, 12). Nor is it cost-effective unless it prevents a significant number of fetal injuries, neonatal intensive care

unit (NICU) admissions, or prolonged hospitalizations of newborns. Data that address these questions suggest that it may not (6–8, 12).

In contrast, protocols for managing patients selectively allow for liberal use of CS but only for specific indications. Correctly applied, we believe that use of such protocols will increase benefits of CS and minimize risks to both mother and fetus resulting from exclusive use.

External Cephalic Version

One way of countering intrapartum breech presentation is to reduce incidence. Van Dorsten and co-workers and others have shown the effectiveness of external version, using terbutaline sulfate (Brethine, Bricanyl) and, more recently, ritodrine hydrochloride (Yutopar) tocolysis, in late gestation (13, 14). Nonstress testing and real-time ultrasound B-scans have enhanced safety.

Version has been less successful intrapartum because tocolysis, which allows gentle manipulation, becomes increasingly difficult as labor advances. Version has also been attempted, with limited success, for transverse lie and to convert second twins at vaginal delivery (15).

Rupture of membranes precludes any such attempt. Also, engagement of the breech invariably occurs when version fails late in gestation. Thus far, with limited numbers, we have been successful in fewer than half our attempted intrapartum versions.

Selective Trial of Labor

The single largest group of breech fetuses in labor are at term and in frank breech presentation. When Collea and co-workers conducted a prospective randomized trial comparing elective CS with protocol-managed labor, they found significant maternal morbidity among patients delivered by CS but no dramatic improvement in neonatal outcome (6). Among 60 of 208 infants delivered vaginally, there were two instances of mild brachial plexus injury. In both cases, nuchal arms complicated delivery. The investigators felt that maternal morbidity resulting from cesarean section balanced fetal morbidity associated with vaginal delivery.

In another trial, using a slightly different protocol,

O'Leary noted one injury in 81 vaginal deliveries (7). It occurred during a breech extraction for fetal distress, done at full dilation. In the control group of 69 patients (delivered vaginally but without strict adherence to protocol), there were four birth injuries, eight low Apgar scores, one neonatal death, and one stillbirth. The investigator concluded that use of the protocol dramatically improved outcomes.

A retrospective study of all types of breech presentations—nonfrank, complete, incomplete, and footling—suggested that selective management by protocol of nonfrank term breeches gave results superior to those seen at vaginal births managed randomly (8). Outcomes for protocol-managed breeches delivered vaginally were essentially identical with those for breeches delivered by elective section and vertex infants delivered vaginally. The protocol used, based on observations made in the 1950s and 1960s, has since been updated to incorporate recent advances in perinatology (Table 59.1). The same authors subsequently found the selective-protocol approach successful in a prospective study (9).

Preliminary Evaluation

When selecting patients who may be candidates for a trial of labor, careful evaluation of fetopelvic spatial relationships is mandatory. X-rays provide this information and also document that the skull is normal in appearance and attitude (Table 59.2).

Hyperextension of the head—an angle of more than 105 degrees between the mandible and the main axis of the cervical spine—is an absolute contraindication to labor, as there is high risk of lethal spinal cord injury during vaginal delivery. Adequate incisions at CS and careful attention during abdominal delivery will virtually eliminate neonatal death resulting from spinal cord injury in these cases.

Assessment of the pelvis by x-ray is essential to exclude the woman with a so-called "borderline" contracture or "moderate degree of disproportion," as well as the woman with an "inadequate" pelvis. X-rays do not guarantee perfect safety; however, such is not their purpose (8, 15, 16).

Table 59.1 Protocol and Nonprotocol Results

	Protocol Group	Nonprotocol Group	Control Group 1	Control Group 2
Type of Delivery	Vaginal	Vaginal	Spontaneous vaginal	Elective CS
Presentation	Breech	Breech	Vertex	95% vertex 5% breech
Mean Birthweight (g) (range)	3,125 (2,001–4,080)	3,025 (2,000–4,210)	3,170 (2,470–4,010)	2,980 (2,350–4,100)
No. Deliveries	130	78	130	130
Ward/Private	59/41	62/38	60/40	58/42
Mean 5-min Apgar	8.6	8.1	8.7	8.6
Neonatal Morbidity	4/130	12/78	3/130	2/130
Intrapartum Mortality	0	1	0	0
Perinatal Mortality★	0	12.8	0	0

★Corrected to exclude congenital anomalies incompatible with life.

From Gimovsky ML, Petrie RH, Todd WD. Neonatal performance of the selected term vaginal breech delivery. Obstet Gynecol 1980;56:687.

Rather, they assist in providing objective pelvic measurement and thus help to select the pelvis most likely to be adequate for a breech delivery. Since 1984, we have converted to computed tomographic measurement (CT), as we have found digital radiography easier to interpret, safer, and probably more accurate than conventional techniques (17).

Continuous Fetal Surveillance

Umbilical cord prolapse, although unlikely before second-stage labor, is a potential hazard, especially during the second stage. We feel that labor and delivery after full dilation is best managed in the delivery room and that the physician in charge should watch the fetal heart rate (FHR) pattern closely. In 1973, Rovinsky and co-workers showed that vertex fetuses had the same risk of intrapartum death from overt prolapse as frank breech fetuses and that both were at greater risk than footling and complete breech presentations (18). Because continuous monitoring was not routine in 1973, perhaps labor room personnel paid unusually close attention to this potential problem in nonfrank breech fetuses.

In 1981, Nishijima and co-workers compared nulliparas' and multiparas' FHR patterns in labor for breech and vertex presentations and found no essential difference (19). Others have suggested that periodic accelerations are more frequent in breech babies, presumably due to a difference in vagal stimulation.

Fetal blood sampling may be used to complement EFM, just as in vertex presentations. A pH below 7.20 or a decreasing trend is felt to confirm serious fetal distress. Our data on umbilical cord gases confirm that fetal acid-base status is normal when FHR patterns are also normal (8, 9 15). Acid-base status at birth after normal FHR findings is no different for breech than for cephalic fetuses (20).

Anesthesia

"Standby" anesthesia support is vital. Although we routinely use pudendal nerve block in trials of labor, we find that supplemental general anesthesia is needed in about 10% of cases to expedite delivery. Regional anesthesia, when available, may offer a further advantage, especially for the small breech or the footling, where it can lessen maternal bearing down until the cervix is fully dilated and so decrease risk of cord or body prolapse. Finally, an anesthesiologist's presence assures immediate recourse to cesarean section, if necessary.

Neonatal Support

The final perinatal requirement is excellent neonatal support. To assure good outcome, regardless of delivery route, we use a "resuscitation team" consisting of a NICU nurse, respiratory therapist, and pediatric house officer or neonatologist. Because breech presentation involves high risk, neonatal resuscitation, when required, must be expert and readily available.

Technique for Delivery

Vaginal delivery of a breech requires watchful waiting and gentle manipulation. An assisted breech delivery requires a sense of relative force and of the vectors of applied force. An obstetrician weighing 100–200 lbs can exert great force on a 7-lb newborn. Rotation of the fetal body to effect delivery of the arms exceeding 90 degrees may compromise vertebral blood supply to the central nervous system.

Maintaining flexion is crucial. During assisted delivery, a gowned and gloved assistant should apply just enough suprapubic (Kristeller) pressure to keep the head flexed, as well as the fetal arms in place across the chest. Loss of flexion of the fetal head or formation of nuchal arms will complicate vaginal delivery immensely.

The Piper forceps was designed to act as a lever, not a tractor. The purpose of suprapubic pressure is not to effect delivery but to maintain flexion during descent. If the obstetrician fails to "follow" the head by exerting pressure on the uterus itself, flexion may be lost, making it more difficult to deliver the following head.

Haste is dangerous and generally unnecessary. We have found essentially normal cord gases in infants for up to six minutes between emergence of the umbilicus and final delivery (12). In our current studies, we compared umbilicus-to-delivery time with incision-to-delivery time at cesarean section. Interestingly, in two-thirds of cases, delivery of the infant by cesarean took markedly longer than vaginal delivery (9).

Table 59.2 Term Breech Outcomes for Different Managements

	Cesarean Section	Vaginal Delivery	Vaginal Delivery Protocol
Patients	512	235	499
Corrected Perinatal Mortality	0	18/1,000	4/1,000
Low Apgar Scores	9	29	13
Birth Injury	4	6	4
Lethal Congenital Anomaly	3	4	2

Data are from References 6, 7, 8, and 12, as well as patients seen and delivered 1983–1987 at White Memorial Medical Center, Los Angeles.

Earlier Recommendations Justified

Results of several recent studies comparing term breech infants delivered vaginally by protocol and by cesarean section confirm by and large the advice given by an earlier generation of obstetricians (6–8, 12). These later findings strongly suggest that radiologic confirmation of pelvic adequacy in conjunction with careful assessment of labor and continuous electronic fetal monitoring can produce outcomes in infants born vaginally comparable to those for their peers delivered by section, while holding the cesarean section rate far below the national average (55% versus 80%–90%) (Table 59.2).

Perhaps the most difficult breech baby to manage, the low-birthweight infant, has up to one chance in five of having a congenital malformation (21). In many cases, labors are complicated by other obstetric problems, such as placenta previa, abruptio placentae, and multiple gestation. There is also a serious risk of cord prolapse and body prolapse through an incompletely dilated cervix.

Recent evidence suggests improved outcome for breech infants weighing between 1,000 and 2,000 g delivered by cesarean section (21, 22). Below this weight, most authorities concur, benefits of section are unclear, regardless of presentation.

We agree with other investigators that, for the breech fetus weighing more than 2,000 g, a trial of labor is a reasonable alternative under appropriate conditions (certainly for frank or complete breech). Our chief problem is inability to differentiate precisely the fetus who will weigh about 1,200 g at birth from one who will weigh about 1,800 g. Between these two, there may be a crucial difference in likelihood of success at vaginal delivery. Until we have greater expertise, we would deliver both by CS.

Factors in Decision-Making

Clearly, liberal use of CS can lessen the potential for hypoxia and trauma in breech delivery. However, because section has greater maternal costs than vaginal birth, we feel achieving optimal outcome for both requires individual assessment. Where facilities (anesthesia, neonatology, and an in-house operating room staff) allow for expeditious section, one can offer selected patients a trial of labor. Obstetricians must be committed to thorough evaluation of both pelvis and labor and understand principles of assisted breech delivery. When the obstetrician has adequate expertise and full patient consent, external cephalic version may also be an alternative.

Many principles regarding safe vaginal delivery apply also to CS. In addition, adequate incisions in both the abdominal wall and uterus are necessary to avoid the trauma that abdominal delivery was chosen in order to avoid. The safe delivery of a breech-presenting fetus was once the hallmark of a well-trained obstetrician-gynecologist. The desire to avoid birth trauma and asphyxia, the advent of the well-equipped NICU, and new treatments for congenital anomalies have resulted in an enormous increase in the use of cesarean section to effect delivery in breech presentation—so much so that some of the classic manual maneuvers used in breech delivery are no longer being taught to physicians in training. Indeed, some teachers themselves feel inadequate in passing on these techniques.

Summary

It is crucial to remember that the safe delivery of a breech fetus at CS requires a total breech extraction, an inherently

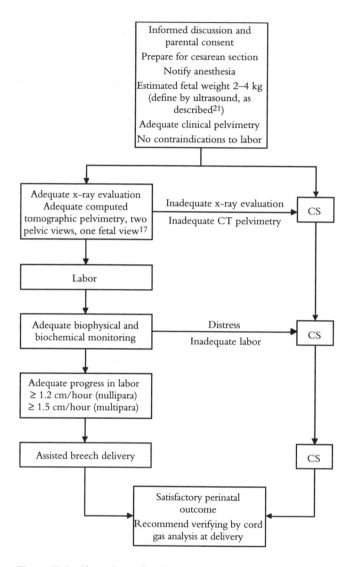

Figure 59.2 Flow chart of authors' protocol.

more dangerous procedure than a spontaneous breech delivery. To deliver a breech fetus safely at CS is also a testament to the operator's skill. CS is the type of delivery now used for the majority of breech fetuses; it is at CS that the necessary appreciation of how to conduct a safe breech delivery can, and should, be taught.

CASE 59.1 Using Authors' Protocol

Select gestations between 36 and 42 weeks (estimated fetal weight 2 to 4 kg), regardless of specific type of breech presentation (see Figure 59.2). Careful fetal ultrasound for anomalies should help estimate weight (23). (We are currently evaluating such ultrasound measurements as biparietal diameter, abdominal circumference, and femur length to increase objective patient selection.)

We use the standard Friedman curve to follow labor. The minimal acceptable progress in active labor is 1.2 cm/h in the nullipara and 1.5 cm/h in the multipara. In his analysis of breech labor, Friedman noted characteristics almost identical to those of vertex labors, except for differing rapidity of descent, since vertex labor tends to start descent at a lower station (24).

Breech labors tend to begin at higher stations. Most investigators currently agree that parity plays almost no role in outcome. However, there may be some increase in fetal injury to the following head among multiparas because of rapid descent during final delivery stages. We have noted that use of oxytocin for induction in selected cases has not prejudiced outcome.

We support, as do most obstetricians, the use of CS in response to arrest in active-phase labor. A recent detailed review showed that oxytocin augmentation rarely achieved safe delivery of a breech infant after arrest (13). This finding confirms Friedman's conclusion that fetopelvic disproportion is the most likely cause of active-phase arrest (24). Friedman, in his study of breech deliveries, noted that three-fourths of women who were delivered of infants weighing 3,500 g or more developed dysfunctional labor and that all infants weighing 4,000 g or more were products of dysfunctional labor. We have set the lower limits of satisfactory progress in labor at 1.2 cm hourly or more for nulliparas and 1.5 cm hourly or more for multiparas. ∎

References

1. Wright RC. Reduction of perinatal mortality and morbidity in breech delivery through routine use of cesarean section. Obstet Gynecol 1959;14:748.

2. Hall JE, Kohl S. Breech presentation. A study of 11,456 cases. Am J Obstet Gynecol 1960;15:158.

3. Potter MG, Heation CE, Douglas GW. Intrinsic fetal risk in breech delivery. Obstet Gynecol 1960;15:158.

4. Goethals TR. Cesarean section as the method of choice in management of breech delivery. Am J Obstet Gynecol 1956;71:536.

5. Gimovsky ML, Petrie RH. Management of breech presentation. Contemp Ob/Gyn 1983;21(April):201.

6. Collea JV, Chein CC, Quilligan EJ. The randomized management of term frank breech presentation. A study of 208 cases. Am J Obstet Gynecol 1980;137:235.

7. O'Leary JA. Vaginal delivery of the term breech. A preliminary report. Obstet Gynecol 1979;53:341.

8. Gimovsky ML, Petrie RH, Todd WD. Neonatal performance of the selected term vaginal breech delivery. Obstet Gynecol 1980;56:687.

9. Gimovsky ML, Wallace RL, Schifrin BS, et al. Randomized management of the nonfrank breech presentation at term. A preliminary report. Am J Obstet Gynecol 1983;146:34.

10. Green JE, McLean F, Smith LP, et al. Has an increased cesarean section rate for term breech delivery reduced the incidence of birth asphyxia, trauma, and death? Am J Obstet Gynecol 1982;142:643.

11. Pitkin RM. Breech delivery: some thoughts on a continuing predicament. Contemp Ob/Gyn 1982;19(March):119.

12. Gimovsky ML, Paul RH. Singleton breech presentation in labor—experience in 1980. Am J Obstet Gynecol 1982; 143:733.

13. Van Dorsten JP, Schifrin BS, Wallace RL. Randomized controlled trial of external cephalic version with tocolysis in late pregnancy. Am J Obstet Gynecol 1981;141:417.

14. Seling E, Muller-Holve W. External cephalic version under tocolysis. J Perinatol Med 1975;3:115.

15. Chervenak F, Johnson RE, Youcha S. Intrapartum management of twin gestation. Obstet Gynecol 1985;65:119.

16. Todd WD, Steer CM. Term breech: review of 1,006 term breech deliveries. Obstet Gynecol 1963;22:583.

17. Gimovsky ML, Wellard K, Neglio M. X-ray pelvimetry and breech protocol: a comparison of digital radiography and conventional methods. Am J Obstet Gynecol 1985;153: 887.

18. Rovinsky JJ, Miller JA, Kaplan S. Management of breech presentation at term. Am J Obstet Gynecol 1973;115:497.

19. Nishijima N, Tatsumi H, Amano K, et al. Differences of fetal heart rate patterns between cephalic and breech presentation in induced labor. J Perinatol Med 1981;9(suppl):129.

20. Gimovsky ML, Nishiyama M, Halle J. Umbilical cord gas parameters as a reflection of acid-base status of birth: a comparison of clinical risk factors. Society of Perinatal Obstetricians, 9th Annual Meeting, 1989. Abstract.

21. Kauppila O, Gronross M, Aro P, et al. Management of low-birthweight breech delivery: should cesarean section be routine? Obstet Gynecol 1981;57:289.

22. Gimovsky ML, Petrie RH. Optimal method of delivery of the low-birthweight breech fetus: an unresolved issue. J Perinatol 1988;8:141.

23. Shepard MJ, Richards VA, Berkowitz RL, et al. An evaluation of two operations for predicting fetal weight by ultrasound. Am J Obstet 1982;142:47.

24. Friedman EA. Labor: clinical evaluation and management, ed 2. New York: Appleton-Century-Crofts, 1978.

60

Aspiration Pneumonitis

J. Antonio Aldrete, M.D.
Evelyn G. Santos, M.D.

WHEN foreign solid or liquid materials enter the respiratory tract, an immediate reflex response closes the glottis and elicits a cough. The response may not appear if the reflex mechanism is depressed or the mass of foreign matter is excessive. Instead, food particles can obstruct major airways, and inhaled acidic gastric contents may injure the tracheobronchial mucosa and produce pneumonitis.

Although aspiration pneumonitis has long been recognized, Mendelson's classic report in 1946 linked the degree of gastric acidity with the severity of pneumonitis (1). The critical pH appeared to be 2.5. The volume is also important: approximately 25 mL in the average parturient. However, aspiration of gastric contents causes severe pulmonary dysfunction even if the pH is greater than 2.5.

Pregnant patients are at high risk for aspiration that may follow vomiting or regurgitation of gastric contents when excessive sedation or effects of anesthetic agents depress their laryngeal reflexes. Pain, anxiety, and narcotics administered during labor and anatomic displacement of the stomach delay gastric emptying, which is already prolonged during pregnancy.

High levels of progesterone relax the gastroesophageal sphincter and make it relatively incompetent. The gravid uterus increases intragastric pressure, which is further aggravated by the lithotomy of Trendelenburg position. The presence of a high gastric content volume or a low pH in any patient, cannot be excluded, irrespective of the time between the last meal and either onset of labor or delivery. Thus, it appears reasonable to consider all pregnant patients as having full stomachs.

Incidence of Aspiration

The true frequency of aspiration is unknown because many cases are subclinical and others may be misdiagnosed. Aspiration while the patient is under anesthesia is a sequel to regurgitation or vomiting. Regurgitation is a passive process that depends on a pressure gradient between the stomach and the esophagus. Vomiting is an active reflex that usually occurs during light anesthesia.

Silent aspiration may occur in 14%–26% of patients given inhalation anesthesia (2). Investigators noted regurgitation in 7.8% of 900 surgical patients; 8.6% of those who regurgitated subsequently aspirated (3). In obstetric patients, aspiration is the leading cause of anesthesia-related mortality. This complication accounts for about 30%–50% of maternal deaths due to anesthesia (4). The increased use of regional anesthetic techniques for both vaginal and cesarean deliveries prevents this problem, but does not totally preclude aspiration.

Predisposing Factors

Most physicians consider patients admitted with trauma as full-stomach patients. Stress and emotional upset increase gastric acid production and gastric volume. Pain and anxiety delay gastric emptying because of the high plasma levels of catecholamines that produce gastric hypotonia and pyloric spasm.

An analysis of gastric contents after induction of anesthesia in adult nonobese outpatients undergoing elective surgery showed a significant proportion at potential risk for the acid aspiration syndrome (patients with gastric pH below 2.5 or volume greater than 25 mL) (5).

The frequency of hiatal hernia in the obese undoubtedly predisposes them to regurgitation. Morbidly obese patients are at risk of aspiration pneumonitis when gastric volume exceeded 25 mL (77% of patients) and pH below 2.5 (85% of patients). It has been postulated that obese patients may have delayed gastric emptying and that the prolonged distension of the stomach may stimulate increased production of acid by the parietal cells.

The high intragastric pressure accompanying cirrhosis, intraabdominal tumors, ascites, and pregnancy favors regurgitation. Similarly, patients with posttonsillectomy bleeding or upper gastrointestinal (GI) hemorrhage are likely to vomit.

Intravenous (IV) alcohol, formerly used to arrest premature labor, may place the patient in jeopardy on several counts should general or regional anesthesia become necessary. Alcohol is a potent secretagogue of highly acidic juice. The obtundation achieved with therapeutic levels may render the patient susceptible to vomiting and aspiration.

Sedatives and narcotics given during labor also delay gastric emptying. If fundal pressure is applied to the uterus, the pyloric sphincter may contract, intragastric pressure may

rise, and regurgitation may result. Generally, intragastric pressure must exceed 25–30 cm H_2O before passive regurgitation can occur.

Anesthesia and Surgical Factors

Most of the halogenated anesthetic agents have little propensity for producing postoperative vomiting. A nasogastric tube is no guarantee of an empty stomach. Routine use of nasogastric tubes during major surgery is associated with unwarranted risks of aspiration through at least three mechanisms:

- Hypersalivation, by allowing secretions to pool in the hypopharynx;
- Laryngeal and pharyngeal abnormalities, which are frequently caused by nasogastric tubes, leading to an inability to handle secretions and protect the airway; and
- Patency between the lower esophagus and the fundus of the stomach.

Other factors that favor regurgitation and aspiration during surgery, when using general or regional anesthesia, include:

- Severe and uncorrected hypotension that occurs as a result of sympathetic blockade from regional anesthesia or a very high level of blockade, producing hypotension, vomiting, or loss of consciousness;
- Excessive fundal pressure during delivery;
- Trendelenburg position;
- Increased intragastric pressure from muscle fasciculations caused by succinylcholine (Anectine, Quelicin);
- Partial upper airway obstruction, forcing air into the stomach; and
- Excessive sedative and analgesic drugs to supplement regional blocks.

Pathophysiology of Aspiration

Depending on the patients' degree of central nervous system (CNS) depression and the alertness of the anesthesia personnel, aspiration may go unrecognized (that is, silent aspiration) or it may lead to pulmonary complications. The crucial factors that relate to the development of pulmonary complications are pH, volume, and character of the aspirate. Toxic fluids (acid, alcohol, mineral oil, blood, and bile) are capable of producing chemical pneumonitis; bacterial pathogens can lead to bacterial infection; and inert substances (particulate matter) can obstruct the airway.

Clinical Presentation of Aspiration Pneumonitis

The complex clinical syndrome, popularly known as Mendelson's syndrome, consists of abrupt onset of cyanosis, tachycardia, dypsnea, and expiratory wheezing. Mendelson noted that hydrochloric acid, rather than bile or pancreatic enzymes, was responsible for aspiration pneumonitis (1). In the anesthetized but nonparalyzed patient, aspiration may be signaled by breath holding and hypotension, followed by labored respiration and wheezing as a result of severe brochospasm.

Pink, frothy, blood-stained fluid may indicate pulmonary edema. Increased airway resistance will necessitate high airway pressures, and high oxygen concentrations will be required to combat severe hypoxemia (Figure 60.1). In some silent episodes, aspiration may be misdiagnosed a number of hours later as atelectasis or pneumonia.

Carefully conducted studies in animals have shown that, within two minutes of aspiration, arterial blood pressure falls by 25% and a similar rise occurs in pulmonary artery pressure (6). Arterial PO_2 decreases, and PCO_2 increases with a concomitant fall in pH. A rapid increase in pulmonary shunting is evident with a diminution of minute volume. Intravascular volume is depleted by a shift of fluid into the interstitial space in an attempt to neutralize the offending acidity. Awe and co-workers reported that pH was raised from 4 to 5 in 15 minutes after instillation of 0.1 ammonium chloride (7).

The copious outpouring of pinkish exudate at the bronchiolar and alveolar levels causes a ventilation–perfusion imbalance, exacerbating the already existent hypoxemia. The lungs become edematous and heavy. The resulting pulmonary edema has been attributed to a blockade of lymphatics produced by thickening of alveolar walls and septal tissues. The great loss of plasma-derived transudate into the alveoli results in hypovolemia. Strangely enough, in chemical pneumonitis, there is only minimal alteration in

the amount of pulmonary surfactant. Some authors have also found that increased alveolar capillary permeability causes acute pulmonary edema (6–8).

Aspiration of Pathogenic Bacteria

Bacterial sources could originate from oropharyngeal secretions or from gastric contents. Potential pulmonary pathogens are the anaerobic streptococci, fusobacteria, *Bacteroides melaninogenicus*, and gram-negative bacilli (*Escherichia coli, Klesiella*), *Pseudomonas*, or *Staphylococcus aureus*). The initial lesion is a pneumonitis that has hallmarks of fever and purulent sputum. Onset is insidious, and symptoms are mild. After 8–14 days, it may lead to tissue necrosis, with abscesses or extension to the pleural space.

Aspiration of Inert Substances

Fluids such as saline solution, water, barium, and neutralized gastric contents produce no distinctive pulmonary lesions. If aspirated in small quantities, they cause only transient respiratory distress.

Particulate matter causes variable degrees of mechanical respiratory obstruction. Large objects lodge in the upper airways and cause sudden respiratory distress, cyanosis, and death. Smaller objects reach peripheral airways and cause complete or partial obstruction.

Diagnostic Aids

In any episode of regurgitation, aspiration should be suspected even if no typical fluid can be suctioned from the tracheobronchial tree. An unexplained increase in the alveolar arterial oxygen gradient or radiologic suggestion of pulmonary infiltrate within 24 hours of the suspected event also strongly suggests aspiration. A sudden episode of "choking," coughing, or temporary cyanosis may sometimes be the only indication of aspiration of foreign material. This is more likely to occur in semicomatose patients or in those recovering from general anesthesia.

In cases of frank aspiration, the marked deterioration of arterial blood gas values (hypoxemia and hypercarbia), accompanied by respiratory or metabolic acidosis, confirms the diagnosis. The degree of dysfunction may serve as a guide to the degree of aggressiveness necessary in therapy. A severe de-

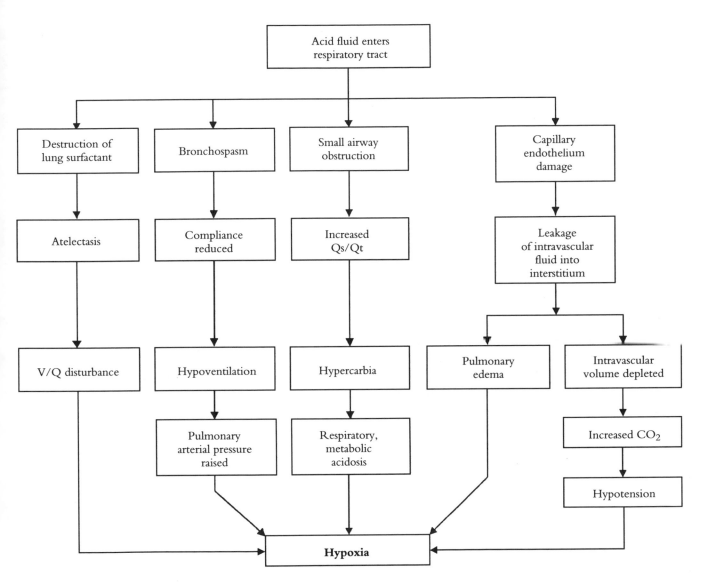

Figure 60.1   Mechanisms that lead to hypoxia.

crease in compliance, mostly at the expense of lung recoil and elasticity, further confirms aspiration or may be one more indication in otherwise unsuspected cases. A massive, diffuse, cloudy, patchy infiltrate seen radiologically in patients in acute respiratory failure is strong evidence of aspiration.

Postmortem examination may show food particles in the tracheobronchial tree; however, if only gastric juice was inhaled, patchy atelectasis, hemorrhagic areas, and perialveolar air leaks may be demonstrated in the most extreme cases (8). Microscopically, a peribronchial infiltrate may be accompanied by structural alveolar damage and hyaline exudate.

Prevention Strategies

As with many other complications, prevention is preferable to treatment. The choice of anesthetic agents and techniques and the skill and judgment exercised by the anesthesiologist are crucial. Highly trained and competent anesthesia personnel need to be available for 24-hour obstetric coverage if this preventable complication is to be avoided.

When anesthesia in a patient presumed to have a full stomach is contemplated, regional techniques are indicated if the surgery is to take place in the extremities, lower abdomen, or perineum. Pregnant patients should always be considered as having a full stomach. Depending on the urgency of the surgical procedure, they would benefit from regional anesthesia. This does not preclude the possibility of regurgitation and aspiration if a spinal and epidural block is excessively high or if patients are oversedated or placed in positions that make them unable to swallow or spit out the pharyngeal content.

Intubation with the patient awake does not guarantee that aspiration will not occur, but it may be the safest technique in patients who have a full stomach or a difficult airway. Although intubation while awake is an uncomfortable procedure for the patient, it can be made more tolerable by spraying the palate and pharynx with a topical anesthetic or giving the patient a small dose of a sedative. Fiberoptic intubation or oral intubation while the patient is awake can be accomplished by experienced anesthesia personnel. The sensory and motor integrity of the vocal cords must be maintained until the endotracheal tube is in place and the cuff inflated to separate the airway from the GI tract.

An alternative is "rapid sequence" or "crash" intubation. The patient is placed in the slight reverse Trendelenburg position and preoxygenated for at least 3–5 minutes. A drug such as thiopental 4 mg/kg; ketamine 0.5 to 1.0 mg/kg; or etomidate 0.1 to 0.2 mg/kg is given IV, followed by succinylcholine 1.0 to 1.5 mg/kg. As soon as the patient becomes unconscious, a trained assistant compresses the esophagus posteriorly between the cricoid ring and the cervical spine (Sellick's maneuver). Application of cricoid pressure while the patient is awake may induce coughing and subsequent regurgitation, or vomiting may occur. To prevent muscle fasciculations, a small dose of nondepolarizing muscle relaxant (usually 3 mg of d-tubocurarine) may be given three minutes before the depolarizing muscle relaxant. As soon as signs of muscle relaxation are evidenced by the cessation of the train-of-four in the nerve stimulator pattern, intubation is performed gently but

promptly, and the cuff is inflated. Only after this sequence is completed should positive pressure ventilation be initiated.

Regardless of the method used, effective suction should be available to the anesthesiologist. The anesthesiologist should be alert to such symptoms as sudden oxygen desaturation, increasing end-tidal CO_2, and increasing airway pressures, which may herald impending catastrophe.

Since the pH and the volume of gastric aspirate were considered as main determinants of the severity of aspiration pneumonitis, several pharmacologic regimens were developed to increase gastric pH or decrease gastric volume. Dewan and co-authors demonstrated that 64% of nonpremedicated patients scheduled to have elective cesarean section have a gastric pH below 2.5 and gastric volume greater than 25 mL (9). No patients showed these risks if they received sodium citrate within 60 minutes of the procedure, whereas 50% showed the risks if sodium citrate was given within more than 60 minutes of the procedure. Hence, the author concluded that sodium citrate effectively raises gastric pH when given less than 60 minutes prior to induction of anesthesia.

Prior ingestion of antacid may reduce the effects of aspiration. However, it is evident that differences exist among various antacids. The potential for lung damage after particular antacids such as magnesium and aluminum hydroxide has been demonstrated in several animal studies, ranging from histologic changes of acute inflammation to severe bronchopneumonia. Moreover, significantly greater lung weights and lower arterial oxygen tension followed the particulate compared with the nonparticulate antacid aspiration. There has also been a report of a case in which the administration of a magnesium and hydroxide suspension was followed by severe hypoxia, decreased compliance, and bilateral pulmonary infiltrates, lasting up to seven days (10).

H_2 receptor antagonists such as cimetidine (Tagamet) and ranitidine (Zantac) have shown promising results in reducing the acidity and volume of gastric contents. Manchikanti and co-workers noted no significant differences between the groups given cimetidine (300 mg) and ranitidine (150 or 300 mg) with respect to gastric pH and mean gastric volume (11). Ranitidine has gained popularity for aspiration prophylaxis because of its longer duration of action. It may also lack some of the side effects that can occur with the former agent. Newer H_2-receptor antagonists are being investigated, including Roxatidine acetate (12), omeprazole (13) and famotidine (14).

Dopaminergic antagonists such as metoclopramide (Reglan) have been shown to accelerate gastric emptying and improve lower esophageal sphincter tone in both elective and emergency surgery patients. The drug also appears to have no adverse effect on the baby. It is probably of benefit to parturients at high risk for aspiration (obese patients with a history of heartburn, peptic ulcer, those undergoing elective general anesthesia, and patients with a difficult airway). In a study of elective surgery patients, a two-drug regimen of cimetidine and metoclopramide raised gastric pH above 2.5 and lowered gastric volume to below 25 mL in all patients receiving both drugs (19).

Preventing aspiration pneumonitis by such measures as esophageal intubation and production of emesis are uncomfortable for the patient, not fully effective, and potentially harmful. In semicomatose and unconscious patients, prophylactic endotracheal intubation should be performed while they are in the lateral decubitus position. In patients recovering from general anesthesia, the cuffed endotracheal tube should be left in place until the patient is fully awake and has recovered laryngeal and pharyngeal reflexes. It is advisable to empty the stomach while the patient is intubated to reduce the possibility of aspiration of gastric contents after extubation.

Therapy Options

Appropriate and systematic plans to manage a difficult airway should be followed to decrease the incidence of aspiration during induction. The reader is referred to the algorithm developed for managing problematic airways (16). Once aspiration is confirmed, intubation of the trachea with immediate suctioning should be performed. Lavage with large quantities of saline tends to distribute the material further into the periphery of the lungs and may further decrease compliance and increase pulmonary shunting. Bronchoscopy is indicated whenever large particles occlude major airways.

Repeated determinations of arterial blood gases provide a guide for a more aggressive approach to respiratory therapy. If the PaO_2 is greater than 60 mm Hg, supplemental oxygen and chest physiotherapy may be all that are needed. With greater degrees of pulmonary impairment, endotracheal intubation with mechanical ventilation should be undertaken immediately. Often, high inflation pressures to deliver adequate tidal volume are necessary. One may need positive-end expiratory pressure (PEEP) whenever adequate oxygen tensions are not maintained with intermittent positive pressure ventilation on volume cycled ventilators. Studies in dogs demonstrated that 10-day mortality could be reduced from 80% to 0% by the immediate institution of PEEP for eight hours. When this was delayed for 24 hours, the dogs died. Pulmonary angiograms demonstrated vasospasm and thrombosis in branches of the pulmonary arteries of untreated animals, but these changes did not occur in animals treated with six hours of positive pressure ventilation.

Bronchodilator agents may be useful in relieving the reflex constriction that immediately follows aspiration and that may continue for several days. IV aminophylline, 1.6 mg/kg given in a bolus followed by maintenance infusion of 2.5 mg/kg per hour, appears to be the most effective. It must be kept in mind that aminophylline can augment any associated tachycardia or dysrhythmia. Pharmacologic vasodilation of the pulmonary arterioles is currently under investigation using nitric oxide inhalation.

The tachycardia and hypotension seen after aspiration reflect hypovolemia, but volume replacement must be judiciously undertaken by the infusion of plasma or plasma substitutes. Excessive volumes of crystalloid or colloid agents may worsen the pulmonary edema. Monitoring should include central venous pressure, urinary output, and pulse and blood pressure as well as O_2 saturation. In the critically ill patients, pulmonary capillary wedge pressure obtained by Swan-Ganz catheterization may be a more reliable guide to fluid management.

Restoring volume is of paramount importance when mechanical ventilation with PEEP is contemplated. In the hypovolemic patient, PEEP can retard venous return, thereby decreasing cardiac output and accentuating hypoxemia.

Intermittent mandatory ventilation may be used instead of controlled ventilation. It has been shown to decrease continuous intrapleural pressures, thus decreasing the possibility of barotrauma to the lungs; it also has less drastic effects on cardiac output.

The value of steroids in treating aspiration pneumonitis appears controversial. Sukumaran and co-workers, in a controlled clinical trial, evaluated corticosteroid treatment in patients with neurologic disorders and young patients who had drug overdoses with aspiration of gastric contents (17). Although the corticosteroid treatment reduced the time for x-ray and arterial blood-gas normalization in the neurologic patients, they remained in the intensive care unit longer. There was no significant difference in the occurrence of complications or mortality between treatment and control groups. Other investigators who reported beneficial effects from steroid therapy may have misinterpreted the more rapid clearing of roentgenograms and higher arterial tensions as resulting from the steroids instead of from positive pressure ventilation, which was used when necessary.

The role of prophylactic antibiotics is also controversial. In an investigation of 43 patients with clinical evidence of aspiration, the majority were drug overdose cases, nine followed massive trauma, and four were related to induction of anesthesia (18). All trauma patients were being treated with antibiotics for their wounds, and samples from these patients grew mixed flora on culture. Staphylococci were found primarily in the patients suffering from drug overdoses. Yeast and *Pseudomonas* appeared later. Of those clearly associated with anesthesia, two were negative, one grew *Staphylococcus aureus*, and the last cultured predominantly gram-negative organisms. This study strongly supports the concept that patients who aspirate should receive prophylactic antibiotics only if there is another infective focus. Frequent cultures of tracheobronchial secretions should dictate therapy, and only when cultures are positive should antibiotics be instituted.

Precautions in Order

Aspiration pneumonia remains an important cause of morbidity and mortality in anesthesia. The parturients are especially at risk because of increased intraabdominal pressure, delayed gastric emptying, high gastric acidity, increased gas-

tric acid production, pain, and anxiety. Provided that there are no contraindications, properly administered regional anesthesia remains preferable to general anesthesia. Pharmacologic regimens such as nonparticulate antacids are available. When administered within 60 minutes of induction of anesthesia, they will raise the pH of gastric juice in all susceptible patients. H_2 receptor antagonists (cimetidine or ranitidine), which decrease gastric acidity and gastric volume, should be considered. Metoclopromide, by decreasing gastric emptying time and increasing lower esophageal sphincter tone, may play an increasing role in the prevention of aspiration pneumonitis.

However, despite antacid, H_2 blockers, and cricoid pressure, aspiration pneumonitis may still occur. While precautions may ameliorate the effects of gastric acid in the stomach, they will not eliminate it.

CASE 60.1 A Case of Pneumonia

A 22-year-old primigravida was admitted in labor at 39 weeks' gestation. An emergency cesarean section was decided on because of apparent acute fetal distress. Past medical history included a seizure disorder as a result of head trauma six months earlier. The patient was given Shohl's solution (30 mL orally), metoclopramide (Reglan) (10 mg), and ranitidine (Zantac) (50 mg IV) a few minutes prior to induction of anesthesia. A rapid sequence induction was carried out with thiopental (Pentothal) and succinylcholine (Anectine, Quelicin, Sucostrin), followed by cricoid pressure. However, while this last procedure was being performed, a large amount of gastric fluid oozed from the patient's mouth and nose. After this was suctioned, a tube was inserted into the trachea without difficulty. More gastric contents were removed. But her oxygen saturation dropped to 60%, and she became progressively bradycardic. She was given 100% oxygen, followed by IV epinephrine. Her heart rate and oxygen saturation rapidly returned to normal limits. Surgery was begun.

A baby girl was delivered in two minutes with Apgar scores of 3 and 7, at one and five minutes, respectively. Maternal arterial blood revealed pH, 7.18; PO_2, 48; PCO_2, 32; O_2SO_2, 71.4%; HCO_3, 11.6; and BE, -15. The pH of aspirated material was 5.5. Mechanical ventilation was administered with a tidal volume of 550, respiratory rate of 8, PEEP of 15 cm, and airway pressure of 35–40 cm H_2O. Vital signs remained stable throughout surgery while the oxygen saturation was maintained between 90% and 97%.

A pulmonary artery catheter was inserted postoperatively (Figure 60.2). Arterial blood gases deteriorated. PEEP was increased up to 35 cm H_2O, and airway pressures reached as high as 90 cm H_2O over several days. She developed several pneumothoraces that were treated with chest tube drainage. She also developed *Pseudomonas* pneumonia and received antibiotics for several weeks. The rest of her organ systems remained normal. She had a tracheostomy six weeks postoperatively. She eventually showed marked improvement in her arterial blood gases and pulmonary function. She was discharged from the hospital nine weeks postoperatively. ■

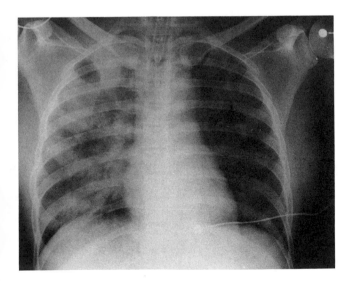

Figure 60.2 Roentgenogram findings noted three hours after massive aspiration include bilateral consolidation in both lungs and superimposed pulmonary edema.

References

1. Mendelson CL. The aspiration of stomach contents into the lungs during obstetric anesthesia. Am J Obstet Gynecol 1946;52:191.
2. Berson W, Adriani J. Silent regurgitation and aspiration during anesthesia. Anesthesiology 1954;15:644.
3. Butt D, Gutman HL, Cohen PD, et al. Silent regurgitation and aspiration during general anesthesia. Anesth Analg 1970;49:707.
4. Tomkins J, Turnbull A, Robson G, et al. Report on confidential enquiries into maternal deaths in England and Wales, 1976–1978. London: Her Majesty's Stationery Office, 1982.
5. Ong BV, Palahniuk RJ, Cumming M. Gastric volume and pH in outpatients. Can Anaesth Soc J 1978;25:38.
6. Bosomworth PP, Coyer J, Bryant LR. Aspiration of gastric juice: physiologic alterations. Anesthesiology 1965;26:241.
7. Awe WC, Fletcher WJ, Jacob SW. The pathophysiology of aspiration pneumonitis. Surgery 1966;60:232.
8. Bartlett J, Gorbach S. The triple threat of aspiration pneumonia. Chest 1975;68:560.
9. Dewan D, Floyd H, Thistelwood J, et al. Sodium citrate pretreatment in elective cesarian section patients. Anesth Analg 1985;64:34.
10. Bond VK, Stoelting RK, Gupta CD. Pulmonary aspiration syndrome after inhalation of gastric fluid containing antacids. Anesthesiology 1979;51:452.
11. Manchikanti L, Colliver J, Roush. Evaluation of ranitidine as an oral antacid in outpatient anesthesia. Southern Med J 1985;78:818.
12. Murdoch D, McTavish D. Roxatidine Acetate. A review of its pharmacodynamic and pharmacokinetic properties, and its therapeutic potential in peptic ulcer disease and related disorders. Drugs 1991;42(22):240–60.
13. Ewart MC, Yaw G, Gin T, Rotor CF, Oh TA. Comparison of the effects of omeprazole and ranitidine on gastric secretion in women undergoing elective caesarean section. Anaesthesia 1990;45:527–30.
14. Jahr JS, Barckart G, Smith SS, Shapiro J, Cook DR. Effects of Famotidine on gastric Ph and residual volume in pediatric surgery. Acta Anaesthesia Scand 1991;35:457–60.
15. Capan LM, Rosenberg AD, Carni A. Effect of cimetidine-metoclopramide combination on gastric fluid volume and acidity. Anesthesiology 1983;59(suppl):A402.
16. Benumof JL. Management of the difficult adult airway with special emphasis on awake tracheal intubation. Anesthe-

siology 1991;75:1087–110.

17. Sukumaran M, Granada M, Beyer, et al. Evaluation of corticosteroid treatment in aspiration of gastric contents. A controlled clinical trial. Mt Sinai J Med 1980;47:35.

18. Aldrete JA, Liem ST. Carrow DJ. Pulmonary aerobic bacterial flora after aspiration pneumonitis. J Trauma 1975;15:1014.

61

Epidural Anesthesia

William C. Wright, M.D.

IDEAL obstetric anesthesia isn't achieved easily. Whereas primary concern formerly tended to be for maternal welfare, in today's era of electronic fetal heart rate monitoring and antenatal testing, the fetus has achieved equality.

It's now axiomatic that anesthesia should provide pain relief without posing harm to either mother or fetus or interfering with progress of labor. Easy conversion to a surgical anesthetic when cesarean section is necessary is also important, as is providing effective nonstuporous postpartum pain relief.

Unique Characteristics of the Obstetric Patient

The healthy obstetric patient is physiologically different from other "normal" healthy patients in being subject to illnesses unique to, or complicated by, pregnancy, such as gestational diabetes or eclampsia. In addition, the fetus's condition may dictate the course of pregnancy, including labor and delivery, as well as the choice of anesthesia. Further, unlike the usual surgical patient, admission is unscheduled, so that the mother may arrive with a full stomach or otherwise be unprepared for anesthesia.

To minimize these problems, anesthesiologists should ideally become involved with patients earlier than the time of delivery. As participants in prenatal education classes, anesthesiologists have been very effective in counteracting misinformation that has made many women fearful of anesthesia.

Also important is the anesthesiologist's role as a medical consultant. Such activity will assure that patients with cardiac disease, pregnancy-induced hypertension, or diabetes will never find the anesthesiologist unprepared. Moreover, anesthetizing the very obese patient, who has special requirements, can be planned well in advance of confinement. Finally, anesthesiologists can teach obstetricians the value of anesthesia's early involvement with high-risk patients.

Unlike most general surgical patients, couples awaiting childbirth usually wish to participate in management decisions. Most women prefer to remain alert and to have the father present at vaginal or cesarean delivery.

Method of Choice

The anesthetic technique that seems best to meet the needs of mother, fetus, and obstetrician is continuous lumbar epidural block. By placing a catheter into the epidural space, the discomfort of both labor and delivery can be relieved without markedly affecting progress of labor or dulling the patient's consciousness.

When properly managed, this approach can be safe for mother, fetus, and newborn. It also allows the patient to participate actively in the second stage of labor and delivery.

Bupivacaine (Marcaine, Sensorcaine), an amide local anesthetic, provides increased safety for fetuses of mothers receiving epidurals. Its affinity for binding to tissues of the epidural space, as well as to maternal plasma proteins, considerably reduces the amount of free drug passing the placenta and entering the fetus. Thus, the ratio of umbilical-to-maternal blood levels of local anesthetic is markedly lower than with lidocaine and mepivacaine, other amide local anesthetics that have been commonly used.

The enhanced capacity of bupivacaine to bind to epidural space tissues prolongs its action on nerve fibers crossing this space. Therefore, it produces blockade more effectively than equivalent doses of lidocaine or mepivacaine.

Continuous infusion of dilute bupivacaine through the epidural catheter is gaining in popularity. It has the advantage of either eliminating the need for "top-ups" or increasing the interval between them. Besides improved comfort, there may be a salutory effect on labor and fetal well-being through avoidance of the periodic catecholamine surges that occur when an interval dosage wears down.

Recently, solutions combining Marcaine with lipid-soluble opiates have been found to work more effectively than either alone. The total dosages required, as well as the onset of action, were decreased. Duration of action was lengthened and the overall quality of analgesia improved without decreasing maternal or neonatal safety.

Should labor fail to progress and abdominal delivery become necessary, the same continuous epidural catheter can convert analgesia to surgical anesthesia by increasing the local anesthetic drug concentration and volume. The patient, remaining awake and comfortable, can see and hear her child during the first seconds of its life.

Postoperative Morphine

Postoperative pain relief can be achieved by injecting 3.5–5 mg of preservative-free morphine through the epidural catheter as surgery is being completed. The pain relief is superior to and longer acting than that provided by parenteral injections. Relief averages 20 hours and leads to the patient's experiencing a more motivated attitude, earlier walking, and the probability of earlier discharge.

Side effects are few and seem to be dose-related. The most common is pruritus. The most serious, delayed respiratory depression, is avoided if dosage is kept low and parenteral narcotics not given concurrently. Urinary retention is not uncommon and can be avoided by allowing the urinary catheter to remain in the bladder for the first 24 hours after surgery. Naloxone (Narcan), a narcotics antagonist, is effective for treating side effects if they are severe but may shorten analgesia.

Alternative Approaches

Extreme emergencies requiring immediate surgical intervention might be better managed by a technique, such as general or spinal anesthesia, that has a shorter onset to complete surgical anesthesia than the 10–15 minutes required by epidural block. Therefore, precautions against aspiration of stomach contents, which might occur with emergency inhalation anesthesia, are required for all patients.

Paracervical, pudendal, subarachnoid, and caudal techniques have been used, singly or in combination, to achieve the same results as those of epidurals. However, none compares in overall ability to provide first- and second-stage pain relief, convert readily into a surgical anesthetic, if necessary, and deliver prolonged postoperative analgesia.

Subarachnoid Block

Although subarachnoid block continues to be widely used, such use is primarily late in the second stage, just before delivery. If given sooner, motor blockade hinders pushing, prolonging the second stage, and may necessitate the use of forceps. Small amounts of drug provide excellent, almost immediate pain relief for delivery, as well as good perineal relaxation via the motor blockade that accompanies sensory loss.

Interruption of sympathetic impulses to blood vessels can cause hypotension, especially if the patient is in the supine position. This potential is far greater with spinal than with epidural anesthesia.

Saddle block, a more localized variation of subarachnoid block, has fewer adverse cardiovascular effects and therefore remains popular for delivery. However, it has been associated with an approximately 10% incidence of postspinal headaches.

Such side effects are less common and severe with epidurals, which have the added advantage of providing relief earlier in labor without affecting its progress. Mothers who have undergone both procedures generally prefer epidural analgesia since they retain motor control and are able to comfortably push the baby out.

Minidose morphine (0.25 mg) deposited into the subarachnoid space has been shown to provide good pain relief during first-stage labor. However, relief is inadequate for the second stage.

This problem might be resolved by using a conventional Tuohy needle positioned in the epidural space as an introducer through which a newly developed spinal needle (manufactured by Vigon Corp., Rutherford, N.J.) can be inserted into the subarachnoid space to deposit medication. A conventional catheter can then be threaded through the Tuohy into the epidural space to give local anesthetic for second-stage pain relief or for surgical anesthesia and postpartum pain relief if needed. The method shows great promise since it should greatly reduce drug exposure, as well as potential for headache and cardiovascular compromise.

Other Block Techniques

Besides lumbar epidural and subarachnoid blocks, only caudal block can provide both first- and second-stage pain relief. A caudal is an epidural given at a lower location: the sacral hiatus. It is rarely used today since it requires considerably more local anesthetic to achieve first-stage pain relief than does the lumbar epidural, and it tends to prolong the second stage by blocking the sacral nerve roots before full cervical dilation, thus eliminating the urge to push. The once-popular paracervical block is rarely used any more for first-stage pain relief owing to the frequent incidence of fetal bradycardias occurring after its administration.

The pudendal block, taught to all obstetric residents, remains popular as a method of numbing the vaginal outlet. Its advantage is that it does not interfere with the patient's ability to feel her contractions or push effectively. It also provides adequate pain relief for placement of outlet forceps, if needed.

Collaboration

To achieve best results, the obstetrician and anesthesiologist must work as a team during labor and delivery. In choosing an anesthetic method, they should together consider preexisting medical conditions, important prenatal history, fetal gestational age, and course of labor. Having the obstetrician introduce the patient to the anesthesiologist while she is in early labor will decrease her anxiety about a long, painful experience and make it easier to bear transient discomfort.

To provide service, an anesthesiologist must be available 24 hours a day exclusively for obstetrics. Since few delivery services have sufficient patient volume to provide such coverage, consolidating small units of fewer than 150 deliveries into larger centralized ones seems a desirable alternative.

Effect on Labor

To avoid having an anesthetic possibly impede the progression of labor, we place a catheter early in labor so as to provide immediate relief when needed, but encourage the patient to go as far as she can without medication. Provided hypotension is avoided, small incremental doses or a continuous controlled infusion of dilute local anesthetic will make the patient comfortable without slowing labor.

Comfortably relaxed patients are less likely to have elevated catecholamine titers or surges that might interfere with labor progress. Accordingly, it is not unusual for efficiency of labor to be enhanced.

When delivery is imminent, we sit the patient up and inject a dose of local anesthetic solution through the catheter sufficient to produce perineal anesthesia. A catheter placed between L-2 and L-4 provides good pain relief during labor, as well as the perineal relaxation and anesthesia necessary for delivery. Most patients are aware of pressure at delivery but rarely seem to find it very uncomfortable.

It is best to tailor drug concentration to the task at hand. Many patients receive good first-stage pain relief with 0.125% bupivacaine repeated at 60- and 90-minute intervals. Bupivacaine in a 0.25% concentration works well for both first- and second-stage pain and can be used to augment a 0.125% concentration during the second stage. A combination of 6–8 mL of 0.25% bupivacaine with 50 μg of fentanyl citrate (Sublimaze) gives superior analgesia during labor for two hours or more and frequently carries the patient through delivery. At delivery, or if forceps are necessary, 10 mL of 3% chloroprocaine hydrochloride (Nesacaine) provides good relief.

Our effort is not to abolish all sensation, as with a subarachnoid block, but to ameliorate pain while retaining some feeling, which mothers often prefer. After delivery, the uterus can be explored and any repairs performed without causing discomfort.

Reducing Aspiration Risk

Nearly all anesthesia-related deaths are preventable. For example, aspiration of stomach contents, as well as intubation problems, contribute importantly to hypoxic cardiac arrest of mothers during childbirth. However, since both complications are associated primarily with inhalation anesthesia, they are far less likely to occur with epidural block.

Nevertheless, because each obstetric patient is a potential candidate for general anesthesia, all should be directed in advance not to eat or drink after going into labor (N.P.O.) since food ingested shortly before or during labor can be retained in the stomach for 12 or more hours after ingestion. More important than the food itself is the fact that it stimulates increased secretion of hydrochloric acid, which, if aspirated, may cause fatal gastric aspiration.

A cuffed endotracheal tube is mandatory, as is cricoid pressure by an assistant before and during insertion. This pressure, which prevents the silent regurgitation of stomach contents, should not be released until tube placement is assured and the cuff inflated.

Minimizing Hypotension

Marked hypotension is less frequent, severe, and quick in onset with epidural than with spinal anesthesia. Nevertheless, one can and should avoid it at all costs. Women in labor are frequently volume-depleted. Having not eaten or drunk, as instructed, and undergoing considerable fluid loss through perspiration and hyperventilation while in labor, most tend to be quite dehydrated. Superimposing sympathetic blockade produced by epidural anesthesia on this volume-depleted state creates the potential for a tragic outcome.

Intravenous fluid infusion of 150–200 mL hourly for all healthy patients in active labor, as well as a bolus fluid load of 500–1,000 mL of Ringer's lactate just before epidural administrations, should prevent dangerous falls in blood pressure. In addition, preventing patients in labor from lying supine reduces the incidence of aortocaval compression. Such compression, combined with sympathetic blockade, greatly impedes venous return to the heart, causing systemic hypotension and decreased perfusion to the fetus. When the supine position becomes necessary, as it generally does at delivery or during cesarean section, a hip wedge that tilts the uterus laterally "off" of the vena cava is helpful.

Although fluid loading and uterine displacement usually prevent hypotension, refractory cases may require β-active vasopressors, such as ephedrine or mephentermine (Wyamine), to return pressure to normal. A 20% fall merits treatment.

Conclusion

Besides providing long-term comfort for the mother with small doses of drug, use of catheters for continuous lumbar epidural block has allowed obstetricians to avoid hurriedly requesting a last-minute, single-shot epidural. Also, because nursing personnel can monitor patients after the cardiovascular system has stabilized, several patients can be under epidural block simultaneously.

As noted, the epidural catheter should be inserted before the patient needs analgesia since it assures cooperation. Further, this approach allows ample time to observe the test dose's effect, evaluate the analgesic dose, and correct any spottiness or unilaterality in the block.

After 21 years of service with exclusively obstetric anesthesia, we believe epidural block is the best method of pain relief for uncomplicated labor and delivery. Responses of patients, neonatologists, and obstetricians support this opinion. However, despite the technique's intrinsic merits, safety depends on the individual anesthesiologist's skills.

Suggested Reading

Abouleish EI, Rawal N, Fallon K, et al. Combined intrathecal morphine and bupivacaine for cesarean section. Anesthesiology 1987;67(A):619.

Ahuja BR, Strunen L. Respiratory effects of epidural fentanyl. Anaesthesia 1985;40:959.

Bader AM, Ray N, Datta S. Continuous epidural infusion of alfentanil and bupivacaine for labor and delivery. Int J Obstet Anesth 1992;1:187–90.

Bogod DG, Rosen M, Reese G, et al. Extradural infusion of 0.125% bupivacaine at 10 mL/hr to women during labour. Br J Anaesth 1987;59:325.

Borgeat A, Wilder-Smith OHG, Saish M, Rifat K. Subhypnotic doses of propofol relieve pruritus induced by epidural morphine. Anesthesiology 1992;678:510–12.

Breen TW, Janzen JA, et al. Epidural fentanyl and caesarean section: when should fentanyl be given? Can J Anesth 1992; 39:317–22.

Celleno D, Capogna G. Epidural fentanyl plus bupivacaine 0.125% for labour: analgesic effects. Can J Anaesth 1988; 35:375.

Coates MB. Combined subarachnoid and epidural techniques. Anaesthesia 1982;37:89.

Hicks JA, Jenkins JG, Newton MC, et al. Continuous epidural infusion of 0.075% bupivacaine for pain relief in labour. Anaesthesia 1988;43:289.

Howell CJ, Chalmers I. A review of prospectively controlled comparisons of epidural with nonepidural forms of pain relief during labor. Int J Obstet Anesth 1992;1:93–110.

Knapp RM, Writer D. Epidural narcotics in obstetrics: survey of SOAP members (Abstract). SOAP 1988:66.

Leighton BL, DeSimone CA, Norris MC, et al. Intrathecal narcotics for labor revisited: fentanyl 25 μg and morphine 0.25 mg provide rapid, profound analgesia. Anesthesiology 1988;69(A):680.

Li DF, Rees GA, Rosen M. Continuous extradural infusion of 0.0625% or 0.125% bupivacaine for pain relief in primigravida labour. Br J Anaesth 1985;57:264.

Lomessy A, Magnin C, Viale JP, et al. Clinical advantages of fentanyl given epidurally for postoperative analgesia. Anesthesiology 1984;61:466.

Scanlon JW, Ostheimer GW, Lurie AO, et al. Neurobehavioral responses and drug concentrations in newborns after maternal epidural anesthesia with bupivacaine. Anesthesiology 1976;45:400.

Shnider SM, Levinson G, eds. Anesthesia for obstetrics. Baltimore: Williams & Wilkins, 1979:113.

Wang BC, Hiller JM, Simon EJ, et al. Distribution of 3-H Morphine after epidural administration in unanesthetized rabbits. Regional Anesth 1992;17:334–9.

PART EIGHT Neonatal Considerations

62

Assessing Maturity

Larry N. Cook, M.D.

IN the past decade, it has become increasingly evident that birthweight is a poor determinant of gestational age. As many as 25% of low-birthweight infants (less than 2,500 g) are victims of deviant fetal growth or intrauterine growth retardation (IUGR). Under usual circumstances, fetal growth and gestational age are directly related to and reflected in measures of height, weight, and head circumference.

Gestational age is the quantitator of fetal growth. Neonates of less than 37 weeks' gestation are designated "preterm" or "premature;" those between 38 and 42 weeks, "term" or "mature;" and those beyond 42 weeks, "postterm" or "postmature." The quality of fetal growth is expressed by birthweight percentile. At a given gestational age, a newborn less than the 10th percentile for weight is designated small for gestational age; between the 10th and 90th, appropriate for gestational age; and greater than the 90th, large for gestational age.

Many conditions can result in deviant fetal growth. Maternal chronic hypertension, for example, can cause marked intrauterine growth retardation.

Fetal wastage correlates strongly with intrauterine growth retardation, whereas neonatal mortality correlates more with prematurity. The prognosis of IUGR is distinctly different from that of prematurity. Morbidity and mortality are directly proportional to both birthweight and gestational age. Morbidity for the term infant, approximately 4%, is due mainly to congenital malformations, infection, and such obstetric accidents as perinatal asphyxia. Premature morbidity rates are inversely related to gestational age and weight and are much higher than term rates. For the perinatologist and neonatologist, the problems and management of the growth-regarded fetus or neonate are completely different from those of the preterm counterpart (Table 62.1).

Prenatal Assessment of Maturity

A system of assessing the maturity, or gestational age, of the fetus and neonate is essential. The assessment of neonatal maturity actually begins prenatally with the obstetrician. The various approaches to prenatal assessment include the following:

Table 62.1 Problems of the Growth-retarded versus the Premature Infant

Growth-retarded Infant	Premature Infant
1. Fetal distress with or without death in utero	1. Respiratory: hyaline membrane disease, bronchopulmonary dysplasia
2. Asphyxia neonatorum and sequelae	2. Gastrointestinal: immature gut function, necrotizing entero-colitis
3. Meconium aspiration syndrome	
4. Perinatal hyperthermia	3. CNS: intraventricular/periventricular hemorrhage, long-term sequelae
5. Polycythemia and hyperviscosity	
6. Temperature instability	4. Patent ductus arteriosus
7. Hypoglycemia	5. Immature renal function
8. Pulmonary hemorrhage	6. Metabolic: hypoglycemia, hypocalcemia, hyperbilirubinemia, labile electrolyte concentration
9. Congenital malformations	
10. Nutrition: hypermetabolic state	7. Infection
11. Congenital infection	8. Temperature instability
12. Persistent pulmonary hypertension	9. Regulatory instability: apnea and bradycardia
13. Long-term consequences in growth and development	10. Oxygen toxicity including retinopathy
	11. Neurodevelopmental sequelae

Calculation of Gestational Age

This involves estimation of the date of confinement from the first day of the last normal menstrual period as related by the mother.

Prenatal Clinical Evaluation

When the woman participates in early and regular prenatal care, the early signs of pregnancy (nausea, vomiting, fatigue, breast changes), as well as increasingly sophisticated pregnancy tests, become helpful in defining conception. Perception of fetal movement, recognition of fetal heartbeat, and palpation of the uterine fundus at the umbilicus are helpful 20-week milestones. Maternal habitus, fetal size, and quantity of amniotic fluid are possible sources of error in clinically assessing fetal maturity.

Prenatal Laboratory Assessment

The use of ultrasound to measure the crown-rump length in the first trimester and the biparietal diameter, head circumference, and femur length in the second trimester provides reliable correlation of these measurements with gestational age. Generally, ultrasound measurements in the third trimester are less reliable predictors of gestational age because of the biologic variation in normal fetuses later in pregnancy. The accuracy of determining gestational age by ultrasound measurement is diminished in certain conditions, notably maternal diabetes and multiple gestations. Although their clinical applicability has been largely replaced by ultrasound, measurements in amniotic fluid, such as of creatinine, protein concentration, optical density at 450 nm, percentage of fat-laden fetal cells, the lecithin/sphingomyelin ratio, and the phospholipid profile, have been shown to correlate with gestational age. While the ability to predict fetal weight accurately continues to improve, gestational age continues to be the best guideline for pregnancy management. Keeping a fetus in utero for the two weeks from 26 to 28 weeks will improve survival from 50% to 85% and result in substantial reductions in costs of care.

Postnatal Assessment of Maturity

Physical Characteristics

In the past decade, investigators have demonstrated correlation between certain physical characteristics and gestational age. Early work by Usher, Dubowitz, and Amiel-Tison has been combined into a clinically useful and simple scoring system by Ballard and co-workers. None of these is absolute for a given period of gestation. Many are influenced by intrauterine events, and, in a given infant, not all indications may agree. If they are taken collectively, however, they yield a reliable estimate of gestational age (Table 62.2). When a discrepancy with prenatal assessment of more than two weeks is found, a decision in favor of the postnatal exam is advised.

Vernix tends to appear at about 24 weeks, covers the fetus between 25 and 38 weeks, decreases in amount from 39 to 41 weeks, and tends to disappear when gestation is prolonged past 42 weeks.

Fetal breast tissue tends to be absent up to 34 weeks and increases in amount as gestation advances. The breast nodule measures 1–2 mm at 36 weeks, 4 mm at 38 weeks, and 7 mm after 39 weeks. Since IUGR is frequently accompanied by loss of subcutaneous fat, the breast nodule may be diminished. Nipples are barely visible up to 31 weeks, are well defined and have a flat areola from 32 to 36 weeks, and are well defined and have a raised areola at 37 weeks and beyond.

Transverse creasing of the soles is one of the most reliable physical findings. Up to 31 weeks, the bottom of the foot is smooth. Creases are found on the anterior third of the sole until 36 weeks, on the anterior two-thirds of the sole from 36 to 39 weeks, and on the entire sole after 39 weeks.

Just as bone deposition increases throughout pregnancy, so does the definition and strength of cartilage. Up to 33 weeks, ear cartilage is soft and the pinna stays folded when bent. From 34 to 37 weeks, the ear returns slowly from folding; from 37 to 39 weeks, it springs back vigorously; and from 39 weeks on, the ear is firm and remains erect from the side of the head. There is similar maturation of ear form.

In the male neonate, the testicles are undescended before 30 weeks. From 31 weeks to 35 weeks, they are high in the inguinal canal; from 36 to 39 weeks, they descend into the scrotum, which becomes progressively rugated; and by 39 weeks, the testes are present in the pendulous rugated scrotum.

Before 35 weeks in the female neonate, the labia majora are wide apart and the clitoris is prominent. To an inexperienced observer, the genitalia may appear ambiguous. From 36 to 39 weeks, the labia majora begin to cover the clitoris, and by 39 weeks, the clitoris is usually not visible. In a clinical situation such as maternal diabetes, where there are altered amounts of fat, the appearance will vary according to the amount of adipose tissue present.

Hair first appears on the fetal head around the 20th week. From 24 to 30 weeks, eyebrows and eyelashes develop. Up to 37 weeks, the hair has a fine woolly texture, after which it becomes more silky and separable into single strands. Lanugo appears at 20 weeks, covers the body from 24 to 27 weeks, is present only on the shoulders by 37 weeks, and is absent beyond that time.

The skin is extremely thin from 24 to 34 weeks; it becomes thicker up to 41 weeks, after which it frequently desquamates. Up to 36 weeks, the skin is plethoric and translucent, and vessels are easily seen beneath it. The skin is pink from 37 to 39 weeks and pale pink to white beyond 39 weeks. Black infants take on a darker pigmentation after 39 weeks' gestation.

Up to 34 weeks, the cranial bones are soft up to 1 inch from the anterior fontanelle. By 38 weeks, the bones are hard, but the sutures can be displaced. Beyond 41 weeks, the bones are hard and the sutures cannot be displaced.

Neurologic Examination

The neurologic development of the neonate correlates strongly with gestational age (Table 62.3). The central nervous system (CNS) seems to mature at a steady rate, and its maturity is reflected in muscular tone and pattern of reflexes. The development of tone, in contrast to all other neurologic functions, begins in the lower extremities and pro-

Table 62.2 Physical Signs of Maturity

	24–31 Weeks	32–35 Weeks	36–37 Weeks	38–42 Weeks
Vernix	Tends to appear at about 24 weeks. Covers fetus between 25 and 38 weeks.			Decreases from 39 to 41 weeks; tends to disappear beyond 42 weeks.
Breast/Nipples	Fetal breast tissue absent; nipples barely visible.	Fetal breast tissue tends to be absent up to 34 weeks and increases in amount as gestation advances; nipples well defined with a flat areola from 32 to 36 weeks.	Fetal breast nodule measures 1–2 mm at 36 weeks; nipples well defined with a raised areola at 37 weeks and beyond.	Fetal breast nodule measures 4 mm at 38 weeks, 7 mm after 39 weeks; nipples well defined with a raised areola.
Sole Creases	Bottom of foot smooth.	Creases on anterior third of sole of foot.	Creases on anterior two-thirds of sole from 36 to 39 weeks.	Creases on entire sole after 39 weeks.
Ear Cartilage	Up to 33 weeks, ear cartilage is soft; pinna stays folded when bent.	From 34 to 37 weeks, the ear returns slowly.	From 37 to 39 weeks, the ear springs back vigorously.	From 39 weeks on, the ear is firm and stands out from the side of the head.
Genitalia	*Male*: Testicles undescended before 30 weeks. *Female*: Labia majora wide apart; clitoris prominent.	*Male*: From 31 to 35 weeks, testicles high in inguinal canal. *Female*: Labia majora wide apart; clitoris prominent.	*Male*: From 36–39 weeks, testicles descend into the scrotum, which becomes progressively rugate. *Female*: From 36 to 39 weeks, the labia majora begin to cover the clitoris.	*Male*: By 39 weeks, the testes are present in a pendulous rugate scrotum. *Female*: By 39 weeks, the clitoris is usually not visible.
Hair and Lanugo	Hair and lanugo appear around the 20th week; from 24 to 30 weeks, eyebrows and eyelashes develop; hair has a fine woolly texture; lanugo covers the body from 24–27 weeks.	Hair has a fine woolly texture.	Hair has a fine woolly texture; lanugo is present only on the shoulders by 37 weeks.	After 37 weeks, hair becomes more silky and separable into single strands; lanugo is absent beyond 37 weeks.
Skin	Skin is extremely thin up to 34 weeks. Up to 36 weeks, skin is plethoric and translucent; vessels are easily seen beneath it.		Skin becomes thicker; color is pink from 37 to 39 weeks.	After 41 weeks, the skin frequently desquamates; color is pale pink to white beyond 39 weeks (black infants take on darker pigmentation).
Skull Firmness	Up to 34 weeks, cranial bones are soft up to 1 inch from the anterior fontanelle.			By 38 weeks, bones are hard but sutures can be displaced; beyond 41 weeks, bones are hard and sutures cannot be displaced.

Table 62.3 Neurologic Signs of Maturity

	24–31 Weeks	32–35 Weeks	36–37 Weeks	38–42 Weeks
Posture	At 24 weeks, lateral decubitus position is assumed; up to 30 weeks, there is complete hypotonia.	From 30 to 33 weeks, there is slight increase in tone of lower extremities.	At 34 to 36 weeks, frog position is assumed.	After 37 weeks, there is maximum flexion of upper and lower extremities.
Recoil	Recoil absent up to 30 weeks.	From 30 to 34 weeks, recoil slight in lower extremities.	From 37 to 38 weeks, recoil appears in the arms.	Beyond 39 weeks, recoil is strong in both upper and lower extremities.
Popliteal Angle	Popliteal angle at 28 weeks is 180 degrees.		By 37 weeks, popliteal angle is 90 degrees.	
Heel-to-Ear Maneuver		Heel-to-ear maneuver difficult by 34 weeks.	Heel-to-ear maneuver impossible by 37 weeks.	
Scarf Maneuver		Up to 34 weeks, there is no resistance and a true "scarf" is formed.		By 38 weeks, the scarf maneuver is difficult.
Neck Extensors	Ability to lift the chin off the chest is absent at 30 weeks; strength of the neck flexors is absent until 32 weeks.	Ability to lift the chin off the chest is slight from 30 to 34 weeks and fair from 34 to 36 weeks.	Ability to lift the chin off the chest is good beyond 36 weeks; strength of the neck flexors is minimal to 37 weeks.	Strength of the neck flexors is fair beyond 38 weeks (term infants may hold their heads erect).
Moro Embrace Reflex	Barely apparent at 26 weeks.	Becomes increasingly well defined with increasing gestational age.		
Grasp Reflex	Fair at 31 weeks.	Solid from 32 to 36 weeks.	After 36 weeks, it may be strong enough to allow infant to be lifted off mattress.	

gresses cephalad. As with the physical examination, absolute gestational correlation cannot be made from a particular reflex or state of tone. The neurologic examination can be altered by stress at birth and is often unreliable for high-risk infants during the first 48 hours of life, when it is most critical to determine gestational age. Some neurologic indexes useful in assessing gestational age include posture, recoil, muscle tone, and grasp reflex.

Posture is defined as the position that the neonate assumes when supine. At 24 weeks, the lateral decubitus position is assumed, and up to 30 weeks, there is complete hypotonia. From 30 to 33 weeks, there is a slight increase in the tone of the lower extremities, so that at 34 to 36 weeks, the frog position is assumed. After 37 weeks, there is maximum flexion of the upper and lower extremities.

Recoil—the magnitude with which the arm or leg returns after stretching—is absent up to 30 weeks. From 30 weeks to 34 weeks, it is slight in the lower extremities; from 37 to 38 weeks, it appears in the arms; and beyond 39 weeks, it is strong in both the upper and lower extremities. At term, recoil of the arm almost causes the neonate to strike himself in the face.

Measurement of muscle tone is provided by the degree of the angle when the leg is extended at the knee. At 28 weeks, the popliteal angle is 180 degrees, and by 37 weeks, it is 90 degrees. Increasing muscle tone makes the heel-to-ear maneuver difficult by 34 weeks and almost impossible by 37 weeks. The scarf maneuver involves draping the arm under the chin and pulling it across the chest. Up to 34 weeks, there is no resistance, and a true "scarf" is formed. By 38 weeks, this has become difficult.

The ability to lift the chin off the chest is absent at 30 weeks, slight from 30 to 34 weeks, fair from 34 to 36 weeks, and good beyond 36 weeks. Similarly, the strength of the neck flexors is absent until 32 weeks, minimal to 37 weeks, and fair beyond 38 weeks. Many term infants have the ability to hold their heads erect. The startle reflex, although barely apparent at 26 weeks, becomes increasingly well-defined with increasing gestational age.

Grasp reflex is fair at 31 weeks, solid from 32 to 36 weeks, and often strong enough after 36 weeks to allow the infant to be lifted off the mattress. Many other reflexes can be distinguished during early periods of gestation but lose their definition afterward. For example, pupillary reactivity to light is established at 30 weeks. Rooting is minimal as early as 24 to 26 weeks and well established beyond 31 weeks in the healthy premature infant. Sucking is present from 24 weeks on, strong by 32 weeks, and synchronous with swallowing at 34 weeks—an important event with regard to feeding.

Regrettably, few specific neurologic or physical indicators exist to allow specific gestational age discrimination at the extremes of prematurity (24 to 28 weeks), where increasing numbers of very-low-birthweight infants challenge our perinatal care system. Hittner and co-workers have proposed the orderly disappearance of the anterior vascular capsule of the lens as a means of accurately assessing gestational age in this range. Recently the Ballard Maturational Score was refined and expanded into a new Ballard Score (NBS), achieving a better tool for the assessment of the extremely premature infant, as well as greater accuracy at more conventional gestational ages (range 20–44 weeks).

Behavioral Indications of Maturity

Important clues to the maturity of the neonate can be obtained by studying his or her behavior in the nursery. There is a direct relationship between ability to maintain body temperature and gestational age; small premature infants are susceptible to thermal stress and require support.

The ability to take nipple feedings, the percentage of birthweight loss initially, and the number of days required to regain weight are all related to gestational age. The small-for-dates baby frequently eats voraciously and gains weight rapidly. The mean peak in bilirubin levels secondary to physiological factors is directly proportional to the degree of prematurity. The occurrence of certain conditions, such as retrolental fibroplasia, patent ductus arteriosus, necrotizing enterocolitis, or intraventricular hemorrhage, can be used retrospectively to assess or confirm the degree of neonatal maturity. The ability of multiple forms of fetal stress to promote mature behavior, including pulmonary, out of relationship to gestational age is well known.

Laboratory Indications of Maturity

Our natural human desire for simplicity and certainty will probably keep us searching for a single test that correlates with gestational age. As yet, this goal has not been achieved, but some laboratory procedures give important clues to gestational age. As shown by Dreyfus-Brisac and co-workers, specific electroencephalogram (EEG) patterns correlate with gestational age, particularly when used in conjunction with a neurologic exam. Motor nerve conduction is related to the degree of myelinization of the CNS and, thus, is also related to advancing gestational age. Similarly, hemoglobin values generally show a progressive rise from 20 weeks to maturity. Levels of serum proteins and calcium are directly proportional to gestational age. Incubation of reticulocytes from cord blood has shown a greater percentage of fetal hemoglobin when synthesized by cells from premature infants than when synthesized by cells from mature controls

Conclusion

Assessment of fetal maturity requires a multidisciplinary approach, including combined pre- and postnatal evaluations. Prenatal evaluation leads to optimal management of the fetus, such as referral to a high-risk center for delivery while postnatal assessment makes it possible to provide care that is appropriate to the gestational age rather than the size of the neonate.

Suggested Reading

Amiel-Tison C. Neurological evaluation of the maturity of newborn infants. Arch Dis Child 1968;43:89.

Amiel-Tison C. Neurologic evaluation of the small neonate: the importance of head straightening reactions. In: Gluck L, ed. Modern perinatal medicine. Chicago: Year Book Medical Publishers, 1974:347–57.

Ballard JL, Khoury JC, Wedig K, Wang L, Eilers-Walsman BL, Lipp R. New Ballard Score, expanded to include extremely premature infants. J Pediatr 1991;119:417–23.

Ballard JL, Novak KZ, Driver M. A simplified score for assessment of fetal maturation of newly born infants. J Pediatr 1979; 95:769.

Constantine NA, Kraemer HC, Kendall-Tackett KA, Bennett FC, Tyson JE, Gross RT. Use of physical and neurologic observations in assessment of gestational age in low birth weight infants. J Pediatr 1987;110:921–8.

Cook LN. Intrauterine and extrauterine recognition and management of deviant fetal growth. Pediatr Clin North Am 1977; 24:431.

Dreyfus-Brisac C, Flescher J, Plassart E. The electroencephalogram: criterion of conceptual age for full-term and premature newborn. Biol Neonate 1962;4:154.

Dubowitz LMS, Dubowitz V. The neurological assessment of the preterm and fullterm infant. London: Spastics International Medical Publisher, 1981.

Hittner HM, Hirsch NJ, Rudolph AJ. Assessment of gestational age by examination of the anterior vascular capsule of the lens. J Pediatr 1977;91:455.

Lubchenco LO. Assessment of gestational age and development at birth. Pediatr Clin North Am 1970;17:125.

Lubchenco LO, Searls DT Brazie JV. Neonatal mortality rate: relationship to birth weight and gestational age. J Pediatr 1972;81:814.

Usher R, McLean F. Intrauterine growth of liveborn caucasian infants at sea level: standards obtained from measurements in 7 dimensions of infants born between 25 and 44 weeks of gestation. J Pediatr 1969;74:901.

Usher R, McLean F, Scott KE, et al. Judgment of fetal age. II Clinical significance of gestational age and an objective method for its assessment. Pediatr Clin North Am 1966; 13:835.

63

Thermoregulation

K.N. Sivasubramanian, M.D.

MAN, like all mammals, is homeothermic. Whereas the body temperature of poikilotherms (reptiles) drifts toward that of the environment (and is the reason they are termed cold-blooded), homeotherms maintain body temperature by increasing heat production in a cold environment. A newborn homeotherm must undergo a series of biological adjustments in order to adapt to extrauterine life. The inability to accommodate this cold stress has long been recognized as a major difference between the preterm and the term neonate. The fact that the preterm infant is unable to maintain body temperature in an environment that is cooler led to the development of incubators.

Thermoregulation of the Fetus

The fetus is metabolically active and generates a significant amount of heat that must be dissipated. Even though the fetus remains inside the mother's womb with fluid insulation, the basal heat generated by its metabolic activity (almost twice that of an adult) needs to be transferred. In order to dissipate this heat, a gradient must exist between the fetus and the pregnant woman. By measuring in utero and immediately after delivery, it has been established that gradient of 0.5°C exists between the fetus and the pregnant woman (1–5). Thus the accumulated heat in the fetus is transferred to the mother primarily via the umbilical arteries and placenta. Any changes in the maternal temperature are closely followed in the fetus to maintain this gradient. This is called heat clamp (6).

The maternal arterial temperature is the single most important factor in thermoregulation of the fetus. The fetus does not independently regulate its body temperature. If the pregnant woman develops prolonged and high fever, reduces the efficiency of the placenta in dissipating the heat generated by the fetus (7). This causes hyperthermia of the fetus which could result in spontaneous abortion, stillbirth or premature delivery. Maternal fever early in pregnancy could be potentially teratogenic. It is also important to note that since the amount of heat generated by the fetus during pregnancy is significant, the removal of the fetus at delivery could be a factor in maternal postpartum shivering (8).

Thermal Regulation After Birth

The term infant has all of the mechanisms for body temperature regulation, albeit in a narrow range. On the other hand, the preterm infant—physiologically and physically—can maintain body temperature only in a neutral thermal environment. Ill-term and preterm infants have even greater difficulty maintaining body temperature.

The mortality rate of newborn infants increases when deep core body temperature is outside the optimal body temperature (36°C–37.8°C) (9). The normal axillary and rectal temperatures range from 36.5° to 37.5°C. The gradient between the core and the mean skin surface temperature is called internal thermal gradient (ITG) and the gradient between the mean skin temperature and the environmental temperature called the external thermal gradient (ETG) (10). The ETG is not a constant but varies with the size and postnatal age of the infant, being narrow for smaller and wider for bigger, older infants (11).

In order to maintain body temperature, homeotherms need a basal metabolic rate several times higher than that of poikilotherms. This requires a steady state in which heat production and heat loss is balanced.

Heat Loss

The loss of heat by the infant to the environment occurs by four methods: (1) radiation, (2) convection, (3) evaporation, and (4) conduction. Under thermoneutral conditions, heat losses by radiation and convection are significant and heat losses by conduction are minimal. The evaporative losses, on the other hand, depend on such varying physiological and environmental conditions as velocity of airflow, difference in temperature between the infant and the environment, and relative humidity (12).

Radiation

Radiant heat loss is related to the ETG and the total radiating surface area of the infant. Since an infant's surface area per kilogram body weight is greater than that of an adult, the radiant heat loss is also greater. This is especially true of the preterm infant. This radiant heat loss is independent of the characteristics of the intervening medium, but is dependent upon the total surface as it relates to the infant's posture and the temperature of the surrounding surfaces (13).

Convection

Heat loss occurs by movement of air around the infant. The flow of air rising from the warm skin surface of the infant to the surrounding gas is called natural convection. Forced convection is attributed to the convective losses above and beyond the natural, such as when an air stream, created by the diffusers of air conditioners and heaters, blows over the body surface of the infant. Wheldon et al. (14) studying premature infants estimated that the convective heat losses were at approximately 40% of nonevaporative heat losses in an incubator and 50% of the non–evaporative heat losses under a radiant warmer.

Evaporation

Evaporation of water occurs at the skin's surface and through the mucus membranes of the respiratory tract. The skin acts as a barrier in adults and to some extent in term infants. The skin of the preterm infant, however, is thin and allows evaporation of water. Under thermoneutral conditions, this insensible water loss is approximately 25% of heat losses in newborns. Each gram of water loss by evaporation results in a heat loss of 540 calories. The evaporative loss in infants in inversely related to the humidity of the ambient air.

Conduction

Heat loss through a medium in contact with the body surface depends on the thermal conductivity of the material in contact, thickness of the material, thermal gradient across the top and bottom portion of the material, and area of the conducting surface. Hey et al. (15) have estimated that approximately 10% of the infant's surface area is in contact with the mattress. The thickness of mattresses used in nurseries is usually one inch. Mattresses that are used in incubators and radiant warmers usually have minimal thermal gradient. Therefore, the conductive heat losses in infants maintained in the standard incubators and radiant warmers are minimal.

Thermogenesis or Heat Production

Warm-blooded animals have two means of increasing heat production in the cold: a physical method of muscular contraction (shivering), and a chemical method capable of increasing heat production in the absence of muscular activity. The latter is often referred to as nonshivering, or chemical, thermogenesis. Studies in adult experimental animals (16–18) and in humans (19) suggest that, quantitatively, shivering is the more important mechanism; in the newborn, however, the reverse is true. Thus, the newborn of most species of mammals—humans included—do not shiver readily in the cold. Yet they show an increase in both oxygen consumption and heat production when exposed to a cool environment, suggesting not only that chemical thermogenesis is functioning, but also that it is of paramount importance in maintaining thermal stability.

This difference in the major mechanism of heat production in newborns and adults has resulted in a good deal of effort directed at identifying the activating mediator and the intermediary mechanism of the neonatal nonshivering system. Although the system appears to be catecholamine-dependent, the nature of the mediator in the adult differs from that in the newborn. Epinephrine appears to be the mediator of chemical thermogenesis in human adults (20), newborn infants exposed to cold (with resultant increases in oxygen consumption and metabolic activity) show large increases in norepinephrine excretion and little change in urinary epinephrine levels (21). Thus, the newborn utilizes a heat-generating system that is mediated differently from that of the adult.

The exogenous infusion of either norepinephrine (22) or epinephrine (23) results in increased levels of nonesterified fatty acid (NEFA) in plasma. The infusion of norepinephrine in the newborn infant results in an increase in oxygen consumption (24). Studies have demonstrated a rise in both NEFA levels and body temperature following norepinephrine infusion, and a rise in vivo in both NEFA and norepinephrine with a subsequent adequate defense of the body temperature when newborn infants are exposed to cold (25). From these observations, one can conclude that the human newborn's defense against cold is mediated via increased norepinephrine and the effect this increase has on intermediary lipid metabolism.

The catecholamines (both epinephrine and norepinephrine) regulate NEFA by activating an adipose-tissue lipase (26). Brown fat (brown because of its rich vascular supply) appears to be implicated in this reaction as the site of heat production (27, 28). Brown adipose tissue can be found in most newborn animals. Its existence has been verified anatomically in the human newborn, where it has been demonstrated both internally and at the body surface (29, 30).

Dawkins and Hull (27) showed that brown adipose tissue from newborn rabbits has a rate of oxygen consumption in vitro 20 times that of the predominantly white fat of adult rabbits. In vitro, the overall rate of lipolysis in brown adipose tissue was found to be 3 times greater than that in white adipose tissue. Dawkins and Hull suggested that thermogenesis is largely a local phenomenon, occurring within the brown fat itself. Under the influence of the catecholamines, triglycerides are split into glycerol and NEFA; NEFA is either oxidized, re-esterified to triglycerides, or released into the circulation. In their view, 30% of the NEFA is oxidized directly, 60% is re-esterified, and 10% is released into the circulation. The oxidized fraction represents an obvious thermogenic reaction. In addition, Ball and Junges (31) have pointed out that the apparently purposeless hydrolysis and resynthesis of triglycerides is potentially a highly exothermic process. It thus appears that the increase in plasma NEFA mirrors, rather than causes, chemical thermogenesis in response to cold, and reflects the much greater lipolytic activity that occurs within the adipose tissue itself.

An intriguing observation regarding the ontogeny and function of brown adipose tissue in the human neonate has been made by Heim, Kellemayer, and Dani (32). Infants who die in the first months of life, and who have suffered from inanition but have not been exposed to cold, show depleted stores of white fat but relatively intact stores of brown fat. By contrast, infants who die well-nourished but who have been exposed to cold show depleted stores of brown fat and relatively intact stores of white fat. It is also interesting that the gradual disappearance of brown fat stores within the first year of life correlates well with the time when the infant's mechanisms of thermogenesis convert from nonshivering to shivering.

Thermal Environment

When there is thermal equilibrium, heat storage is near zero and heat loss is equal to the heat production. The physical conditions of the environment that influence direction of heat flow toward heat loss or heat storage are the temperature of the air, the temperature of the surrounding radiative and contact surfaces, the relative humidity and the air velocity.

The neutral thermal environment is defined as "the range of ambient temperature within which metabolic rate is at minimum and within which temperature regulation is achieved by nonevaporative physical processes alone, the individual being in thermal equilibrium with the environment (33).

The homeothermic model depicts the range of thermal conditions from cold to heat stress and their physiological consequences (34). The thermoneutral zone has an upper critical temperature above which the body temperature begins to increase. Below the lower critical temperature, chemical regulation is initiated to produce heat. Further exposure to cold will result in decreased body temperature and eventual death.

Hey (35) pointed out the possibility that a thermoneutral environment is not always optimal. It is possible that exposure to slight cold stress may be necessary for the development of adequate thermoregulatory capabilities in newborns. Also, since temperature regulation is affected by a host of factors other than ambient temperature, a neutral thermal environment can be defined only if all other variables are constant. Skin temperature has been shown to correlate with the metabolic rate of infants nursed in incubators and under radiant warmers. To maintain the thermal environment, newborn infants are cared for in open bassinets, single- or double-walled incubators, or radiant warmers. Term infants can maintain their body temperature if they are cared for in an open bassinet, wrapped in one or two cotton blankets at an environmental temperature of 25°C to 26°C.

Incubators

Silverman et al. (36), Day et al. (37), and Buetow (38) demonstrated an improved survival rate in premature infants who were cared for in convectively heated incubators with a radiant roof panel and whose skin temperature was maintained at 36°C. At present, single- and double-walled incubators with forced convective heated air are commonly used in the care of both preterm and term infants. To provide thermoneutral conditions, incubators can either be adjusted manually or by an air temperature to skin temperature servo-control mechanism. A higher air temperature should be used in the care of preterm infants. In addition, use of heat shields, blankets, and hats from stockinets helps reduce heat loss in preterm infants. Humidity of about 50% to 60% is appropriate. Opening and closing of incubators disturbs the stability of the thermal environment. Double-walled incubation may be advantageous in maintaining body temperature of preterm infants, especially during transport. The recent incubator models have proportional control units that allow for maintaining a constant temperature at the control point.

Radiant Warmers

Rapid, safe warming of hypothermic infants can be accomplished with radiant warmers (39, 40). These heating devices maintain body temperature by providing radiant heat. Radiant warmers allow for easy accessibility to the infant and are used predominantly in the delivery room and in the care of ill infants who need intensive monitoring and frequent intervention. The optimal skin temperature for the control of radiant heaters is undetermined, but radiant warmers should be used only with a servo-control and an abdominal skin temperature set at 36.5°C. Such constraints as possible dislodgement of the probe and the need for the thermistor to be covered by an aluminum patch should be clearly understood by those who operate radiant warmers.

It should be noted that there are some disadvantages to radiant warmers. Radiant warmers significantly increase insensible water loss (41–44), especially in preterm infants (50% or more). This can result in rapid dehydration unless there is sufficient water replacement. The increase in the water requirement can be met by frequent and close monitoring of the infant's biochemical status, weight, and urine output. Devices such as heat shields made of rigid Plexiglass are not recommended. Use of Saran wrap (45) or polyurethane blankets (46) may help decrease convective and evaporative loss and help decrease insensible water loss. In addition, hyperthermia and burns (47) have been reported in newborn infants when the thermistor has been accidentally dislodged. Finally, because skin temperature can be influenced by air currents, decreased evaporation, and the infrared energy directly heating the thermistor, the temperature control may be unstable.

Consequences of Thermal Imbalance

Hyperthermia

Maternal fever, especially if high and prolonged, will increase the temperature of the fetus (heat clamp) and the newborn may be born with a fever (48). Infection in term infants could also cause fever. A core to foot difference of >1.7°C in a term infant may suggest infection. Improper use of radiant warmers or placement of incubators near windows with incidental sunlight exposure could result in hyperthermia (greenhouse effect) (49). Phototherapy could also cause fever because of its radiant energy (49). Maternal fever could result in central nervous system and facial defects as well as an increase in the frequency of spontaneous abortions, still births and prematurity.

Once diagnosed with hyperthermia, systematic, rapid cooling with careful monitoring of vital signs and temperature should be effected. Use of tepid water baths and reduction of environmental temperature (room air) is recommended in severe hyperthermia.

Hypothermia

Maintaining an adequate thermal environment and protecting against excessive heat loss enhances the premature infant's prospects for survival (36–38). Accidental lowering of the environmental temperature for pronged periods may result in physical cold injury. But even short of obvious tissue destruction, progressive reduction of the infant's heat content may ultimately become incompatible with life. Mann and Elliott (50) reported their experience in treating 14 hypothermic infants whose deep body temperature had fallen to between 27°C and 32°C. Fewer than half of these infants survived.

A number of physiologic derangements result from hypothermia. Since these are the newborn's attempts to compensate for the stress of a cold challenge, they represent a beneficial response of the organism. Nevertheless, these responses may seriously compromise the integrity of functioning systems and thereby place the infant at further risk, reducing its chances for survival.

Blood vessels in the skin constrict in response to cold, both in term and in preterm infants (51). The effect of this peripheral vasoconstriction is an increase in ITG and, consequently, maximum insulation of the tissues. This response is more effective in the term infant, due to its greater soft-tissue mass. Even when blood vessels are maximally constricted, however, the tissue-insulation effect in a low-birthweight infant is small compared to that in the term infant. In addition, it is smaller in both preterm and full-term infants than in older infants and adults. This defect in tissue insulation is essentially a function of body size and is not significantly modified by gestational age (52).

The obligatory increase in metabolic rate that results from a cold environment may have serious consequences for the infant. The baby already in respiratory difficulty must increase oxygen consumption, something that can be accomplished only at the expense of increasing minute ventilation. An infant with respiratory distress syndrome (RDS), already breathing at a rate of 80 to 100 times/minute, may be unable to meet his challenge, since to do so in the face of a relatively fixed tidal volume involves an obligatory increase in respiratory rate. The demand itself may be the final precipitating event in the onset of irreversible respiratory failure. To an extent, hypoxia has a partially protective effect in such a situation. Evidence in both newborn infants and experimental animals has shown that moderate acute hypoxia has no effect on minimal oxygen consumption, but it does reduce the metabolic response to cold (53). Elevating arterial PO_2 by oxygen administration can restore the depressed human newborn's ability to increase its metabolic rate in the cold (54). But the phenomenon may be a double-edged sword; while reducing the hypoxic infant's obligatory increase in metabolic demand, it may also make it more difficult to maintain thermal equilibrium when cold-stressed. In contrast to acute hypoxia, chronically low P_{O_2} does not interfere with metabolic responses to cold even when P_{CO_2} is elevated (55). The reasons for this difference are unknown, but they may involve a process of adaptation and adjustment to a chronically unfavorable situation.

Hypothermia effects changes in acid–base homeostasis that favor the development of metabolic acidosis (56). Several factors combine to promote this trend: prolonged increase in the metabolic rate in response to cold stress; persistent vasoconstriction, with reduction in tissue perfusion and metabolism, leading to the accumulation of ketone bodies; and an altered relationship of glucose to free fatty acids, with hypoglycemia and the accompanying inability to utilize glucose as a primary metabolic source. Overall, the trend is toward acidemia and a fall in pH.

Not only does acidosis impose its own demand for counterregulatory homeostatic mechanisms, but it may also play a major role in perpetuating the cycle of pulmonary deterioration in infants already suffering from respiratory disorders. Acting as a potent pulmonary vasoconstrictor, the acidosis can, by reducing pulmonary perfusion, materially influence the ability of the organism to oxygenate itself. The resultant hypoxemia further increases the acidosis, establishing a vicious cycle of progressive deterioration and increasing impairment. Such a view of the pathophysiology of the respiratory distress syndrome focuses on factors that maintain the adequacy of the pulmonary circulation (57) as crucial both to the development of the disease and to its management. Moreover, because synthesis of surfactant, which appears to be diminished in RDS, must be re-established if recovery is to ensue, and seems to depend on pulmonary blood flow (58–60), control of the pulmonary vasculature emerges as a major problem in managing the disease. Challenges that tend to impair surfactant synthesis become serious pathophysiologic factors. Stephenson and associates (61) have demonstrated a fall in arterial P_{O_2} in hypothermic full-term newborn infants without any change in pH. The mechanism of this fall is not known, but has been postulated to involve the action of norepinephrine released as a result of hypothermia. Norepinephrine increases pulmonary vascular resistance (62, 63), which could increase right-to-left shunting through the still-patent ductus arteriosus and the functionally open foramen ovale (64).

The increased resistance of the pulmonary vessels may also change ventilator-perfusion relationships in the lung. Both of these effects would lower arterial oxygen tension.

Here again is a vicious cycle: Hypothermia-induced acidemia and hypoxemia increase respiratory distress, while temperature loss ensues from the disease itself via increased evaporation of water from the lungs due to the affected infant's increased respiratory rate and ventilator efforts. Not only may hypothermia worsen RDS, but RDS itself may increase the hypothermia. The cycle must be broken by efforts to maintain total homeostasis of multiple parameters throughout the course of RDS.

Hypoglycemia

Hypothermia results in a fall in blood glucose; as a consequence, the hypothermic infant is hypoglycemic as well (50). The hypoglycemia results from elevation of NEFA in the cold (25), which in turn leads to a fall in blood glucose, an effect consistent with the known inverse relationship between blood glucose and NEFA levels (65). In practice, two precautions should therefore be taken. The infant exposed to cold may be profoundly hypoglycemic and requires determinations of blood glucose levels and energetic provision of supplemental parenteral glucose. Conversely, a true index of glucose homeostasis cannot be obtained in a hypothermic baby. Therefore, neonatal glucose metabolism should be studied only in a neutral thermal environment or after a cold infant has been warmed.

Thermal Regulation Under Special Circumstances

The Delivery Room

At delivery, newborn infants rapidly lose heat by evaporative, radiant, and convective heat losses. Heat losses by conduction are minimal unless the infant is placed on a cold surface. Dahm and James (66) have demonstrated that the infant's abdominal skin temperature falls rapidly within minutes of delivery and this fall can be significantly minimized by immediately drying the baby with dry, prewarmed towels, wrapping the infant and placing him or her under radiant warmer. Their studies also showed that the fall of mean deep body temperature could be decreased by treating the newborns in the same manner as above. The drop in temperature in the delivery room corresponds to a loss of 100 cal/kg/min resulting in hypoglycemia and acidosis. Breech deliveries may be at high risk for a significant drop in body temperature immediately after delivery.

Infants whose mothers have received Demerol (67) may have a greater fall in temperature, and infants of mothers who received Diazepam (68) show impaired metabolic responses to cold stress. Preterm infants, asphyxiated infants, small for gestational age infants, infants of mothers receiving maternal sedation or anesthesia, and infected newborns may have even greater difficulties in maintaining body temperature after delivery.

The delivery room should be kept reasonably warm (>25°C) and both term and preterm infants should be dried with prewarmed blankets, wrapped and placed under a radiant warmer. If additional resuscitative effort is anticipated, the infant should be placed in a warmer infant resuscitation room or special care nursery. Even healthy term infants left with the mother (skin to skin) should be wrapped or covered with prewarmed blankets. Circumcision or bathing should never be done in the delivery room.

Transport

Newborn infants, especially those that are preterm, are at risk of hypothermia while being transported from delivery room to nursery, from one hospital to another, or to and from the operating room. Using a prewarmed double-walled transport incubator or a single-walled transporter with the infant dressed and/or covered by a blanket or silver swadler will help prevent a fall in body temperature. Transport by aircraft increases the risk of hypothermia by radiant heat loss, so the use of a double-walled transporter is recommended to decrease the loss of body temperature. For procedures, the infant should be placed under a radiant warmer with servo-control on a continuously warmed mattress, in a draft-free, humidified (50%) room to minimize heat loss. Transporting the infant to and from the operating room should also be done with the precautions outlined earlier.

Author's Note: I have retained significant portions of the text previously written by the late Dr. Leo Stern.

References

1. Galletti G. Environmental temperature of human fetus. Surg Gynecol Obstet 1960;110:524.
2. Wood C, Beard RW. Temperature of human fetus. J Obstet Gynaecol Br Common 1964;71:768.
3. Adamsons K Jr, Towell ME. Thermal homeostasis in the fetus and newborn. Anesthesiology 1965;26:531.
4. Mann TP. Observations on temperatures of mothers and babies in the perinatal period. J Obstet Gynaecol Br Common 1968;75:316.
5. Peltonen R, et al. The difference between fetal and maternal temperatures during delivery (abstract), p. 188. Uppsala Sweden: Fifth European Conferences of Perinatal Medicine, June 1976.
6. Power GG (ed). Fetal thermoregulation: animal and human zinc. In: Fetal and Neonatal Physiology. Polin RA and Fox WW, eds. p. 47. Philadelphia: Saunders, 1992.
7. Abrams RM. Thermal physiology of fetus. In: Sinclair JC, ed. Temperature Regulation and Energy Metabolism in the Newborn. New York: Grunne Stratton, 1978, p. 87.
8. Clapp JF, Abrams RM. Possible metabolic and thermal basis for post-partum shivering. J Med Sci 1976; 12:1131.
9. Yashiro K, Adams FH, Emmanonilides GC, et al. Preliminary studies on the thermal environment of low birthweight infants. Pediatrics 1973;82:994–999.
10. Burton AC. The application of the theory of heat flow to the study of energy metabolism. J Nutrition 1934;7:497.
11. Swyer P. Heat loss after birth. In: Sinclair JC, ed. Temperature Regulation and Energy Metabolism in the Newborn. New York: Grunne Stratton, 1978, p. 100.
12. Okken AC, et al. Effect of forced convection of heated air on insensible water loss and heat loss in premature infants in incubators. Pediatrics 1982;101:108.
13. Sinclair JC. Metabolic rate and temperature control. In: Smith AC and Nelson NM, eds. The Physiology of the Newborn Infant, Fourth Edition. Charles Thomas, 1976, p. 373.
14. Wheldon AE, Rutter N. The heat balance of small babies nursed in incubators and underradiant warmers. Early Human Dev 1982;6:1331.
15. Hey ED, et al. The total thermal insulations of the newborn baby. J Physiol 1970;207:683.
16. Davis TRA, Johnston DR, Bell FC, et al. Regulation of shivering and nonshivering heat production during acclimation of rats. Am J Physiol 1980;198:471.

17. Hart JS, Heroux O, Depogas F. Cold acclimation and the EMG of unanesthetized rats. J Appl Physiol 1956;9:404.

18. Hsieh ACL, Carlson LD, Gray G. Role of the sympathetic nervous system in the control of chemical regulation of heat production. Am J Physiol 1957;190:247.

19. Davis TRA, Johnson DR. Seasonal acclimatization to cold in man. J Appl Physiol 1961;16:231.

20. Arnett EL, Watts DT. Catecholamine excretion in the newborn infant. Proc R Soc Med 1960;15:499.

21. Stern L, Lees MH, Leduc J. Environmental temperature, oxygen consumption, and catecholamine excretion in newborn infants. Pediatrics 1965;36:367.

22. Abboud FM, Wendling MG, Eckstein JW. Effect of norepinephrine on plasma FFA. Am J Physiol 1963;205:57.

23. Gordon RS Jr, Cherkes A. UFA in human blood plasma. J Clin Invest 1956;35:206.

24. Karlberg P, Moore RE, Oliver TK Jr. The thermogenic response of newborn infants to noradrenaline. Acta Paediatr Scand 1963; Supp140:53.

25. Schiff D, Stern L, Leduc J. Chemical thermogenesis in newborn infants; catecholamine excretion and the plasma non-esterified fatty acid response to cold exposure. Pediatrics 1966;37:577.

26. Rizack MA. Activation of epinephrine-sensitive lipolytic activity from adipose tissue by adenosine 3,5-phosphate. J Biol Chem 1964;239:392.

27. Dawkins MJ, Hull D. Brown adipose tissue and the response of newborn rabbits to cold. J Physiol (Lond) 1964; 172:216.

28. Smith RE. Thermoregulation by brown adipose tissue in the cold. Fed Proc 1962;21:221.

29. Aherne W, Hull D. The site of heat production in the newborn infant. Proc R Soc Med 1964;57:1172.

30. Silverman W, Zamelis A, Sinclair JC, et al. Warm nape of the newborn. Pediatrics 1964; 33:984.

31. Ball EG, Junges RL. On the action of hormones which accelerate the rate of oxygen consumption and fatty acid release in rat adipose tissue in vitro. Proc Natl Acad Sci USA 1961; 47:932.

32. Heim T, Kellermayer M, Dani M. Thermal conditions and the mobilization of lipids from brown and white adipose tissue in the human neonate. Acta Paediatr Acad Sci Hung 1968;9:109.

33. Bligh J, Johnson KG. Glossary of terms for thermal physiology. J Appl Physiol 1973;35:941–961.

34. Brody S. Bioenergetics and Growth. New York: Reinhold, 1945.

35. Hey EN, O'Connell B. Oxygen consumption and heat balances in the cot-nursed baby. Archives of Diseases of Children 1970; 45:335–343.

36. Silverman WA, et al. The influence of the thermal environment upon the survival of the newly born premature infant. Pediatrics 1958;22:876.

37. Day RL, et al. Body temperature and survival of premature infants. Pediatrics 1964;34:171.

38. Buetow KC, Klein SW. Effect of maintenance of "normal" skin temperature on survival of infants of low birthweight. Pediatrics 1964;34:163.

39. Friedman WF, et al. Regulation of body temperature of premature infants with low-energy radiant heat. Pediatrics 1967;70:270.

40. Yashiro K, et al. Preliminary studies on the thermal environment of low birthweight infants. Pediatrics 1973;82:991.

41. Marks KH, et al. Oxygen consumption and insensible water loss in premature infants under radiant heaters. Pediatrics 1980;66:228.

42. Jones RWA, et al. Increased insensible water loss in newborn infants nursed under radiant heaters. Br Med J 1976;2:1347.

43. Wu PYK, Hodgman JE. Insensible water loss in preterm infants: changes with postnatal development and non-iodizing radiant energy. Pediatrics 1974;54:704.

44. Williams PR, Oh W. Effects of radiant warmer on insensible water loss in newborn infants. Am J Dis Child 1974;128:511.

45. Baumgart, S, et al. Effect of heat shielding on convective and evaporative losses and on radiant heat transfer in the premature infant. Pediatrics 1981;99:948.

46. Baumgart S. Reduction of oxygen consumption, insensible water loss and radiant heat demand with use of plastic blanket for LBW infants under radiant warmers. Pediatrics 1984;76:1022.

47. Anonymous. Infant radiant warmers. Health Devices 1975; 4:128.

48. Abrams RM. Thermal physiology of the fetus. In: Sinclair JC, ed. Temperature Regulation and Energy Metabolism in the Newborn. New York: Grunne Stratton, 1978;p. 87.

49. Marks KH. Thermal and caloric balance. In: Nelson NM, ed. Current Therapy in Neonatal-Perinatal Medicine-2. Philadelphia: Decker, 1990, p. 368.

50. Mann TP, Elliot RI. Neonatal and cold injury due to accidental exposure to cold. Lancet 1957;1:229.

51. Bruck K. Temperature regulation in the newborn infant. Biology of the Neonate 1961;3:65.

52. Sinclair JC. Heat production and thermoregulation in the

small for date infant. Pediatr Clin North Am 1970;17:147.

53. Hill J. The oxygen consumption of newborn and adult mammals; its dependence on the oxygen tension in the inspired air and on the environmental temperature. J Physiol (Lond) 1959;149:346.

54. Adamsons K Jr, Gandy GM, James LS. The effects of higher oxygen environment upon the oxygen consumption of the newborn baby. Obstet Gynecol 1963;21:264.

55. Bruck K, Adams FH, Bruck M. Temperature regulation in infants with chronic hypoxemia. Pediatrics 1962;30:350.

56. Gandy GM, Adamsons K Jr, Cunningham N, et al. Thermal environment and acid base homeostasis in human infants during the first few hours of life. J Clin Invest 1964; 43:751.

57. Chu J, Clements JA, Cotton E, et al. The pulmonary hypoperfusion syndrome. Pediatrics 1960;26:42.

58. Bozic C. Pulmonary hyaline membrane and vascular anomalies of the lung: description of a case. Pediatrics 1963; 32:1094.

59. Cohen MM, Weintraub DH, Lilienfeld AM. The relationship of pulmonary hyaline membranes to certain factors in pregnancy and delivery. Pediatrics 1960;26:42.

60. Tooley WH, Gardner R, Thung N, et al. Factors affecting the surface tension of lung extracts. Fed Proc 1961;20:428.

61. Stephenson JM, Du JN, Oliver TK Jr. The effect of cooling on blood gas tensions in newborn infants. Pediatrics 1970; 76:848.

62. Cassin S, Dawes GS, Ross BB. Pulmonary flow and vascular resistance in immature foetal lambs. J Physiol (Lond) 1964; 171:80.

63. Dawes GS, Mott JC. The vascular tone of the foetal lung. J Physiol (Lond) 1962;164:465.

64. Lind J, Stern L, Wegelius C. Human Fetal and Neonatal Circulation. Springfield, IL: Thomas, 1964, p. 37–44.

65. Dole VP. A relation between non-esterified fatty acids in plasma and the metabolism of glucose. J Clin Invest 1956; 35:150.

66. Dahm KS, James LS. Newborn temperature: heat loss in the delivery room. Pediatrics 1972;49:504–513.

67. Burnard ED, Cross KW. Rectal temperature in the newborn after birth asphyxia. Br Med J 1958;2:1197–1199.

68. Owens JR, Evans SF, Blair AW. Effect of Diazepam administered to mothers during labor in temperature regulation of neonates. Am J Dis Child 1972;47:107–110.

64

Hypoxemia

Roger J. Harris, M.D.

IN recent years, the perinatal mortality rate in the developed world has fallen. Much of the improvement in perinatal care has been due to increased awareness of the dangers of hypoxemia during this critical phase of life. Also, there is better management of postnatal conditions that could lead to chronic hypoxemia.

The most disastrous effects of perinatal hypoxemia are seen in the developing brain. The outcome may range from no change in normal morphology to severe brain swelling and total cerebral necrosis, depending on the degree and duration of oxygen deprivation.

In both antenatal and postnatal hypoxemia, the brain relies on anaerobic glycolysis for survival. As time goes by, the rate of energy supply by glycolysis becomes inadequate. There are two main limiting factors: first, exhaustion of substrate and, second, a fall in intracellular pH, which inhibits the metabolism of all cells, including those in the brain. The initial histologic change is mitochondrial swelling; ultimately, self-destruction proceeds.

Patterns of morphologic change in the brain differ in total and partial asphyxia. Total asphyxia results in damage to brain stem structures, whereas partial asphyxia causes cortical damage. In clinical practice, total asphyxia is rarely encountered and is usually seen only if maternal cardiac arrest occurs. Even if there is a prolapsed cord, some blood usually reaches the fetus, and the asphyxia is partial.

Brain swelling is the mildest change observed. If it becomes severe, there may be compression of the cerebellum and herniation of the vermis and tonsils through the foramen magnum. Gradual impairment of blood circulation, due to compression of the capillary lumen by surrounding tissues, is associated with this edema. Impairment of circulation is first regional, then general (1). Although the entire brain may be affected, softening and necrosis in specific areas are more common. Frequent sites are the middle third of the paracentral region and posterior parietal cortex, the basal nuclei, especially the caudate nucleus and putamen, the nuclei of the inferior colliculus, other brain stem nuclei, especially the gracile and medial cuneate, and the cerebellum and thalamic nuclei if the asphyxia is prolonged. The areas of softening may be hemorrhagic, depending on the fetal circulatory state. Recent work has focused on autoregulation of cerebral blood flow, and has shown that there is a fall in mean cerebral blood flow velocities, which increases further the risk of brain damage (2).

Periventricular leukomalacia, which has attracted considerable attention, refers to cerebral infarctions occurring near the lateral ventricles (3). It is believed to be a result of hypoperfusion, secondary to asphyxia or hemorrhage, in an area where circulation is hazardous: the junction between ventriculopetal and ventriculofugal circulations (4). Although not necessarily fatal, it interrupts the descending long tracts and may result in spastic quadriplegia and/or mental retardation.

Animal studies have shown that involvement of the cerebral cortex as a result of acute birth asphyxia is unusual. It is seen only when recovery from asphyxia is complicated by prolonged resuscitative measures over several hours.

During prolonged partial asphyxia, compensatory vasoconstriction in vessels supplying the limbs and abdominal viscera may be sufficient to support brain metabolism, but this leads to temporary or permanent damage to the viscera involved. Thus, renal damage, including renal cortical necrosis, papillary necrosis, medullary hemorrhage, and renal vein thrombosis, has been described (5), as have acute gastric perforation and functional intestinal obstruction.

Fetal Hypoxemia

The partial pressure of oxygen in fetal blood (PO_2)—normally about 30 mm Hg—depends predominantly on maternal placental blood flow. Any reduction will reduce fetal oxygenation (Table 64.1).

Fetal causes of hypoxemia are rare, with prolapsed cord the chief one. In rhesus monkeys, brain injury does not occur until the PO_2 falls to 9–14 mm Hg (1). Assuming that a similar situation occurs in the human fetus, indirect evidence of hypoxemia is sought during labor. Although it is now possible to measure subcutaneous PO_2 in the fetus, the electrodes are fragile and difficult to calibrate; thus, it is not currently appropriate for routine use.

The principal methods of assessing fetal well-being are continuous electronic monitoring and use of the biophysical profile. Continuous fetal heart rate (FHR) recordings can be obtained by applying a fetal skin electrode to the presenting part to record the fetal electrocardiogram (ECG), or indirectly by using a Doppler ultrasound transducer on the maternal abdomen. Radiotelemetry allows women in labor to move around rather than be confined to bed for monitoring. The FHR is normally 120–160 bpm, with "beat-to-beat" variability of 10 bpm and long-term oscillations of 10–25 bpm at intervals of 10–20 seconds. Different FHR patterns have been described as indicators of fetal distress.

There is often profound bradycardia associated with vagal stimulation in a severely stressed fetus, and this is ominous. Fetal tachycardia is less ominous and can be seen in preterm babies; it is associated with maternal pyrexia. Loss of beat-to-beat variation and late or variable decelerations are similarly features of fetal hypoxemia, and may indicate the need for prompt delivery.

Fetal scalp pH measurements are used to evaluate whether an abnormal FHR pattern indicates the need for immediate delivery. A pH of less than 7.2 indicates severe acidosis, and immediate delivery is the rule. If the pH is between 7.2 and 7.25, it should be repeated within one hour, while a pH of greater than 7.25 is probably normal, and labor can be allowed to continue (6).

Use of the fetal electroencephalogram (EEG) has been advocated (7). The fetal EEG closely resembles the EEG

Table 64.1 Causes of Reduced Placental Blood Flow
Obstetric Conditions
Preeclampsia, antepartum hemorrhage, multiple pregnancies, extreme prematurity, postmaturity, maternal hypertension
Transient Hypotension
Patients receiving strong analgesics IV, or after epidural analgesia
Hypovolemia
Maternal dehydration
Myometrial Activity
Increased resting tone of the uterus and prolonged duration of contraction
Placental Edema
Erythroblastosis fetalis and intrauterine infections such as toxoplasmosis, cytomegalovirus, and syphilis, hydrops fetalis

immediately after birth, and it has been acclaimed as a sensitive indicator of the responses of the fetal brain to events and stresses during labor. Major difficulties of the fetal EEG are due to artifacts. Earlier suggestions that the cerebral function monitor may be more useful in monitoring fetal brain activity have not been realized, and it remains primarily a research tool (8).

Biophysical methods of assessing fetal well-being have become more popular. Breathing movements, fetal movements, fetal tone, and amniotic fluid volume are measured, together with FHR, and a biophysical profile score is determined; the higher the score, the healthier the fetus (9). Contraction tests have been more popular in North America than in the United Kingdom.

Birth Asphyxia

Even with precautions, some babies fail to breathe spontaneously at birth and may suffer hypoxemic damage. Asphyxia is defined as hypoxemia, mixed acidosis and hypercapnea. Birth asphyxia, the commonest cause of hypoxemia in perinatal life, must be dealt with quickly and efficiently. In a fetal rhesus monkey that was delivered without anesthesia, the following sequence of events in initiation of respiration at birth was observed (10):

> Initial "struggling" respirations;
> Primary apnea, lasting 30–60 seconds;
> Gasping, increasing in frequency;
> Sudden cessation of gasping—secondary or terminal apnea—and death.

The period of primary apnea is short but can be extended by anesthetics or analgesics, especially morphine derivatives, given to the mother. In that part of primary apnea not caused by drugs, tactile stimulation induces a gasp. When a gasp occurs, adequate respiration little different from that of the adult ensues (if the lungs are filled with air and not saline). In secondary apnea, however, active resuscitation of the newborn is required.

Although the human infant appears to follow a sequence of events similar to the rhesus monkey, it is important to realize that intrapartum asphyxia is an infrequent cause of delayed onset respiration at birth or birth injury.

Only 8 to 10% of cerebral palsy can be attributed to intrapartum asphyxia (i.e., 1–2% per 10,1000 live births (11, 12). In a recent study of over 3,000 neonates, an umbilical arterial pH of <7.2 correlated only very poorly with neonatal apnea, seizures, or death (13). If a pH of 7.0 was used, the correlation was strengthened; however, two-thirds of those infants were admitted to the normal newborn nursery with no apparent neurologic sequelae!

An infant who has reached the stage of secondary apnea is usually pale and hypotonic. There is little reflex activity, and the heart rate is less than 100 bpm. Skin color depends on peripheral circulation. A pale baby may be cold, shocked, or anemic, and still be suffering primary apnea. Thus, although skin color can be used as a guide to the baby's state, it is not a reliable indicator of the degree of asphyxia. And no matter what the baby's color, if there is no respiration, the P_{O_2} is nearly zero. Similarly, muscle tone and reflex activity are readily influenced by maternal sedation, fetal maturity, or preceding cerebral damage, and therefore are unreliable.

The Apgar score (14) is unreliable in assessing clinical status at such a birth and, at most, should be used as a guide only. In deciding the amount of resuscitation required, the heart rate and respiration are the most important criteria. Figure 64.1 shows the scheme followed at The Royal London Hospital.

Table 64.2 Causes of Delayed Onset of Respiration

Antenatal or intrapartum hypoxemia

Drugs given mother during labor

Prolonged or difficult labor and delivery

Fetal immaturity

Lung abnormalities preventing adequate respiration

Compression of lungs

Pneumothorax

Aspiration of meconium or ingested amniotic fluid

Obstructed upper airways

Major congenital abnormalities

Severe cerebral injury

Resuscitation

Resuscitation ensures adequate oxygenation of all organs to prevent asphyxial damage. Skill in resuscitation techniques is essential. Allowing an inexperienced person to attempt neonatal resuscitation can only result in failure at a vital stage.

Anticipation of birth asphyxia is vital. At The Royal London Hospital, a pediatrician attends the delivery of every at-risk infant. In general, this includes all operative and instrumental deliveries, including breech extraction. A pediatrician is also present at the delivery of all preterm and suspected small-for-gestational-age infants, as well as infants whose mothers' obstetrical and medical complications are known to place the fetuses at some risk (such as preeclampsia, antepartum hemorrhage, diabetes mellitus, multiple pregnancies). A pediatrician attends the birth of infants known to be affected with erythroblastosis fetalis. Moreover in case of unexpected birth asphyxia, a pediatrician is always immediately available.

The resuscitation carts must be equipped with an overhead heater, switched on in readiness at all times. Before the baby is born, the resuscitator must check all parts of the cart, especially oxygen cylinders and suction apparatus, to make sure that all the instruments are present and in working order. An endotracheal tube should be available for immediate insertion, if indicated. Drugs likely to be used should be drawn up into a syringe beforehand. If these measures are not carried out, the resultant delay can have serious consequences for the baby.

The baby must be dried and placed in a warm, dry towel on the resuscitation cart. The airways should be cleared by suction. Then the resuscitation scheme is used. This scheme gives working rules only. The experienced resuscitator will vary his or her technique, depending on the baby's responses.

It is recommended that all high-risk infants be delivered in an obstetric unit that provides facilities for fetal monitoring and the presence of pediatricians skilled in resuscitation techniques. Our hospital contains a regional intensive care unit for the newborn, and many high-risk pregnancies are referred to our obstetric department from peripheral hospitals for management of pregnancy, labor, delivery, and the newborn infant.

Bag and Mask Ventilation

This is a useful technique that can be followed in units where experienced pediatricians are not readily available. Some form of pressure-release valve must be incorporated into the system, since pressures can be generated in excess of 60 cm H_2O. Such pressures can damage the infant's lungs. The same rule applies to the masks traditionally used to supply facial oxygen. They, too, should incorporate a pressure-release valve, as very high pressures can arise if the mask fits the infant's face tightly.

Drugs

Naloxone should be used if an opiate has been given to the mother within six hours of birth. It should be given IV in a dose of 0.1 mg/kg (15, 16).

Intermittent Positive Pressure Ventilation (IPPV)

There are many instruments designed to administer IPPV via an endotracheal tube. The basic principle is the delivery of oxygen at pressures of up to 30 cm H_2O; above this pressure, a release valve opens. No evidence indicates that administration of 100% oxygen for a short while is harmful, but it should be used with extreme caution if resuscitation is prolonged. The rate of intermittent positive pressure ventilation should usually be 40–60 per minute, although slower or faster rates are probably just as effective. After initiation of regular respirations, the neonate may receive hood humidified oxygen.

Correction of Acidosis

The hypoxemic infant has a metabolic acidosis secondary to the accumulation of pyruvic and lactic acid. If, after 30–60 seconds of IPPV, the infant's heart rate does not improve, external cardiac massage should be administered. The depressed state may be the result of poor cardiac output, continuing acidosis, or severe cerebral depression caused by trauma or drugs. Inflating the lungs with oxygen combats the acidosis, but administering 8.4% sodium bicarbonate at 1 meq/kg in 10 mL of 10% dextrose can dramatically improve the infant's clinical state. Sodium bicarbonate is used when the neonate has persistant metabolic acidosis that is unresponsive to treatment.

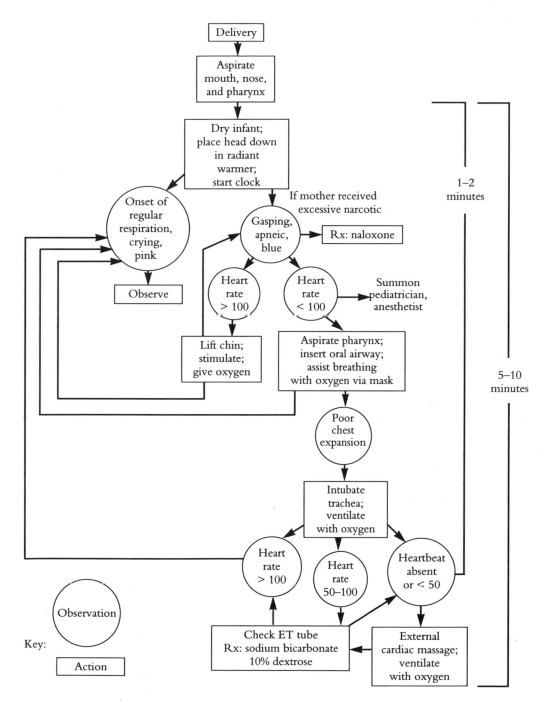

This resuscitation scheme is used at The Royal London Hospital, University of London, for infants with birth asphyxia.

Figure 64.1   Infant resuscitation chart.

Failure to Respond

An occasional infant does not respond to the measures described here. In this event, the baby should be checked to see that both sides of the chest move with each inflation. If they do not, an immediate x-ray to look for diaphragmatic hernia, bilateral pneumothorax, or other intrathoracic pathology should be arranged. In pneumothorax, immediate drainage is often life-saving.

If the infant's chest is moving adequately, the likely cause is profound cerebral depression. The mother should be checked again for use of opiates; naloxone may be given if indicated, but not if already administered. Otherwise, continuous artificial ventilation is necessary until respirations are established or the infant dies. Such an infant usually has major cerebral pathology and will never respond. The decision to stop attempting resuscitation is a difficult ethical problem; however, it seems likely that, if a period of 30 minutes has elapsed and the baby has not shown signs of spontaneous respiration, the prognosis is extremely poor, with the survivors having severe neurodevelopment problems (17).

Management of Asphyxiated Newborn Infants

After resuscitation, a number of infants become neurologically abnormal over the next 48 hours. This is referred to as hypoxic-ischemic encephalopathy and is usually classified as mild, moderate, or severe (18). Mildly affected babies are irritable, have poor sucking, and are hypotonic. Moderately affected babies are lethargic, with appreciably abnormal tone, and most will have convulsions. Severely affected babies are comatose, with prolonged seizures and respiratory failure.

Supportive Care

This should include the maintenance of adequate temperature, ventilation, perfusions, and stable glucose. Most babies drop their temperature slightly after birth, but this is compounded by the lower metabolic rate of the asphyxiated newborn. Any baby must be dried immediately after birth and wrapped in warm blankets if these are available. All resuscitation carts must be equipped with overhead heat sources, which should not be switched off at any time.

Hypoxemia should be prevented by adequate ventilation if there is any evidence of respiratory depression, or by adequate FiO_2 if the baby is breathing well. It is essential that continuous PO_2 monitoring, either intraarterial or transcutaneous, be available. It has been suggested that hyperoxia can be dangerous in reducing cerebral blood flow (19), but there is no supportive evidence available. Similarly, hypercapnia should be avoided, as it results in tissue acidosis and seems to be linked to focal cerebral ischemia due to "intracranial steal" and increased cerebral blood flow and hemorrhage (20). Hypocapnia certainly seems to help adults with cerebral edema, but the evidence for its effectiveness in neonates is less certain, and in some circumstances it may be harmful (21). Nevertheless, it is still usual to hyperventilate asphyxiated newborn babies, as there has been no controlled trial of hyperventilation in the asphyxiated newborn.

The combination of raised intracranial pressure and low blood pressure is particularly devastating to the brain. Hypovolemia can occur in an asphyxiated newborn and is characterized by peripheral vasoconstriction, metabolic acidosis, and an arterial blood pressure of below 40 mm Hg. If the clinical picture suggests hypovolemia, it is essential to infuse colloid at 10–20 mL/kg before carrying out other measures of cerebral protection.

The effects of peripheral vasoconstriction on other organs will also be minimized by colloid as soon as there are signs suggestive of hypovolemia. If arterial blood pressure remains low despite colloid replacement, any remaining metabolic acidosis can be corrected with sodium bicarbonate, and perfusion may be improved with inotropic support, such as dopamine at 5 µg/kg/min, increasing by 5-µg/kg increments to 20 µg/kg/min, to maintain a mean arterial blood pressure of 40 mm Hg. However, at higher infusion rates, renal perfusion may be compromised, and dobutamine, starting at 10 µg/kg/min, and increasing in 10-µg/kg increments, may be better if an inotropic effect alone is being sought.

Maintenance of Blood Glucose Levels

The maintenance of correct blood glucose levels is important. Too low a level may compromise brain adenosine triphosphate production and the availability of glucose to the brain. Conversely, too high a glucose level could be harmful in an asphyxiated newborn because of excess lactic acid production (22). Ideally, blood glucose should be maintained between 60 and 100 mg/100 mL.

Other Metabolic Consequences of Birth Asphyxia

The hypoxemic infant is more likely to develop hyperbilirubinemia than a normal infant. This may be due in part to resorption of hematoma following a traumatic delivery, but hypoxemia itself increases red cell breakdown and impairs bilirubin conjugation in the liver cell. Other consequences of birth asphyxia are hypocalcemia and hyponatremia from inappropriate antidiuretic hormone production.

In addition to consumption coagulopathy, hemorrhage may occur because hypoxemia and acidosis interfere with the production of various coagulation factors by the liver. All asphyxiated babies should be given vitamin K_1 immediately after birth, and, if there is any continuing evidence of hemorrhage, fresh frozen plasma should be transfused.

Control of Seizures

Generalized tonic-clonic seizures may occur and must be treated, as they can lead to further hypoxemia and the potential for more severe hypoxic-ischemic damage. Phenobarbital is the drug of first choice, in a dose of 20-mg/kg IV loading dose, and 5–10 mg/kg IV/24 hours as maintenance. It used to be thought that barbiturates exerted some independent cerebral protective effect, but this is no longer thought to be true (23). Phenytoin, 20 mg/kg IV, may also be effective, continuing with a maintenance dose of 5–10 mg/kg/24 hours. Refractory seizures may be controlled by lorazepam 0.05–0.1 mg/kg IV or paraldehyde 0.3 mL/kg IV or rectally, provided that the dose is diluted with glycerol.

Cerebral Protection

The maintenance of correct metabolic homeostasis, oxygenation, and control of convulsions all contribute significantly to cerebral protection. However, additional measures should be used in an attempt to reduce the degree of cerebral edema that can occur.

Oliguria is likely because of inappropriate antidiuretic hormone secretion and renal dysfunction, and consequently fluids should be restricted to 30–40 mL/kg/24 hours. Fluid balance should be assessed by regular measurements of urine output, electrolytes, and osmolarity; plasma electrolytes, urea, creatinine, and osmolarity; blood pressure; and weight.

Many babies recover over the course of a few days, and, once urine output and osmolarity are adequate, liberalization of fluids may be allowed. Gradually, normal reflex activity, including sucking, returns, and the baby can be treated as normal. Continuing sedation beyond the first week is seldom necessary, although anticonvulsant therapy may need to be continued longer. The time sequence of recovery varies; the longer abnormal features persist, the more likely that the baby has suffered some degree of permanent brain damage. In a good many asphyxiated babies, however, the abnormal clinical features are only transient, and, within a few hours of birth, these babies are acting normally. The use of intracranial pressure monitoring has shown that the more sustained the intracranial pressure, the worse the prognosis (24).

Continuing Hypoxemia

The pathologic and metabolic effects of continuing hypoxemia are similar to those outlined above. The major cause is hyaline membrane disease in the preterm infant due to lack of pulmonary surfactant.

Recently there has been an improvement in the ventilatory support and postnatal surfactant therapy for affected infants. With antenatal prediction of at-risk infants using the amniotic fluid lecithin-to-sphingomyelin (L/S) ratio and phosphatidyl glycerol test (25) and administration of corticosteroids to women with low L/S ratios (26), the disease can often be prevented. In term neonates with continuing hypoxemia secondary to PPHN newer strategies such as high frequency ventilation, ECMO and nitric oxide have all been used with success.

Role of Ultrasound

Ultrasound scanning of the newborn brain through the

anterior fontanelle has become the method of choice, not only for assessing the presence or absence of periventricular or intraventricular hemorrhage in preterm infants, but also for assessing the severity of birth asphyxia. Serial scans allow observation of the location and extent of hypoxic-ischemic lesions in the brain. Ultrasound can detect diffuse changes by a generalized increase in cerebral parenchymal echoes (27) and is helpful in the recognition of focal areas of ischemia. Areas of leucomalacia, either periventricular or subcortical, can be seen, giving parents a clearer prognosis at an earlier stage.

Conclusion

Of paramount importance in consideration of perinatal hypoxemia is the survivor's fate. Unfortunately, babies who suffer hypoxemia before birth have a worse prognosis than do babies with birth asphyxia. Indeed, recent evidence suggests that perinatal asphyxia accounts for under 10% of all cases of cerebral palsy in term infants and that the cause of the cerebral palsy is more often the result of nonasphyxial disorders (27).

The prognosis for babies who are suffering from birth asphyxia worsens with the presence of convulsions, apathy, apneic or cyanotic attacks, feeding difficulty, irritability, hypothermia, and vomiting. If only one of these symptoms is present, then the prognosis is good. If clonic convulsions are the only feature, the prognosis is also good. Tonic convulsions carry a uniformly bad prognosis (28).

Attempts have been made to find predictions of outcome. Somatosensory-evoked potentials (29) and phosphorous magnetic resonance spectroscopy (30) have both been used to assess prognosis and show some promise but are only available in a few centers. Good quality ultrasound with Doppler is probably still the best predictor over and above the clinical features mentioned earlier (31).

CASE 64.1 Infant with Asphyxia

A 26-year-old gravida 1, para 0, was admitted at term in early labor. Late decelerations were noted on FHR traces, but labor progressed rapidly, and the baby was delivered before an emergency cesarean section could be performed. Heavy meconium staining of the amniotic fluid was noted during the second stage of labor.

At birth, the baby made no respiratory effort. Pharyngeal aspiration was carried out, and the baby was intubated. The one-minute Apgar score was 4, rising to 6 at five minutes. The baby was breathing spontaneously by 10 minutes and was extubated. Birthweight was 2.9 kg.

In the first six hours of life, the baby became tachypneic and irritable and was screaming continuously. Blood glucose was recorded at 35 mg/100 mL. Phenobarbitone was commenced, but the baby remained jittery. Possible convulsions were seen on the second day, and a cranial ultrasound on the same day showed very small ventricles with no pulsation of the anterior cerebral artery, confirming the presence of cerebral edema. Mannitol was given at this time, resulting in a good diuresis and a lessening of the irritability. However, the baby was noticed to be increasingly stiff over the next two or three days, and an EEG showed very little cerebral activity. Over the next two weeks, the increase in muscle tone in the limbs was maintained. The baby made rather feeble attempts to suck, but much of the time he was crying and restless. A repeat ultrasound scan showed areas of subcortical leucomalacia, and a further EEG showed some returning cerebral activity, although this was very abnormal, with an epileptiform pattern. At four weeks of age, obvious multifocal clonic convulsions were seen. At this time, the baby was feeding a little better, but remained stiff. Head circumference was 36.5 cm, having been 34.5 cm at birth.

At one year of age, the baby had generalized rigidity, was unresponsive, cried most of the time, slept poorly, and had difficult-to-control seizures. Feeding had remained difficult. The head circumference was 38.2 cm, with overlapping sutures.

This case illustrates how unexpectedly a baby may become asphyxiated and how important it is that pediatricians be available at all times. However, despite our efforts, the baby is very severely handicapped, with no prospect of improvement.

This case also illustrates the value of the ultrasound scan in assessing the progress of the hypoxic–ischemic damage. The presence at one month of extensive subcortical leucomalacia gave the parents a reliable, but gloomy prognosis. The outcome of this baby was predictable, in that babies who have areas of subcortical leucomalacia are usually very severely handicapped, have uncontrollable fits, and, most upsetting for the parents, are constantly crying inconsolably.

It is difficult to know whether the outcome could have been influenced in any way, as labor progressed so rapidly that a cesarean section could not be performed before delivery took place. ■

CASE 64.2 Birth Asphyxiation with Hypoglycemia

A 27-year-old gravida 2, para 0, had an uneventful pregnancy and was admitted to a peripheral unit at 38 weeks' gestation with spontaneous onset of labor. No FHR monitoring was carried out, and meconium staining of the liquor was noticed at the onset of the second stage of labor. At no time had auscultation detected any abnormalities of the fetal heart.

Following a spontaneous vertex delivery, the Apgar score was 3 at one minute. Aspiration of the pharynx was carried out under direct vision, but, before intubation could be performed, the baby commenced spontaneous respira-

tions. At 30 minutes of age, the baby was breathing normally with no signs of cerebral irritability. At two hours of age, the temperature was 35°C, but this rose rapidly after the baby was placed in an incubator. At seven hours of age, the baby was feeding, but two hours later was noted to be pale and floppy, with a blood glucose recording of <10 mg/100 mL. A review of the observation charts revealed that the BMstix had been noted to be unrecordable three hours earlier by the nursing staff, but this had not been brought to the attention of the medical staff. Intravenous glucose was given immediately, but the baby remained cyanosed and hypotonic. The baby became apneic and required intubation and ventilation. The baby then became increasingly hypertonic, with fisting and generalized jitteriness. Plasma sodium was 128 mM/L, and she was given phenobarbitone and mannitol, and IPPV was continued. Following the mannitol, there was a brisk diuresis, but she remained hypertonic. Cranial ultrasound was normal, but the EEG showed an asymmetrical pattern with an epileptiform pattern.

At five days, the baby was extubated, and she made good feeding attempts. She remained hypertonic, however, and developed multifocal seizures during the fourth week of life, necessitating the use of sodium valproate as an anticonvulsant. Serial ultrasound assessment failed to reveal any obvious areas of leucomalacia, even though the earlier scans had shown evidence of a diffuse hypoxic–ischemic insult.

Subsequently, the baby has made very slow developmental progress, with a slowly growing head circumference (41.5 cm at one year of age, compared with 34 cm just after birth). There were variable alterations of tone in all four limbs, and, by three years, she was only just sitting with support and had no language development. Her handling was complicated by the presence of severe atopic eczema.

This case is difficult in that there seem to have been two insults to the brain: namely, birth asphyxia and hypoglycemia. There seems to be no doubt that there was a prolonged period of hypoglycemia that was unreported to the medical staff, and this can, of course, be devastating to an already compromised brain. What is impossible to answer is whether the baby would have been as severely damaged had the hypoglycemia been detected and treated more efficiently earlier, but the outcome would probably have been more favorable had this been managed appropriately. The importance of correct maintenance of metabolic homeostasis is illustrated by this case. ■

References

1. Adamsons K, Myers RE. Perinatal asphyxia: causes, detection, and neurologic sequelae. Pediatr Clin North Am 1973;20: 465.

2. Van Bel F, Walther FJ. Myocardial dysfunction and cerebral blood flow velocity following birth asphyxia. Acta Paediatr Scand 1990;79:756.

3. Armstrong D, Norman MG. Periventricular leucomalacia in neonates. Complications and sequelae. Arch Dis Child 1974;49:367.

4. Van den Bergh R, Vander Eecken H. Anatomy and embryology of cerebral circulation. In: Cerebral circulation, progress in brain research, vol 3. Amsterdam: Luyendijk, 1968.

5. Renal vascular damage after birth. Br Med J 1974;3:295.

6. Knox Ritchie JW. Obstetrics for the neonatologist. In: Roberton N RC, ed. Textbook of neonatology. Edinburgh: Churchill Livingston 1986:79.

7. Sokol RJ, Rosen MG, Borgstedt AD, et al. Abnormal electrical activity of the fetal brain and seizures of the infant. Am J Dis Child 1974;127:477.

8. Prior PF, Maynard DE, McDowall DG. Fetal monitoring. In: Monitoring cerebral function. Amsterdam: Elsevier, 1979.

9. Manning FA, Morrison I, Lange IR, et al. Antepartum determination of fetal health: composite biophysical profile scoring. Clin Perinatol 1982;9:285.

10. Dawes GS. Fetal and neonatal physiology. Chicago: Year Book Medical Publishers, 1968.

11. Freeman JM, Nelson KB. Intrapartum asphyxia and cerebral palsy. Pediatrics 1988;82:240–9.

12. Blair E, Stanley FJ. Intrapartum asphyxia: a rare cause of cerebral palsy. J Pediatr 1988;112:515–9.

13. Goldaber KG, Gilstrap LC, Leveno KJ, et al. Pathologic fetal academia. Obstet Gynecol 1992;78:1103–7.

14. Apgar V. Proposal for a new method of evaluation of the newborn infant. Anesth Analg 1953;32:260.

15. American Academy of Pediatrics Committee on Drugs. Emergency drug doses for infants and children and naloxone use in newborns: clarification. Pediatrics 1989;83:803.

16. Standards and guidelines for cardiopulmonary resuscitation (CPR) and emergency cardiac care (ECC). JAMA 1992.

17. Levene MI. Management of the asphyxiated full term infant. Arch Dis Child 1993;68:612.

18. Levene MI, Kornberg J, Williams THC. The incidence and severity of postasphyxial encephalopathy in full term infants. Early Hum Dev 1986;11:21.

19. Barmada MA, Moossy J, Painter M. Pontosubicular necrosis and hyperoxemia. Pediatrics 1980;66:840.

20. Volpe JJ. Neurology of the newborn. Philadelphia: WB Saunders, 1981.

21. Whitelaw A. Intervention after birth asphyxia. Arch Dis Child 1989;64:66.

22. Vannucci RC, Mujsce DJ. Effect of glucose on perinatal hypoxic-ischaemic brain damage. Biol Neonate 1992;62: 215.

23. Eyre JA, Wilkinson AR. Thiopentone induced coma after severe birth asphyxia. Arch Dis Child 1986;61:1084.

24. Levene MI, Evans DH, Forde A, Archer LNJ. Value of intracranial pressure monitoring of asphyxiated newborn infants. Dev Med Child Neurol 1987;29:311.

25. Gluck L, Kulovich MV, Borer RC, et al. Diagnosis of the respiratory distress syndrome by amniocentesis. Am J Obstet Gynecol 1971;109:440.

26. Liggins GC, Howie RN. A controlled trial of antepartum glucocorticoid treatment for prevention of the respiratory distress syndrome in premature infants. Pediatrics 1972;50: 515.

27. Naeye RL, Peters EC, Bartholomew M, et al. Origins of cerebral palsy. Am J Dis Child 1989;143:1154.

28. Brown JK. Convulsions in the newborn period. Dev Med Child Neurol 1973;15:823.

29. Gibson NA, Graham M, Levene MI. Somatosensory evoked potentials and outcome in perinatal asphyxia. Arch Dis Child 1992;67:393.

30. Moorcraft J, Bolas NM, Ives NK, et al. Global and depth resolved phosphorus magnetic resonance spectroscopy to predict outcome after birth asphyxia. Arch Dis Child 1991; 66:1119.

31. Levene MI, Fenton AC, Evans DH, et al. Severe birth asphyxia and abnormal cerebral blood-flow velocity. Dev Med Child Neurol 1989;31:427.

65

Neonatal Hypocalcemia

Sergio Demarini, M.D.
Reginald C. Tsang, M.D.

MANY newly born infants have total serum calcium concentrations below 7 mg/dL. We consider such neonatal hypocalcemia to be "early" when it appears within the first 2 days of life, and we regard it as being "late" when it occurs after the first 2 days (Table 65.1).

Early hypocalcemia is believed to be caused by factors such as prematurity, birth asphyxia, and maternal diabetes or hypoparathyroidism. This condition is found in 30% of preterm infants (37 weeks' gestational age or less), 89% of very-low-birthweight infants (less than 1,500 g), 35% of infants with one-minute Apgar scores of 6 or below, and 50% of infants of insulin-dependent diabetic mothers (1–4). In contrast, late neonatal hypocalcemia is believed typically to result from dietary calcium-phosphate imbalance.

New insights into calcium homeostasis have been made possible by the development of specific ion electrodes for ionized calcium. Improved measurement of radioimmunoassays (RIAs) for parathyroid hormone and calcitonin and of the radioassay for vitamin D metabolites has also contributed to such understanding. Consequently, researchers have uncovered a number of possible pathogenetic factors (Table 65.2).

Calcium Supply

Radioactive calcium studies of pregnant women indicate rapid transfer of calcium from mother to fetus and marked avidity of fetal bone for calcium. The greatest accumulation occurs during the third trimester, when 140–280 mg of calcium daily are transferred to the fetus. Serum total, diffusible, and ionized calcium concentrations are higher in fetal than in maternal blood. Active maternal-fetal calcium transfer occurs by means of a placental "calcium pump" and appears to occur against a marked fetal-to-maternal calcium gradient (5).

Pregnancy itself seems to have little influence on overall maternal bone mineral content (6). For this reason, it appears probable that maternal calcium metabolism remains well regulated during gestation. Both serum parathyroid hormone and $1,25(OH)_2$ vitamin D concentrations are elevated. Presumably, enhanced intestinal calcium absorption and retention maintain overall calcium economy.

At birth, however, this situation changes. With the

Table 65.1 Nature and Treatment of Hypocalcemia

Diagnosis

Total serum calcium level <7.0 mg/dL

Early hypocalcemia

(First two days) thought to be caused by decreased postnatal calcium supply, low magnesium status, increased endogenous phosphorus load, temporary functional hypoparathyroidism (in infants of diabetic mothers), increased calcitonin concentrations (asphyxia, preterm infants), and 1,25 (OH)$_2$ vitamin D resistance (very-low-birthweight infants).

Late hypocalcemia

(After the first two days) can occur with increased exogenous phosphorus load, intestinal malabsorption of calcium and magnesium, and postacidotic tetany. Maternal vitamin D deficiency may be a predisposing factor.

Treatment

Asymptomatic: 10% calcium gluconate (9.4 mg of elemental calcium per mL) given orally at a rate of 75 mg of elemental calcium/kg daily, divided in six equal doses.

Symptomatic: 10% calcium gluconate should be given IV at a dose of 2 mL/kg over 10 minutes. Monitor the heart rate closely. If the newborn becomes bradycardic, the infusion must be immediately stopped.

Hypomagnesemia: 50% magnesium sulfate should be given IM or IV at a dose of 0.20–0.25 mL/kg.

maternal calcium supply terminated, the offspring may require several days before its postnatal calcium intake becomes adequate. Since exogenous postnatal calcium intake is comparatively low, it has been estimated that, for monkeys and sheep at birth, an immediate increase of about 15%–20% in the calcium supply from endogenous fetal stores is required to maintain postnatal calcium homeostasis in the exchangeable pool (7). In human infants who have

Table 65.2 Pathogenetic Factors in Neonatal Hypocalcemia

	Early	Late
Biochemical		
Calcium	Decreased supply	Intestinal malabsorption
Magnesium	Hypomagnesemia in infants of diabetic mothers	Intestinal malabsorption
Phosphate	Increased endogenous production	Increased exogenous ingestion
Acid-base balance	Base correction of acidosis?	Postacidotic tetany
Endocrine		
Parathyroid	Decreased function (some cases)	———
Vitamin D	Resistance to 1,25(OH)$_2$ vitamin D in VLBW infants	Decreased vitamin D status
Calcitonin	Increased	———

VLBW: very-low-birthweight.

shown signs of perinatal distress, oral intake is even more sharply curtailed since, conventionally, calcium-free IV solutions are prescribed until sufficient milk intake can be tolerated. Thus, in all newborns, especially sick ones, the possibility arises that serum calcium concentrations may fall precipitously.

Late neonatal hypocalcemia can result from decreased intestinal calcium absorption. For example, decreased calcium absorption occurs with steatorrhea, chronic diarrhea, or when an infant ingests milk with a high fat content.

Magnesium Deficiency

Hypomagnesemia can result in hypocalcemia through end-organ unresponsiveness to, or decreased production of, parathyroid hormone. In addition, since homeostatic control mechanisms for magnesium and calcium may be similar, changes in magnesium and calcium homeostasis can result because of a common primary disturbance.

Often, infants with birth asphyxia and infants of diabetic mothers who develop early neonatal hypocalcemia also suffer from hypomagnesemia (3, 8). Even without specific therapy, both hypocalcemia and hypomagnesemia in these infants appear to resolve spontaneously within a few hours or days.

Hypomagnesemia in infants of diabetic mothers is related to the severity of the maternal condition and appears to be associated with decreased parathyroid function (9). Thus, decreased parathyroid function may act to cause neonatal hypocalcemia in these particular infants (10).

An isolated low serum magnesium concentration on the first day of life has been associated with neonatal hyperexcitability in otherwise normal full-term infants (11). Rarely, hypomagnesemia can cause hypocalcemic seizures that do not respond to calcium therapy alone or to anticonvulsants, but do respond to magnesium administration.

In rare instances, hypomagnesemia can cause hypocalcemia in later infancy. The best-described cases have involved hypomagnesemia secondary to intestinal magnesium malabsorption resulting from either specific intestinal magnesium absorption defects or surgically induced malabsorption syndromes (12).

Excess Phosphate

An excess of phosphate in extracellular fluid may decrease calcium through three theoretic mechanisms: 1) increased deposit of calcium in bone and soft tissues through an increased calcium-phosphate concentration product; 2) decreased response of bone to parathyroid hormone; and 3) increased response of bone to the hypocalcemic effect of calcitonin.

Hyperphosphatemia is associated with hypocalcemia in the following circumstances: prematurity, maternal diabetes, birth asphyxia, and intrauterine growth retardation (IUGR) (1, 3, 13–16). In preterm infants and infants of diabetic mothers, relatively high early neonatal serum phosphate concentrations correlate with subsequent low serum calcium concentrations, suggesting a possible causal relationship. During the first three days of life, before dietary phosphate intake becomes significant, there is increased serum phosphate concentration but no alteration in phosphate excretion (3, 13, 14). These data are consistent with increased endogenous phosphate production.

After the first few days of life, increased exogenous phosphate loading occurs, as milk feeding is established. Some infant formulas, such as those made with evaporated milk, supply phosphate intake greatly exceeding that of human milk. With use of such cow milk-derived formulas, late infantile hypocalcemia can occur.

Serum phosphate concentrations are less elevated and serum calcium values relatively normal in infants receiving modern "adapted proprietary formulas," in which phosphate content is closer to that of human milk (17). Nevertheless, cases of late neonatal tetany have recently occurred even in healthy full-term infants fed such formulas (18).

Symptomatic hypocalcemia can result after administering phosphate to correct low serum phosphate concentrations in infants with rickets of prematurity (19). Finally, early addition of cereals to newborns' diets raises phosphate intake and may be an aggravating factor in late hypocalcemia (20).

Acid-Base Effects

Chronic alkalosis shifts calcium from extracellular fluid into bone and slows its release from bone into extracellular fluid. In contrast, chronic acidosis causes calcium to move from bone to extracellular fluid. In bone culture studies, increasing the pH in the culture medium decreased the release of calcium from bone and increased the rate of bone calcification (21).

Low serum calcium concentrations have been correlated with relatively large amounts of bicarbonate administered to correct acidosis in infants who had birth asphyxia or IUGR or were preterm, born to diabetic mothers, or of low birthweight (1, 3, 13–16). However, it's uncertain whether the low serum calcium was caused by the bicarbonate or the underlying conditions.

In later infancy, correction of diarrhea-induced acidosis with bicarbonate has been implicated as a cause of hypocalcemia, or "postacidotic tetany" (20, 21). One study showed decreases in total serum calcium concentrations of infants given sodium bicarbonate (21). However, it is possible that such underlying factors as malnutrition, diarrhea, dehydration, and prematurity may have set the stage for hypocalcemia by causing mineral depletion before the administration of bicarbonate.

Other Factors

In newborns, as in children and adults, oral ingestion of glucose results in decreased serum calcium, phosphorus, and magnesium concentrations (22). Phototherapy may be an additional factor associated with neonatal hypocalcemia, especially in preterm infants (23). The precise mechanism is unknown.

Parathyroid Function

Parathyroid hormone raises serum calcium concentration mainly by moving calcium from bone into extracellular fluid and partly by increasing renal tubular reabsorption of calcium. It decreases serum phosphate concentrations largely through its phosphaturic effect. Consequently, hypoparathyroidism results in decreased serum calcium and increased serum phosphate.

Hypoparathyroidism has long been suspected as the cause of early neonatal hypocalcemia. Theoretically, it could result from either decreased parathyroid hormone production or decreased end-organ responsiveness to the hormone.

Decreased parathyroid hormone production has been

suspected to cause hypocalcemia of prematurity. Some studies cite low serum concentrations of the hormone in hypocalcemic preterm infants and increasing concentrations with increasing gestational age (24, 25). However, in other studies, hypocalcemia was accompanied by an appropriate elevation of parathyroid hormone in small premature infants; increase in serum calcium, induced by IV infusion, resulted in a decline in serum parathyroid hormone (26). Another report showed a rapid postnatal increase in serum parathyroid hormone in the first three days of life to be more pronounced in hypocalcemic than in normocalcemic preterm infants (27).

Our data suggest that infants of diabetic mothers have impaired parathyroid hormone production during the first few days of life associated with marked falls in serum calcium postnatally (28–38). Neonatal magnesium deficiency caused by maternal magnesium losses during pregnancy may lead to functional hypoparathyroidism in infants of diabetic mothers (28, 29). Tight management of maternal diabetes during pregnancy apparently reduces the incidence of neonatal hypocalcemia (30).

Infants who have birth asphyxia also show decreased parathyroid hormone responses to hypocalcemia (3). However, these data do not take gestational age into account.

Rarely, maternal hyperparathyroidism due to parathyroid adenoma has caused neonatal hypocalcemia. The postulated mechanism is maternal hypercalcemia leading to fetal hypercalcemia through placental transfer of calcium (31). Fetal hypercalcemia then suppresses fetal parathyroid function. The infant's suppressed parathyroid glands presumably cannot maintain adequate serum calcium concentrations.

Phosphaturic response to parathyroid hormone may be decreased in newborns. Nevertheless, end-organ unresponsiveness to parathyroid hormone seems to play, at best, a minor role in neonatal hypocalcemia (3, 13, 14, 32, 33).

Parathyroid function in late neonatal hypocalcemia appears adequate. Investigations have shown that hyperplasia of the parathyroid glands is associated with increased serum parathyroid hormone concentrations (24, 34).

Vitamin D

$1,25(OH)_2$ vitamin D is necessary for parathyroid hormone action on bone, intestinal absorption of calcium and phosphate (and, indirectly, bone formation), and probably renal calcium reabsorption. Hence, vitamin D deficiency can cause hypocalcemia.

Recent data have established the following sequence for vitamin D metabolism:

1. After production in the skin or ingestion, vitamin D is absorbed in the duodenum and jejunum and transported to the liver for 25-hydroxylation to 25-hydroxycholecalciferol [25(OH) vitamin D].

2. 25(OH) vitamin D is transported to the kidneys for conversion to 1,25-dihydroxycholecalciferol [1,25 (OH)$_2$ vitamin D]. This latter metabolite is the final active metabolite of vitamin D.

3. The final step of the conversion process from 25(OH) vitamin D to 1,25(OH)$_2$ vitamin D is expedited by parathyroid hormone, hypocalcemia, and hypophosphatemia (35).

25(OH) vitamin D is the major circulating vitamin D metabolite and reflects vitamin D nutritional status. Placental transfer of both vitamin D3 and 25(OH) vitamin D has been shown in rats and in humans: 25(OH) vitamin D values in cord blood correlate with maternal values. English studies have suggested that maternal vitamin D deficiency may predispose infants to late neonatal hypocalcemia (36, 37).

Serum concentration of the active form, 1,25(OH)$_2$ vitamin D appears to be tightly regulated. Reports vary as to whether there is a correlation between maternal and cord blood 1,25(OH)$_2$ vitamin D concentrations (38). Little, if any, placental transfer of 1,25 (OH)$_2$ vitamin D seems to take place unless the mother receives very high doses (39).

In full-term infants, cord 1,25(OH)$_2$ vitamin D is low at birth but rises to normal adult concentrations by 24 hours of age. This rise is probably due to the decrease in serum calcium and subsequent increase in serum parathyroid hormone concentration that usually occurs during this time (38).

In preterm infants (32–37 weeks' gestation), 1,25 (OH)$_2$ vitamin D is higher in newborns who are given supplements of vitamin D (2,100 units daily for 5 days) than in those not supplemented. Therefore, renal 1α–hydroxylase, and hence 25-hydroxylase, appear functional in preterm infants (40).

Vitamin D disturbance doesn't appear to have a role in early neonatal hypocalcemia in full-term and moderately preterm infants and in offspring of diabetic mothers (30, 41). However, in very-low-birthweight (VLBW) infants (less than 1,500 g), hypocalcemia is refractory to large oral doses of 1,25(OH)$_2$ vitamin D and responsive only to very high parenteral doses, which cause elevation of diastolic blood pressure (42). Therefore, in VLBW infants, this apparent end-organ resistance to 1,25(OH)$_2$ vitamin D may contribute to hypocalcemia.

Calcitonin

Disturbances in calcitonin function can disrupt calcium-phosphate homeostasis. The principal action of calcitonin on bone is to inhibit the mobilization of calcium and phosphate induced by parathyroid hormone. For this reason, excessive calcitonin production can lower serum calcium and phosphate concentrations. Production of calcitonin is increased by acute increases in serum calcium and magnesium concentrations.

Calcitonin does not appear to cross the placenta (43). Serum calcitonin concentrations in umbilical venous blood are significantly higher than maternal serum concentrations. Serum concentrations in pregnancy appear to be higher than those in nonpregnant women (44).

After birth, serum calcitonin concentrations in nearly all infants increase sharply to a peak at 12–26 hours (45). Preterm infants appear to have higher serum calcitonin concentrations than full-term ones, and calcitonin is higher in hypocalcemic than in normocalcemic preterm infants (27). Serum calcitonin concentrations are also higher in asphyxiated than in nonasphyxiated full-term infants (46). Since neonatal serum calcium concentrations are inversely related to calcitonin values in preterm and asphyxiated infants, it's likely that increased calcitonin concentrations play a role in neonatal hypocalcemia in these two groups.

In infants of diabetic mothers, plasma calcitonin concentrations rise after birth to values comparable to those of term infants (45). Therefore, there doesn't appear to be a specific disturbance in calcitonin function in infants of diabetic mothers. However, the increase in plasma calcitonin concentrations theoretically aggravates the infant's "ordinary" tendency to hypocalcemia.

Calcitonin doesn't appear to have any role in the development of late neonatal hypocalcemia. This condition is usually accompanied by hyperphosphatemia, not hypophosphatemia.

C A S E 6 5 . 1 Hypocalcemia with Maternal Diabetes

A baby born at 34 weeks' gestation weighed 2,700 g and showed development appropriate for gestational age. The mother, a 26-year-old gravida 2, para 1, was a class C insulin-dependent diabetic. Labor was spontaneous, with partial abruption of the placenta and prolapse of the umbilical cord. The Apgar score was 1 (for heart rate) at one minute, 4 at five minutes, and 8 at 10 minutes. The infant received endotracheal intubation and positive pressure ventilation with 100% oxygen. A total of 30 mL of a blood volume supporter (Plasmanate) was infused through an umbilical venous catheter.

The infant arrived in the neonatal intensive care unit (NICU) 15 minutes after delivery and was pink and in no distress. The endotracheal tube was removed and supplemental oxygen discontinued. The staff began IV fluids with 10% dextrose at 100 mL/kg per day. Serial serum glucose determinations ranged from 48 to 98 mg/dL.

At 12 hours of age, the infant had serum calcium concentration of 6.7 mg/dL; at 24 hours, it was 6.2 mg/dL. The infant's arms were noted to "twitch" at 24 hours. He was given 10% calcium gluconate (9.4 mg of elemental calcium per milliliter) by nasogastric tube initially, and orally after 36 hours of age. The dose was 4 mL every four hours.

The serum calcium concentrations were 7.8 mg/dL at 36 hours and 8.0 mg/dL at 48 hours of age. By 48 hours, no signs of neuromuscular hyperactivity were present. The calcium gluconate dose was therefore halved to 2 mL every four hours. IV fluids were also discontinued.

At 100 hours of age, the infant had a serum calcium level of 8 mg/dL, and calcium supplementation was discontinued. At this age, the infant was already ingesting 50 mL of infant formula (Similac) every three hours. ∎

References

1. Tsang RC, Oh W. Neonatal hypocalcemia in low-birthweight infants. Pediatrics 1970;45:773.

2. Venkatamaran PS, Tsang RC, Steichen JJ, et al. Early neonatal hypocalcemia in extremely preterm infants. Am J Dis Child 1986;140:1004.

3. Tsang RC, Chen I, Hayes W, et al. Neonatal hypocalcemia in infants with birth asphyxia. J Pediatr 1974;84:428.

4. Tsang RC, Kleinman LI, Sutherland JM, et al. Hypocalcemia in infants of diabetic mothers. J Pediatr 1972;80:384.

5. Whitsett JA, Tsang RC. Calcium uptake and binding by membrane fractions of human placenta; ATP-dependent calcium accumulation. Pediatr Res 1980;14:769.

6. Pitkin RM. Calcium metabolism in pregnancy and the perinatal period: a review. Am J Obstet Gynecol 1985;151:99.

7. Ramberg CF Jr, Delivora-Papadopoulos M, Crandall ED, et al. Kinetic analysis of calcium transport across the placenta. J Appl Physiol 1973;35:682.

8. Tsang RC, Hartman C, Brown D, et al. Hypomagnesemia in infants of diabetic mothers: perinatal studies. J Pediatr 1976; 89:115.

9. Tsang RC, Chen I-W, Friedman MA, et al. Parathyroid function in infants of diabetic mothers. J Pediatr 1975;86:399.

10. Noguchi A, Eren M, Tsang RC. Parathyroid hormone in hypocalcemic and normocalcemic infants of diabetic mothers. J Pediatr 1980;97:112.

11. Nelson N, Finnstrom O, Larsson L. Neonatal hyperexcitability in relation to plasma ionized calcium, magnesium, phosphate and glucose. Acta Paediatr Scand 1987;76:579.

12. Tsang RC, Neonatal magnesium disturbances. Am J Dis Child 1972;126:282.

13. Tsang RC, Light IJ, Sutherland JM, et al. Possible pathogenetic factors in neonatal hypocalcemia of prematurity: the role of gestation, hyperphosphatemia, hypomagnesemia, urinary calcium loss and parathormone responsiveness. J Pediatr 1973;82:423.

14. Tsang RC, Kleinman LI, Sutherland JM, et al. Hypocalcemia in infants of diabetic mothers—studies in Ca, P, and Mg metabolism and parathormone responsiveness. J Pediatr 1972;80:384.

15. Bergman L, Kjellmer I, Selstam U. Calcitonin and parathyroid hormone: relation to early neonatal hypocalcemia in infants

of diabetic mothers. Biol Neonate 1974;24:151.

16. Tsang RC, Gigger M, Oh W, et al. Studies in calcium metabolism in infants with intrauterine growth retardation. J Pediatr 1975;86:936.

17. Oppe TE, Redstone D. Calcium and phosphorus levels in healthy newborn infants given various types of milk. Lancet 1968;1:1045.

18. Venkataraman PS, Tsang RC, Greer FR, et al. Late infantile tetany and secondary hyperparathyroidism in infants fed humanized cow milk formula. Am J Dis Child 1985;139:664.

19. Kovar IZ, Mayne PD, Robbe I. Hypophosphatemic rickets in the preterm infant: hypocalcemia after calcium and phosphorus supplementation. Arch Dis Child 1983;58:629.

20. Pierson JD, Crawford JD. Dietary-dependent neonatal hypocalcemia. Am J Dis Child 1972;123:472.

21. Rapport S, Dodd K, Clark M, et al. Postacidotic state of infantile diarrhea. Am J Dis Child 1947;73:391.

22. Venkataraman PS, Blick KE, Rao R, et al. Decline in serum calcium, magnesium and phosphorus values with oral glucose in normal neonates. studies of serum parathyroid hormone and calcitonin. J Pediatr 1986;108:607.

23. Romagnoli C, Polidori G, Cataldi L, et al. Phototherapy-induced hypocalcemia. J Pediatr 1979;94:815.

24. David L, Anast CS. Calcium metabolism in newborn infants: the interrelationship of parathyroid function and calcium, magnesium, and phosphorus metabolism in normal, "sick," and hypocalcemic newborns. J Clin Invest 1974;54:287.

25. Tsang RC, Chen I-W, Friedman MA, et al. Neonatal parathyroid function: role of gestational age and postnatal age. J Pediatr 1973;83:728.

26. Cooper LJ, Anast CS. Circulating immunoreactive parathyroid hormone levels in premature infants and the response to calcium therapy. Acta Paediatr Scand 1985;74:669.

27. Romagnoli C, Zecca E, Tortorolo G, et al. Plasma thyrocalcitonin and parathyroid hormone concentrations in early neonatal hypocalcemia. Arch Dis Child 1987;62:580.

28. Shaul PW, Mimouni F, Tsang RC, et al. The role of magnesium in neonatal calcium homeostasis: effects of magnesium infusion on calciotropic hormones and calcium. Pediatr Res 1987;22:319.

29. Mather HM, Nisbeth JA, Burton GH, et al. Hypomagnesemia in diabetes. Clin Chim Acta 1979;95:235.

30. Steichen JJ, Tsang RC, Ho M, et al. Perinatal magnesium, calcium and 1,25(OH)$_2$D in relation to prospective randomized management of maternal diabetes. Calcif Tissue Int 1981;33:317.

31. Wilson DT, Martin T, Christensen R, et al. Hyperparathyroidism in pregnancy: case report and review of the literature. Can Med Assoc J 1983;129:986.

32. Connelly JP, Crawford JD, Watson J. Studies of neonatal hyperphosphatemia. Pediatrics 1962;30:425.

33. Linarelli LG. Newborn urinary cyclic AMP and developmental responsiveness to parathyroid hormone. Pediatrics 1972;50:14.

34. Gardner LI. Tetany and parathyroid hyperplasia in the newborn infant: influence of dietary phosphate load. Pediatrics 1952;9:534.

35. Tsang RC. The quandary of vitamin D in the newborn infant. Lancet 1983;1:1370.

36. Roberts SA, Cohen MD, Fortar JO. Antenatal factors associated with neonatal hypocalcemic convulsions. Lancet 1973;2:809.

37. Watney PJ, Change GW, Scott P, et al. Maternal factors in neonatal hypocalcemia: a study in three ethnic groups. Br Med J 1971;2:432.

38. Steichen JJ, Tsang RC, Gratton T, et al. Vitamin D homeostasis in the perinatal period. N Engl J Med 1980;302:315.

39. Marx SJ, Swart EG, Hamstra AJ, et al. Normal intrauterine development of a fetus of a woman receiving extraordinarily high doses of 1,25 dihydroxy vitamin D3. J Clin Endocrinol Metab 1980;51:1138.

40. Glorieux FH, Salle BL, Delvin EE, et al. Vitamin D metabolism in preterm infants: serum calcitriol values during the first five days of life. J Pediatr 1981;99:640.

41. Chan GM, Tsang RC, Chen IW, et al. The effect of 1,25 dihydroxy vitamin D3 supplementation in premature infants. J Pediatr 1978;93:91.

42. Koo WK, Tsang RC, Poser JW, et al. Elevated serum calcium and osteocalcin levels from calcitriol in preterm infants. Am J Dis Child 1986;140:1152.

43. Wezeman FH, Reynolds WA. Stability of fetal calcium levels and bone metabolism after maternal administration of thyrocalcitonin. Endocrinology 1971;89:445.

44. Samaan NA, Anderson GD, Adam-Mayne ME. Immunoreactive calcitonin in the mother, neonate, child, and adult. Am J Obstet Gynecol 1975;121:622.

45. David L, Salle B, Chopard P, et al. Studies on circulating immunoreactive calcitonin in low-birthweight infants during the first 48 hours of life. Helv Paediatr Acta 1977;32:39.

46. Venkataraman PS, Tsang RC, Chen IW, et al. Pathogenesis of early neonatal hypocalcemia: studies of serum calcitonin in gastrin and plasma glucagon. J Pediatr 1987;110:599.

66

Extracorporeal Membrane Oxygenation

Martin Keszler, M.D.
K.N. Sivasubramanian, M.D.

DESPITE continued advances in obstetric and neonatal care over the past decade, hundreds of term or near-term newborns continue to die each year of acute, potentially reversible respiratory failure. Extracorporeal membrane oxygenation (ECMO), the prolonged use of extracorporeal circulation and an artificial membrane lung, has emerged over the past few years as an effective treatment (1). This invasive technique facilitates recovery by avoiding continued exposure of the lungs to the damaging effects of high ventilator pressures and oxygen concentrations.

Initial attempts at ECMO in neonates date back to 1971 (2). While these early efforts were unsuccessful because of intracranial bleeding associated with prematurity, they demonstrated the basic feasibility of the technique. The first successful use of ECMO in a newborn was reported in 1975, and a few moribund newborns were rescued over the next five years (3). By 1993, more than 90 centers in the U.S. and abroad had ECMO capabilities (4).

Despite rapid growth in popularity, ECMO technology has yet fully to establish its niche. Concerns about possible long-term effects of carotid artery ligation continue to impede acceptance. Recent reports question the appropriateness of aggressive hyperventilation and suggest that babies meeting ECMO criteria can be saved with better conventional management (5).

These claims, however, fail to recognize that most babies who ultimately require ECMO are initially managed at outlying hospitals and arrive at the ECMO center already failing on maximal therapy. In the eight years since our program's inception, we have never had a patient with meconium aspiration born at our institution who required ECMO. At the same time, it is probably true that at least some instances of ECMO are preventable.

For example, we have observed a substantial number of babies born by elective repeat cesarean delivery among our outborn ECMO population (6). These full-term infants had good Apgar scores and appeared well at birth. However, they developed pulmonary hypertension, perhaps as a result of altered levels of circulating prostaglandins. When this is not recognized promptly and treated effectively, severe, life-threatening illness can result.

Indications for Selection

Because of the need to ligate the right common artery and the risk of major hemorrhage from systemic heparinization, ECMO is reserved for neonates who are failing despite maximal conventional support and have a less than 20% chance of survival. Because of the high risk of intracranial hemorrhage in babies born before 34 weeks' gestation, ECMO is currently applicable only to term or near-term infants. In general, to be considered for ECMO therapy, a baby must have completed 34 weeks of gestation, weigh at least 2 kg, and suffer from a reversible cause of pulmonary or cardiac failure.

Meconium aspiration syndrome is the most frequent cause of respiratory failure leading to ECMO. Other conditions are perinatal asphyxia, sepsis, congenital pneumonia, respiratory distress syndrome, and diaphragmatic hernia. Persistent pulmonary hypertension is almost always a major contributing factor, usually accompanied by varying degrees of myocardial dysfunction. Primary cardiac failure is a less common indication for ECMO, and the success of the procedure in these patients is limited.

Many of the criteria traditionally used to identify patients with 80% predicted mortality are outdated, influenced by therapeutic strategies or by altitude above sea level. Therefore, it is important for each center to review its own recent experience with similar patients and establish criteria representative of 80% mortality in the institution.

The ECMO program at Georgetown University Medical Center has been active since February 1985 (7). Our eligibility criteria for the procedure derive from a retrospective review of 31 term infants who required maximal support (fraction of inspired oxygen [FiO_2] 1.0, peak inspiratory pressure [PIP] > 34 cm H_2O) over a two-year period just before we began the ECMO program. The following criteria were identified as predicting an 80% or higher mortality:

- Acute deterioration: PO_2 < 50 mm Hg (or alveolar-arterial oxygen difference [$AaDO_2$] > 630) for more than two hours on maximal pharamacologic and ventilatory support (PIP > 40 cm H_2O; FiO_2, 1.0).

- Failure to respond: PO_2 < 60 (or $AaDO_2$ > 620) for eight consecutive hours despite maximal therapy.

In addition, pH below 7.15 for two hours or below 7.20 for eight hours as associated with nonsurvival was also considered a criterion to initiate ECMO. Our concept of what constitutes maximal therapy is rigorous. As long as ECMO requires systemic heparinization and the potential of ligation of a carotid artery, we continue to avoid ECMO until we are certain that conventional therapy and usually high frequency ventilation have failed. As a consequence, our patients generally progress well beyond the given criteria before ECMO is instituted (mean PIP pre-ECMO = 45.9 cm H_2O; mean PO_2 = 33.4 mm Hg). This reflects our belief that management of critically ill newborns continues to improve, affecting the reliability of predicted mortality data based on experience of 8–10 years ago. As a result of this approach, fewer than half the patients referred to us for the procedure actually require ECMO.

The procedure is usually carried out in the intensive

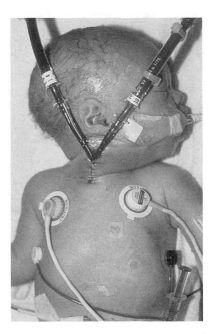

Figure 66.1   The procedure is usually carried out in the NICU where all babies are screened by echocardiography.

care nursery. All patients are screened by echocardiography to rule out cyanotic heart disease and by cranial ultrasound to ensure that no important preexisting intracranial hemorrhage is present (see Figure 66.1).

Preparing the Circuit

After the ECMO circuit is assembled, it is flushed with CO_2 to remove all nitrogen and filled with crystalloid containing 40 mL of 25% human albumin (10 g). This solution is recirculated for 20–30 minutes to make sure it completely coats the internal surface in order to minimize fibrin deposits. Finally, the crystalloid prime is displaced with packed red blood cells reconstituted with plasma, heparin, calcium and tris (hydroxymethyl) aminomethane/tromethamine/trisaminomethane (THAM), aiming for a final hematocrit of 40%, normal pH, and electrolyte composition. Proper electrolyte and acid–base balance are important because the priming volume of about 400 mL is greater than the infant's entire blood volume.

Surgical Technique

Cannulation for ECMO is performed at the bedside using a radiant warmer with temperature servocontrol. The infant's head is hyperextended by placing a roll of towels under the shoulders. Turning the head fully to the left exposes the right side of the neck. The skin of this area is cleansed with povidone-iodine solution, and drapes are applied using sterile technique. Morphine sulfate (0.2 mg/kg) or fentanyl citrate (2 μg/kg) is given for analgesia and sedation. Pancuronium bromide is administered to relax muscles and to prevent spontaneous respiratory effort. This is essential, since any spontaneous inspiration during venous cannulation could cause massive embolization of air into the central venous system.

Before making the incision, the skin and subcutaneous tissue overlying the sternocleidomastoid muscle are infiltrated with 0.5% xylocaine. A small incision, minimal dissection, and liberal use of electrocautery will ensure hemostasis and minimize bleeding during ECMO. Venoarterial bypass is accomplished using the internal jugular vein and the common carotid artery for vascular access. Venous cannulation is performed using a 10F, 12F, or 14F beveled polyethylene catheter with multiple side holes over the distal 5 cm.

Initially, modified chest tubes were used. In 1986, specially designed Elecath ECMO cannulas with superior flow characteristics became available (Electro Catheter Corporation, Rahway, New Jersey). A further refinement occurred with the development of thin-walled wire reinforced catheters manufactured by Bio-Medicus, Inc. (Eden Prairie, MN). Arterial cannulas of 8F, 10F, or 12 F are identical but without side holes.

The internal jugular vein, readily identified between the two heads of the sternocleidomastoid muscle, is mobilized, controlled, and elevated proximally and distally with loops of 3-0 or 4-0 sutures. The common carotid artery is found slightly deeper than and just medial to the internal jugular vein and is controlled in an identical fashion.

Before beginning cannulation, the proper depth of insertion is estimated by measuring the distance from the insertion site to the aortic arch and lower one-third of the right atrium for arterial and venous cannulas, respectively. Either the artery or the vein can be cannulated first. The largest cannula that can be inserted safely is used to provide maximal venous drainage.

Careful, meticulous, gentle technique is necessary to avoid intimal dissection or disruption of the vessel. Resistance to smooth passage usually signifies that the cannula is too large or that there is angulation or narrowing of the vessel. Once the cannula is in position, sutures are tied snugly around the vessel. So they can be identified easily, two sutures are used around the arterial cannula, leaving the ends 1.0–1.5 cm long. Traction on them will provide control of both vessels. The neck wound is closed with vertical mattress sutures, making sure the skin is tightly closed around the cannulas. The cannulas are securely sutured to the skin, and povidone-iodine is applied to the operative site.

After the cannulas are inserted and secured, they are carefully connected to the ECMO circuit to avoid air bubbles. At this time, a chest x-ray is obtained to confirm optimal cannula position, and bypass is ready to commence (8).

ECMO Circuit

The ECMO system consists of a roller head perfusion pump, a membrane artificial lung (Sci-Med Life Systems,

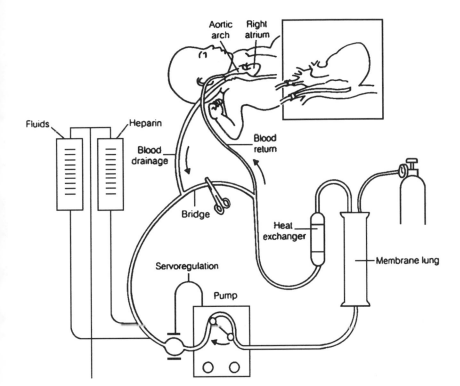

Figure 66.2   The ECMO circuit. After the circuit is assembled, it is flushed with CO_2 and filled with crystalloid. This solution is recirculated for about half an hour. Then, the crystalloid is replaced by packed red blood cells reconstituted to achieve proper electrolyte and acid–base balance. Venoarterial bypass is achieved using the internal jugular vein and the common carotid artery for vascular access. (Reproduced with permission from the University of Michigan ECMO Technical Specialist Manual, 1984.)

Avecor Inc., Minneapolis, Minnesota), a heat exchanger with a heat source, and a 1/4-inch Tygon tubing circuit with polycarbonate connectors. Blood drains by gravity from the right atrium through a cannula inserted into the internal jugular vein and is pumped through the membrane oxygenator, where gas exchange takes place. The oxygenated blood then passes through a heat exchanger, where it is rewarmed to body temperature and returns to the baby through the carotid artery cannula advanced into the aortic arch (Figure 66.2).

The pump is servo-controlled by a microswitch sensor in contact with a 50-mL, soft-walled Silastic reservoir. When venous drainage is insufficient to keep the reservoir filled, the switch breaks contact, power to the pump is interrupted, and an alarm alerts the operator to adjust pump flow.

The core of the ECMO system is the Kolobow membrane lung, which consists of a large silicone rubber envelope wound around a spool and enclosed in a watertight jacket. Ventilating gas flows on the inside of the envelope in one direction, and blood passes on the outside in the opposite direction between the turns of the coil. Fresh gas and blood thus come into close contact across a large surface area, much as they do in the natural lung. Because the blood and gas are separated by a semipermeable membrane, hemolysis in the artificial lung is effectively eliminated.

Control of Gas Exchange

A precise flow meter and an air–oxygen blender allow accurate adjustments of ventilating gases to the membrane lung. The FiO_2 to the oxygenator can be adjusted to maintain postoxygenator PO_2 at 120–150 mm Hg. The patient's PaO_2 is determined by the proportion of fully saturated blood returning from the artificial lung to that of desaturated blood shunting through the nonfunctioning natural lungs. For full support, bypass flow of 70%–80% of cardiac output is required. Thus, to improve oxygenation, the operator has only to increase bypass flow, thereby decreasing the admixture of desaturated blood returning from the damaged lungs. Once the natural lungs begin to recover, blood in the pulmonary circulation becomes oxygenated and blood flow can gradually be transferred from the artificial back to the natural lung. To control $PaCO_2$, ventilating gas flow rate is adjusted within the manufacturer's recommended range (1.0–2.4 L/minute), and CO_2 is added to the ventilating gas as necessary to avoid hypocarbia.

Anticoagulation and Hemostasis

Controlled heparinization is maintained throughout the procedure by means of a loading dose of 75–100 U of heparin/kg, followed by a continuous infusion adjusted to maintain an activated clotting time at 200–230 seconds. Platelets are maintained above 100,000/mL with platelet transfusions as necessary. Hematocrit is kept above 40%. All blood sampling (except patient blood gases) and all infusions (except platelet transfusion) are performed via ECMO circuit to avoid venipuncture and heel stick.

To enhance hemostasis, fibrin polymer "glue" is applied before closing the wound and whenever it needs to be reexplored for bleeding. Using two separate syringes, 10 mL of single-donor cryoprecipitate and 5 mL of 10% $CaCl_2$ combined with 5 mL of bovine thrombin (1,000 U/mL) are mixed to create a gelatinous material to fill the wound interstices.

Reexploration of the cannulation site is indicated if blood loss is greater than 10 mL/hour over four hours. The use of fibrin glue for hemostasis at the cannulation site has dramatically reduced the amount of bleeding during the procedure and decreased the need for reexploration and blood transfusion.

Conduct of ECMO

Cardiopulmonary bypass is initiated at a low flow, to mix in the prime volume gradually. Over the next 10–15 minutes, pump flows are increased to match the maximum available venous drainage, and the baby's blood volume is adjusted as needed. Since drainage is passive, by gravity, the flow is limited by the diameter of the venous cannula, the vertical distance from the baby to the pump and systemic venous return.

Once adequate bypass flow is established, ventilator settings are rapidly reduced over 15–30 minutes. The PIP is adjusted to 18–22 cm H_2O, intermittent mandatory venti-

lation (IMV) to 10 breaths/minute, FiO_2 to 0.21–0.30, and inspiratory time is set at 0.5 to 0.8 seconds. PEEP has traditionally been maintained at 3–5 cm H_2O. However, data from our institution have shown that positive end-expiratory pressure (PEEP) of 12–14 cm H_2O accelerates lung recovery and shortens the duration of ECMO (9, 10).

Strict aseptic technique is maintained throughout. Prophylactic antibiotics (methicillin, ampicillin, and gentamicin) are used for the duration of the procedure, and daily blood cultures are also taken. Spontaneous breathing is encouraged during the procedure, and frequent pulmonary toilet is provided. Inotropic agents are usually discontinued, although dopamine is frequently maintained at a low dose to optimize renal perfusion. ECMO support is typically required for 3–7 days. Total parenteral nutrition, including fat emulsion, provides the substrate and calories needed for optimal healing.

Weaning

When pulmonary function begins to recover, as evidenced by improving oxygenation, clearing of pulmonary infiltrates on chest x-ray, and better lung compliance, blood flow through the ECMO circuit is gradually decreased. This allows more blood to flow through the infant's lungs. In this manner, as pulmonary function continues to improve, the burden of gas exchange is gradually transferred to the natural lungs. When adequate blood gases are achieved with low ventilator support and minimal ECMO flows, a four- to six-hour trial off ECMO is attempted. If blood gases remain stable during this period, the cannulas are removed and the vessels permanently ligated. Although reconstruction of the carotid artery is, in principle, feasible, the procedure is still under evaluation.

Outcome, Complications, Follow-up

The survival rate of ECMO patients listed in the Extracorporeal Life Support Organization central registry based at the University of Michigan was 81.4% as of January 1990. For the years 1973 to 1979, survival was 47%, rising to 71% in 1980–84, and to 82% in 1985–1993. Our 150 patients treated in 1985–1992 had a survival rate of 89.3%. The

Table 66.1 ECMO Patient Diagnoses

	Total Patients	Survived ECMO (No.)	(%)	Overall Survival (No.)	(%)
Meconium aspiration	77	76	99	75	97
Other aspiration syndromes	6	6	100	5	83
Respiratory distress syndrome	18	17	94	17	94
Primary PPHN	12	11	92	11	92
Diaphragmatic hernia	16	14	88	9	56
Sepsis/pneumonia	16	13	81	12	75
Pulmonary hypoplasia	3	3	100	3	100
Other	2	2	100	2	100
Total	150	142	95	134	89

prognosis for survival depends mainly on birthweight, gestational age, and the underlying diagnosis (Table 66.1).

Another useful predictor of outcome appears to be pre-ECMO arterial pH. In our patients, pH below 6.9 was associated with a poor outcome (death, central nervous system damage) in four of five cases. This is not surprising, since the development of severe metabolic acidosis signals ultimate failure of oxygen delivery at the tissue level. Low pH was also found to be a negative predictor of survival in an analysis of 3528 cases from the central ECMO registry (11).

The typical duration of ECMO support is five days, and the infants are usually able to be weaned from the ventilator within 1–3 days of decannulation. The hospital stay is approximately one month. The total cost of hospitalization is substantially less than for comparably ill surviving patients not treated with ECMO. This is so because those who reached ECMO criteria and survived without ECMO in the past suffered major respiratory and central nervous system morbidity, leading to prolonged hospitalization (Table 66.2). The use of high PEEP shortens the duration of ECMO therapy and thus further improves its cost effectiveness (10).

Serious complications of ECMO are not frequent but can be devastating. Of greatest concern are those related to systemic heparinization and to the ligation of the carotid and perhaps jugular vessels. Intracranial hemorrhage occurs in approximately 16% of patients and is more frequent in babies of 34–35 weeks' gestation. Other complications include internal hemorrhage, renal failure, and seizures. More recently, cerebral infarction, predominantly involving the right hemisphere, has been recognized as an occasional occurrence in patients who were hypotensive at the time of carotid artery ligation (12). Accidental air embolism is a rare but potentially catastrophic complication. An air bubble detection system should virtually eliminate this occurrence.

Follow-up data suggest that, despite extreme severity of their neonatal illness, most ECMO graduates survive the experience without apparent neurologic or developmental impairment. The group with the longest follow-up period was reported in 1985 and represents the earliest survivors of ECMO (13). Of 18 survivors, 13 were free of marked handicap at 4–11 years of age. Other investigators have reported normal growth and development in 50%–85% of patients (14–16). These results are similar to those observed in comparably ill survivors not treated with ECMO (17).

Future Directions

Several key developments are likely to change the practice of ECMO radically over the next few years. The perfection of techniques designed to avoid systemic heparinization—heparin-bonded circuits or enzymatic heparin removal—could make the technique safer, possibly allowing its use in babies born before 34 weeks' gestation.

The recent introduction into clinical practice of single-cannula veno-venous techniques avoids sacrifice of the

Table 66.2 Hospital Cost Analysis

Conventional Treatment	ECMO
Mortality: 80%	Mortality: 10%
Mean hospital stay (survivors): 108 days	Mean hospital stay (survivors): 29 days
Mean cost of initial hospitalization: $135,000	Mean cost of initial hospitalization: $57,000

carotid artery, making ECMO safer and more widely accepted. Other important benefits of veno-venous perfusion are: infusion of possible emboli into the pulmonary, rather than systemic circulation, perfusion of the pulmonary vascular bed with oxygenated blood, possibly leading to more rapid fall in pulmonary vascular resistance, preservation of pulsatile blood flow, maintenance of pulmonary blood flow and improved myocardial oxygen delivery. Lack of direct cardiac support, partial recirculation of oxygenated blood and lower systemic PO_2 are among the important disadvantages of this approach.

Two approaches to VV ECMO are currently utilized. In one method, a double lumen cannula drains blood through one lumen while reinfusing oxygenated blood via the other. With the second method, blood is alternately drained and reinfused in the manner of tidal flow through a single lumen cannula. Studies in our laboratory have demonstrated that the single lumen tidal flow technique is capable of safely providing long-term full respiratory support (18). Durandy et al. recently reported successful clinical use of an innovative tidal flow system using the Colin Cardio® pump in newborns (19). This device is a roller pump with a distensible, compliant segment of tubing stretched around its rollers. This eliminates the need for an arterial and venous reservoir of the standard tidal flow VV system thereby simplifying the tidal flow technique and adding to its safety. The device, unfortunately, is not available in the United States at this time.

In the meantime, the ultrathin-walled Kendall double lumen catheter (Kendall Healthcare Products Co., Mansfield, MA) has been developed at the University of Michigan (20) and has now been successfully used in hundreds of babies. While its effectiveness is limited by considerable recirculation and by catheter size considerations (currently only size 14 Fr. is available) its major advantage is simplicity—no new equipment is required. In order to be successful in the majority of babies, the VV techniques will probably require some relaxation of ECMO eligibility criteria. This is because infants meeting rigorous ECMO criteria often have significant myocardial dysfunction and may require the cardiac assist of veno-arterial ECMO.

The use of high PEEP and low peak pressures with 5–10 sigh breaths/minute preserves the gas-exchange func-

tion of the lungs, allowing much of the O_2 requirement to be met by essentially apneic oxygenation, while still providing lung rest. This approach uses the artificial lung primarily for CO_2 removal, which requires only 20%–30% of the cardiac output to be diverted through the extracorporeal circuit. The term "extracorporeal CO_2 removal" ($ECCO_2R$) has been applied to this technique, which has been shown to be effective in experimental animals and in adults (21). The lower flow requirements of this approach would facilitate the use of less invasive cannulation techniques such as single-cannula veno-venous or arterio-venous perfusion via the umbilical vessels. However, pulmonary oxygen uptake in newborns with pulmonary hypertension is often limited by decreased pulmonary blood flow, rather than parenchymal lung disease. This may, in fact, prove to be the limiting factor in any extracorporeal technique relying on the natural lungs for O_2 uptake.

The likely scenario for the near future is that a combination of a heparinless circuit and less invasive cannulation techniques will justify earlier application of ECMO technology. It will thus become practical to intervene much earlier in the course of the disease. ECMO will become recognized as safer than aggressive mechanical ventilation and will be used primarily to remove CO_2, while low-amplitude/high-PEEP ventilation safely allows adequate O_2 uptake through the natural lungs. On the other hand, the recent discovery of nitric oxide (22), the first effective vasodilator specific to the pulmonary circulation is an exciting new development in the management of newborn pulmonary hypertension and may substantially reduce (though not eliminate) the need for ECMO in the future. Regardless of the specific scenario, a substantial decrease in mortality and morbidity of newborns with respiratory failure will likely follow.

References

1. Bartlett RH, Toomasian JM, Roloff DW, et al. Extracorporeal membrane oxygenation (ECMO) in neonatal respiratory failure: 100 cases. Ann Surg 1986;204:236.
2. White JJ, Andrews HG, Risenberg H, et al. Prolonged respiratory support in newborn infants with a membrane oxygenator. Surgery 1971;70:288.

3. Bartlett RH, Andrews AF, Toomasian JM, et al. Extracorporeal membrane oxygenation for newborn respiratory failure: forty-five cases. Surgery 1982;92:425.

4. Extracorporeal Life Support Organization Registry. Ann Arbor, Michigan: January, 1993.

5. Dworetz AR, Fernando MR, Sabo B, et al. Survival of infants with persistent pulmonary hypertension without extracorporeal membrane oxygenation. Pediatrics 1989;84:1.

6. Keszler M, Carbone MT, Cox C, Schumacher RE. Severe persistent pulmonary hypertension after elective Cesarean section—a potentially preventable condition leading to ECMO. Pediatrics 1992;89:670–72.

7. Moront MG, Katz NM, Keszler M, et al. Extracorporeal membrane oxygenation for neonatal respiratory failure. A report of fifty cases. J Thorac Cardiovasc Surg 1989;97:706.

8. Siva Subramanian KN, Keszler M, Hoy G. ECMO for severe neonatal respiratory failure. Contemp Ob/Gyn 1986;28 (Technology):21.

9. Keszler M, Siva Subramanian KN, Smith YA, et al. Pulmonary management during extracorporeal membrane oxygenation. Crit Care Med 1989;17:495.

10. Keszler M, Ryckman F, McDonald JV, et al. Pulmonary management during extracorporeal membrane oxygenation (ECMO). Pediatr 1992;120:107–113.

11. Stolar CJH, Snedecor SM, Bartlett RH. Extracorporeal membrane oxygenation and neonatal respiratory failure: experience from the Extracorporeal Life Support Organization. J Pediatr Surg 1991;26:563–71.

12. Schumacher RE, Barks JDE, Johnston MV, et al. Rightsided brain lesions in infants following extracorporeal membrane oxygenation. Pediatrics 1988;82:155.

13. Towne BH, Lott IT, Nicks DA, et al. Long-term follow-up of infants and children treated with extracorporeal membrane oxygenation (ECMO). J Pediatric Surg 1985;20:410.

14. Andrews AF, Nixon CA, Cilley RE, et al. One to three year outcome for 14 neonatal survivors of extracorporeal membrane oxygenation. Pediatrics 1986;78:692.

15. Glass P, Miller M, Short B. Morbidity for survivors of extracorporeal membrane oxygenation: neurodevelopmental outcome at 1 year of age. Pediatrics 1989;83:72.

16. Rosenberg EM, Wilkerson SA, Cook LN. Three years of follow-up of extracorporeal membrane oxygenation (ECMO) patients. Proceedings of the 5th Annual ECMO Symposium, Snowmass, Colorado, Feb. 1989.

17. Cohen RS, Stevenson KD, Malachowski N, et al. Late morbidity among survivors of respiratory failure treated with tolazoline. J Pediatr 1980;97:644.

18. Keszler M, Moront MG, Cox C, et al. Oxygen delivery with a tidal flow veno-venous system for ECMO. Clin Res 1988;36:49A.

19. Chevalier JY, Durandy Y, Batisse A, et al. Preliminary report: extracorporeal lung support for neonatal acute respiratory failure. Lancet 1990;335:1364–66.

20. Anderson HL, Otsu T, Chapman RA, Bartlett RH. Venovenous extracorporeal life support in neonates using a double lumen catheter. Trans Am Soc Artif Intern Org 1989;35:650–3.

21. Gattinoni L, Pesenti A, Macheroni D, et al. Low frequency positive pressure ventilation with extracorporeal CO_2 removal in severe acute respiratory failure: clinical results. JAMA 1986;256:881.

22. Roberts JD, Polaner DM, Lang P, Zapol WM. Inhaled nitric oxide in persistent pulmonary hypertension of the newborn. Lancet 1992;340:818–19.

Index